Coronavirus Disease-19 (COVID-19): A Perspective of New Scenario

(Volume 1)

COVID-19: Epidemiology, Biochemistry, and Diagnostics

Edited by

Kamal Niaz

Department of Pharmacology and Toxicology
Faculty of Bio-Sciences, Cholistan University of Veterinary
and Animal Sciences
Bahawalpur-63100
Pakistan

&

Muhammad Farrukh Nisar

Department of Physiology and Biochemistry
Faculty of Bio-Sciences, Cholistan University of Veterinary
and Animal Sciences (CUVAS)
Bahawalpur-63100
Pakistan

Coronavirus Disease-19 (COVID-19): A Perspective of New Scenario

(Volume 1)

COVID-19: Epidemiology, Biochemistry, and Diagnostics

Editors: Kamal Niaz & Muhammad Farrukh Nisar

ISBN (Online): 978-981-4998-93-2

ISBN (Print): 978-981-4998-94-9

ISBN (Paperback): 978-981-4998-95-6

need for a court order if at any point you breach any terms of this License Agreement. In no event will any delay or failure by Bentham Science Publishers in enforcing your compliance with this License Agreement constitute a waiver of any of its rights.

3. You acknowledge that you have read this License Agreement, and agree to be bound by its terms and conditions. To the extent that any other terms and conditions presented on any website of Bentham Science Publishers conflict with, or are inconsistent with, the terms and conditions set out in this License Agreement, you acknowledge that the terms and conditions set out in this License Agreement shall prevail.

Bentham Science Publishers Pte. Ltd.
80 Robinson Road #02-00
Singapore 068898
Singapore
Email: subscriptions@benthamscience.net

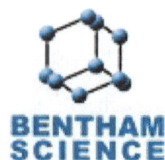

BENTHAM SCIENCE

CONTENTS

FOREWORD

The connection between human health, animals, and the environment has been widely recognized as important for the ecosystem we inherit and intend to improve for the generations to come. This of course is not a responsibility of a region or a country, rather its responsibility of all of us. Efforts have to be collaborative and transboundary in approach. Of the many types of challenges, respiratory diseases have emerged as a real threat in the recent past. Scientists have been working to reduce their load and easily spread it from animals to human beings. Newly emerging respiratory diseases such as severe acute respiratory syndrome-coronavirus (SARS-CoV), Middle East respiratory syndrome (MERS), and severe acute respiratory syndrome-coronavirus-2 (SARS-CoV-2) posing a serious threat to the human population and reported in the year 2003, 2012, and 2019, respectively.

This book is very relevant in this connection. The volume-1 of this book consists of three key modules. The first module provides clearly defined progression and entry of SARS-CoV-2 to the human population. The learning outcomes of this module are developing knowledge, skills, and competencies in scientists, students, employers, and human resource specialists. The other modules of this book focus on developing a detailed set of guidelines regarding epidemiology, genetic alteration, a structural protein, quantitative analysis, and diagnostic approaches of SARS-CoV-2 and will give step-by-step awareness to the researchers about SARS-CoV-2. This book will be adopted to give reliable knowledge to all scientists globally. I hope that this book will be distributed widely in Pakistani higher institutions in the near future for thorough implementation at all levels of postgraduate studies.

Muhammad Sajjad Khan
Cholistan University of Veterinary and Animal Sciences
Bahawalpur-63100
Pakistan

PREFACE

Since the outbreak of novel coronavirus (CoVs), the first patient was related to seafood in Wuhan city, Hubei Province, China, on 12th December 2019. A new type of coronavirus was found in the patient's sample having pneumonia-like signs and symptoms via unbiased high-throughput sequencing. This new coronavirus was found in the patient's epithelial cell, which falls in the subgenus of the *Sabevirus* of the subfamily Coronavirus. Later, on 11th February 2020, the World Health Organization (WHO) officially announced and named "Coronavirus Disease-19 (COVID-19)" and the International Committee on Taxonomy of Viruses named it severe acute respiratory syndrome-coronavirus-2 (SARS-CoV-2). This virus is different from the previous isolated Middle East respiratory syndrome coronavirus (MERS-CoV) and severe acute respiratory syndrome coronavirus (SARS-CoV) which is the seventh one that can infect humans. SARS-CoV-2 spread rapidly and infected many of the population in Wuhan city then to other territories of China epidemically and abruptly abroad. Due to pandemic occurrence, on 31st January 2020, the WHO declared as "Global Health Emergency" as there is no effective drug and/or vaccine available for this infection till now. According to WHO and InfoGraphics CNA 31st March, there are 786,228 confirmed cases, 37,820 reported deaths, and 166,041 recovers from COVID-19. In the current scenario, the United States of America, Italy, and Spain are the most affected countries globally due to the COVID-19 pandemic, which is increasing day-by-day globally.

With this book proposal, we consolidate the various evolutionary domains, genetic techniques, and diagnostic methodologies widely used in the global emergency of COVID-19. Since SARS-CoV-2 is the closest to SARS-CoV and MERS-CoV, the approaches brought here will be similar and/or varying with a slight degree. It is cleared that in the last 17-18 years, this is the third outbreak of the same coronavirus with a small mutation that shock the whole world. The chapters in this book should be prioritized as up-to-date literature of techniques used in the study SARS-CoV-2 and will act as a suitable reference if any such wary appear soon.

The 1st volume of the proposed book proposal has been classified into three parts: *Part I: Evolution and Entry of SARS-CoV-2, Part II: Genetic Alteration and Structural Determination of SARS-CoV-2 Proteins, and Part III: Quantitation Analysis of SARS-CoV-2.*

With the emergence of new coronavirus variants, epidemiology, different host tropism permits a thorough analysis of their evolution and acquired adaptability to their host. Thus in Part I, we start the book with chapters' dealing with evolutionary epidemiology, evolutionary adaptation and genetics, and its entrance pathways. To keep in mind how the virus enters a host cell to provoke an infection is essential to design techniques to avoid it. Furthermore, chapters describing various methodologies regarding SARS-CoV-2 entrance pathways and characterizing the important proteins employed by the virus to achieve. In part II, a critical analysis of the virus involves the potential to mutate its genome by opposite genetics and to get better recombinant viruses with described mutations. Such processes will help study the capabilities of particular genes and their effects on virus survival and pathogenesis. These strategies can help determine checkpoints inside the virus genome growth and proliferation that give therapeutics strategies. We also added to know the biochemical characterization of spike glycoprotein and structural elucidation of viral proteins of SARS-CoV-2. Due to the emergence of COVID-19, a possible available diagnostic tool is employed in the medical setting to identify this virus and further prevent the infection. In part III, we added a chapter that helps detect antigen via virus loaded using enzyme-linked immunosorbent assay (ELISA) and quantitative real time-polymerase chain reaction (qRT-PCR) based techniques. To measure host immune parameters, techniques such as microneutralization, pseudovirus neutralization assay, and COVID-19 specific antibodies using ELISA chapters are presented. The second last chapter is given to know the lung's condition via CT scan. In contrast, the last chapter describes the nucleic acid-based assays for COVID-19, which is a more precise and sophisticated technique.

This book will appear as a baseline for academicians, scientists, and health professionals as still, research will overcome this outbreak of COVID-19 and find effective diagnostic techniques. However, just a single book proposal like this wouldn't have flourished without enthusiasm and determined publishers' and investigators' strength to take time from their busy schedule and subsidize on time. We thank the whole investigators who contributed, directly and indirectly, to bring it to reality.

Kamal Niaz
Department of Pharmacology and Toxicology
Faculty of Bio-Sciences, Cholistan University of Veterinary and Animal Sciences
Bahawalpur-63100
Pakistan

&

Muhammad Farrukh Nisar
Department of Physiology and Biochemistry
Faculty of Bio-Sciences, Cholistan University of Veterinary and Animal Sciences
(CUVAS)
Bahawalpur-63100
Pakistan

List of Contributors

Abdul Basit
Department of Microbiology, Faculty of Life Sciences, University of Okara, Pakistan

Abhinav Anand
School of Pharmaceutical Sciences, Lovely Professional University, Phagwara, Punjab, India

Amjad Islam Aqib
Department of Medicine, Faculty of Veterinary Science, Cholistan University of Veterinary and Animal Sciences, Bahawalpur-Pakistan-63100

Amar Nasir
Department of Clinical Sciences, University of Veterinary and Animal Sciences Lahore Sub-campus Jhang-Pakistan

Ankush Sharma
School of Pharmaceutical Sciences, Lovely Professional University, Phagwara-144411, Punjab, India

Arbab Sikandar
Department of Anatomy and Histology, University of Veterinary and Animal Science, Lahore Sub-campus Jhang-Pakistan

Asif Javaid
Department of Animal Nutrition, Cholistan University of Veterinary and Animal Sciences, Bahawalpur, Pakistan

Devesh Tewari
School of Pharmaceutical Sciences, Lovely Professional University, Phagwara, Punjab, India

Faisal Siddique
Department of Microbiology, Cholistan University of Veterinary and Animal Sciences (CUVAS), Punjab, Bahawalpur 63100, Pakistan

Firasat Hussain
Department of Microbiology, Cholistan University of Veterinary and Animal Sciences (CUVAS), Punjab, Bahawalpur 63100, Pakistan

Haroon Ahmed
Department of Biosciences, COMSATS University Islamabad (CUI) 45550, Pakistan

Hayat Khan
Department of Microbiology, University of Swabi, Khyber Pakhtunkhwa 23561, Pakistan

Ihtisham Ulhaq
Department of Biosciences, COMSATS University Islamabad (CUI) 45550, Pakistan

Ijaz Ali
Department of Biosciences, COMSATS University Islamabad (CUI) 45550, Pakistan

Imran Ahmad Khan
Faculty of Pharmacy and Alternative Medicine IUB Bahawalpur, Pakistan

Jinbiao Zhan
Department of Biochemistry, and Cancer Institute of the Second Affiliated Hospital, Zhejiang University, School of Medicine, Hangzhou 310058, China

Kamal Niaz
Department of Pharmacology & Toxicology, Faculty of Bio-Sciences, Cholistan University of Veterinary and Animal Sciences, Bahawalpur-63100, Pakistan

Kashif Prince
Department of Medicine, Faculty of Veterinary Science, Cholistan University of Veterinary and Animal Sciences, Bahawalpur-63100, Pakistan

Kashif Rahim
Deaprtment of Microbiology, Faculty of Veterinary Science, Cholistan

	University of Veterinary and Animal Sciences, Bahawalpur-63100, Pakistan
Maher Darwish	Department of Pharmaceutical Chemistry and Drug Control, Faculty of Pharmacy, Wadi International University, Homs, Syria
Maida Manzoor	Institute of Microbiology, University of Agriculture, Faisalabad, Pakistan
Muhammad Adil	Department Pharmacology and Toxicology, University of Veterinary and Animal Sciences Lahore Sub-campus Jhang-Pakistan
Mohammad Ejaz	Department of Microbiology, The University of Haripur, Haripur, Pakistan
Muhammad Ali Syed	Department of Microbiology, The University of Haripur, Haripur, Pakistan
Muhammad Farooq	Faculty of Veterinary Medicine, University of Teramo, Italy
Muhammad Farrukh Nisar	Department of Physiology and Biochemistry, Cholistan University of Veterinary and Animal Sciences, Bahawalpur, Pakistan
Muhammad Kalim	Department of Biochemistry, and Cancer Institute of the Second Affiliated Hospital, Zhejiang University, School of Medicine, Hangzhou 310058, China
Muhammad Saeed	Department of Poultry Sciences, Cholistan University of Veterinary and Animal Sciences, Bahawalpur, Pakistan
Muhammad Shuaib	School of Ecology and Environmental Science, Yunnan University, Kunming, China
Muhammad Usman	Institute of Biochemistry, Biotechnology & Bioinformatics (IBBB), The Islamia University of Bahawalpur, Punjab, Pakistan
Muhammad Yasir Waqas	Department of Physiology & Bio-Chemistry, Faculty of Bio-Sciences, Cholistan University of Veterinary and Animal Sciences, Bahawalpur-63100, Pakistan
Naman Wahal	Sardar Patel Medical College, Bikaner, Rajasthan, India
Navneet Khurana	School of Pharmaceutical Sciences, Lovely Professional University, Phagwara, Punjab, India
Neha Sharma	School of Pharmaceutical Sciences, Lovely Professional University, Phagwara, Punjab, India
Noor Muhammad Khan	Department Physiology, University of Veterinary and Animal Sciences Lahore Sub-campus Jhang-Pakistan
Pooja Patni	School of Pharmaceutical Sciences, Lovely Professional University, Phagwara-144411, Punjab, India
Samina Ejaz	Institute of Biochemistry, Biotechnology & Bioinformatics (IBBB), The Islamia University of Bahawalpur, Punjab, Pakistan
Shafi Ullah	Cardiology Unit, Khyber Teaching Hospital (KTH), Peshawar, Pakistan
Shahzad Ali	Department of Wildlife and Ecology, University of Veterinary & Animal Sciences, Lahore, Pakistan

Shaukat Hussain Munawar	Department of Pharmacology and Toxicology, Faculty of Bio-Sciences, Cholistan University of Veterinary and Animal Sciences, Bahawalpur-63100, Pakistan
Sneha Joshi	Department of Pharmaceutical Chemistry, PCTE Group of Institutions, Ludhiana, Punjab, India
Sonali Bajaj	School of Pharmaceutical Sciences, Lovely Professional University, Phagwara, Punjab, India
Tahir Shah	Department of Animal Science, Faculty of Agriculture, Ege University, İzmir, Turkey
Umair Younas	Department of Livestock Management, Faculty of Animal Production and Technology, Cholistan University of Veterinary and Animal Sciences, Bahawalpur-63100, Pakistan
Uzma Karamat	Institute of Biochemistry, Biotechnology & Bioinformatics (IBBB), The Islamia University of Bahawalpur, Punjab, Pakistan
Waqas Nazir Malik	Institute of Biochemistry, Biotechnology & Bioinformatics (IBBB), The Islamia University of Bahawalpur, Punjab, Pakistan
Yasir Hameed	Institute of Biochemistry, Biotechnology & Bioinformatics (IBBB), The Islamia University of Bahawalpur, Punjab, Pakistan
Zahid Ali	Department of Biosciences, COMSATS University Islamabad (CUI) 45550, Pakistan
Zahid Manzoor	Department of Pharmacology and Toxicology, Faculty of Bio-Sciences, Cholistan University of Veterinary and Animal Sciences, Bahawalpur-63100, Pakistan
Zia Ullah	Institute of Microbiology, University of Agriculture Faisalabad, Pakistan
Zia-ud-Din	Department of Community Medicine, Kohat Institute of Medical Sciences (KIMS), Kohat, Pakistan

Part I: Evolution and Entry of SARS-CoV-2

CHAPTER 1

Coronavirus Disease-2019 (COVID-19) Epidemiology

Ihtisham Ulhaq[1], Abdul Basit[2], Ijaz Ali[1], Firasat Hussain[3], Zahid Ali[1], Faisal Siddique[3], Haroon Ahmed[1], Amjad Islam Aqib[4] and Kashif Rahim[3,*]

[1] *Department of Biosciences, COMSATS University Islamabad (CUI) 45550, Pakistan*

[2] *Department of Microbiology, Faculty of Life Sciences, University of Okara, Pakistan*

[3] *Department of Microbiology, Cholistan University of Veterinary and Animal Sciences (CUVAS), Punjab, Bahawalpur-63100, Pakistan*

[4] *Department of Medicine, Faculty of Veterinary Science, Cholistan University of Veterinary and Animal Sciences, Bahawalpur, Pakistan-63100*

Abstract: At the end of December 2019, patients were diagnosed with a pneumonia-like infection in the Wuhan wholesale market of seafood, Hubei Province, China. Laboratory diagnosis revealed a novel coronavirus named severe acute respiratory syndrome-coronavirus-2 (SARS-CoV-2), that causes coronavirus disease-19 (COVID-19). Initially, t he novel virus was reported in bats. Due to the highly contagious nature of pathogens and the susceptibility of every human the virus spread rapidly across China then Globally. Respiratory droplets of infected patients played a significant role in the transmission of COVID-19 from human to human. Wuhan being a transport hub, and the crowd of people during New Chinese Year played a considerable role in the virus spread across the country. In link with earlier coronaviruses, the SARS-CoV-2 was noticed with a more contagious nature, and it quickly spread throughout the world. It was declared a pandemic by the World Health Organization (WHO) on March 12, 2020. In March 2021, the spread of infection decreased in China but increased globally, mainly in Europe. In April 2020, the disease burden increased in the USA. Till April 17 2020, China reported 84,149 cases with 4642 deaths, while worldwide cases reached 2,074,5279 with 139378 deaths. Europe reported confirmed cases 1,050,871 with 93,480 deaths, 743,607 patients in USA regions, Western Pacific regions with 127,595 patients, Eastern Mediterranean Regions reached 115,824 cases, and South-East Asia Regions reported 23,560 cases while African regions had 12,360 cases. The below figure illustrates the analysis of the epidemiological studies of COVID-19 (Fig. **1**).

Keywords: Bats, COVID-19, Host Susceptibilities, Morbidity, Mortality, Pandemic, SARS-CoV-2, Virology.

---

* **Corresponding author Kashif Rahim:** Department of Microbiology, Faculty of Veterinary Science, Cholistan University of Veterinary and Animal Sciences (CUVAS), Punjab, Bahawalpur 63100, Pakistan; E-mail: kashifrahim@cuvas.edu.pk

Kamal Niaz & Muhammad Farrukh Nisar (Eds.)

INTRODUCTION

A patient with respiratory signs and symptoms was diagnosed in Wuhan city, Hubei Province, China at the end of December 2019 [1]. The patients were diagnosed having pneumonia infection-like symptoms. Still, after genomic analysis by next-generation sequence (NGS) and real-time reverse transcription-polymerase chain reaction (RT-PCR) of the throat, samples revealed a pathogen like a coronavirus [2]. Hence a novel coronavirus was identified and initially named novel coronavirus-2019 (nCOV-19) by World Health Organization (WHO) on January 7, 2020 [1, 3]. However, because of genetic similarity with previous SARS-CoV (severe acute respiratory syndrome coronavirus), the nCoV-19 was renamed as severe acute respiratory syndrome coronavirus-2 (SARS-Co--2) by the International Committee on Taxonomy of Viruses (ICTV) [4]. The disease caused by SARS-CoV-2 was officially named coronavirus disease-19 (COVID-19) by WHO on February 11, 2020 [5]. The severe acute respiratory syndrome-coronavirus-2 (SARS-CoV-2) appeared to be more pathogenic in comparison with other coronaviruses, till January 2nd, 2020, it affected 42 individuals in China [6]. On January 13, 2020, the first COVID-19 disease case was reported in Thailand, which was the first case outside China [7]. First death due to COVID-19 disease outside China was reported in the Philippines [8]. The COVID-19 disease affects the human's respiratory tract, and disease symptoms include fever, cough, flu, sneezing, and fatigue. In contrast, the production of sputum, lymphopenia, dyspnoea, and diarrhea is observed in severe clinical conditions of patients [6, 9 - 11]. Additionally, the other severe symptoms include acute kidney failure, dysfunction of various organs, and even mental confusion is also expected [12]. The COVID-19 disease incubation period is almost two weeks [13], with a median of 4-5 days [14, 15]. However, the incubation period fluctuates in proportion to the patient's age, immune status and shorter old patients younger than 70 years [16]. The COVID-19 emergence in China was then rapidly expanded to various provinces and later to the globe, resulting in the declaration of a pandemic on March 12 2020 by the WHO [17]. Because of the highly contagious nature of SARS-CoV-2, non-availability of vaccines and antiviral drugs COVID-19 disease rapidly and as of April 7 2020, the disease affected 1,349,660 people worldwide in more than 190 countries with almost 74,816 deaths [18].

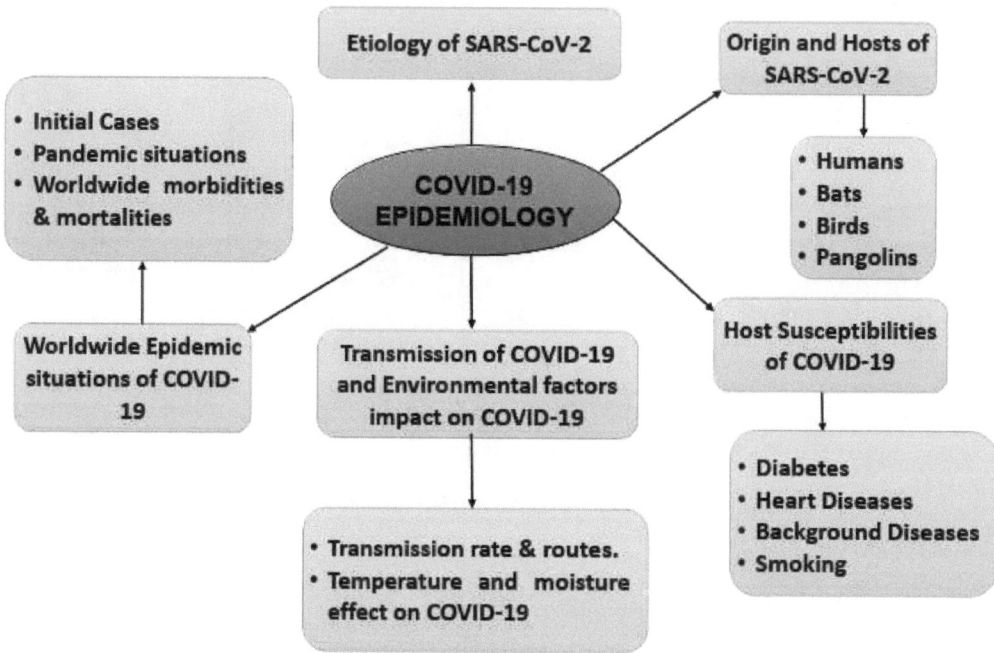

Fig. (1). Graphical abstract of the spread of Coronavirus.

Besides humans, coronaviruses are also reported to infect other animals, including birds and fishes [19]. So far, three different human pathogenic coronaviruses are reported. The first two had caused minor outbreaks; however, SARS-CoV-2 had become the basis for the notoriety of the coronaviruses in the scientific community [20]. The International Committee on the Taxonomy of Viruses established the family of *Coronaviridae* in 1975 [21]. Among RNA viruses, the most giant virus is coronavirus [22]. The coronaviruses are non-segmented enveloped viruses with a genome of positive-sense RNA, belong to the *Coronaviridae* family, and are classified into an order of Nidovirales [23]. Among *Nidovirales* order, the most prominent family is *Coronaviridae* which comprises two subfamilies, Orthocoronavirinae and Letovirinae [24]. The Orthocoronavirinae family accommodated four genera. Two genera are instigated in birds, such as *deltacoronavirus* and *gammacoronavirus* while the other two were found in mammals that are *alphacoronavirus* and *betacoronavirus* [24]. The members of betacoronavirus have got the zoonotic potential that essentially infects bats, camels, and humans [25 - 28]. The size of the *betacoronaviruses* is about 60-140 nm in diameter with round shape manifestation. The genome ranges from 26 to 32-kilobases in size that encodes both structural and non-structural proteins [29 - 31]. The SARS-CoV-2 RNA isolated from Wuhan patients entirely consists of almost 29844-29891 coding nucleotides while lacking the gene of hemagglutinin-esterase [23]. Lipids and proteins form the virus's envelope with a function to protect the nucleocapsid [32]. The viral genome and capsid are collectively known as the nucleocapsid. The envelope, capsid, and structural proteins ensure virus protection in the environment [33]. The coronavirus nucleocapsid is helical in symmetry. It is only thought to be present in negative-sense RNA and exceptional in the genome of positive-sense RNA viruses [20]. The coronavirus represents the crown (crown shape structure was observed under an electron microscope), spike glycoproteins give around, and pleiomorphic exterior forms like a crown to the virus [20]. Spikes protrusions of the coronaviruses are considered an essential characteristic prompting the coronavirus name [34]. Additionally, spikes glycoproteins of coronaviruses also play a role in the recognition and binding to host cell receptors during entry for replication and survival [35]. Two subunits are found in the spike proteins, the SI unit containing the receptor binding domain while the S2 domain is linked with the viral envelope [36].

SARS-CoV-2 was found to be novel *betacoronavirus* and genetically more parallel to SARS coronavirus than MERS coronavirus [37, 38]. SARS coronavirus and SARS coronavirus-2, both coronary viruses, used a similar cellular receptor in humans that is an angiotensin-converting enzyme-2 (ACE-2) while binding at the cell surface [36, 39]. However, the SARS-CoV-2 binds more weakly in comparison to SARS-CoV [37]. COVID-19 disease consequently causes alarming situations worldwide that pose a cluster of questions for the scientific community. Itinquired contemporaneous exploration of epidemiological studies such as the origin of the emerging coronavirus, its nature, mode and routes of transmission, host susceptibilities, and epidemic situations throughout the world. It also needs the purpose of valid and utmost awareness concerning circumstances and updates intercessions. The purpose of this comprehensive study was to report the updated epidemiological factors regarding COVID-19 to deduce all valuable tall parameters to fill gaps primarily.

Origin of SARS-CoV-2

Emergence and re-emergence of viral infectious diseases occur periodically in various countries globally, and some are moderate. At the same time, many are life-threatening, posing severe clinical conditions [40]. The sudden and unusual outbreaks of SARS-CoV-2 representing impulsive nature were started at the end of 2019 [1] with the deficiency of deliberate and consistent epidemiological studies to summarize the SARS-CoV-2 source decisively. The SARS-CoV-2 source has remained a hot topic of great discussion after initial reports of pneumonia-like infections with unknown etiology [41]. Meanwhile, analyzing the risk factors and other associated features of the hospital enrolled infected patients, they were revealed to have epidemiologically associated with supermarkets and exposed them to seafood and wet animals [42]. Mammals include rodents and bats, had been an origin of the previous human pathogenic coronaviruses [43]. Retrospectively, SARS-CoV, which was reported in 2002, Guangdong Province, China, a wide variety of wild and domestic animals were examined to trace the virus origin. The most likely animals involved in virus transmission were raccoon dogs and Himalayan palm civets [44]. Unpredictably, genetically similar coronavirus to SARS-CoV was identified in bats [45, 46]. After a decade of SARS-CoV outbreak, another coronavirus Middle East Respiratory Syndrome (MERS), emerged in KSA (Kingdom of Saudi Arabia). The disease signs and symptoms were similar to the SARS CoV [47]. However, without any past exposure history and serological evidence, the disease initiated the keen hunt for suspected animal origin [25, 47 - 49].

Primarily bats were considered as the origin of the MERS-CoV. However, after a brief analysis of suspected animals, the camels were also identified as host MERS-CoV along with bats [50]. About 90% of the camels are found with the MERS-CoV in the Middle East regions [51]. Recently, SARS-CoV-2 emerged in China with an unknown origin; however, the affected people had an association epidemiologically with seafood and wet animals in the wholesale market, indicating zoonotic origin [52, 53]. During early investigations, genomic analysis of various patient specimens revealed 99.9% genomic similarity among them, giving the clue of a very new host genetic shift into patients [9, 39]. Like the other two previous coronaviruses, such as SARS and MERS, those animals of the market were postulated as an intermediate host between virus and human, even though the particular animal is still not identified [6]. The zoonotic origin of SARS-CoV-2 was predicted from the exposure of the infected population to the live animals in the wholesale market of Wuhan [42].

The exact origin and location of SARS-CoV-2 is still unexplored. Yet, bats were suggested as culprits due to genomic sequence similarity of SARS-CoV-2 to the other coronaviruses. SARS-CoV-2was isolated from bats [54] during the serological investigations of other animals with direct or indirect links with the affected patients. It is thought that after escaping from origin (bats), SARS-CoV-2 faced evolution and mutated on exposure to different environmental conditions and got the potential to infect humans [55]. Consequently, it was the adaptation of coronavirus to a pathogenic state under the influence of nature. Southern China, Europe, Asia, and Africa are abundant with the species of bats species of *Rhinolophus affinis* [56]. Human interference in natural territories and recurrent incorporation of different species in markets is one of the leading causes of novel 'viruses' emergence and re-emergence [23]. However, 96% of the genetic similarity was found between bat coronavirus and SARS-CoV-2 [40]. Bats are natural hosts of the coronaviruses, and because of mutation, several viruses had experienced evolutionary phases inside bats [57, 58].

Furthermore, the other indicated animals with having the potential of intermediate hosts were snakes, cat civets, and pangolins [59]. Considerably, coronaviruses similar to SARS-CoV-2 were found in the *Manis javanica* (Malayan pangolins) that were shipped to Guangdong province of China without authorization [60]. Surprisingly, the identified genes of SARS-CoV-2 were identical to the partial spike genes of other coronaviruses. Another coronavirus isolated from pangolins [61 - 63] had a potential linkage with SARS-CoV-2 [64].

Above and beyond all recent research innovations and breakthroughs, there are still certain issues that need to be addressed, along with the questions of evolution patterns. The forces that drive the SARS-CoV-2 outbreak precisely need to be answered [65]. The emergence of novel coronavirus signified the unique challenges to biological/medical sciences and stimulate the researcher's interest in tracing the exact viral origin.

Host Susceptibilities

During an early epidemic of COVID-19 presumed the susceptibility of every individual. However, vulnerability increase with certain risk factors and underlying conditions like diminished immunity, older age, renal disorders, smoking, cardiovascular diseases, and hypertension [56]. The host's susceptibility to SARS-CoV-2 is determined by the presence of a particular receptor ACE-2 on SARS-CoV-2 binds to enter its genome inside the host cell [66]. Previous SARS-CoV that emerged in 2002 was using the same receptor ACE-2 during pathogenesis [67], though the SARS-CoV-2 binds more weakly in comparison with the SARS-CoV [37]. The SARS-CoV-2 mainly targets the respiratory tract of humans [68]. The lower airways cells have been reported as target sites of SARS-CoV-2. The evidence of radiology graphs confirms the replication of SARS-CoV-2 in that site, although no apparent clinical symptom appears in infected patients [69]. The motive behind the targeting of the respiratory tract by SARS-CoV-2 is an ACE-2 receptor that facilitates its genetic materials entry of pathogen inside the cells. ACE-2 is primarily expressed in the human respiratory tract [70 - 72]. The individuals are at a higher risk for COVID-19 disease with a high magnitude of ACE-2 receptors on the cell surfaces. Based on some theories, the expression of the ACE-2 receptor might be associated with race as an early report suggested males from Asian countries had major proportions of cells that express ACE-2 receptors than African people, white people, and Americans [73].

Moreover, the expression of the ACE-2 gene is considerably high in smokers, suggesting smokers are more susceptible to COVID-19 [74]. Additionally, the

ACE-2 receptor is also expressed in the epithelial cells and type2 pneumonocytes of the submucosal glands of ferrets and cats [75]. Thus, these animals facilitate the efficient replication of SARS-CoV-2 and make the ferrets a suitable candidate to be utilized for evaluating vaccines and antiviral drug trials or other therapeutic strategies against COVID-19 as an animal model. Finally, the susceptibility of Egyptian fruit bats is also reported to be infected by SARS-CoV-2, although disease symptoms were not observed nor capably spread the infection to other animal members [76].

Inhaling the SARS-CoV-2 containing aerosols is the most probable cause of COVID-19 disease [77 - 80]. Initially, the SARS-CoV-2 penetrates in the nasal opening and binds with the ACE-2 receptor on epithelial cells, where its replication started [81]. *In vitro* study of the SARS coronavirus indicates that the ciliated cells in the conducting airways to be infected primarily by the virus [83]. In this phase, because of limited, inadequate responses of innate immunity, the virus propagates locally and diagnosed with nasal swabs. However, the viral load is low but still infectious [84]. Furthermore, the virus propagation continues besides conducting airways and reaches the lower region of the respiratory system, and infection symptoms become visible, representing typical clinical symptoms of the disease. The virus triggers innate immunity response robustly; early markers of inherent immunity virus yield should be present in the sputum and nasal swabs. The innate immunity response in cytokines, like the intensity of CXCL10, may be predictive of the consequent clinical course [85]. However, in the infections of SARS coronaviruses, the reported valuable disease marker is the CXCL10 gene [86]. Approximately 20% of patients progress to the next phase of COVID-19 characterized by pulmonary infiltrates development, while some develop severe type disease with a 2% fatality rate [87]. Initial research findings of demographic and clinical distinctiveness of laboratory-confirmed COVID-19 patients in China revealed the susceptibilities of all individuals of both sexes, male and female of all ages, with ranges of 0 to >90 [88]. The people at the highest risk to get COVID-19 infection those with underlying diseases and abnormal health conditions like hypertension, diabetes mellitus, cardiac, renal, malfunctioned immune system, and elders individuals [89, 90]. Especially the elders with underlying diseases like renal, lung, coronary infections, and high blood pressure can slow down the immune system processes, increasing their vulnerability for COVID-19 [87]. During an early outbreak of SARS-CoV-2 till January 2, 2020, in China, among initial 42 hospitals admitted laboratory-confirmed patients, 30 patients were male with the 49 years age median, fewer than half were noticed with background diseases like hypertension, diabetes, and cardiovascular disease [6]. These comorbidities like diabetes, cardiovascular diseases, and hypertension are rarely observed among children compared to adults [91]. There are mild immunological reactions in children due to less prevalence of

C-reactive proteins result in reduced immunity or less minor immune damage in children. There is a greater chance of immune damage in adults due to a higher prevalence of increased C-proteins [92]. Untilmid-March 2020, reported confirmed cases of COVID-19 reached 169,930 confirmed COVID-19 cases worldwide, among which 73% of patients were 40+ in age and the fatality rate of patients younger than 40 years was 2.6%. Notably, no fatalities were reported among children of less than ten years [93]. According to the COVID-19 reports of the different countries, the older patients presented the highest case fatalities [94]. In Italy, the highest fatality rate is reported in older people with age ranges of 70-80 years. However, based on reports of statistics, China and Italy reported similar fatalities in older people in age ranges of 0-69 years [95]. The aged male population with hypertension is more susceptible to developing the severe type of COVID-19 with the renin-angiotensin system (RAS) that helps maintain the blood pressure homeostasis and the salt balance and fluids [96].

Furthermore, due to the critical immune system of the aged individuals and weakening capability to heal damage, the epithelium is particularly higher at risk of getting COVID-19. The virus may spread efficiently to gas exchange units of the lungs as a result of reducing mucociliary clearance in this population [97]. For aged people, the COVID-19 can be life-threatening and devastating. Raise the concentration of myocardial enzymes indicates that COVID-19 has a striking effect on other vital organs like the heart other than lungs which are thought to be remarkable characteristics of COVID-19 infection in humans. Though, these circumstances of increased myocardial enzymes are observed in both children and adults [6]. Moreover, a case study of COVID-19 disease was conducted on infants with age ranges of 45 days to 1 year, all patients were noticed with mild symptoms, and the requirement of intensive care was not observed [98]. Conversely, a WHO report noticed the infected children group that was rarely affected with mild symptoms of COVID-19 disease, and the infection percentage of the children and teenagers was 2.4%. At the same time, the other patients that were above 60 years and those with underlying diseases were appeared to develop the COVID-19 disease with severe symptoms; even death is also reported [99]. The COVID-19 disease is less prevalent in children attributable to limited outdoor activities and less exposure to the potential source. Moreover, according to some scholars, due to less exposure to outdoor, they did not experience hazardous pollutants, and their respiratory tract is healthier. Furthermore, the cytokines storm develops with less intensity in the immune system of children [100]. However, the symptoms progress is accelerated with background diseases and co-infections like influenza virus and bacterial infection (*Klebsiella*) that lead the disease to be poorly diagnosed. Additionally the significant deterministic feature of the severity of the symptoms is age and those underlying disease [101]. Although according to the study's findings conducted in Singapore, the infected patient could too build up severe disease without background diseases. Additionally, they need to be facilitated with intensive care [102]. Furthermore, postoperative patients with COVID-19 disease are noticed with severe complications and included death. According to Wang *et al.* [103], 138 COVID-19 confirmed patients were hospitalized, among which 34 patients undergo surgery. Later on, seven operative patients with severe complications of COVID-19 disease were died. However, this fatality rate of operative patients is much higher than the general mortality rate of 2.3% COVID-19 [87]. It is also higher than fatalities of 7.9% of the other noncardiac postoperative ICU admitted patients without COVID-19 disease [104]. In another surgery-linked study of COVID-19 patients, 34 postoperative patients quickly manifested the COVID-19 symptoms and subsequently confirmed by laboratory diagnosis as well. However, priorsurgery, they were not observed with the signs of COVID-19.They had been exposed directly to the city of Wuhan [105]. It was believed that earlier than enduring surgeries, those patients were in the incubation period of COVID-19 infection that time. It is evident that the severity and exacerbation of the COVID-19 disease progression lead by surgical pressure during the incubation period [104]. Moreover, besides surgeries majority of patients were aged and suffering from other diseases. Postoperative patients were found with immune malfunctioning [106]. In addition to immune malfunctioning, the systemic inflammatory response is also induced due to surgery [107]. If a patient recently recovered from viral infection if got COVID-19 disease, he could have severe challenges while combating COVID-19 as his immune system is down due to that recent viral infection [108]. In a viral infection, the immune cells are diminished in body fluids, and cytokine levels become high, which leads to a condition termed cytokine release syndrome (CRS). It is sensitive systemic inflammatory patterns in which patients suffer from fever and malfunctions of numerous organs dysfunctions [109]. According to the review, Amir ad colleagues [66] has gathered the clinical data of 76993 COVID-19 patients, the most common background disease found among the COVID-19 affected population was hypertension (16.37%), the fraction of the affected population with cardiovascular disease was 12.11%, diabetic patients were 7.87%. In contrast, the lowest susceptible population was 7.63% smokers [66]. Individuals with pre-existing cardiovascular conditions are at risk of developing COVID-19 infection; the pro-inflammatory cytokines are decreased due to cardiovascular diseases that lead the immune system to become weak [110, 111]. The ACE-2 receptors in smokers are unregulated in remodeled cell types. However, smoking amount, duration, and cessation also play a role [66].

Previously, the receptor of MERS coronavirus dipeptidyl peptidase 4 (DPP4) was reported with high expression in smokers [112]. Notably, the consequences of the COVID-19 have been noticed more severe in people with smoking habits and chronic obstructive pulmonary diseases (COPD) [113]. This is a significant point that needs to be considered. People with tumors are also more vulnerable to COVID-19 disease than those without tumors as they can become immunosuppressed by taking chemotherapy, surgery, and other anti-cancerous treatments [114]. Therefore, the people with the aforementioned therapies, conditions and risk factors should be examined thoroughly. The concerned authorities are responsible for screening the travelers and immediately isolating the confirmed COVID-19 patients, providing a protective mechanism, guiding the local people, and instructing the population with the highest susceptibilities [115, 116]. Travel restrictions are essential for the patients with those underlying diseases. They must be conscious about their vulnerability, equipped with the basic fundamental knowledge of COVID-19 disease prevention like the covering of nose and mouth, frequent hand washing with a sanitizer, and social distancing [117]. A study investigated comparing blood groups among infected patients. Interestingly, the individuals with the A-blood group are significantly higher at risk of getting COVID-19 disease, while individuals with the O-blood group are lower at risk for the disease [118]. However, females are noticed to have a lower chance of developing severe and critical illness. At the same time, the male is comparatively higher at risk of developing the severe and critical disease [119], of developing severe and critical acute disease [119], the exact reason is unknown. However, the probable cause may be smoking and underlying conditions contributing to the worsening of males [120].

Transmission Routes

The SARS-CoV-2 has emerged in China in a particular population who were exposed to seafood and wet animals in the Huanan wholesale market of Wuhan city [6]. Early investigations of the bats were postulated as the origin of the SARS-CoV-19. Patently, there was 88% of the genomic similarity among SARS-CoV-2 and the two SARS-like coronaviruses that were isolated from bats during early investigations of SARS-CoV-2 origin [37, 121]. It is revealed that only that population could be infected with COVID-19 who have experienced the reservoir or eaten the infected animals. Although SARS-CoV-2 needs to be spread resourcefully to cause large extended transmission from human to human-like previous SARS coronavirus reported in Guangdong province, China 2002 [6, 122]. Based on two previous coronavirus epidemics, such as SARS and MERS experiences, the initially proposed mechanism for transmission of SARS-CoV-2 was human to human by respiratory secretions through close contact [123]. In the beginning, the transmission from bat origin and other suspected infected wilds animals were considered the reason for early outbreaks of COVID-19, whereas human-to-human transmission was not highlighted. Surprisingly the SARS-Co--2 spread from humans to humans was appeared by a cluster of COVID-19 cases among members of the same family through close contact between them [124 - 127]. Hence this was the first report which describes the SARS-CoV-2 transmission among humans. Surprisingly, after the first outbreak in China, SARS-CoV-2 spread worldwide by close contact of human-to-human in a month [6]. After the initial symptoms onsets of COVID-19 infection, the highest virus load was found in nasal secretions instead of the throat [56]. The nasal secretions start spreading the virus in almost one week of infection, and then within four days, the outflow and transmission rate reaches peak [12, 129]. Besides nasal secretions, the virus is also found in the stool, but nasal secretions are thought to be the primary mode of transmission [130]. In comparison with other animal viruses the particular conditions of the environment required for the SARS-CoV-2 endurance and spread are fewer and limited but obvious to some extent [131], included humidity and temperatures that are noticed for having the potential to affect the SARS-CoV-2 transmissibility. Moreover, the most probable route of COVID-19 infection transmission is human to human that is supported by family members cases that did not expose to wet animals but developed COVID-19 infection [132, 133]. Besides the family cases, additional evidence made known the person-to-person transmission with the particular staff of the hospital, such as physicians, nurses, and support staff. Notably, the room's condition in the hospital where the COVID-19 infected patients were quarantined was noticed with extensive contamination [56, 134]. Eventually, virus transmission from human-t--human due to close contact was officially recognized by scientists and health professionals as the disease spread rapidly [103]. Furthermore, some other persons were diagnosed with COVID-19, and they have not even visited the seafood market or contacted wet animals. Shockingly transmission of SARS-CoV-2 *via* person to person noticed from asymptomatic carriers as well [103, 125] while having peak viral loads like symptomatic individuals without revealing any symptom of COVID-19 [135]. MERS coronavirus transmission from person to person was also reported in the primary healthcare settings and the same transmission route and mechanism as by coughs and sneezes [136]. The same route and mode of transmission as SARS CoV-2 and MERS were observed in the SARS outbreaks in 2002 as well, although, in comparison with COVID-19, the SARS coronavirus was not that much quickly transmitting. Additionally, the other less common transmission methods include handling the wild animals, transmission by feco-oral route, and fomites [137]. The transmission of SARS Coronavirus was reported using fecal-containing materials and broken sewage pipes [138]. Human-to-human transmission occurred by respiratory secretions through coughs and sneezes. Those who are most frequently involved in COVID-19 spread and do not be confused with transmission through the air [139]. Because due to the large size of droplets, it has a propensity to go down on the ground around the infected person within 2 meters instead of remain in the air.

However, due to direct and indirect contact, the SARS-CoV-2 can transmit to other humans from the landed droplets of the infected population. Meanwhile, before or after landing, any close human is present nearer to the infected person [93]. From the droplets of the infected person, the virus attached to the host cell receptor by spikes containing receptor binding proteins while facilitating the viral entry inside the cells. Furthermore, the complement host cell receptor is determined by species range and tissue tropism of the virus [140, 141]. However, in the case of humans infection, the SARS-CoV-2 binds to ACE2 present on their cells [142]. Infection transmission from infected patients was more probably observed in the early stages of infection meanwhile peak viral loads in the nasal cavity [135].

However, the SARS-CoV-2 is also isolated from a stool sample of COVID-19 infected patients that suggests the alternative mode with transmission potential by route of feco-oral, although official transmission is not documented yet [128, 129, 143, 144]. Furthermore, the SARS-CoV-2 was also found in the serum samples [145, 146], blood samples [6], saliva samples, urine samples, and rectal swabs [147]. Interestingly no vertical transmission of COVID-19 by sexual intercourse and during breastfeeding is reported so far. However, in a couple of COVID-19 infections in infected mothers, the infant was perceived with adverse health results, including death [14, 149]. There were 1252000, and 1423 healthcare officials reported in China and Italy, respectively, on March 17, 2020 [150, 151]. The transmission of COVID-19 infection through blood is not recognized yet. However, precautionary procedures were made active by the National Blood Center of the National Institute of Health (ISS) for blood transfusion practices [152]. Under another Chinese published study, 8.7% of patients were reported to get infection directly from the potential source (Huanan fish market). In comparison, the human-to-human transmission was reported in 41% of patients, 12.3% were family cases, and 29% were healthcare officials [103]. Until April 1, some countries like Nepal, Bhutan, Angola, Namibia, Sudan, Somalia, Mongolia, and Papua New Guinea did not report the infection spread due to local transmission. Therefore, infection remains limited to imported cases [153]. However, some countries, such as the Holy See, Timor-Leste United Republic of Tanzania, where transmission classification is under investigation [153].

Environmental Factors Influence on SARS-CoV-2

SARS-CoV-2 was broke out in China in late December 2019 [154], while the virus emerged in humans most probably during the second week of November 2019 [155]. These two months (November and December 2019) in China are the coldest months of the winter season [156]. Additionally, during these months, severe drought season was observed in Wuhan for almost 40 years with 5.5mm precipitation in December 2019 [157, 158]. Coincidently, the outbreak of the first SARS-CoV was observed in the same country and same season in Guangdong Province, 2002 [159] with similar weather patterns like Wuhan [160], while the precipitation was 0 mm in Foshan, Guangdong in December 2002 [161]. According to the study of Chan and colleagues [162], the humidity and low temperatures may have a positive impact on the SARS-CoV-2 spread. Usually, low temperatures provide a conducive environment for the virus, while in the moist temperate areas, the virus would not spread proficiently [163]. The summer and monsoon periods can decrease the transmission of SARS-CoV-2 effectively [164]. Indirectly low temperatures can significantly enhance the viral pathogenesis because of reduced blood supply that causes immune cells provision to the nasal route. At the same time, cilia cells can eliminate particles of the virus from the airway reduced in low humidity, which can facilitate viral pathogenesis and survival [165]. An experimental study was conducted on airborne human coronavirus 229E (HCV/229E) similar to SARS-CoV-2 as a representative, which shows that at 30 and 50% humidity, the half-life of the virus was 27 and 67 hours respectively.

In contrast, the half-life of the virus was reduced to only 3 hours at 80% humidity [166]. The temperature harm the survival of SARS Coronavirus, the optimal environmental temperature during the cases of SARS Coronavirus was from 16°C to 28°C [167], and the virus quickly inactivated at 20°C in the *in vitro* comparison with the lower temperature less than 5°C on surfaces [168]. According to another laboratory study, the viability of coronavirus rapidly lost at higher temperatures while at 22-25°C temperature virus can remain stable for more than 5 days on smooth surfaces [123]. Furthermore, the viability and survivability of *betacoronaviruses* depend on the nature of the surface on which nasal secretions of the patient landed. Founded on previous coronaviruses, SARS, and MERS, on glass, plastic, metals, or other inanimate surfaces, viruses remain viable and infectious from 2 hours to 9 days. However, this period can increase colder and dry environments [169 - 171]. Similarly, the MERS virus was also susceptible to high temperatures, and less stability was observed at high temperatures [170]. Most of the studies have revealed the sensitivity of the coronaviruses (SARS and MERS) to high temperatures.

Correspondingly, SARS-CoV-2 was also expected to be denatured at the start of outbreaks. Still, according to Zhu and co-workers' laboratory study, the negative consequence of high temperature could not observe on COVID-19 infection [172]. The survival of human coronavirus 229E (HCoV-229E) was evaluated by infecting human hands revealed that 45% of viruses remain viable following 60 minutes. This experiment was performed as a substitute for SARS-CoV-2 due to its similarity. The deliberate infection of COVID-19 is not permissible because of safety and ethical considerations [173]. Following another study, washing hands with water reduced 70% viral concentration of HCoV-229E, while with hand sanitizer, the virus was declined by 99.99% within half a minute [174].

Additionally, the common disinfectants like sodium hypochlorite and ethanol were reported effective and inactivate the coronaviruses within 1 min contact [169]. In comparison with the other pathogenic viruses, all the three coronaviruses SARS, MERS, and SARS-CoV-2, are at higher risk influence by environmental factors [175]. According to scientific reports, the high temperatures have depress the SARS-CoV-2 survival. Therefore, infectivity is reduced with high temperatures as the droplets containing SARS-CoV-2 nuclei evaporated with high temperatures [176, 177]. Although, ultraviolet light has been reported to have the potential to denature the viruses, the susceptibility of previous SARS coronavirus to ultraviolet light has already been reported. Still, it is not exclusively analyzed against SARS-CoV-2 [178].

Worldwide Epidemics of COVID-19 Disease

Outbreaks of COVID-19. The earliest cases of COVID-19 with the distress of respiratory system was reported at the end of December 2019, in the population of Wuhan city, Hubei Province, China during the last dates of the month [179], during the period of December 18, to December 29, one patient died among the enrolled patients in hospital [9]. Further till January 2, 2020, a total of 41 other laboratories confirmed patients reported with the COVID-19 disease in Wuhan, China [6]. The mode of transmission of the SARS-CoV-2 was similar to the influenza virus by coughing, sneezing, and exhaling droplets of the respiratory tract [180]. Wuhan, a being transport hub and movement of the Chinese population for preparation of Chunyun (Chinese New Year), played a substantial role in the spread of COVID-19 disease throughout China [181]. The people who visit Wuhan from other cities and regions experience exposure to potential COVID-19 sources, and the infected population included asymptomatic carriers. However on the way back to their destinations, they imported the infection, then the virus spread rapidly by population transmission after their arrival [181]. Later on, till January 22, 2020, the pathogen COVID-19 extended to the 25 other regions, *i.e.,* districts and cities of China, infecting 571 patients in those regions [182]. Shortly, on January 24, 2020, the cases of COVID-19 disease reached 878 across China, while there were only 17 other cases in 6 countries [183]. Human-to-human transmission of infection contributed to the rapid distribution and increased cases of COVID-19 disease like outbreaks of previous two coronaviruses such as SARS and MERS [184].

In a while, till January 25, the cases were then reached to 1975 cases, whereas the 56 patients of them had lost their lives as said by the Chinese National Health Commission (CNHC) [185]. According to another study, the estimated growing incidence of COVID-19 disease reached 5502 cases till January 24, 2020, according to the study of Nishiura and co-workers [186].

Initial Episode in the USA

The US evaluated the initial confirmed case of the nCoV-19 with mild symptoms related to pneumonia for diagnosis and treatment first case of nCoV-19 [187]. On January 30, 2020, the United States of America (USA) first reported the SARS-CoV-2 transmission by human-to-human [188]. At the end of January 2020, the incidence of infected patients were reached 7734 and 90 cases with a 2.2% fatality rate in China other countries that include Japan, Vietnam, Finland, Philippines, Malaysia, Thailand, Australia, India, Singapore, United States, France, Taiwan, Republic of Korea, Nepal, Canada, Germany, Sri Lanka, UAE, and Cambodia respecively [189].

Epidemic in Diamond Princess (Cruise Ship)

Regrettably, a cruise ship (Diamond Princess) with 3711 travelers was reported positive with the outbreak of COVID-19. Furthermore, a traveler from Hong Kong who boarded in Yokohama port and landed in Hong Kong on January 25, 2020. Later on, on February 1 he was daignosed positive with COVID-19 infection, although earlier than boarding, he has coughs [190]. Furthermore, after ship arrival on February 4, in Yokohama port, 10 more cases were confirmed, and the ship was then quarantined for two weeks before departure to Japan. Till February 16, 355 ship individuals reported positive with COVID-19 infection [190]. Later on, the positive cases reached 696 with 7 fatalities [191].

On February 7, 2020, the cases of infected patients in the Chinese population were reached 31,161, with 630 deaths, accomplished by health authorities in China, published in Nature Scientific Reports [192]. As of February 16, 2020, 70548 COVID-19 cases were reported in China [193]. The COVID-19 disease has affected 1775 individuals with a 2.8% fatality rate [194]. Iran reported the initial confirmed cases of COVID-19 on February 19, 2020, in the province of Qom [195]. However, both had died after that day, following reports of the Ministry of Health and Medical Education [196]. Afterward, according to the health authorities of Iran, the confirmed cases of COVID-19 reached 9000, including 354 deaths; this was the first highest incidence in Western Asia and the globally third highest incidence of COVID-19 faced by Iran after China and Italy [197]. Several higher-ranking Iranian Government officials were diagnosed positive of COVID-19, including Mr. Iraj Harirchi (Deputy Health Minister) [198], Mr.

Masoumeh Ebtekar, who is the Vice President for Women and Family Affairs and Mr. Mojtaba Zolnour, the Parliament's Chairman of Foreign Affairs Committee and National Security [199].

Italy

In Italy, the initial outbreak of COVID-19 was noticed in two regions, Codogno, Lombardy, and Vo Euganeo, Veneto [200]. In Italy February 25, 2020, 243 cases were reported in regions, 240 in Lombardy and 43 in Veneto, which were then spread rapidly, and on the March 31, the cases of Lombardy reached 1520 and 307 in Veneto [201]. At the end of February, the COVID-19 infection reached 66 countries. Overall, reported worldwide cases were 89,068 with 3,046 deaths, and most affected countries were China, Korea, Italy, and Iran with infection cases of 80,134, 42,212,1689, and 978 respectively [202].

Worldwide Cases since March

The frequency of new cases was nine times higher than in China, leading the various countries to bans the entry of arriving travelers. They apply forceful quarantine measures included closures of schools and other educational institutes, shutting of public transports, and avoiding social gatherings consecutively to limited and prevent the spread of COVID-19 infection [203, 204]. However, the acclamation about the school closing condition was released by CDC [100]. Until March 2, 2020, the new cases acceleration of COVID-19 has decreased considerably in China due to confrontational control and preventive approaches like complete lockdown and other safety measures. However, outside of China across the world, the acceleration of COVID-19 cases increased significantly. The asymptomatic individuals were responsible for this rapid emergence, they might spread the infection during the incubation period, and the transmission chain remains unnoticed [205]. However, according to the study of Cascella and colleagues [206], there were 79,968 COVID-19 patients who are diagnosed clinically and confirmed by the laboratory are documented in China by March 3, 2020. Overall worldwide cases reached 87,317, among which 2,977 patients recovered from the COVID-19 [206]. The greater part of the COVID-19 cases (92%) has been reported from mainland China and the highest fatality rate of 96.5% of 2,873 deaths. Next to China, the COVID-19 affected 59 different countries worldwidely, with 7,169 reported cases [207]. Approximately, every continent is affected by COVID-19 globally [208].

The COVID-19 Turning into Pandemic

By mid of March 2020, the COVID-19 disease extended to 117 countries, affected almost every continent of the world, and WHO declared the COVID-19 as pandemic [209], with overall cases of COVID-19 of 126,277 with the highest incidence rates in China (Mainland), Italy, Iran, and South Korea [210]. Later in March 2020, the highest incidence of COVID-19 disease was reported in Italy, with 24,747 confirmed cases after China which is mainland. On the other hand, Iran reported 13,938, and worldwide deaths were 6522 with a 3.83% case fatality rate, among which 3212 deaths were reported from China [93]. Thus, till March 20, 2020, the overall worldwide reported cases were reached 270,069 with 11,271 fatalities, whereas the recovered patients were 90,603. Among which 4,032 deaths were reported from Italy, 3,248 from China, 1,433 from Iran, and Spain reported 1,1044 deaths [211].

The Robust Spread of COVID-19 in European Countries

On March 22, 2020, the COVID-19 infection reached 189 countries, and 292,142 individuals were affected, while death cases were 12,784 [6]. The prevalence of COVID-19 disease was higher among adults and elders, men are slightly predominant compared to women, and the infection incidence was low in pediatrics [87, 212]. However, the fatality rate was significantly high in older people and the people diagnosed late and did not get isolation and supportive treatment as they remain unnoticed for a long time [213]. Moreover, more severe symptoms and critical conditions were noticed in people with pre-existing background diseases such as diabetes, cardiovascular, and respiratory distress [213]. Since March 25, 2020, the worldwide reported cases of COVID-19 reached 467,593, and Italy, which has become the hot spot of the COVID-19 pandemic, reported 74,386 cases with 7,503 deaths [214]. However, as of April 7 2020, the worldwide confirmed cases reach 1,349,660 with 74,816 deaths while affecting the 190 countries and territories [215].

WHO Reports

According to WHO report that published on January 20, the COVID-19 affected 282 individuals, and 258 in Hubei Province, 20 from other provinces with the majority of cases, 14 from Guangdong Province, while 4 cases reported from other countries. On the same date, 1 from Japan, and Korea, respectively, and 2 cases from Thailand were reported. All the cases reported outside of China were connected with the travel history of China [216]. Later on, the confirmed cases of other countries were adruptly reached to 683 [217]. On the WHO website, the worldwide documented cases of COVID-19 disease were reached 71,429 by February 17, 2020 [218]. Out of 71,429, 70,635 were reported from China and the remaining 794 cases were reported from 24 other different countries, including Vietnam, Malaysia, Singapore, Thailand, Japan, Philippines Republic of Korea, Canada, France, Australia, Belgium, Cambodia, Nepal, Finland, India, Sri Lanka,

USA, Italy, the UK, UAE, Russian Federation, Sweden, Germany, and Spain [218].

Table 1. The COVID-19 incidence among Chinese Provinces till February 22 [219].

Province/Regions	Positive Confirmed Patients	Fatalities
Hubei Province	62662	2144
Guangdong Province	1333	05
Henan	1267	19
Zhejiang	1203	01
Hunan	1011	04
Anhui	988	06
Jiangxi	934	01
Shandong	748	04
Jiangsu	631	0
Chongqing	567	06
Sichuan	525	03
Heilongjiang	479	12
Beijing Province	396	04
Shanghai Province	334	02
Hebei Province	308	05
Fujian	293	01
Guangxi	246	02
Shaanxi	245	01
Yunnan	174	2
Total	75769	2239

According to WHO Situation Report-32 (February 22, 2020), the worldwide cases of COVID-19 reached 76,769, among which 75769 cases were reported from China with 2239 fatalities [219] (Table **1**). The rest 1200 cases outside of China with 8 deaths reported from various areas of Western Pacific, South-East Asia, United States America, Europe, and Eastern Mediterranean regions (Fig. **2**) [219].

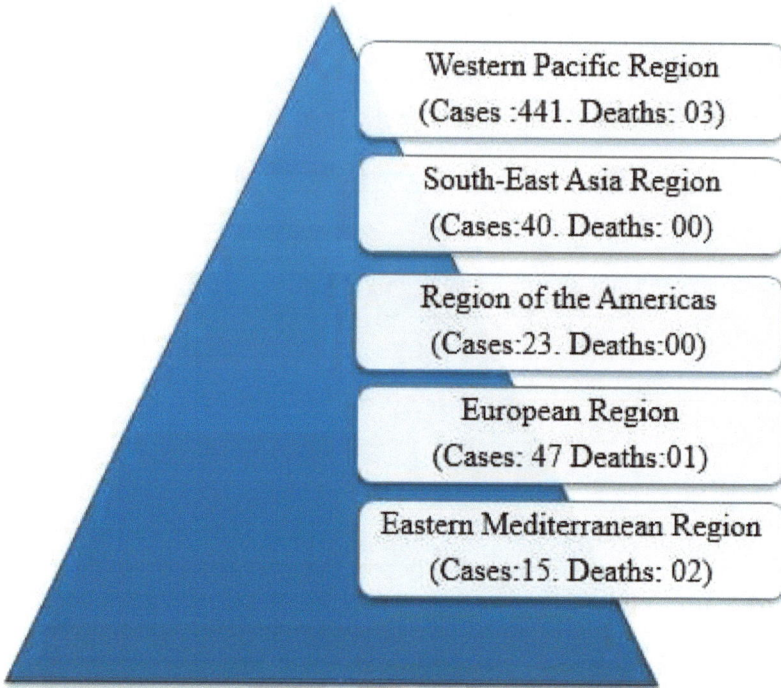

Fig. (2). The Worldwide cases of COVID-19 across different regions February 22, 2020 [219].

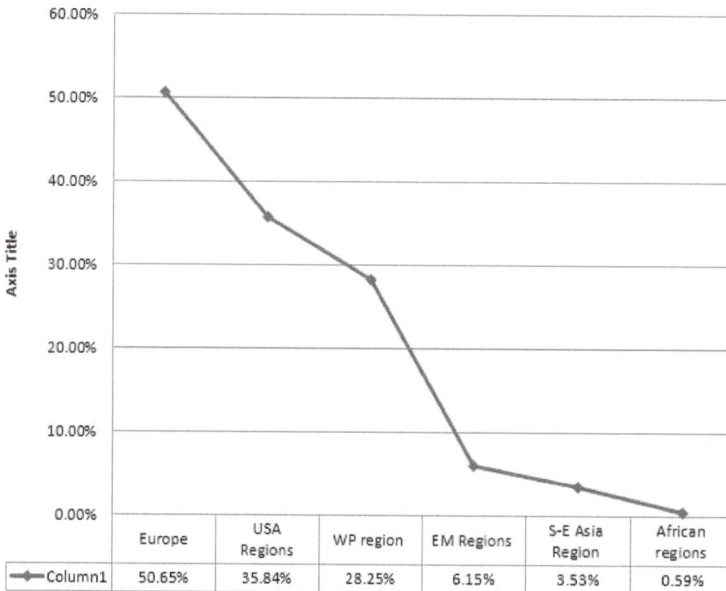

Fig. (3). WP= Western Pacific, EM= Eastern Mediterranean, S-E= South-East Worldwide Prevalence of COVID-19 until April 17.

According to the WHO report of March 31, 2020, the total worldwide cases were 693,224 with 33,106 deaths [220]. European Region was more prevalent with 392,757 infection cases and 29,962 fatalities. Region of the Americas reported 142,081 cases with 2457 deaths. The reported cases of the Western Pacific region were 103,775 with 3649 fatalities, Eastern Mediterranean 46,329 cases with 2813 fatalities, South East Asia 40,84, 158 cases with fatalities while Africa 3486 cases with 60 fatalities [220]. WHO published situation report-72 on April 1 2020, which states that overall worldwide cases reached 823,626 with 40,598 fatalities [221]. The disease burden has been increased in European regions as highest cases 464,212 found in the European regions with 30,089 deaths, second highest cases numbers found in the regions of America 188,751 with 3400 deaths. Western Pacific region reported 106,422 cases with 3701 deaths, Eastern Mediterranean 54,281 cases with 3115 deaths, South-East Asia 5175 cases with 195 deaths. In comparison, African regions reported 4073 cases with 91 deaths [221]. Afterward, on April 17 2020, another report of WHO states that worldwide cases reached 2,074,5279 with 139378 deaths [222]. European regions reported the highest cases 1,050,871 with 93,480 deaths, USA 743,607 cases with 33,028 deaths, Western Pacific 127,595 cases with 5558 deaths, Eastern Mediterranean 115,824 cases with 5662 deaths, South-East Asia 23,560 cases with 1,051 deaths. In comparison, African regions reported 12,360 cases with 586 deaths (Fig. **3**) [222].

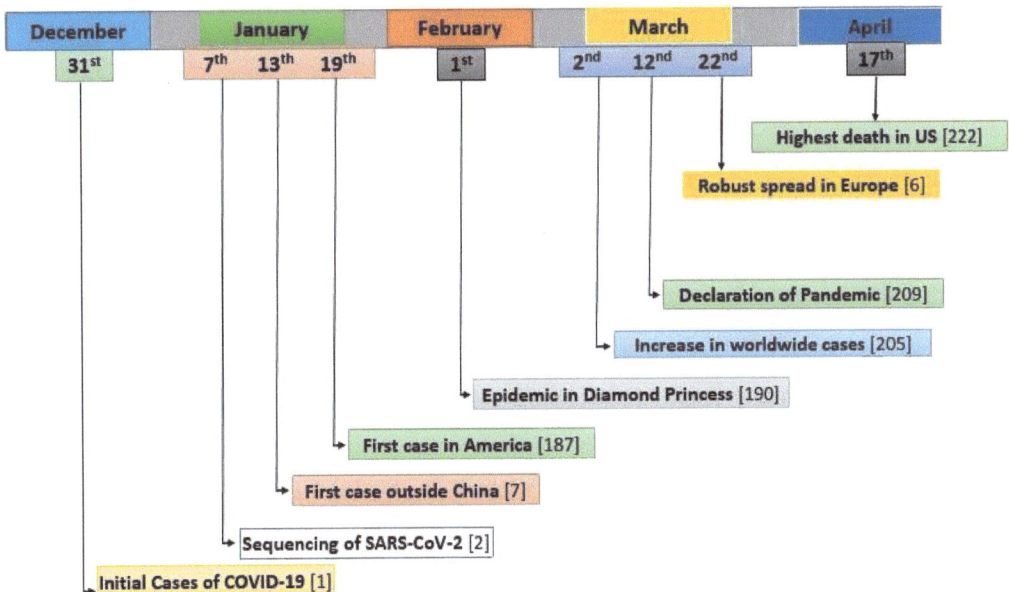

Fig. (4). Important events have occurred during the COVID-19 outbreak from December 31 to April 17.

Table 2. The infection and death cases of COVID-19 disease in most affected countries.

European Regions				
	Countries	Total Cases	Deaths	Mortality Rate
	Spain	182816	19130	10.46%
	Italy	168941	22172	13.12%
	Germany	133830	3868	2.89%
	France	107778	17899	16.60%
	UK	103097	13729	13.31%
	Turkey	74193	1643	1.65%
	Belgium	34809	4857	13.95%
	Russian Federation	32008	273	0.85%
	Netherlands	29214	3315	11.34%
	Switzerland	26651	1016	3.81%
	Portugal	18841	629	3.33%
	Austria	14448	410	2.83%
	Ireland	13271	486	3.66%
	Israel	12591	140	1.11%

(Table 2) cont.....

Americas Regions				
	USA	632781	28221	4.45%
	Canada	28884	1048	3.62%
	Brazil	28320	1736	6.12%

Americas Regions			
Peru	11475	254	2.21%
Chile	8807	105	1.19%
Ecuador	8225	403	4.89%
Mexico	5847	449	7.67%
Dominican Republic	3755	196	5.21%
Panama	3751	103	2.74%
Colombia	3105	131	4.21%
Argentina	2598	115	4.42%
Cuba	862	27	3.13%
Costa Rica	626	4	0.63%
Uruguay	493	9	1.82%
Bolivia	441	29	6.57%

(Table 2) cont.....

Western Pacific Region			
China	84149	4642	5.51%
Republic of Korea	10635	230	2.16%
Japan	9167	148	1.61%
Australia	6468	63	0.97%
Philippines	5660	362	6.39%
Malaysia	5182	84	1.62%
Singapore	4427	10	0.22%
New Zealand	1086	11	1.01%
Viet Nam	268	0	00
Brunei Darussalam	136	1	0.73%
Cambodia	122	0	00
Mongolia	31	0	00
Lao People's Democratic Republic	19	0	00
Fiji	17	0	00
Papua Ne	07	0	00

COVID-19
Table 2) cont.....

Eastern Mediterranean Region			
Iran (Islamic Republic of)	77995	4869	6.24%
Pakistan	7025	135	1.92%
Saudi Arabia	6380	83	1.30%
UAE	5825	35	0.60%
Qatar	4103	7	0.17%
Egypt	2673	196	7.33%
Morocco	2283	130	5.69%
Bahrain	1700	7	0.41%
Kuwait	1524	3	0.19%
Iraq	1434	80	5.57%
Oman	1069	5	0.46%
Afghanistan	845	30	3.55%
Tunisia	822	37	4.50%
Lebanon	663	21	3.16%
Djibouti	591	2	0.33%
Jordan	402	7	1.74%

Table 2) cont.....

South-East Asia Region			
India	13387	437	3.26%
Indonesia	5516	496	8.99%
Thailand	2700	247	9.14%
Bangladesh	1572	60	3.81%
Sri Lanka	238	7	2.94%
Myanmar	85	4	4.70%
Maldives	23	0	00
Timor-Leste	18	0	00
Nepal	16	0	00
Bhutan	5	0	00

COVID-19
(Table 2) contd....

African Region			
	South Africa	2605	48	1.84%
	Algeria	2268	348	15.34%
	Cameroon	855	17	1.98%
	Côte d'Ivoire	688	6	0.87%
	Ghana	641	8	1.24%
	Niger	609	15	2.46%
	Burkina Faso	543	32	5.89%
	Guinea	438	1	0.22%
	Nigeria	373	11	2.94%
	Senegal	335	2	0.59%
	Mauritius	324	9	2.77%
	Republic of Congo	287	23	8.01%
	Kenya	234	11	4.70%
	Mali	171	13	7.60%
	Rwanda	138	0	00
	Congo	117	5	4.27%

The highest cases were reported in United States America, 632781 with 28221 deaths. In the European regions, Spain reported the highest cases 182816 with 5183 deaths. In the Western Pacific region, China reported 84149 cases with 4642 deaths. In comparison, in Eastern Mediterranean region, Iran reported 7795 cases with 4869 deaths. There were 13387 cases with 437 deaths reported in India, while in the African region, South Africa had the highest cases, 2605 cases with 48 deaths (Table **2**) [222]. Conclusively, the critical events took place from December 31, 2019, to April 17, 2020 (Fig. **4**).

CONCLUSION

This book chapter evaluated the updated epidemiological factors of COVID-19. The SARS-CoV-2 is originated from bats and then quickly spread among humans through respiratory droplets. All the human population appeared to be susceptible to it; however, susceptibility increases with background diseases like cardiovascular diseases, diabetes, and hypertension. The environmental temperature role on the transmission of COVID-19 is not found yet. Initially, SARS-CoV-2 grabbed China, and then in very little time, it spread throughout the world and declared a pandemic in the second week of March. In March, the Chinese Government controlled the COVID-19, but outside China, infection acceleration increases significantly in Europe and the America.

CONSENT FOR PUBLICATION

Not Applicable.

CONFLICT OF INTEREST

The author confirms that this chapter contents have no conflict of interest.

ACKNOWLEDGEMENT

Declared none.

REFERENCES

[1]   Novel coronavirus (2019-nCoV) - who.int. Available at: https://www.who.int/docs/default-source/coronaviruse/situation-reports/20200121-sitrep-1-2019-ncov

[2]   Zhu N, Zhang D, Wang W, *et al.* China Novel Coronavirus Investigating and Research Team. A novel coronavirus from patients with pneumonia in China 2019. N Engl J Med 2020; 382(8): 727-33. [http://dx.doi.org/10.1056/NEJMoa2001017] [PMID: 31978945]

[3]   WHO Clinical management of severe acute respiratory infection when Novel coronavirus (nCoV) infection is suspected: interim guidance. Available from https://www.who.int/internal -publication--detail/clinical-management-of-severe-acute-respiratory-infection-when-novel-coronav-rus-(ncov)-infection-is-suspected

[4]   David R. A Mini-review of the 2019 Novel Coronavirus, SAR S-CoV-2. AJBSR. Ms 2020; 8: 1.

[5]   WHO. Novel Coronavirus (2019-nCoV) Situation Report-22 2019. https://www.who.int/docs/default source/coronaviruse/situation-reports/20200211-sitrep-22-ncov

[6]   Huang C, Wang Y, Li X, *et al.* Clinical features of patients infected with 2019 novel coronavirus in Wuhan, China Lancet 2020; 395(10223): 497-506.
        [PMID: 3952020]

[7]   World Health Organization. Novel coronavirus (2019-nCoV) situation report - 13. 2020. Available from: https://www.who.int/docs/default-source/coronaviruse/situationreports/20200202-sitrep-13

[8]   Hui DS, I Azhar E, Madani TA, *et al.* The continuing 2019-nCoV epidemic threat of novel coronaviruses to global health - The latest 2019 novel coronavirus outbreak in Wuhan, China. Int J Infect Dis 2020; 91(26): 264-6.
        [http://dx.doi.org/10.1016/j.ijid.2020.01.009] [PMID: 31953166]

[9]   Ren LL, Wang YM, Wu ZQ, *et al.* Identification of a novel coronavirus causing severe pneumonia in human: a descriptive study. Chin Med J (Engl) 2020; 133(9): 1015-24.
        [http://dx.doi.org/10.1097/CM9.0000000000000722] [PMID: 32004165]

[10]   Wang W, Tang J, Wei F. Updated understanding of the outbreak of 2019 novel coronavirus (2019-nCoV) in Wuhan, China. J Med Virol 2020; 92(4): 441-7.
        [http://dx.doi.org/10.1002/jmv.25689] [PMID: 31994742]

[11]   Carlos WG, Dela CC, Cao B, *et al.* Novel wuhan (2019-nCoV) coronavirus. Am J RespirCrit Care Med 2020; 201(4): P7.

[12]   Wang D, Hu B, Hu C, *et al.* Clinical characteristics of 138 hospitalized patients With 2019 novel coronavirus-infected pneumonia in wuhan, china. JAMA 2020; 323(11): 1061-9.
        [http://dx.doi.org/10.1001/jama.2020.1585] [PMID: 32031570]

[13]   World Health Organization, World Health Organization. Report of the WHO-China Joint Mission on Coronavirus Disease 2019 (COVID-19) 2020.

[14]   ECDC. Outbreak of acute respiratory syndrome associated with a novel coronavirus, China:first local transmissions in the EU/EEA-third update. 2020. Availablefrom: https://www.ecdc.europa.eu/sites/default/files/documents/novel-coronavirus-risk-assessmentchina

[15]   ECDC. Outbreak of novel coronavirus disease 2019. Available from: https://www.ecdc.europa.eu /sites/default/files/documents/RRA

[16]   Li Q, Guan X, Wu P, *et al.* Early transmission dynamics in Wuhan, China, of novel coronavirus-infected pneumonia. N Engl J Med 2020; 382(13): 1199-207.
        [http://dx.doi.org/10.1056/NEJMoa2001316] [PMID: 31995857]

[17]   WHO Director-General's opening remarks at the media briefing on COVID-19-11 March 2020. World Health Organization 2020.

[18]   World meter April 7 2020. Available from: www.worldometers.info

[19]   Song Z, Xu Y, Bao L, *et al.* From SARS to MERS, thrusting coronaviruses into the spotlight. Viruses 2019; 11(1): 59.
        [http://dx.doi.org/10.3390/v11010059] [PMID: 30646565]

[20]   Richman DD, Whitley RJ, Hayden FG, Eds. Clinical virology. John Wiley & Sons 2016.
        [http://dx.doi.org/10.1128/9781555819439]

[21]   Cowley JA, Dimmock CM, Spann KM, Walker PJ. Gill-associated virus of Penaeus monodon prawns: an invertebrate virus with ORF1a and ORF1b genes related to arteri- and coronaviruses. J Gen Virol 2000; 81(Pt 6): 1473-84.
        [http://dx.doi.org/10.1099/0022-1317-81-6-1473] [PMID: 10811931]

[22]   Schoeman D, Fielding BC. Coronavirus envelope protein: current knowledge. Virol J 2019; 16(1): 69.

[http://dx.doi.org/10.1186/s12985-019-1182-0] [PMID: 31133031]

[23] Chan JF, To KK, Tse H, *et al.* Interspecies transmission and emergence of novel viruses: lessons from bats and birds. Trends Microbiol 2013; 21(10): 544-5.
[http://dx.doi.org/10.1016/j.tim.2013.05.005]

[24] Woo PC, Huang Y, Lau SK, *et al.* Coronavirus genomics and bioinformatics analysis. viruses 2010; 2(): 20-1804.

[25] Woo PC, Wang M, Lau SK, *et al.* Comparative analysis of twelve genomes of three novel group 2c and group 2d coronaviruses reveals unique group and subgroup features. J Virol 2007; 81(4): 1574-85.
[http://dx.doi.org/10.1128/JVI.02182-06] [PMID: 17121802]

[26] Lau SK, Woo PC, Yip CC, *et al.* Isolation and characterization of a novel Betacoronavirus subgroup A coronavirus, rabbit coronavirus HKU14, from domestic rabbits. J Virol 2012; 86(10): 5481-96.
[http://dx.doi.org/10.1128/JVI.06927-11] [PMID: 22398294]

[27] Lau SK, Poon RW, Wong BH, *et al.* Coexistence of different genotypes in the same bat and serological characterization of Rousettus bat coronavirus HKU9 belonging to a novel Betacoronavirus subgroup. J Virol 2010; 84(21): 11385-94.
[http://dx.doi.org/10.1128/JVI.01121-10] [PMID: 20702646]

[28] Zhang W, Zheng XS, Agwanda B, *et al.* Serological evidence of MERS-CoV and HKU8-related CoV co-infection in Kenyan camels. Emerg Microbes Infect 2019; 8(1): 1528-34.
[http://dx.doi.org/10.1080/22221751.2019.1679610] [PMID: 31645223]

[29] Liu DX, Fung TS, Chong KK, Shukla A, Hilgenfeld R. Accessory proteins of SARS-CoV and other coronaviruses. Antiviral Res 2014; 109: 97-109.
[http://dx.doi.org/10.1016/j.antiviral.2014.06.013] [PMID: 24995382]

[30] Narayanan K, Huang C, Makino S. SARS coronavirus accessory proteins. Virus Res 2008; 133(1): 113-21.
[http://dx.doi.org/10.1016/j.virusres.2007.10.009] [PMID: 18045721]

[31] Dong N, Yang X, Ye L, *et al.* Genomic and protein structure modelling analysis depicts the origin and infectivity of 2019-nCoV, a new coronavirus which caused a pneumonia outbreak in Wuhan, China BioRxiv 2020.
[http://dx.doi.org/10.1101/2020.01.20.913368]

[32] Lai MM, Cavanagh D. The molecular biology of coronaviruses. Adv Virus Res 1997; 48: 1-100.
[http://dx.doi.org/10.1016/S0065-3527(08)60286-9] [PMID: 9233431]

[33] Neuman BW, Kiss G, Kunding AH, *et al.* A structural analysis of M protein in coronavirus assembly and morphology. J Struct Biol 2011; 174(1): 11-22.
[http://dx.doi.org/10.1016/j.jsb.2010.11.021] [PMID: 21130884]

[34] Fehr AR, Perlman S. Coronaviruses: an overview of their Replication and pathogenesis. In: coronaviruses; 2015; pp. 1-23.
[http://dx.doi.org/10.1007/978-1-4939-2438-7_1]

[35] Wu A, Peng Y, Huang B, *et al.* Genome composition and divergence of the novel coronavirus (2019-nCoV) originating in China 2020; 27(3): 325-8.

[36] Chan JF, Kok KH, Zhu Z, *et al.* Genomic characterization of the 2019 novel human-pathogenic coronavirus isolated from a patient with atypical pneumonia after visiting Wuhan. Emerg Microbes Infect 2020; 9(1): 221-36.
[http://dx.doi.org/10.1080/22221751.2020.1719902] [PMID: 31987001]

[37] Lu R, Zhao X, Li J, *et al.* Genomic characterisation and epidemiology of 2019 novel coronavirus: implications for virus origins and receptor binding. Lancet 2020; 395(10224): 565-74.
[http://dx.doi.org/10.1016/S0140-6736(20)30251-8] [PMID: 32007145]

[38] Letko M, Marzi A, Munster V. Functional assessment of cell entry and receptor usage for SARS-Co-

-2 and other lineage B betacoronaviruses. Nat Microbiol 2020; 5(4): 562-9.
[http://dx.doi.org/10.1038/s41564-020-0688-y] [PMID: 32094589]

[39] Zhou P, Yang XL, Wang XG, *et al.* A pneumonia outbreak associated with a new coronavirus of probable bat origin. Nature 2020; 579(7798): 270-3.
[http://dx.doi.org/10.1038/s41586-020-2012-7] [PMID: 32015507]

[40] Shaila R, Tamanna B. COVID-19: The New Threat. Int J Infect 2020; 7e102184

[41] Wu F, Zhao S, Yu B, *et al.* A new coronavirus associated with human respiratory disease in China. Nature 2020; 579(7798): 265-9.
[http://dx.doi.org/10.1038/s41586-020-2008-3] [PMID: 32015508]

[42] Rothan HA, Byrareddy SN. The epidemiology and pathogenesis of coronavirus disease (COVID-19) outbreak. J Autoimmun 2020; 109102433
[http://dx.doi.org/10.1016/j.jaut.2020.102433] [PMID: 32113704]

[43] Fan Y, Zhao K, Shi ZL, Zhou P. Bat Coronaviruses in China. Viruses 2019; 11(3): 210.
[http://dx.doi.org/10.3390/v11030210] [PMID: 30832341]

[44] Guan Y, Zheng BJ, He YQ, *et al.* Isolation and characterization of viruses related to the SARS coronavirus from animals in southern China. Science 2003; 302(5643): 276-8.
[http://dx.doi.org/10.1126/science.1087139] [PMID: 12958366]

[45] Lau SK, Woo PC, Li KS, *et al.* Severe acute respiratory syndrome coronavirus-like virus in Chinese horseshoe bats. Proc Natl Acad Sci USA 2005; 102(39): 14040-5.
[http://dx.doi.org/10.1073/pnas.0506735102] [PMID: 16169905]

[46] Li W, Shi Z, Yu M, *et al.* Bats are natural reservoirs of SARS-like coronaviruses. Science 2005; 310(5748): 676-9.
[http://dx.doi.org/10.1126/science.1118391] [PMID: 16195424]

[47] Woo PC, Lau SK, Li KS, *et al.* Molecular diversity of coronaviruses in bats. Virology 2006; 351(1): 180-7.
[http://dx.doi.org/10.1016/j.virol.2006.02.041] [PMID: 16647731]

[48] Woo PC, Lau SK, Li KS, *et al.* Genetic relatedness of the novel human group C betacoronavirus to Tylonycterisbat Coronavirus HKU4 and Pipistrellusbat coronavirus HKU5. Emerg Microbes Infect 2012; 1: 1-5.
[http://dx.doi.org/10.1038/emi.2012.45]

[49] Lau SK, Li KS, Tsang AK, *et al.* Genetic characterization of Betacoronavirus lineage C viruses in bats reveals marked sequence divergence in the spike protein of pipistrellus bat coronavirus HKU5 in Japanese pipistrelle: implications for the origin of the novel Middle East respiratory syndrome coronavirus. J Virol 2013; 87(15): 8638-50.
[http://dx.doi.org/10.1128/JVI.01055-13] [PMID: 23720729]

[50] Raj VS, Osterhaus AD, Fouchier RA, Haagmans BL. MERS: emergence of a novel human coronavirus. Curr Opin Virol 2014; 5: 58-62.
[http://dx.doi.org/10.1016/j.coviro.2014.01.010] [PMID: 24584035]

[51] Raj VS, Smits SL, Provacia LB, *et al.* Adenosine deaminase acts as a natural antagonist for dipeptidyl peptidase 4-mediated entry of the Middle East respiratory syndrome coronavirus. J Virol 2014; 88(3): 1834-8.
[http://dx.doi.org/10.1128/JVI.02935-13] [PMID: 24257613]

[52] Bogoch II, Watts A, Thomas-Bachli A, *et al.* Pneumonia of unknown etiology in Wuhan, China: potential for international spread *via* commercial air travel. J Trav Med 2020.

[53] Lu H, Stratton CW, Tang YW. Outbreak of pneumonia of unknown etiology in Wuhan, China: The mystery and the miracle. J Med Virol 2020; 92(4): 401-2.
[http://dx.doi.org/10.1002/jmv.25678] [PMID: 31950516]

[54] Perlman S. Another decade, another coronavirus. N Engl J Med 2020; 382(8): 760-2.
[http://dx.doi.org/10.1056/NEJMe2001126] [PMID: 31978944]

[55] Kuba K, Imai Y, Rao S, *et al.* A crucial role of angiotensin converting enzyme 2 (ACE2) in SARS coronavirus-induced lung injury. Nat Med 2005; 11(8): 875-9.
[http://dx.doi.org/10.1038/nm1267] [PMID: 16007097]

[56] Gabutti G, d'Anchera E, Sandri F, Savio M, Stefanati A. Coronavirus: Update related to the current outbreak of COVID-19. Infect Dis Ther 2020; 8: 1-13.
[PMID: 32292686]

[57] Cui J, Li F, Shi ZL. Origin and evolution of pathogenic coronaviruses. Nat Rev Microbiol 2019; 17(3): 181-92.
[http://dx.doi.org/10.1038/s41579-018-0118-9] [PMID: 30531947]

[58] Li X, Song Y, Wong G, Cui J. Bat origin of a new human coronavirus: there and back again. Sci China Life Sci 2020; 63(3): 461-2.
[http://dx.doi.org/10.1007/s11427-020-1645-7] [PMID: 32048160]

[59] Amodio E, Vitale F, Cimino L, Casuccio A, Tramuto F. Outbreak of Novel Coronavirus (SARS-Co--2): First Evidences From International Scientific Literature and Pending Questions. Healthcare (Basel) 2020; 8(1): 51.
[http://dx.doi.org/10.3390/healthcare8010051] [PMID: 32120965]

[60] Zhang T, Wu Q, Zhang T. Pangolin homology associated with 2019-nCoV BioRxiv 2020.

[61] Wong MC, Cregeen SJ, Ajami NJ, *et al.* Evidence of recombination in coronaviruses implicating pangolin origins of nCoV-2019 BioRxiv 2020.
[http://dx.doi.org/10.1101/2020.02.07.939207]

[62] Xiao K, Zhai J, Feng Y, *et al.* Isolation and Characterization of 2019-nCoV-like Coronavirus from Malayan Pangolins BioRxiv 2020.
[http://dx.doi.org/10.1101/2020.02.17.951335]

[63] Lam TT, Shum MH, Zhu HC, *et al.* Identification of 2019-nCoV related coronaviruses in Malayan pangolins in southern China bioRxiv 2020.
[http://dx.doi.org/10.1101/2020.02.13.945485]

[64] Cyranoski D. Did pangolins spread the China coronavirus to people? Nature 2020.
[http://dx.doi.org/10.1038/d41586-020-00364-2] [PMID. 33547428]

[65] Wu CI, Poo MM. Moral imperative for the immediate release of 2019-nCoV sequence data. Nat Sci Rev 2020; pp. 719-20.

[66] Emami A, Javanmardi F, Pirbonyeh N, Akbari A. Prevalence of underlying diseases in hospitalized patients with COVID-19: A systematic review and meta-analysis. Arch Acad Emerg Med 2020; 8(1)e35
[PMID: 32232218]

[67] Zhou P, Yang XL, Wang XG, *et al.* Discovery of a novel coronavirus associated with the recent pneumonia outbreak in humans and its potential bat origin BioRxiv 2020.
[http://dx.doi.org/10.1101/2020.01.22.914952]

[68] WMHC. Wuhan Municipal Health and Health . Commission's Briefing on the Current Pneumonia Epidemic Situation in Our City. February 4 2020. Available from: http://wjw.wuhan.gov.cn/front/web/showDetail/2019123108989

[69] Heymann DL, Shindo N. WHO Scientific and Technical Advisory Group for Infectious Hazards. COVID-19: what is next for public health? Lancet 2020; 395(10224): 542-5.
[http://dx.doi.org/10.1016/S0140-6736(20)30374-3] [PMID: 32061313]

[70] Yan R, Zhang Y, Li Y, Xia L, Guo Y, Zhou Q. Structural basis for the recognition of SARS-CoV-2 by full-length human ACE2. Science 2020; 367(6485): 1444-8.

[http://dx.doi.org/10.1126/science.abb2762] [PMID: 32132184]

[71]   Letko M, Marzi A, Munster V. Functional assessment of cell entry and receptor usage for SARS-Co-
         -2 and other lineage B betacoronaviruses. Nat Microbiol 2020; 5(4): 562-9.
         [http://dx.doi.org/10.1038/s41564-020-0688-y] [PMID: 32094589]

[72]   Team TC. Cell editorial team. Embracing the Landscape of Therapeutics. Cell 2020; 181(1): 1-3.
         [http://dx.doi.org/10.1016/j.cell.2020.03.025] [PMID: 32243785]

[73]   Zhao Y, Zhao Z, Wang Y, *et al.* Single-cell RNA expression profiling of ACE2, the putative receptor
         of Wuhan 2019-nCov BioRxiv 2020.

[74]   de Wit E, van Doremalen N, Falzarano D, Munster VJ. SARS and MERS: recent insights into
         emerging coronaviruses. Nat Rev Microbiol 2016; 14(8): 523-34.
         [http://dx.doi.org/10.1038/nrmicro.2016.81] [PMID: 27344959]

[75]   van den Brand JM, Haagmans BL, Leijten L, *et al.* Pathology of experimental SARS coronavirus
         infection in cats and ferrets. Vet Pathol 2008; 45(4): 551-62.
         [http://dx.doi.org/10.1354/vp.45-4-551] [PMID: 18587105]

[76]   Liu S, Zhang M, Yang L, *et al.* Prevalence and patterns of tobacco smoking among Chinese adult men
         and women: findings of the 2010 national smoking survey. J Epidemiol Community Health 2017;
         71(2): 154-61.
         [http://dx.doi.org/10.1136/jech-2016-207805] [PMID: 27660401]

[77]   Paules CI, Marston HD, Fauci AS. Coronavirus infections-more than just the common cold. JAMA
         2020; 323(8): 707-8.
         [http://dx.doi.org/10.1001/jama.2020.0757] [PMID: 31971553]

[78]   Li W, Sui J, Huang IC, *et al.* The S proteins of human coronavirus NL63 and severe acute respiratory
         syndrome coronavirus bind overlapping regions of ACE2. Virology 2007; 367(2): 367-74.
         [http://dx.doi.org/10.1016/j.virol.2007.04.035] [PMID: 17631932]

[79]   Cao Y, Li L, Feng Z, *et al.* Comparative genetic analysis of the novel coronavirus (2019-nCoV/SAR-
         -CoV-2) receptor ACE2 in different populations. Cell Discov 2020; 6: 11.
         [http://dx.doi.org/10.1038/s41421-020-0147-1] [PMID: 32133153]

[80]   Press information Novel Coronavirus SARS-CoV-2: Fruit bats and ferrets are susceptible, pigs and
         chickens are not First results of studies conducted at the Friedrich-Loeffler-Institut 2020.

[81]   Wan Y, Shang J, Graham R, Baric RS, Li F. Receptor recognition by novel coronavirus from Wuhan:
         An analysis based on decade-long structural studies of SARS. J Virol 2020; 94(7): e00127-20.
         [http://dx.doi.org/10.1128/JVI.00127-20] [PMID: 31996437]

[82]   Hoffmann M, Kleine-Weber H, Schroeder S, *et al.* SARS-CoV-2 cell entry depends on ACE2 and
         TMPRSS2 and is blocked by a clinically proven protease inhibitor. Cell 2020; 181(2): 271-280.e8.
         [http://dx.doi.org/10.1016/j.cell.2020.02.052] [PMID: 32142651]

[83]   Sims AC, Baric RS, Yount B, Burkett SE, Collins PL, Pickles RJ. Severe acute respiratory syndrome
         coronavirus infection of human ciliated airway epithelia: role of ciliated cells in viral spread in the
         conducting airways of the lungs. J Virol 2005; 79(24): 15511-24.
         [http://dx.doi.org/10.1128/JVI.79.24.15511-15524.2005] [PMID: 16306622]

[84]   Robert J. Mason, National Jewish Health. USA: Dept of Medicine 2020.

[85]   Tang NL, Chan PK, Wong CK, *et al.* Early enhanced expression of interferon-inducible protein-10
         (CXCL-10) and other chemokines predicts adverse outcome in severe acute respiratory syndrome.
         Clin Chem 2005; 51(12): 2333-40.
         [http://dx.doi.org/10.1373/clinchem.2005.054460] [PMID: 16195357]

[86]   Rockx B, Baas T, Zornetzer GA, *et al.* Early upregulation of acute respiratory distress syndrome-
         associated cytokines promotes lethal disease in an aged-mouse model of severe acute respiratory
         syndrome coronavirus infection. J Virol 2009; 83(14): 7062-74.

[http://dx.doi.org/10.1128/JVI.00127-09] [PMID: 19420084]

[87] Wu Z, McGoogan JM. Characteristics of and important lessons from the coronavirus disease 2019 (COVID-19) outbreak in China: summary of a report of 72 314 cases from the Chinese Center for Disease Control and Prevention. JAMA 2020; 323(13): 1239-42.
[http://dx.doi.org/10.1001/jama.2020.2648] [PMID: 32091533]

[88] Park M, Cook AR, Lim JT, Sun Y, Dickens BL. A Systematic review of COVID-19 epidemiology based on current evidence. J Clin Med 2020; 9(4): 967.
[http://dx.doi.org/10.3390/jcm9040967] [PMID: 32244365]

[89] Zhou F, Yu T, Du R, *et al.* Clinical course and risk factors for mortality of adult in patients with COVID-19 in Wuhan, China: a retrospective cohort study. Lancet 2020; 395(10229): 1054-62.
[http://dx.doi.org/10.1016/S0140-6736(20)30566-3] [PMID: 32171076]

[90] Raghupathi V. An empirical investigation of chronic diseases: a visualization approach to Medicare in the United States. Int J Healthc Manag 2019; 12: 327-39.
[http://dx.doi.org/10.1080/20479700.2018.1472849]

[91] Qiu H, Wu J, Hong L, Luo Y, Song Q, Chen D. Clinical and epidemiological features of 36 children with coronavirus disease 2019 (COVID-19) in Zhejiang, China: an observational cohort study. Lancet Infect Dis 2020; 20(6): 689-96.
[http://dx.doi.org/10.1016/S1473-3099(20)30198-5] [PMID: 32220650]

[92] Standage SW, Wong HR. Biomarkers for pediatric sepsis and septic shock. Expert Rev Anti Infect Ther 2011; 9(1): 71-9.
[http://dx.doi.org/10.1586/eri.10.154] [PMID: 21171879]

[93] Rabi FA, Al Zoubi MS, Kasasbeh GA, Salameh DM, Al-Nasser AD. SARS-CoV-2 and Coronavirus Disease 2019: what we know so far. Pathogens 2020; 9(3): 231.
[http://dx.doi.org/10.3390/pathogens9030231] [PMID: 32245083]

[94] Onder G, Rezza G, Brusaferro S. Case-fatality rate and characteristics of patients dying in relation to COVID-19 in Italy. JAMA 2020; 323(18): 1775-6.
[http://dx.doi.org/10.1001/jama.2020.4683] [PMID: 32203977]

[95] World Health Organization, World Health Organization. Coronavirus disease (COVID-19) outbreak. 2020. Available from: https://www.who.int/emergencies/diseases/novel-

[96] Patel VB, Zhong JC, Grant MB, Oudit GY. Role of the ACE2/Angiotensin 1-7 Axis of the Renin-Angiotensin System in Heart Failure. Circ Res 2016; 118(8): 1313-26.
[http://dx.doi.org/10.1161/CIRCRESAHA.116.307708] [PMID: 27081112]

[97] Ho JC, Chan KN, Hu WH, *et al.* The effect of aging on nasal mucociliary clearance, beat frequency, and ultrastructure of respiratory cilia. Am J Respir Crit Care Med 2001; 163(4): 983-8.
[http://dx.doi.org/10.1164/ajrccm.163.4.9909121] [PMID: 11282777]

[98] Wei M, Yuan J, Liu Y, Fu T, Yu X, Zhang ZJ. Novel coronavirus infection in hospitalized infants under 1 year of age in china. JAMA 2020; 323(13): 1313-4.
[http://dx.doi.org/10.1001/jama.2020.2131] [PMID: 32058570]

[99] Report of the WHO-China Joint Mission on Coronavirus Disease 2019 (COVID-19) 2020. Available from: https://www.who.int/docs/defaultsource/

[100] Abduljali JM, Abduljali BM. Epidemiology genome and clinical features of the pandemic SARS-CoV2: a recent view. New Microbes New Infect 2020.100762

[101] Ng LFP, Hiscox JA. Coronaviruses in animals and humans. BMJ 2020; 368: m634.
[http://dx.doi.org/10.1136/bmj.m634] [PMID: 32075782]

[102] Phelan AL, Katz R, Gostin LO. The Novel coronavirus originating in wuhan, china: challenges for global health governance. JAMA 2020; 323(8): 709-10.
[http://dx.doi.org/10.1001/jama.2020.1097] [PMID: 31999307]

[103] Wang D, Hu B, Hu C, *et al.* Clinical characteristics of 138 hospitalized patients with 2019 novel coronavirus - infected pneumonia in Wuhan, China. JAMA 2020; 323(11): 1061-9.
[http://dx.doi.org/10.1001/jama.2020.1585] [PMID: 32031570]

[104] Kumar P, Renuka MK, Kalaiselvan MS, Arunkumar AS. Outcome of noncardiac surgical patients admitted to a multidisciplinary intensive care unit. Indian J Crit Care Med 2017; 21(1): 17-22.
[http://dx.doi.org/10.4103/0972-5229.198321] [PMID: 28197046]

[105] Lei S, Jiang F, Su W, *et al.* Clinical characteristics and outcomes of patients undergoing surgeries during the incubation period of COVID-19 infection. EClinicalMedicine 2020; 21100331
[http://dx.doi.org/10.1016/j.eclinm.2020.100331] [PMID: 32292899]

[106] Amodeo G, Bugada D, Franchi S, *et al.* Immune function after major surgical interventions: the effect of postoperative pain treatment. J Pain Res 2018; 11: 1297-305.
[http://dx.doi.org/10.2147/JPR.S158230] [PMID: 30022848]

[107] Ni Choileain N, Redmond HP. Cell response to surgery. Arch Surg 2006; 141(11): 1132-40.
[http://dx.doi.org/10.1001/archsurg.141.11.1132] [PMID: 17116807]

[108] Young BE, Ong SWX, Kalimuddin S, *et al.* Singapore 2019 Novel Coronavirus Outbreak Research Team. Epidemiologic features and clinical course of patients infected with SARS-CoV-2 in Singapore. JAMA 2020; 323(15): 1488-94.
[http://dx.doi.org/10.1001/jama.2020.3204] [PMID: 32125362]

[109] Mehta P, McAuley DF, Brown M, Sanchez E, Tattersall RS, Manson JJ. HLH Across Speciality Collaboration, UK. COVID-19: consider cytokine storm syndromes and immunosuppression. Lancet 2020; 395(10229): 1033-4.
[http://dx.doi.org/10.1016/S0140-6736(20)30628-0] [PMID: 32192578]

[110] Chen N, Zhou M, Dong X, *et al.* Epidemiological and clinical characteristics of 99 cases of 2019 novel coronavirus pneumonia in Wuhan, China: a descriptive study. Lancet 2020; 395(10223): 507-13.
[http://dx.doi.org/10.1016/S0140-6736(20)30211-7] [PMID: 32007143]

[111] Zheng YY, Ma YT, Zhang JY, Xie X. COVID-19 and the cardiovascular system. Nat Rev Cardiol 2020; 17(5): 259-60.
[http://dx.doi.org/10.1038/s41569-020-0360-5] [PMID: 32139904]

[112] Seys LJM, Widagdo W, Verhamme FM, *et al.* DPP4, the middle east respiratory syndrome coronavirus receptor, is upregulated in lungs of smokers and chronic obstructive pulmonary disease patients. Clin Infect Dis 2018; 66(1): 45-53.
[http://dx.doi.org/10.1093/cid/cix741] [PMID: 29020176]

[113] Zhang JJ, Dong X, Cao YY, *et al.* Clinical characteristics of 140 patients infected with SARS-CoV-2 in Wuhan. China: Allergy 2020.
[http://dx.doi.org/10.1111/all.14238]

[114] Xia Y, Jin R, Zhao J, Li W, Shen H. Risk of COVID-19 for patients with cancer. Lancet Oncol 2020; 21(4)e180
[http://dx.doi.org/10.1016/S1470-2045(20)30150-9] [PMID: 32142622]

[115] Okada P, Buathong R, Phuygun S, *et al.* Early transmission patterns of coronavirus disease 2019 (COVID-19) in travellers from Wuhan to Thailand, January 2020. Euro Surveill 2020; 25(8)2000097
[http://dx.doi.org/10.2807/1560-7917.ES.2020.25.8.2000097] [PMID: 32127124]

[116] Wax RS, Christian MD. Practical recommendations for critical care and anesthesiology teams caring for novel coronavirus (2019-nCoV) patients. Can J Anesth 2020; 1-9.

[117] Jin YH, Cai L, Cheng ZS, *et al.* for the Zhongnan Hospital of Wuhan University Novel Coronavirus Management and Research Team, Evidence-Based Medicine Chapter of China International Exchange and Promotive Association for Medical and Health Care (CPAM). A rapid advice guideline for the diagnosis and treatment of 2019 novel coronavirus (2019-nCoV) infected pneumonia (standard version). Mil Med Res 2020; 7(1): 4.

[http://dx.doi.org/10.1186/s40779-020-0233-6] [PMID: 32029004]

[118]   Zhao J, Yang Y, Huang H, *et al.* Relationship between the ABO Blood Group and the COVID-19 susceptibility medRxiv 2020.
[http://dx.doi.org/10.1101/2020.03.11.20031096]

[119]   Pan A, Liu L, Wang C, *et al.* Association of public health interventions with the epidemiology of the COVID-19 outbreak in wuhan. China: JAMA 2020.

[120]   Vardavas CI, Nikitara K. COVID-19 and smoking: A systematic review of the evidence. Tob Induc Dis 2020; 18: 20.
[http://dx.doi.org/10.18332/tid/119324] [PMID: 32206052]

[121]   Wan Y, Shang J, Graham R, Baric RS, Li F. Receptor recognition by novel Coronavirus from Wuhan: an analysis based on decade-long structural studies of SARS. J Virol 2020; 94(7): e00127-20.
[http://dx.doi.org/10.1128/JVI.00127-20] [PMID: 31996437]

[122]   World Health Organization Novel Coronavirus (2019-nCoV) 2020. Available from: www.who.int/emergencies/diseases/novel-coronavirus-2019

[123]   Chan JF, Yuan S, Kok KH, *et al.* A familial cluster of pneumonia associated with the 2019 novel coronavirus indicating person-to-person transmission: a study of a family cluster. Lancet 2020; 395(10223): 514-23.
[http://dx.doi.org/10.1016/S0140-6736(20)30154-9] [PMID: 31986261]

[124]   Rothe C, Schunk M, Sothmann P, *et al.* Transmission of 2019-nCoV infection from an asymptomatic contact in Germany. N Engl J Med 2020; 382(10): 970-1.
[http://dx.doi.org/10.1056/NEJMc2001468] [PMID: 32003551]

[125]   Phan LT, Nguyen TV, Luong QC, *et al.* Importation and human-to-human transmission of a novel coronavirus in Vietnam. N Engl J Med 2020; 382(9): 872-4.
[http://dx.doi.org/10.1056/NEJMc2001272] [PMID: 31991079]

[126]   Chen N, Zhou M, Dong X, *et al.* Epidemiological and clinical characteristics of 99 cases of 2019 novel coronavirus pneumonia in Wuhan, China: a descriptive study. Lancet 2020; 395(10223): 507-13.
[http://dx.doi.org/10.1016/S0140-6736(20)30211-7] [PMID: 32007143]

[127]   Li Q, Guan X, Wu P, *et al.* Early transmission dynamics in Wuhan, China, of novel coronavirus-infected pneumonia. N Engl J Med 2020; 382(13): 1199-207.
[http://dx.doi.org/10.1056/NEJMoa2001316] [PMID: 31995857]

[128]   Jiang X, Rayner S, Luo MH. Does SARS-CoV-2 has a longer incubation period than SARS and MERS? J Med Virol 2020; 92(5): 476-8.
[http://dx.doi.org/10.1002/jmv.25708] [PMID: 32056235]

[129]   Nishiura H, Linton NM, Akhmetzhanov AR. Serial interval of novel coronavirus (COVID-19) infections. Int J Infect Dis 2020; 93: 284-6.
[http://dx.doi.org/10.1016/j.ijid.2020.02.060] [PMID: 32145466]

[130]   Zhang H, Kang Z, Gong H, *et al.* The digestive system is a potential route of 2019-nCov infection: a bioinformatics analysis based on single-cell transcriptomes BioRxiv 2020.
[http://dx.doi.org/10.1101/2020.01.30.927806]

[131]   Kamel Boulos MN, Geraghty EM. Geographical tracking and mapping of coronavirus disease COVID-19/severe acute respiratory syndrome coronavirus 2 (SARS-CoV-2) epidemic and associated events around the world:how 21st century GIS technologies are supporting the global fight against outbreaks and epidemics. Int J Health Geogr 2020; 19(1): 8.
[http://dx.doi.org/10.1186/s12942-020-00202-8] [PMID: 32160889]

[132]   Carlos WG, Dela Cruz CS, Cao B, Pasnick S, Jamil S. Novel Wuhan (2019-nCoV) Coronavirus. Am J Respir Crit Care Med 2020; 201(4): 7-P8.
[http://dx.doi.org/10.1164/rccm.2014P7] [PMID: 32004066]

[133] Wu P, Hao X, Lau EHY, *et al.* Real-time tentative assessment of the epidemiological characteristics of novel coronavirus infections in Wuhan, China, as at 22 January 2020. Euro Surveill 2020; 25(3)2000044
[http://dx.doi.org/10.2807/1560-7917.ES.2020.25.3.2000044] [PMID: 31992388]

[134] Ong SWX, Tan YK, Chia PY, *et al.* Air, surface environmental, and personal protective equipment contamination by severe acute respiratory syndrome coronavirus 2 (SARS-CoV-2) from a symptomatic patient. JAMA 2020; 323(16): 1610-2.
[http://dx.doi.org/10.1001/jama.2020.3227] [PMID: 32129805]

[135] Zou L, Ruan F, Huang M, *et al.* SARS-CoV-2 viral load in upper respiratory specimens of infected patients. N Engl J Med 2020; 382(12): 1177-9.
[http://dx.doi.org/10.1056/NEJMc2001737] [PMID: 32074444]

[136] World Health Organization,World Health Organization. Middle east respiratory syndrome coronavirus (MERS-CoV). WHO 2014.

[137] Chan-Yeung M, Xu RH. SARS: epidemiology. Respirology 2003; 8 (Suppl.): S9-S14.
[http://dx.doi.org/10.1046/j.1440-1843.2003.00518.x] [PMID: 15018127]

[138] Sampathkumar P, Temesgen Z, Smith TF, Thompson RL. SARS: epidemiology, clinical presentation, management, and infection control measures. Mayo Clin Proc 2003; 78(7): 882-90.
[http://dx.doi.org/10.4065/78.7.882] [PMID: 12839084]

[139] CDC. Coronavirus Disease 2019(COVID-19). 2019. Available from: https://www.cdc.gov/corona virus/2019-ncov/about/transmission

[140] Masters PS. The molecular biology of coronaviruses. Adv Virus Res 2006; 66: 193-292.
[http://dx.doi.org/10.1016/S0065-3527(06)66005-3] [PMID: 16877062]

[141] Cui J, Li F, Shi ZL. Origin and evolution of pathogenic coronaviruses. Nat Rev Microbiol 2019; 17(3): 181-92.
[http://dx.doi.org/10.1038/s41579-018-0118-9] [PMID: 30531947]

[142] Li F, Li W, Farzan M, Harrison SC. Structure of SARS coronavirus spike receptor-binding domain complexed with receptor. Science 2005; 309(5742): 1864-8.
[http://dx.doi.org/10.1126/science.1116480] [PMID: 16166518]

[143] Poon LLM, Peiris M. Emergence of a novel human coronavirus threatening human health. Nat Med 2020; 26(3): 317-9.
[http://dx.doi.org/10.1038/s41591-020-0796-5] [PMID: 32108160]

[144] Xiao F, Tang M, Zheng X, Liu Y, Li X, Shan H. Evidence for gastrointestinal infection of SARS-CoV-2. Gastroenterology 2020; 158(6): 1831-1833.e3.
[http://dx.doi.org/10.1053/j.gastro.2020.02.055] [PMID: 32142773]

[145] Chinese Center for Disease Control and Prevention. Epidemic update and risk assessment of 2019 Novel Coronavirus 2020. Available from: http://www.chinacdc.cn/yyrdgz/202001 /P0202001285233549192922

[146] Backer JA, Klinkenberg D, Wallinga J. Incubation period of 2019 novel coronavirus (2019-nCoV) infections among travellers from Wuhan, China, 20-28 January 2020. Euro Surveill 2020; 25(5)2000062
[http://dx.doi.org/10.2807/1560-7917.ES.2020.25.5.2000062] [PMID: 32046819]

[147] Guan WJ, Ni ZY, Hu Y, *et al.* Clinical characteristics of 2019 novel coronavirus infection in China. medRxiv 2020.
[http://dx.doi.org/10.1101/2020.02.06.20020974]

[148] Chen H, Guo J, Wang C, *et al.* Clinical characteristics and intrauterine vertical transmission potential of COVID-19 infection in nine pregnant women: A retrospective review of medical records. Lancet 2020; 39(5): 9-15.

[149] Zhu H, Wang L, Fang C, *et al.* Clinical analysis of 10 neonates born to mothers with 2019-nCoV pneumonia. Transl Pediatr 2020; 9(1): 51-60.
[http://dx.doi.org/10.21037/tp.2020.02.06] [PMID: 32154135]

[150] Anzolin E, Amante A. Coronavirus outbreak grows in northern Italy, 16 cases reported in one day. Thomson Reuters 2020.

[151] Epidemiology Working Group for NCIP Epidemic Response, Chinese Center for Disease Control and Prevention. The epidemiological characteristics of an outbreak of 2019 novel coronavirus diseases (COVID-19) in China. Zhonghua Liu Xing Bing Xue Za Zhi 2020; 41(2): 145-51.
[PMID: 32064853]

[152] Coronavirus: first case in Milan. What we know about new infections in Lombardy Veneto and Piemount 2020.

[153] Coronavirus disease 2019 (COVID-19) Situation Report -72. Data as reported by national authorities by 10:00 CET April 1 2020.

[154] Lu H, Stratton CW, Tang YW. Outbreak of pneumonia of unknown etiology in Wuhan, China: The mystery and the miracle. J Med Virol 2020; 92(4): 401-2.
[http://dx.doi.org/10.1002/jmv.25678] [PMID: 31950516]

[155] Kock RA, Karesh WB, Veas F, *et al.* 2019-nCoV in context: lessons learned? Lancet Planet Health 2020; 4(3): e87-8.
[http://dx.doi.org/10.1016/S2542-5196(20)30035-8] [PMID: 32035507]

[156] NBSC. National Bureau of Statistics PRC: China Statistical Yearbook 2019 (Chinese-English Edition). Beijing, China: China Statistics Press 2019.

[157] Ding YT. Heavy drought in the middle and lower reaches of Yangtze River. People Net 2019; 7: 2019-11.

[158] The average rainfall in Wuhan in December was 26 millimeters, and there were only scattered light rain on the 3rd. Wuhan Weather News 2020. Available online https://weather.mipang.com /wuhan/news- 1549253.html

[159] Xu RH, He JF, Evans MR, *et al.* Epidemiologic clues to SARS origin in China. Emerg Infect Dis 2004; 10(6): 1030-7.
[http://dx.doi.org/10.3201/eid1006.030852] [PMID: 15207054]

[160] NBSC. National Bureau of Statistics PRC: China Statistical Yearbook 2018 (Chinese-English Edition). Beijing, China: China Statistics Press 2018.

[161] Shi NN, Liu JY, Kuang YL, *et al.* Characteristics and Influences of Precipitation Tendency in Foshan under Environmental variations. J Water Resour 2014; 03: 41-9.
[http://dx.doi.org/10.12677/JWRR.2014.31007]

[162] Chan KH, Peiris JS, Lam SY, Poon LL, Yuen KY, Seto WH. The effects of temperature and relative humidity on the viability of the SARS coronavirus. Adv Virol 2011; 2011734690
[http://dx.doi.org/10.1155/2011/734690] [PMID: 22312351]

[163] Bukhari Q, Jameel Y. Will Coronavirus Pandemic Diminish by Summer? SSRN 355998.2020;

[164] Wang J, Tang K, Feng K, *et al.* High Temperature and High Humidity Reduce the Transmission of COVID-19 SSRN3551767 2020.

[165] Kudo E, Song E, Yockey LJ, *et al.* Low ambient humidity impairs barrier function and innate resistance against influenza infection. Proc Natl Acad Sci USA 2019; 116(22): 10905-10.
[http://dx.doi.org/10.1073/pnas.1902840116] [PMID: 31085641]

[166] Narges NH, Shirbandi K, Rahim F. Environmental concern regarding the effect of humidity and temperature on SARS-COV-2 (COVID-19) survival Fact or Fiction 2020.

[167] Tan J, Mu L, Huang J, Yu S, Chen B, Yin J. An initial investigation of the association between the

SARS outbreak and weather: with the view of the environmental temperature and its variation. J Epidemiol Community Health 2005; 59(3): 186-92.
[http://dx.doi.org/10.1136/jech.2004.020180] [PMID: 15709076]

[168] Casanova LM, Jeon S, Rutala WA, Weber DJ, Sobsey MD. Effects of air temperature and relative humidity on coronavirus survival on surfaces. Appl Environ Microbiol 2010; 76(9): 2712-7.
[http://dx.doi.org/10.1128/AEM.02291-09] [PMID: 20228108]

[169] Kampf G, Todt D, Pfaender S, Steinmann E. Persistence of coronaviruses on inanimate surfaces and their inactivation with biocidal agents. J Hosp Infect 2020; 104(3): 246-51.
[http://dx.doi.org/10.1016/j.jhin.2020.01.022] [PMID: 32035997]

[170] van Doremalen N, Bushmaker T, Karesh WB, Munster VJ. Stability of Middle East respiratory syndrome coronavirus in milk. Emerg Infect Dis 2014; 20(7): 1263-4.
[http://dx.doi.org/10.3201/eid2007.140500] [PMID: 24960335]

[171] Warnes SL, Little ZR, Keevil CW. Human coronavirus 229E remains infectious on common touch surface materials. MBio 2015; 6(6): e01697-15.
[http://dx.doi.org/10.1128/mBio.01697-15] [PMID: 26556276]

[172] Xie J, Zhu Y. Association between ambient temperature and COVID-19 infection in 122 cities from China. Sci Total Environ 2020; 724138201
[http://dx.doi.org/10.1016/j.scitotenv.2020.138201] [PMID: 32408450]

[173] Warnes SL, Little ZR, Keevil CW. Human coronavirus 229E remains infectious on common touch surface materials. MBio 2015; 6(6): e01697-15.
[http://dx.doi.org/10.1128/mBio.01697-15] [PMID: 26556276]

[174] Geller C, Varbanov M, Duval RE. Human coronaviruses: insights into environmental resistance and its influence on the development of new antiseptic strategies. Viruses 2012; 4(11): 3044-68.
[http://dx.doi.org/10.3390/v4113044] [PMID: 23202515]

[175] Zhao D, Yao F, Wang L, *et al.* A comparative study on the clinical features of COVID-19 pneumonia to other pneumonias. Clin Infect Dis 2020; 71(15): 756-61.
[http://dx.doi.org/10.1093/cid/ciaa247] [PMID: 32161968]

[176] Woodward A. High temperatures and muggy weather might make the new coronavirus less contagious, a group of experts says. Business insider India 2020. [cited 2020 March 30].

[177] Bannister-Tyrrell M, Meyer A, Faverjon C, *et al.* Preliminary evidence that higher temperatures are associated with lower incidence of COVID-19, for cases reported globally up to February 29 2020 MedRxiv 2020.
[http://dx.doi.org/10.1101/2020.03.18.20036731]

[178] 2020 COVID-19 Coronavirus Ultraviolet Susceptibility Technical Report 2020.

[179] Du Toit A. Outbreak of a novel coronavirus. Nat Rev Microbiol 2020; 18(3): 123.
[http://dx.doi.org/10.1038/s41579-020-0332-0] [PMID: 31988490]

[180] CDC. Symptoms of Novel Coronavirus (2019-nCoV). U.S. Centers for Disease Control and Prevention 2020.

[181] Report of the WHO-China Joint Mission on Coronavirus Disease 2019 (COVID-19) 2020.

[182] Lu H. Drug treatment options for the 2019-new coronavirus (2019-nCoV). Biosci Trends 2020; 14(1): 69-71.
[http://dx.doi.org/10.5582/bst.2020.01020] [PMID: 31996494]

[183] Geographical Distribution of 2019-nCov Cases.. European Centre for Disease Prevention and Control 2020. Available at: https://www.ecdc.europa.eu/en/geographic aldistribution- 2019-ncov-cases.

[184] First Travel-Related Case of 2019 Novel Coronavirus Detected in United States. Centers for Disease Control and Prevention 2020. Available at: https://www.cdc.gov/media/ releases/2020/p0121-nove--coronavirus-travel-case.html

[185] Wang W, Tang J, Wei F. Updated understanding of the outbreak of 2019 novel coronavirus (2019-nCoV) in Wuhan, China. J Med Virol 2020; 92(4): 441-7.
[http://dx.doi.org/10.1002/jmv.25689] [PMID: 31994742]

[186] Nishiura H, Jung SM, Linton NM, *et al.* The extent of transmission of novel coronavirus in Wuhan, China. J Clin Med 2020; 9(2): 330.
[http://dx.doi.org/10.3390/jcm9020330] [PMID: 31991628]

[187] Holshue ML, DeBolt C, Lindquist S, *et al.* Washington State 2019-nCoV Case Investigation Team. First case of 2019 novel coronavirus in the United States. N Engl J Med 2020; 382(10): 929-36.
[http://dx.doi.org/10.1056/NEJMoa2001191] [PMID: 32004427]

[188] CDC confirms person to person spread of new coronavirus in the United States 2020. Availble at: https://www.cdc.gov/media/releases/2020/p0130

[189] Bassetti M, Vena A, Giacobbe DR. The novel Chinese coronavirus (2019-nCoV) infections: Challenges for fighting the storm. Eur J Clin Invest 2020; 50(3)e13209
[http://dx.doi.org/10.1111/eci.13209] [PMID: 32003000]

[190] Ministry of Health, Labour and welfare of Japan Identification of novel coronavirus infection on cruise ship in quarantine at yokohama port (report 8) 2020. Available from: https://www.mhlw.go.jp/stf/newpage_09425.html

[191] ECDC Outbreak of novel coronavirus disease 2019 (COVID-19): increased transmission globally-fifth update 2020. Available from: https://www.ecdc.europa.eu/sites/default/ files/documents/RRA-outbreak-novel-coronavirus

[192] https://www.cdc.gov/coronavirus/2019-ncov

[193] National health commission of the People's Republic of China. The latest situation of new coronavirus pneumonia
[http://dx.doi.org/10.5582/bst.2020.01020]

[194] Battegay M, Kuehl R, Tschudin-Sutter S, Hirsch HH, Widmer AF, Neher RA. 2019-novel Coronavirus (2019-nCoV): estimating the case fatality rate - a word of caution. Swiss Med Wkly 2020; 150w20203
[http://dx.doi.org/10.4414/smw.2020.20203] [PMID: 32031234]

[195] Iran Reports Its First 2 Cases of the New Coronavirus New York Times February 19 2020.

[196] Two Iranians die after testing positive for coronavirus. CNBC 19 Feb 2020.

[197] Smith J, Stanway D. Germany: heading for epidemic as virus spreads faster outside China. Thomson Reuters 2020.

[198] Iran's deputy health minister tests positive for coronavirus. Middle East Eye February 25 2020.

[199] Jump up to: Iranian Vice President MasoumehEbtekar tests positive for coronavirus: ReportEnglishalarabiyanet February 27 2020.

[200] Grasselli G, Pesenti A, Cecconi M. Critical care utilization for the COVID-19 Outbreak in Lombardy JAMA published online March 13 2020.

[201] Signorelli C, Scognamiglio T, Odone A. COVID-19 in Italy: impact of containment measures and prevalence estimates of infection in the general population. Acta Biomed 2020; 91(3-S): 175-9.
[PMID: 32275287]

[202] European Centre for Disease Prevention and Control. Outbreak of novel coronavirus disease 2019 (COVID-19): increased transmission globally-fifth update. Stockholm: ECDC 2020.

[203] PM Abe Asks All of Japan Schools to Close Over coronavirus Reuters 2020. Available online: https://www.reuters.com/article/us-china-health-japan-idUSKCN20L0BI

[204] Yeung J, Marsh J, Kottasová I, Vera A. Coronavirus News CNN World March 15 2020. Available

online: https://www.cnn.com/world/live-news/coronavirus-outbreak-2-03-15-20-intl-hnk /index.html

[205] CDC Coronavirus Disease 2019 (COVID-19)-Resources for K-12 Schools and Childcare Programs Available online at https://www.cdc.gov/coronavirus/2019-ncov/community/schools-childcare /index.html

[206] Cascella M, Rajnik M, Cuomo A, *et al.* Features, Evaluation and Treatment Coronavirus (COVID-19). Treasure Island, FL: StatPearls Publishing 2020.

[207] Hassan SA, Sheikh FN, Jamal S, Ezeh JK, Akhtar A. Coronavirus (COVID-19): A review of clinical features, diagnosis, and treatment. Cureus 2020; 12(3)e7355
[http://dx.doi.org/10.7759/cureus.7355] [PMID: 32328367]

[208] Coronavirus Update for COVID-19 Wuhan China Virus Outbreak -Confirmed Cases and Deaths by Country. Territory, or Conveyance www.worldometers.info2020.

[209] World Health Organization. WHO Director-General's opening remarks at the media briefing on COVID-19 disease 2020.

[210] Worldmeter. Coronavirus Update for COVID-19 Wuhan China Virus Outbreak 2020. Available at www.worldometers.info

[211] Said Nadeem. Coronavirus COVID-19: Available Free Literature Provided by Various Companies, Journals and Organizations around the World. J OngChem Res 2020; 5: 7-13.

[212] Yang S, Cao P, Du P, *et al.* Early estimation of the case fatality rate of COVID-19 in mainland China: a data-driven analysis. Ann Transl Med 2020; 8(4): 128.
[http://dx.doi.org/10.21037/atm.2020.02.66] [PMID: 32175421]

[213] The Center for Systems Science and Engineering. Coronavirus COVID-19 global cases 2020. https://arcg.is/0fHmTX

[214] Worldometer. Available from: https://www.worldometers.info/coronavirus/

[215] WHO. Situation Report Novel Coronavirus (2019-nCoV). World Health Organization 2020.

[216] WHO. Situation Report-1 Coronavirus disease 2019 (COVID-19). World Health Organization 2020.

[217] WHO. Situation Report-28 Coronavirus Disease 2019 (COVID-19). World Health Organization 2020.

[218] WHO. Situation Report -32Coronavirus disease 2019 (COVID-19) Feb 21 2020.

[219] WHO. Situation reports 2020 Coronavirus disease 2019 (COVID-19). World Health Organization 2020.

[220] WHO. Situation Report-70 Coronavirus disease 2019 (COVID-19). World Health Organization 2020.

[221] WHO. Situation Report-72 Coronavirus disease 2019 (COVID-19). World Health Organization 2020.

[222] WHO. Situation Report-88Coronavirus disease 2019 (COVID-19). World Health Organization 2020.

CHAPTER 2

Studying Evolutionary Adaptation of SARS-CoV-2

Samina Ejaz[1,*], Yasir Hameed[1], Waqas Nazir Malik[1], Muhammad Usman[1] and Uzma Karamat[1]

[1] *Institute of Bio-Chemistry, Bio-Technology & Bioinformatics (IBBB), The Islamia University of Bahawalpur, Punjab, Pakistan*

Abstract: Although the acute respiratory syndromes causing SARS-Coronaviruses are not new to humanity, the recent SARS-CoV-2 based epidemic has spread to almost every part of the world and claimed a large number of human lives without any discrimination of race, gender, and color. However, multiple issues related to its origin, its transfer time in humans, evolutionary patterns, and underlying forces that derived the SARS-CoV-2 outbreak and pandemic remain unclear. Knowing the pathogen is an essential step to devise appropriate strategies for controlling and treating associated infection. This chapter attempts to enhance knowledge regarding the history of SARS-CoV-2 origin, zoonotic transfer events, and related evolutionary adaptions. This manuscript also provides an overview of various factors that contributed to making this virus more compatible with infecting the human cell and evaluated the possibility of its engineered / laboratory-based emergence. Our in-depth literature analysis demonstrated that SARS-CoV-2 was possibly pre-adopted in different animal species. Molecular fingerprints and phylogenetic analysis have confirmed high similarity (96% and 84%, respectively) of SARS-CoV-2 with bats (RaTG13) and pangolins SARS-CoV-like coronavirus. The genomic similarities of SARS-CoV-2 are due to the spike glycoprotein and RBD domain and poly cleavage site with bats and pangolin coronaviruses. It conclusively suggests that it is not a man-made bioweapon but rather emerged naturally through the recombination process. Thus generated information may help develop effective treatment strategies for SARS-CoV-2 and avoid the high risk of its re-emergence in the future.

Keywords: Coronaviruses, Evolutionary Adaptation, Phylogenetic Analysis, Recombination, SARS-CoV-2, SARS-CoV-like Coronavirus, Zoonotic Transfer.

INTRODUCTION

Coronaviruses belong to a group of common viruses that are recognized as a cause of mild or severe acute respiratory syndrome (SARS) in mammalian and avian species [1 - 3]. Coronaviruses are the enveloped viruses having a single-

* **Corresponding author Samina Ejaz:** Institute of Biochemistry, Biotechnology & Bioinformatics (IBBB) The Islamia University of Bahawalpur, Punjab, Pakistan; E-mails: samina.ejazsyed@iub.edu.pk and saminaejazsyed@yahoo.com

stranded, positive-sense RNA genome and belonging to the *Coronaviridae* family [4]. These viruses are classified in the subfamily *Coronaviranae* based on phylogenetic relationships and genomic organization. The Coronoviranae is further comprised of 4 genera, including *alpha, beta, gamma,* and *deltacoronavirus. Alpha* and *beta-coronaviruses* originated from bats and rodents, while gamma and delta from avian species [5].

The emergence of human SARS-coronavirus (SARS-CoV) in Southern China in 2002 increased the scientific interest exponentially to investigate the nature and mechanism of this virus [6, 7]. The SARS-CoV epidemic has led to more than 8000 cases and 774 deaths globally [8]. This virus belongs to the Coronaviridae family, which consists of many coronaviruses (CoVs) naturally found in mammals and birds [8, 9]. In the 1960s, the first few human coronaviruses were characterized and found to be associated with respiratory infections in both adults and children [10]. The human SARS-CoV-like variant was detected initially in Himalayan palm civets [11], which may have served as an amplification host of SARS-CoV. The genome of civet SARS-CoV contained a unique sequence of 29 nucleotides in its open reading frame (ORF) 10 that was not present in other human SARS-CoV isolates previously found responsible for the global epidemic [11]. A similar SARS-CoV virus was later detected in horseshoe bats [12, 13]. An additional region consisting of 29 nucleotides was detected in the ORF 8 of the bat-SARS-CoV genome. The absence of this part in most human SARS-CoVs genomes suggested a common ancestor with civet SARS-CoV [12]. Followed by the SARS epidemic, bats were thought to be a potential reservoir species of SARS-CoV that may be possibly involved in future coronavirus-related pandemics in humans [14]. The Middle East respiratory coronavirus (MERS-CoV) appeared for the first time in Saudi Arabia in 2012 [15, 16] and claimed 919 lives out of 2521 (35%) affected people [16]. The origin of MERS-CoV has been traced to bats [17].

A novel coronavirus known as severe acute respiratory syndrome-coronavirus-2 (SARS-CoV-2) is responsible for the coronavirus disease-2019 (COVID-2019). This virus was initially detected as a newly discovered beta (β) coronavirus (SARS-CoV-2) in the respiratory tract of pneumonia patients from Wuhan city of China in December 2019 [19]. Later on, it has been declared as a pandemic by the World Health Organization (WHO) on March 11, 2020 [18]. A staggering number of deaths are being reported in this ongoing pandemic due to a lack of population-specific herd immunity. The clinical manifestation of COVID-19 may vary from symptomatic and asymptomatic pneumonia to mild upper respiratory infections, acutepneumonia, severe pneumonia and multi-organ failures [20]. No therapeutic techniques are currently available, and prevention includes travel restriction, avoiding social gathering, patient isolation, and supportive treatment [21].

Characterization of this virus is done through throat swabs and bronchi-alveolar fluids [5]. This chapter aims to provide an insight into the evolutionary fingerprints of SARS-CoV-2 and enhance understanding regarding factors regulating the evolutionary adaptation of this virus.

The Zoonotic Origins of SARS-CoV-2 Viruses: Reservoirs and Transmission

Theories of SARS-CoV-2 Origins

The COVID-19 pandemic has changed our daily lifestyle considerably as we know it, but how did this novel coronavirus (SARS-CoV-2) emerge in the first place? The origins of SARS-CoV-2 have become a political issue, as the leaders seek to blame each other for the disease spread. There have been various unproven theories circulating widely regarding the origins of SARS-CoV-2 [22].

One opinion is that the SARS-CoV-2 virus was engineered in a laboratory [23]. After the viral genome was fully sequenced, this idea was disproved by many researchers who extensively studied the viral sequence of SARS-CoV-2. They found no evidence regarding its man-made origin and claimed confidently that the virus had originated naturally [24].

Speculation has also begun to arise concerning a laboratory named Wuhan Institute of Virology (WIV) located in Wuhan, where the virus is thought to have emerged. There were some safety concerns at the laboratory in 2018, but what provoked these concerns is unclear. Still, it was enough for someone to worry that the SARS-CoV-2 virus might accidentally have been released from that laboratory [25]. However, a researcher from the United States (US) working in the facility has rejected that idea saying that WIV scientists follow the proper safety protocols [26].

Shi Zhengli, a scientist, working on the bat coronavirus in WIV, has traced the origin of SARS coronavirus in 2003 from the one population of bats that lived in Yunnan caves in China. When she was informed about the SARS-CoV-2 virus outbreak affecting Wuhan city on December 30, 2019, she and her laboratory promptly started to sequence the SARS-CoV-2 genome to compare them to the genomes of the SARS viruses already stored and studied in their laboratory. The sequencing results revealed that SARS-CoV-2 did not match any virus they had in the laboratory [26]. However, another study conducted by Zhou *et al.* [27] has documented high similarity (96%) of SARS-CoV-2 with bats SARS-CoV-like coronavirus (RaTG13) from *Rhinolophus affinis* bat.

There might be no way to know the exact origin of the SARS-CoV-2 and rule out confusion regarding the source of this virus. However, the following 3 conditions are thought to provide clues regarding SARS-CoV-2 origin [28].

Natural Selection in an Animal Host Before the Zoonotic Transfer

The earlier reported incidences of SARS-CoV-2 were associated with the Huanan market in the Wuhan city of China [27, 29], so there may be an animal source present at that site. The similarities between SARS-CoV-2 and bat SARS-Co-like coronaviruses (RaTG13) exist [29]. However, the spike glycoprotein of bat SARS-CoV-like coronavirus RaTG13 (96% overall similar to SARS-CoV-2) diverges from the SARS-CoV-2 in the RBD, which is essential to bind with human angiotensin-converting enzyme 2 (ACE2). Hence, it is suggested that RaTG13 probably lacked absolute affinity for human ACE2 receptors [30]. Therefore, bats (*Rhinolophus affinis*) probably served as its progenitor's host reservoirs [27].

Illegally smuggled Malayan pangolins (*Manis javanica* to Guangdong province of China were also identified to harbor SARS-CoV-2-like coronaviruses [31]. A few pangolin coronaviruses exhibited high similarity with the SARS-CoV-2 genome, particularly in their RBD region, including six amino acid residues that are essential for its binding with human ACE2 [31]. This observation indicates that the optimization of the spike glycoprotein of SARS-CoV-2 for binding with human-like ACE2 is the outcome of natural selection.

Although a high level of similarities exists among the bats and pangolin coronaviruses withSARS-CoV-2. However, researchers do not find polybasic cleavage sites in bats pangolin coronaviruses spike glycoproteins that help to bind with human ACE2 through RBD regions [32]. The researcher suggested that various genetic alterations might occur in SARS-CoV-2 progenitors near the S1–S2 junction, including mutations, insertions, and deletions [33], and resulted in the formation of polybasic cleavage in SARS-CoV-2 through the natural evolutionary process and made it fit to bind with the human ACE2 [34].

Natural Selection in Humans Following Zoonotic Transfer

A progenitor of SARS-CoV-2 may have jumped directly into humans from animals like pangolins and bats. The presence of similar RBD regions in both SARS-CoV-2and pangolin coronaviruses indicates that this virus possibly jumped into humans. It acquired the polybasic cleavage site insertion during transmission from human-to-human through genetic alterations [27, 29]. This observation helped scientists speculate that the SARS-CoV-2 progenitors went through the unrecognized time of transmission before the initial zoonotic event and the emergence of the polybasic cleavage site [35].

Studies screening samples drawn from initially infected human subjects may provide information to better judge the possibility of any past viral spread event. Considering the usefulness of retrospective serological investigations, many researchers from China investigated the serology of patients. It showed low-level SARS-CoV coronavirus exposures [36]. Moreover, these studies did not help to identify that whether the documented exposure levels were because of previous infections with SARS-CoV, SARS-CoV-2, or other SARS-CoV-like coronaviruses. Hence, all such serological studies are required to be extended with careful measurement of any past exposure [28].

Selection During Passage

For many years worldwide, scientists have been attempting to explore bat SARS-CoV-like coronaviruses' details in animal models and/or cell culture [37] and documented many instances of the SARS-CoV escape from the laboratory [38]. Hence, the probability of an unintentional SARS-CoV-2 laboratory release is an accepted reality. Earlier it was the common perception that the RBD of SARS-CoV-2 have acquired mutation during adaptation to cell passage in cell culture, as found in various SARS-CoV studies [39]. Knowing about the SARS-CoV-2 laboratory escape events, scientists ruled out the possibility that the emergence of both polybasic cleavage sites and O-linked glycans is solely the outcome of the adaptation process of cell cultures. Their speculation was reinforced by observing the generation of polybasic cleavage sites in low pathogenicity avian influenza virus *via in vivo* and *in vitro* models [40]. Furthermore, scientists also concluded that the repeated passage in animals or cell cultures having ACE2 receptors identical to the ones present in humans would be required for the subsequent polybasic cleavage site generation [28].

Silent Evolutionary Features of the SARS-CoV-2 Genome

It was confirmed that there are similarities between human SARS-CoV-2 and bat SARS-CoV-like coronaviruses genome. Bats naturally hosted and evolutionarily shaped the coronaviruses [14, 41]. Although However, it has been previously claimed that most coronaviruses present in humans originated from the bat reservoirs [42]. Following evolutionary signatures of the SARS-CoV-2 genome may serve as the primary supporting factor of the SARS-CoV-2 outbreak [43].

SARS-CoV-2 Spike (S) Glycoprotein Adaptation Evolution: A Unique in COVID-19

Coronavirus spike glycoprotein is a unique, and a self-sufficient molecule that facilitates coronaviruses' entry into the host cells. First of all, the virus binds to a cell surface receptor, and then the viral envelope fuses with host cell plasma membranes [44]. The amino acids sequence of spikes glycoprotein of human SARS-CoV-2 shares 76% similarity with the SARS coronavirus Urban strain (SARS-CoV S Urbani). Furthermore, it contributes 80% identity with *Rinolophus sinicus* (Chinese horseshoe bats), SARS-CoV-like ZXC21, and ZC45 spike glycoproteins [45]. Moreover, Zhou *et al.* [27] reported that SARS-CoV-2 has the closest relation with the bat SARS-CoV (RaTG13) as reflected by the 97% amino acid sequence identity of their spike glycoproteins. Researchers found that SARS-CoV–like RBD, which binds to human ACE2 is less conserved [44]. Evolution in SARS-CoV-2 spike protein has changed the amino acid composition of the RBD domain, which makes it fit to bind with ACE2 properly. Researchers have found 14 different types of spike glycoproteins in other countries worldwide [46]. The altered amino acid pattern in the RBD domain may decide the fate of the host and the role of this virus in a viral outbreak by presenting a species barrier for viral infections [44].

Origin of SARS-CoV-2 Lineage: Recombination

The origin of SARS-CoV-2 through the recombination process is still debatable. Few researchers have proved that SARS-CoV-2 is not a mosaic and has the closest link with the bat SARS-CoV-like coronavirus RaTG13 found in bats in the Yunnan Province, China [47]. Although genetic similarities documented between SARS-CoV-2 and RaTG13, suggest discordant phylogenetic relationships, and most scientists agree that the disease outbreak in humans is not because of the RaTG13 variant. However, SRAS-CoV-2 probably originated from bats, and both SARS-CoV-2 and RaTG13 share a higher degree of homology with the Bat SARS-like coronavirus sequences [48]. The phylogenetic analysis [49] of the bat SARS-CoV-like RaTG13 virus and SRAS-CoV2virus sequences grouped both viruses in different clusters in a phylogenetic tree, thus suggested that they are recombinants [50, 51]. In an earlier codon usage (CU) based study, the researchers indicated that the SARS-CoV-2 possibly acquired spike glycoproteins through the recombination involving unknown coronavirus [50]. In this study, biased CU was observed in the case of the SARS-CoV-2 genome. The codon usage analysis can determine the origin of proteins having deep ancestry and insufficient phylogenetic signals or invented *de novo*. Another study conducted by Paraskevis *et al.* [52] rejected the hypothesis that a recombination event would lead toSARS-CoV-2 emergence. In the study of Paraskevis *et al.* [52], 50% of the

SARS-CoV-2 genome exhibited no close genetic connections to other viruses within the *Sarbecovirus* subgenus. This unique genomic region constitutes half of the spike region and is responsible for encoding a proteinthat facilitates viral entry into the host cells [13, 53]. The unique genetic characteristics of SARS-CoV-2 and their association with potential virulence in humans need to be clarified.

Receptor-binding Domain (RBD) of SARS-CoV-2

Spike (S) glycoprotein is a major coronavirus protein [54] that helps to initiate the viral envelops fusion with cell membrane followed by attachment of the virus to the receptor present on the surface of the host cell. The viral nucleocapsid is then delivered inside the host for successive replication. The spike protein consists of two subunits including S1 and S2. The RBD present within the S1 subunit interacts directly with the host cell receptors [14]. The SARS-CoV-2 structural and functional analysis showed that its RBD binds to the ACE2 receptor located on alveolar cells in humans [30, 43, 55]. Scientists proposed that RBD encoding region is the most variable region of the coronavirus genome [56, 57]. In total, 6 amino acids of RBD were found to be essential for ACE2 receptors binding and determining the host range for SARS-CoV-like viruses [30]. The SARS-CoV-like virus, Y442, L472, N479, D480, T487, and Y4911, are the six essential amino acids present in RBD, which altered and corresponded to L455, F486, Q493, S494, N501, and Y505 in novel SARS-CoV-2 [30]. In total, 5 out of these 6 residues differ between SARS-CoV-2 and SARS-CoV-like viruses. Based on the other structural [45, 58] and experimental biochemical studies [58, 59], the RBD of SARS-CoV-2 seems to be capable of binding more tightly with ACE2 in humans, cats, and other species having higher receptor homology [30]. Scientists proposed that the SARS-CoV-2 spike glycoprotein efficient binding to human ACE2 is most probably due to the natural selection on a human or human-like ACE2 that permitted another optimal binding solution to arise. This scenario provides a substantial piece of evidence that SARS-CoV-2 is not a deliberately manipulated product [30].

Polybasic Furin Cleavage Site and O-linked Glycan SARS-CoV-2

Another remarkable characteristic of the SARS-CoV-2 genome is the polybasic cleavage site, also known as RRAR (Arginine-Arginine-Alanine-Arginine), located at the junction of S1 and S2 subunits of spike glycoprotein [45]. This site allows an efficient cleavage by various proteases, including furin, and plays a role in determining viral infection capacity and the host range [60]. Furthermore, this site in SARS-CoV-2 harbors a proline residue; therefore, the new sequence in SARS-CoV-2 is PRRA instead of RRAR. The effect produced by adding a proline residue has been predicted to promote the addition of O-linked glycans to S673, T678, and S686, which are rare to SARS-CoV-2 flank the cleavage site [45].

Although less is known about the role of O-linked glycans, it is suggested to develop a 'mucin-like domain' that would shield the epitopes or key residues of SARS-CoV-2 spike glycoprotein [61]. Several other viruses use mucin-like domains as glycan shields that facilitate during immunoevasion [61]. The predicted O-linked glycosylation is reliable, but experimental evidence is required to justify their use by SARS-CoV-2.

The scientists also explored the functional impact of a polybasic cleavage site insertion at the junction of S1–S2 in various other SARS-CoV-like viruses through different experiments and concluded the following conclusions [62]. The effective cleavage of MERS-CoV-like coronaviruses spike glycoprotein allows them to infect the human cells more rapidly [63]. Avian influenza viruses contain the poly-basic cleavage sites in their hemagglutinin (HA) protein in chickens [64]. Its function is similar to the S glycoprotein of coronavirus. The polybasic cleavage sites creation in HA protein either through the insertion or recombination process converts low-pathogenic avian influenza viruses into the high pathogenic forms [64].

Replication of SARS-CoV-2

The SARS-CoV-2, like SARS-CoV, targets alveolar macrophages, type I and type II pneumocytes. However, SARS-CoV-2 replicates more efficiently, generating 3.3 folds more viral infectious particles than SARS-CoV. Pathophysiology of this virus resembles SARS-CoV, and an increased secretion of inflammatory particles is associated with disease severity [65]. But Chu *et al.,* 2020 reported fewer vital inflammatory cytokines and interferon are produced followed by SARS-CoV-2 infection than SARS-CoV despite efficient replication [20].

The SARS-CoV-2 replication mechanism has to be deciphered to identify therapeutic targets for this deadly virus [66]. Cell lines and tissue cultures were used to study viral replication. The quantitative real-time polymerase chain reaction (qRT-PCR) was used to determine ongoing replication and indirect immunofluorescence. It was employed as a confirmatory test for SARS-CoV, the virus having more significant similarity with SARS-CoV-2. These methods are also being used to determine the mechanism of replication in the novel COVID-19. Furthermore, the comparative analysis revealed common structural and functional aspects of SARS-CoV and SARS-CoV-2 [66].

Genomic Organization

SARS-CoV-2 contains a positive sense non-segmented enveloped RNA genome of 26 to 32 kb size [1, 4] and consisting of 6 to 11 ORFs which encode 9680 amino acid polyproteins. There are 5′ and 3′ UTRs present at the end of 265 and 358 nucleotides. However, the hemagglutinin esterase (HEs) gene present in coronaviruses with receptor destroying activity is missing in the genome [66]. The RNA of SARS-CoV-2 possesses a 5′ cap and a 3′ poly (A) tail structure that allows it to act as a complete mRNA to produce replicase polyproteins through translation. The 5′ end of the SARS-CoV-2 genome features a leader sequence and several stem-loop structures essential for their transcription and translation.

Additionally, SARS-CoV-2 also contained transcriptional regulatory sequences (TRSs) at the 5′ end of its genome. The TRSs are required for the expression of various structural genes. These *cis*-acting elements modulate both replication and transcription processes in SARS-CoV-2 by forming a complex known as replicase-transcriptase (RCT). The 3′ UTR of SARS-CoV-2 also features different essential elements which are required for replication of its genome. The genome of coronavirus is comprised of 5′-leader-UTR- replicase-S-E-M-N-3′ UTR-poly A tail with interspersed accessory genes present in the region within structural genes located at the 3′ end of the genome [1].

Viral Proteins

ORF1 encodes 16 nonstructural proteins (nsps) and occupies 67% of genome size, while other ORFs encode for structural and accessory proteins [1, 4]. Frameshift in ORF1a and ORF1b produce polyproteins pp1a and pp1b, which are cleaved by viral encoded proteases, main protease (Mpro), Chymotrypsin-like protease (3CLpro), and one or two papain-like proteases into 16 nsps [67]. No significant difference has been documented between the nsps and ORFs of SARS-CoV-2 and SARS-CoV. The nsp3 acts as papain-like protease, nsp5 as chymotrypsin-like protease, nsp12 as RNA-dependent RNA polymerase, and nsp13 functions as helicase. Other nsps may engage in the SARS-CoV-2 transcription and replication. In contrast, structural proteins like N, M, E, and S are encoded by ORFs 10 and 11 (Fig. **1**) in addition to nsps [4, 66].

In tissue culture, the accessory proteins of SARS-CoV-2 were proven completely nonessential for its replication. However, some of them have shown significant roles in SARS-CoV-2 pathogenesis [1]. The SARS-CoV-2 assembly, morphogenesis, and budding require spike glycoprotein along with M and E proteins which are also embedded in the viral envelope [4, 66]. The spike glycoproteins of SARS-CoV-2 and SARS-CoV, are similar in structure as revealed by cloning and the crystallization of ectodomain (1-1208a.a) spike protein [68]. Due to greater affinity (10-20 folds) for human ACE2 receptors, the SARS-CoV-2 spike proteins can cause more severe infection than SARS-CoV and promote the inter-individual spread of disease. The lysine 31 of ACE2 receptor present on the human cell surface can recognize 394 glutamine residue of SARS-CoV-2 spike glycoprotein that corresponds to 479 glutamine residue of SARS-CoV spike protein [68]. The spike glycoprotein of SARS-CoV-2 consists of two different S1 and S2 subunits. The S1 subunit contains an RBD, N-terminal domain (NTD), and signal peptide [4, 66], having a 70% sequence homology with SARS-CoV. Differences have been documented in the external subdomain required for the interaction of viral spike glycoproteins with human ACE2 receptors. The S2 subunit of SARS-CoV-2 has a 90% sequence similarity with human SARS-CoV and bats SARS-CoV-like coronaviruses and contains HR-N and HR-C, two heptad repeat regions. The HRs make a coiled-coil structure occupied by protein ectodomain. A furin-cleavage site, PRRAS'V, which is processed during the biogenesis of the virus, is present in the S- protein at the interface of S1 and S2 subunits [4, 66].

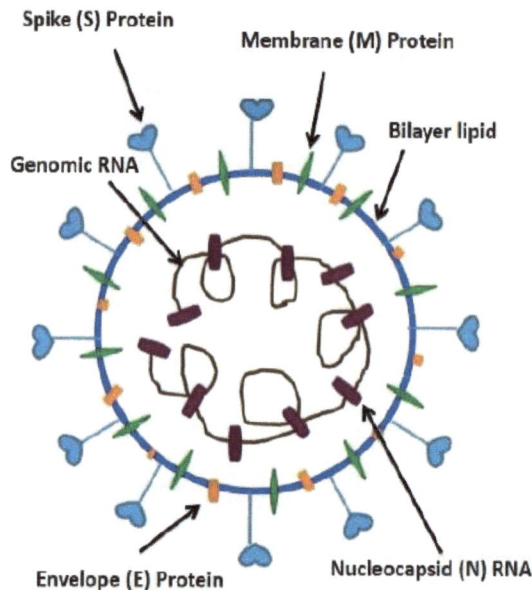

Fig. (1). Structure of SARS-CoV-2. This figure is a modified version of an earlier reported figure [66].

Attachment and Entry

SARS-CoV-2 utilizes RBD of its spike glycoprotein to bind with human ACE2 receptors and enter into human cells. These viruses spread due to higher ACE2 receptor expression in human respiratory tissues [4, 66]. Followed by the binding of spike glycoprotein with ACE2 receptors, host cell TMPRSS2, cathepsin serine protease causes priming of spike glycoprotein, a process required for the spike glycoprotein activation and adherence to the host receptor [67]. The step of priming is a common step observed in the case of both SARS-CoV and SARS-CoV-2 viruses (Fig. **2**). The SARS-CoV-2 spike proteins interact with human ACE2 receptors, and binding leads to the conformational changes in its spike glycoproteins. It helps to fuse viral envelope proteins with the host cell membrane, allowing the virus to enter into the host cells *via* the endosomal pathway [66].

Fig. (2). Replication pathway of SARS-CoV-2. This figure is a modified version of an earlier reported figure [66].

The cathepsin protease, TMPRRS2, stimulates the acid-dependent (Low pH) spike glycoprotein cleavage at two different sites within itsS2 subunit. The first cleavage occurs with acidified viral endosomes and separates the RBD. It also happens when there is the fusion domain of spike glycoprotein. The second cleavage exposes a fusion peptide that inserts into the membrane. Two HRs present in S2 bind with each other and form a six-helix fusion bundle (Fig. **2**). This fusion bundle allows the mixing of host and viral proteins [1], and the viral RNA enters the host cell's cytoplasm [66].

Translation

Virus The virus utilizes RNA pseudoknot structure and a slippery sequence (5′-UUUAAAC-3′) required for the ribosomal frame-shifting from ORF rep1a to rep1b. The ribosome machinery unzips the pseudoknot structure of RNA and keeps elongating the polypeptide chain until the rep1a stop codon is encountered. Occasionally this elongation is interrupted by pseudoknot, which blocks ribosome form continuing elongation bypassing ribosome on slippery sequence before ribosome can unwind pseudoknot structure, thus extending translation into rep1ab generating pp1ab. The next step is the translation of replicase genes related to ORFs, rep1a, and rep1ab, into co-terminal polyproteins, pp1a, and pp1ab, respectively [4, 66]. These polyproteins are cleaved by viral encoded proteases 1 or 2 papain-like proteases, 3CLpro or Mpro, into nsps. The pp1a comprises nsps1 to 11 and pp1ab contains nsps 12 to 16 (Fig. **2**). Many of these nsps combine into replicase- RTC and thus create an environment favorable for RNA synthesis and replication [66].

RNA Synthesis and Replication

The nsps in RTC provide RNA-dependent RNA polymerase, helicase, and proteolytic activities. RNA synthesis and replication of coronaviruses take place at cytoplasmic membranes and involve both continuous and discontinuous transcription [67].

The RNA positive-strand is replicated into a negative strand. This negative-strand RNA is again replicated into a positive-stranded genomic mRNA through a continuous transcription and subgenomicpositive-stranded mRNAs through discontinuous transcription starting from multiple transcriptions start sites (Fig. **2**). The subgenomic mRNAs are then translated to yield viral proteins, *i.e.,* structural and accessory proteins [66].

Assembly and Release

Genomic mRNA synthesized by replication and proteins translated from subgenomic mRNAs interacted at the endoplasmic reticulum and transported to the Golgi complex. These assembled particles are further transported from the Golgi complex to the cell surface in the form of vesicles (Fig. **2**), and thus viral progeny is released *via* exocytosis [66]. The spike glycoproteins, which are not assembled into viral particles, are taken to the cell surface and initiate the fusion of infected cells with adjacent uninfected cells creating a multi-nucleated giant cell that is not detected by virus-specific antibodies; thus, the virus spreads within the host genome [1].

Classification of SARS-CoV-2

SARS-CoV-2 is an RNA virus, and RNA viruses are divided into three different orders, including order Nidovirales. The order Nidovirales is grouped into four families. The Coronaviridae, to which SARS-CoV-2 belongs is categorized into two subfamilies, and the subfamily *Coronavirinae* contains four genera [69]. The recent valid classification of SARS-CoV-2 [70] is shown in Fig. (**3**).

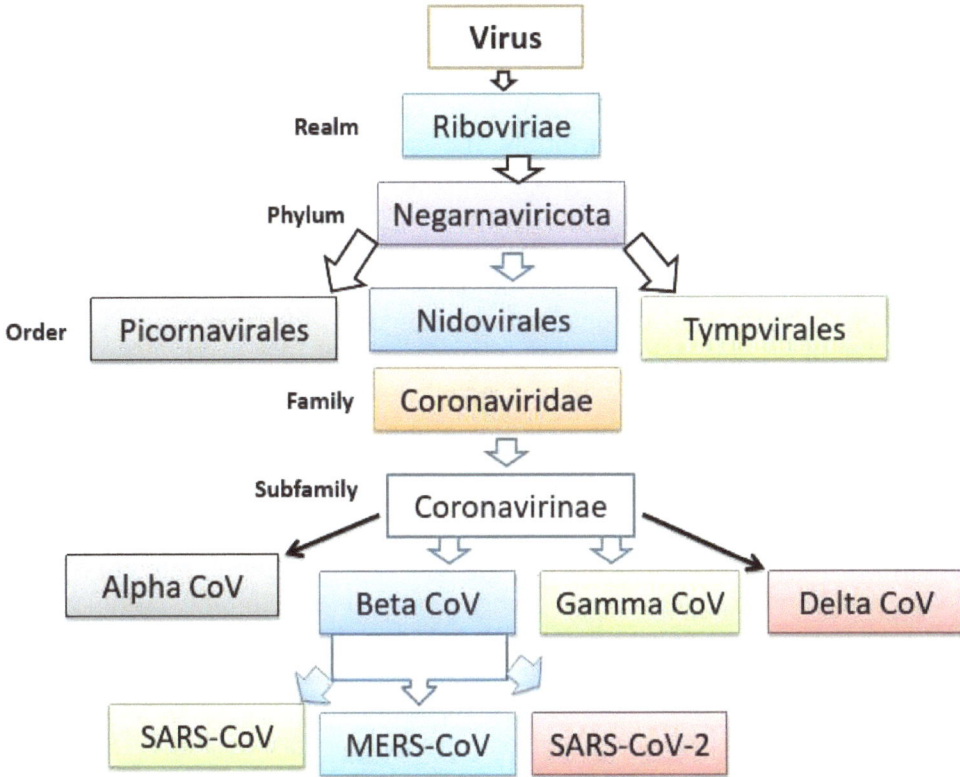

Fig. (3). Classification of SARS-CoV-2. This figure is a modified version of a figure that has been published previously [69].

Molecular Phylogenetic Analysis of SARS-CoV-2

A phylogenetic tree is an illustration that characterizes evolutionary associations among organisms. The inferences regarding the evolutionary relationship are hypotheses, not decisive evidence. The branching configuration of the phylogenetic tree reveals how species evolved from a chain of shared ancestors. It also gives us information regarding the route(s) of viral induction in a specific geographical region. This virus has been placed in the taxonomy group based on the evidence obtained from a sequence-based family classification [71, 72], which is accomplished through phylogenetic analysis. Researchers studying the SARS-CoV-2 emergence faced challenges related to the requirement to describe whether this recently emerged coronavirus belongs to an existing group of viruses or a new species. The present taxonomy and family classification of coronaviruses, developed by Coronaviridae Study Group (CSG) of the International Committee of virus taxonomy (ICVT), distinguishes 39 species into the family *Coronaviridae* in realm *Riboviria* [73].

Evolutionary Phylogenetic Tree Construction Based on Whole-Genome Analysis

The evolutionary rate of SARS-CoV-2 is studied while assessing the utmost topical common ancestor. In a study, Li *et al*. [74], executed transmission networks, phylogenetic, comparative analyses, likelihood-mapping, and split networks of the genomes. They constructed a phylogenetic tree on Bayesian time-scaled using the tip-dating method. The study revealed that there is high similarity of SARS-CoV-2 virus genome with the bat SARS-CoV-like coronavirus rather than the SARS-CoV-like coronavirus of pangolin. Many other phylogenetic analyses based studies have been conducted so far, and most scientists have concluded the same. In another study conducted by Zhou *et al*. [75], revealed that the SARS-CoV-2 genome is 96% similar to a bat SRAS-CoV-like coronavirus. Paraskevis *et al*. [52], proposed a phylogenetic tree based on the whole-genome sequence analysis, inferred it by maximum likelihood and Bayesian method, and concluded that the newly emerged SARS-CoV-2 virus shares 96.3% similarity and clusters with BatCoV RaTG13 (MN996532.1). Large numbers of the coronavirus genomic sequences are being submitted to the biological repositories daily, and their phylogeny is being done. Most of these studies involved the analysis of newly submitted sequences and other SARS-related *betacoronaviruses*. A very few studies are known to involve other genera of coronaviruses in phylogeny. To investigate the intermediate host of SARS-CoV-2, *alphacoronavirus* is the most important candidate to be considered for phylogeny [76].

A phylogenetic tree can be constructed by different methods and using a variety of tools like Bayes Phylogenies, BEAST, Fast Tree 2, IQ-TREE, jModel Test 2, MEGA, PHYLIP, PhyML, Tree-Puzzle. The majority of the tools are based upon multiple sequence alignment (MSA), while others employ alignment-free methods. In sequence alignment methods using Clustal W and MUSCLE algorithms of multiple sequence alignment, either the virus's whole-genome is aligned to whole-genomes of other related viruses [74]. It might be aligned to only coding sequences (CDs), *i.e.,* ORF1ab, S, N, and E genes, can be aligned [77]. The whole-genome sequences and coding sequences of all viruses can be accessed from the virus-related NCBI platform (https://www.ncbi.nlm.nih.gov /labs/virus/vssi/#/).

In the present study, using the maximum-likelihood method, a phylogenetic tree was constructed. The whole-genome sequences of a few representative *betacoronavirus* species (n = 17, Table **1**) and *alphacoronavirus* species (n = 2, Table **1**) retrieved from the NCBI platform were subjected MSA, and the tree was inferred using MEGA X. Node-A is representative of 12 species of genus *betacoronavirus*. In comparison, node B represents the SARS-related *betacoronavirus*. The tree is rooted with species of genus *alphacoronavirus* (Fig. **4**). According to former reports [78, 79], the phylogenetic tree of genus *betacoronavirus* constructed during the present study indicated clustering of SARS-CoV-2 and SARS-CoVs in the common clade (Fig. **4**).

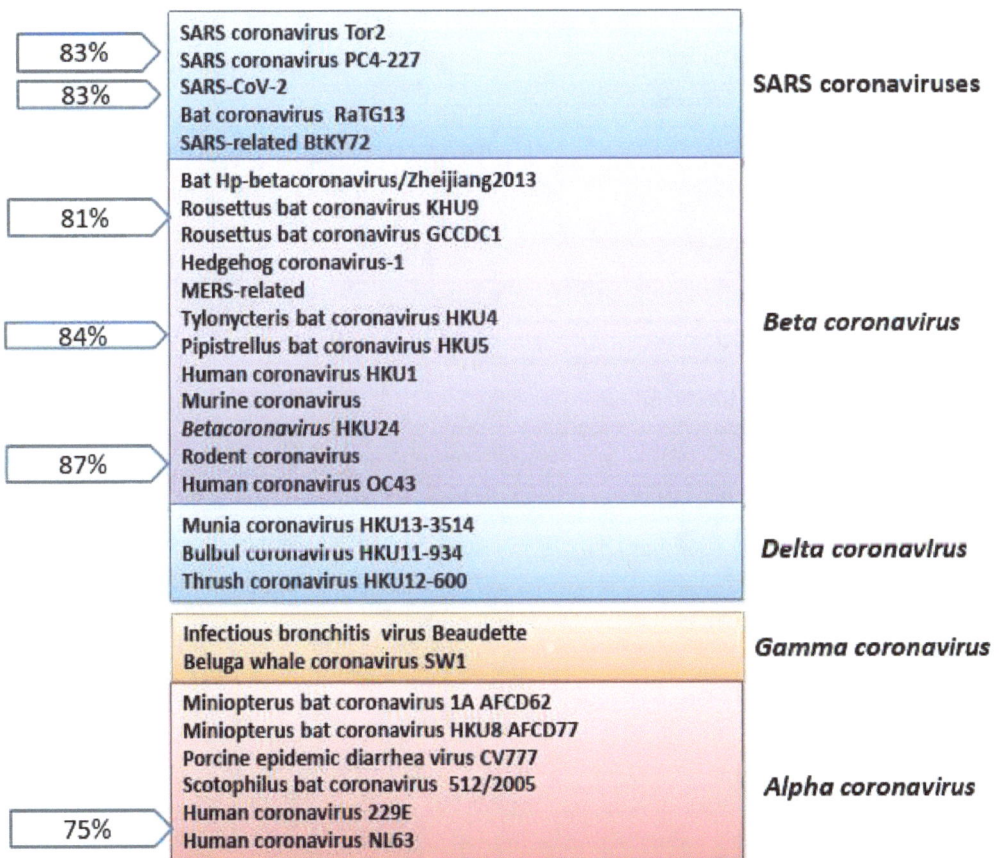

Fig. (4). Evolutionary relationships of *betacoronavirus* and *alphacoronavirus*. The phylogenetic tree is based upon the Neighbor-Joining method and 19 SARS-CoV-2 genomic sequences [80], and the sum of branch length is equivalent to 3.07757254. The evolutionary distance is measured by the number of base substitutions per site through the Maximum Composite Likelihood method [81]. The evolutionary analyses were conducted using MEGA X and involved codon positions 1st+2nd+3rd+Noncoding and removing all ambiguous positions for each sequence pair (pairwise deletion option). The final dataset consisted of a total of 35870 positions [82].

Table 1. Details of viral genomes used for phylogenetic tree construction.

Sr.No.	Type of Virus	GenBank ID	Name
1	*Alphacoronavirus*	KY996417.1	Human coronavirus 229E strain 229E/UF-1/2016, complete genome
2		MG428701.1	Human coronavirus NL63 isolate Kilifi_HH_0512_04-Ju--2010, complete genome
3	*Betacoronavirus*	KY370046.1	Rodent coronavirus isolate RtMruf-CoV-2/JL2014, complete cds
4		MN306036.1	Human coronavirus OC43 strain HCoV_OC43/Seattle/USA/SC0682/2019, complete genome
5		NC_026011.1	Betacoronavirus HKU24 strain HKU24-R05005I, complete genome
6		MK167038.1	Human coronavirus HKU1 strain SC2521, complete genome
7		KP887098.1	Murine coronavirus strain AM2, complete genome
8		MK679660.1	Hedgehog coronavirus 1, complete genome
9		MH454272.1	Middle East respiratory syndrome-related coronavirus strain HCoV-EMC, complete genome
10		NC_009019.1	Bat coronavirus HKU4-1, complete genome
11		NC_009020.1	Bat coronavirus HKU5-1, complete genome
12		MG762674.1	Rousettus bat coronavirus HKU9 isolate Rousettusspp/Jinghong/2009, complete genome
13		NC_025217.1	Bat Hp-betacoronavirus/Zhejiang2013, complete genome
14	SARSr coronavirus	AY274119.3	SARS coronavirus Tor2, complete genome
15		MN908947.3	Severe acute respiratory syndrome coronavirus 2 isolate Wuhan-Hu-1, complete genome
16		KY352407.1	Severe acute respiratory syndrome-related coronavirus strain BtKY72, complete genome
17		AY613950.1	SARS coronavirus PC4-227, complete genome
18		MN996532.1	Bat coronavirus RaTG13, complete genome
19		NC_030886.1	Rousettus bat coronavirus isolate GCCDC1 356, complete genome

Comparative analysis of SARS-CoV-2 Wuhan-Hu 1 and SARS-CoV genomes

The whole-genome sequence of the SARS-CoV22 (NCBI Reference Sequence: NC_045512.2) with SARS-CoV (NCBI Reference Sequence: NC_004718.3) was compared through sequence alignment showed that newly emerged SARS-CoV2 is 79% similar to the SARS-CoV virus [83]. A large fragment (50 bp) insertion was observed at positions 3211-3263 (ORF1ab) in the SARS-CoV-2 genome

(Figs. **5a** and **5b**). Characteristics of both genomes are given in Table **2** while Fig. **5** (**c** and **d**) show the comparative genomic architecture of both viral genomes.

Table 2. Characteristics of SARS-CoV-2 and SARS-CoV genomes.

Sr. No.	Feature	SARS-CoV-2	SARS-CoV
1	Accession No.	NC_045512.2	NC_004718.3
2	Sequence Type	ssRNA, linear	ssRNA, Linear
3	Number of Nucleotide	29903 bp	29751 bp
4	5' UTR	1-265	1-264
5	3' UTR	29675-29903	29389-29751
6	Coding genes	11	13

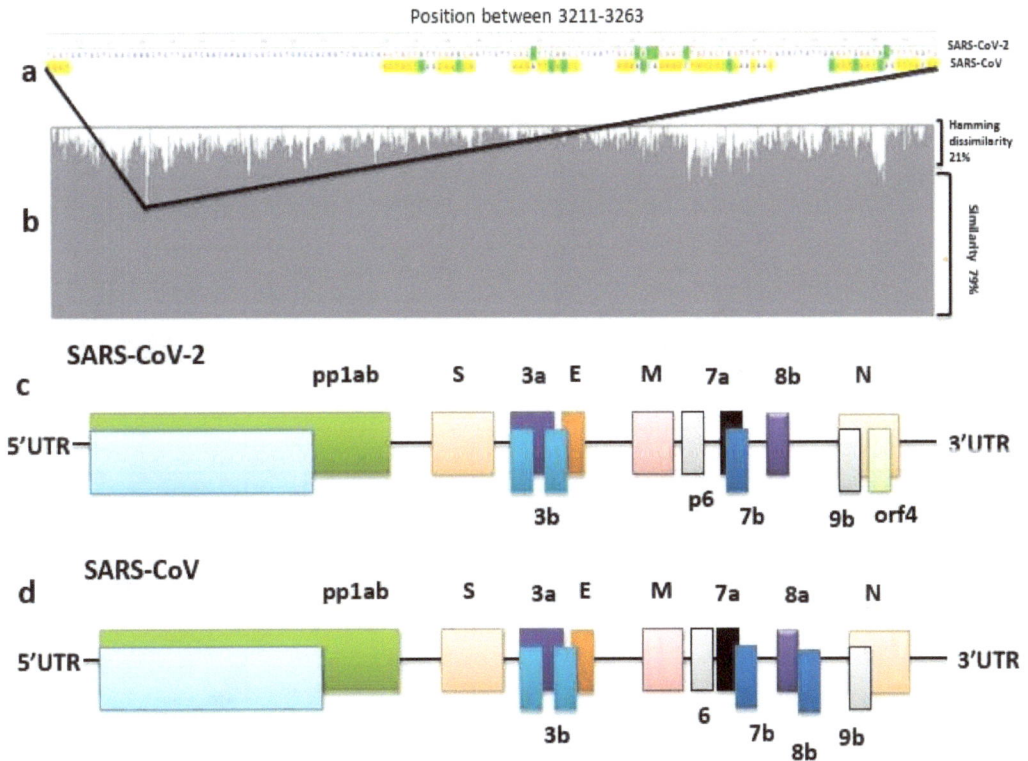

Fig. (5). (a) a long nucleotide (50 bp) sequence insertion in SARS-CoV-2 genome at the position between 3211-3263, (b) represents the sequence alignment of SARS-CoV-2 and SARS-CoV in a graphical view created in UGENE software showing 79% similarity and 21% hamming dissimilarity, (c and d) pictorial diagram of SARS-CoV-2 and SARS-CoV genomic structure respectively, representing the organization of genes coding ORF1ab, S=spike glycoprotein, E=envelope protein, M=membrane protein, and N= nucleocapsid protein, *etc.*

Blastp analysis of proteins encoded by both genomes suggested that both viruses are closely related species. Most of their proteins shared more than 80% identity [83]. However, a few proteins, *i.e.,* encoded by orf8 and orf10, of SARS-CoV-2 have no similar functional counterpart in SARS-CoVs. Moreover, the sequence of orf8 protein in SARS-CoV-2 is different from the sequences of SARS-CoV derived orf8a or orf8b [84]. A detailed comparison of proteins encoded by both genomes are given in Table **3**.

Table 3. Comparative Detail of proteins expressed from viral genomes of SARS-CoV-2 and SARS-CoV.

	SARS-CoV-2		SARS-CoV		
Sr.No	Accession Number	Protein Name	Putative Function/Domain	Accession Number	Mutual Percent Identity
1	YP_009725295.1	orf1a polyprotein	orf1a polyprotein (pp1a)	NP_828850.1	68.34
2	YP_009724389.1	orf1ab polyprotein	orf1ab polyprotein (pp1ab)	NP_828849.2	86.12
3	YP_009724391.1	orf3a protein	Hypothetical protein sars3a	NP_828852.2	72.36
4	YP_009724394.1	orf6 protein	Hypothetical protein sars6	NP_828856.1	68.85
5	YP_009724395.1	orf7a protein	protein 8	ARO76387.1	87.70
6	YP_009725296.1	orf7b protein	Hypothetical protein sars7b	NP_849175.1	81.40
7	YP_009724396.1	orf8 protein	-	-	-
8	YP_009725255.1	orf10 protein	-	-	-
9	YP_009725298.1	nsp2	Nonstructural polyprotein pp1a	ABF65834.1	68.34
10	YP_009725299.1	nsp3	Polyprotein orf1a	AFR58698.1	75.82
11	YP_009725300.1	nsp4	Polyprotein 1a	ARO76381.1	80.00
12	YP_009725302.1	nsp6	nsp6-pp1a/pp1ab (TM3)	NP_828864.1	88.15
13	YP_009725303.1	nsp7	Chain A, Replicase Polyprotein 1ab, Light Chain	2AHM_A	98.80
14	YP_009725304.1	nsp8	Chain E, ReplicasePolyprotein 1ab, Heavy Chain	2AHM_E	97.47
15	YP_009725305.1	nsp9	nsp9-pp1a/pp1ab	NP_828867.1	97.35

(Table 3) cont.....

Sr.No	SARS-CoV-2			SARS-CoV		
	Accession Number	Protein Name	Putative Function/Domain	Accession Number	Mutual Percent Identity	
16	YP_009725306.1	nsp10	Chain A, Non-structural Protein 10	5C8S_A	97.12
17	YP_009725312.1	nsp11	nsp11-pp1a	NP_904321.1	84.62
18	YP_009725311.1	2'-O-ribose methyltransferase	nsp16-pp1ab (2'--MT)	NP_828873.2	93.29
19	YP_009725301.1	3C-like proteinase	Polyprotein 1a	ARO76381.1	96.08
20	YP_009725309.1	3'-to-5' exonuclease	nsp14-pp1ab (nuclease ExoN homolog)	NP_828871.1	95.07
21	YP_009725310.1	endoRNAse	nsp15-pp1ab (endoRNAse)	NP_828872.1	88.73
22	YP_009725297.1	leader protein	nsp1-pp1a/pp1ab	NP_828860.2	84.44
23	YP_009724392.1	envelope protein	E protein	APO40581.1	94.74
24	YP_009724393.1	membrane glycoprotein	Matrix protein	NP_828855.1	90.54
25	YP_009725308.1	Helicase	nsp13-pp1ab (ZD, NTPase/HEL)	NP_828870.1	99.83
26	YP_009724390.1	surface glycoprotein	Spike glycoprotein	ABD72985.1	76.04
27	YP_009724397.2	nucleocapsidphosphoprotein	Nucleocapsid protein	ARO76389.1	90.52
28	YP_009725307.1	RNA-dependent RNA polymerase	nsp12-pp1ab (RdRp)	NP_828869.1	96.35

Recombination Events Documented in Newly Emerged SARS-CoV-2

The emergence of a novel virus through the recombination process usually requires the coexistence of multiple or at least two viruses in a single host cell. Such a condition is supported by most of the viral genomes within infected cells over long periods. In the case of CoVs, this condition has been explained by a study. Scientists from Wuhan city of China analyzed the feces of bats and detected a wide variety of novel coronaviruses with sequences entirely different from the SARS-CoV-1 virus. Thus indicated the role of massive CoVs genomes rearrangements in the emergence of novel coronaviruses [85].

The evolution of SARS-CoV-2 through the recombination process remains a question mark. However, few studies have analyzed the available pieces of evidence regarding SARS-CoV-2 emergence through the recombination process. The results of these analyses demonstrated that the emergence of SARS-CoV-2 through the natural occurred recombination process involving at least two viruses:

a bat SARS-CoV-like coronavirus, RaTG13 (genus *Rhinolophus*), and a pangolin SARS-CoV-like coronavirus. Typically, none of both cause infection in humans [28]. Although the genome of bat coronavirus RaTG13 shares 96% similarity with SARS-CoV-2. It has a diverged RBD (only 60% similar to SARS-CoV-2), due to which its spike protein can bind loosely to the human ACE2 receptor. This makes the entry of this virus into human cells unlikely. The pangolin SARS-CoV-like virus genome is 90% similar to SARS-CoV-2. While the RBD region of both viruses is 99% identical thus, it has a high affinity with human ACE-2 based on the RBD similarity with SARS-CoV-2 [86]. As reported in two recent studies, it has a great affinity to human ACE-2 than the SARS-CoV-1 RBD [30, 87].

Regarding the emergence of SARS-CoV-2, it has been speculated that the bat and pangolin SARS-CoV-like viruses may have infected the same organism (which is unknown), and their genes got recombined in that host. The recombination thus facilitated the acquisition of RBD by the bat SARS-CoV-like coronavirus, RaTG13. The RBD acquired from the pangolin SARS-CoV-like virus helped to boast the infection-causing capability of SARS-CoV-2 because it contains a cleavage site of furin enzyme. The cleavage of spike glycoprotein by furin promotes multiple subtypes of viruses, including influenza and other CoVs, into host cells. The significance of this proteolytic cleavage can better be understood through an earlier experiment that was carried out on bats MERS-CoV. The experimental data suggested that the bats MERS-CoV-like viruses cannot enter into human cells efficiently until a small quantity of trypsin protease was applied to the virion to imitate the furin cleavage of spike glycoprotein [63]. Interestingly, researchers also demonstrated that the ability of spike glycoprotein to get cleaved by furin protease (Cellular, not synthetic) is lost readily when CoVs propagate in cell cultures, as observed in the case of feline CoV. This shows that furin cleavage site acquisition by CoVs might switch on the infection capability, but it is lost as these viruses start amplifying in cell cultures [88].

Factors Contributing to the Evolutionary Adaptation of SARS-CoV-2

The world has experienced three different coronaviruses outbreaks in humans over the last two decades, which contributed to the significantly high morbidity rate around the globe. Currently, the world is facing an ongoing pandemic due to the SARS-CoV-2 based infections. Whole-genome analysis of SARS-CoV-2 revealed that it is the descendant of the Bat SARS/SARS-like CoVs. Recombination and mutations in the different regions of the SARS-CoV-2 genome have been identified as the crucial strategies involved in the evolution of this novel infectious agent. SARS-CoV-2 has four structural proteins, namely spike (S), envelop (E), membrane (M), and nucleocapsid (N) proteins. Wuhan-Hu-1-CoV (Wuhan seafood market pneumonia virus) has more sequence homology with SARS-CoV than the MERS-CoV. However, remarkable genetic diversity has been observed between Wuhan-Hu-1-CoV and SARS-CoV. The percentage of homology and genetic variations in the different regions of the Wuhan-Hu-1-CoVSARS-CoV is given in Table **4**. Nine regions in the Wuhan-Hu-1-CoV were more sensitive for the recombination, and it was suggested that Wuhan-Hu-1-CoV could be a recombinant of SARS (GZ02, Rf1), SARS-like (ZXC21, ZC45, W1V1), and MERS-CoVs. Evidence of recombination provided by the PHI-test was significant (p-value < 0.00001). S protein, mainly towards the 5' end, was found to be closely associated with recombination, and only one recombination event was found to be associated with the RNA-dependent RNA polymerase, ORF3a, and helicase [89].

Table 4. Homology and genetic variations documented in Wuhan-Hu-1-CoV as compared to SARS-CoV (84).

Envelop Protein		Membrane Protein		Nucleocapsid Protein		Spike Protein	
Homology	Genetic Variations	Homology	Genetic Variations	Homology	Genetic Variations	Homology	Genetic Variations
93%	7%	92%	08%	93%	7%	81%	19%

Most frequent recombination breakpoints lie within the spike gene that codes for spike protein, upstream of orf8 that codes for the accessory protein, and ORF3, which codes for ORF3b, a 154 amino acid protein act an interferon antagonist [90]. However, spike protein is more prone to mutations, and it plays a crucial role in the attachment of virus with host cell receptors, fusion with the host cell membrane, and final entry of the virus into the host cell. Moreover, it can also be utilized as a potential target for developing vaccines, antibodies, and entry inhibitors. It was found that in SARS-CoV-2, the recombinant RBD of spike protein-bound more tightly to the human ACE2 receptors as compared to the bat ACE2 receptors. Multiple sequencing (Fig. **6**) of S protein shows that some variable amino acids are present between SARS-CoV-2, SARS-CoV [91].

Role of Traveling in the Spread and Emergence of New SARS-CoV-2 Variants

Coronavirus can fly and the world is facing the third deadly disruptive coronavirus epidemic that has been experienced during the last two decades [21, 92]. The first was SARS occurred in 2002–2003. The second was MERS-CoV that emerged in 2012. The SARS and MERS were linked with the nosocomial transmission process and the super-spreader events, where a single individual infected various other subjects [93]. A pneumonia case-based cluster reported in Wuhan city of China was linked with the seafood market in December 2019. This time the world is facing 2019-nCoV emergence, and the WHO on January 30, 2020, declared it as a Public Health Emergency of International Concern [94].

```
a   331   -NITNLCPFGEVFNATRFASVYAWNRKRISNCVADYSVLYNSASFSTFKCYGVSPTKLND      389
b   318   -NITNLCPFGEVFNATKFPSVYAWERKKISNCVADYSVLYNSTFFSTFKCYGVSATKLND      376
c   377   QAEGVECDFSPLLSG-TPPQVYNFKRLVFTNCNYNLTKLLSLFSVNDFTCSQISPAAIAS      435

a   390   LCFTNVYADSFVIRGDEVRQIAPGQTTGKIADYNYKLPDDFTGCVIAWNSNNLDSKVGGNY    449
b   377   LCFSNVYADSFVKVGDDVRQIAPGQTTGKIADYNYKLPDDFMGCVLAWNTRNIDATSTGNY    436
c   436   NCYSSLILDYFSYPLSMKSDLSVSSAGPISQFNYKQSFSNPTCLILATVPHNLTTITKPL      495

a   450   NYLYRLFRKSNLKPFERDISTEIYQAGSTPCNGVEGFNCYFP-------------LQSYGFQ    498
b   437   NYKYRYLRHGKLRPFERDISNVPFSPDGKPCT-PPALNCYFP-------------LNDYGFY    484
c   496   KYSYINKCSRLLSDDRTEVPQLVNANQYSPCVSIVPS-TVWEDGDYYRKQLSPLEGGGWL     554

a   499   PTNGVGYQPYRVVVLSFELLHAAPAT-----V-------                         524
b   485   TTTGIGYQPYRVVVLSFELLNAAPAT-----V-------                         510
c   555   VASGSTVAMTEQLQMGFGITVQYGTDTNSVCPKL                              588
```

Legends: a: SARS-CoV, b: SARS-CoV, and c: MERS-CoV

Fig. (6). Multiple sequencing alignments of the RBD of SARS-CoV-2, SARS-CoV, and MERS-CoV. Conserved amino acids between SARS-CoV-2, SARS-CoV, and MERS-CoV are represented by yellow, while the variable amino acids between SARS-CoV-2 and SARS-CoV are represented cyan. Periods represent low conserved residues; colons indicate highly conserved residues, and asterisks represent fully conserved residues. This figure is a modified version of a figure that was used in a previous study [91].

Wuhan combines several favorable elements for the worldwide spread and emergence of SARS-CoV-2. Being the largest city in central China (With 11 million populations), it is a central transport hub for industry and commerce. This is the land where two rivers (Yangtze and Han) intersect, and it also in-house Central China's largest train station, airport, and deep-sea port. Many passengers (around 30,000) fly daily from Wuhan to their destinations around the globe. An estimated >24.5 million travelers passed through the Wuhan city airport in 2018. In 2019, China's high-speed bullet trains also handled a huge number (around 2.31 billion) of travelers [95].

An analysis of the 2018 volumes of travelers moving from Wuhan International Airport between January and March showed that Hong Kong, Bangkok, Taipei, and Tokyo had received the biggest volume of travelers [95]. By January 28, 2020, outside of China, the largest confirmed number of 2019 nCoV cases was found in Hong Kong, Thailand, and Japan. All these countries have high Infectious Disease Vulnerability Index (IDVI) scores. IDIV is a validated tool to measure the capacity of any country to respond to outbreaks [96].

A simulation study conducted to assess the effectiveness of safe exit of travelers through the screening process, revealed that >60% of infected travelers would not be adequately detected using plausible assumptions based on the current situation [97]. The simulation was based on incomplete information data but utilized the best estimates available to date. Airports exit and entry screening could detect many infection cases, especially during long flights, because patients have the maximum chances of developing symptoms during this period. Scientists concluded that airport exit or entry screening using a thermal scanner is unlikely to detect a sufficient number of infected travelers to avoid entering new areas to prevent the new infection cases [97].

Travelers have a significant contribution to SARS-CoV-2 spread worldwide. Accurate diagnostic testing is still not available to those who need it. Hence, it is essential to focus on the most vulnerable places, and populations such as among the top 20 received the higher number of travelers from Wuhan, Bali, and Indonesia ranked lowest based on the IDVI score [98]. Accordingly, more support can be provided to countries with low IDVI, considering it a parameter to identify such support needing places [96]. Moreover, the commercial air traffic analysis could also help the cities, towns, and regions most likely to receive infected travelers [98].

CONCLUSION REMARKS

By looking at the global COVID-19 pandemic, it is reasonable to investigate these virus's possible evolutionary adaptations. It is essential to explore the mechanism through which this animal virus acquired the capability to infect humans. The information thus generated can be employed by the scientific community to devise a preventive strategy to inhibit such zoonotic transfer. The development of any strategy is critically valuable considering the high risk of its re-emergence due to the past pre-adaptation history in different animal species. If adaptation and zoonotic transfer of this virus occurred in humans, its ability to infect humans will not be lost eliminated without experiencing the chain of mutations. In the future, the analysis of its closest viral relative present in animals (RaTG13) will provide an insight into its infection mechanism as it helped scientists previously to detect the key RBD mutations and the acquisition of the polybasic cleavage site. The comparative analysis of SARS-CoV-2 with its closest relative also helped determine the possibility of its emergence through the recombination process; however, the conclusions are still conflicting.

Although the genomic features of SARS-CoV-2 described in the present study provided enough pieces of evidence to show that this is not a man-made virus. Like SARS-CoV-2, the presence of an optimized RBD and polybasic cleavage site in SARS and MERS is not possible, that any purposeful laboratory-based scenario of its emergence is plausible.

CONSENT FOR PUBLICATION

Not Applicable.

CONFLICT OF INTEREST

The author confirms that this chapter contents have no conflict of interest.

ACKNOWLEDGEMENT

Declared none.

REFERENCES

[1]   Fehr AR, Perlman S. Coronaviruses: an overview of their replication and pathogenesis. Methods Mol Biol 2015; 1282: 1-23.
[http://dx.doi.org/10.1007/978-1-4939-2438-7_1] [PMID: 25720466]

[2]   Malta M, Rimoin AW, Strathdee SA. The coronavirus 2019-nCoV epidemic: Is hindsight 20/20? EClinicalMedicine 2020; 20100289
[http://dx.doi.org/10.1016/j.eclinm.2020.100289] [PMID: 32154505]

[3]   Millet JK, Whittaker GR. Host cell proteases: Critical determinants of coronavirus tropism and pathogenesis. Virus Res 2015; 202: 120-34.
[http://dx.doi.org/10.1016/j.virusres.2014.11.021] [PMID: 25445340]

[4]   Belser JA. Assessment of SARS-CoV-2 replication in the context of other respiratory viruses. Lancet Respir Med 2020; 8(7): 651-2.
[http://dx.doi.org/10.1016/S2213-2600(20)30227-7] [PMID: 32386570]

[5]   Srivastava N, Baxi P, Ratho RK, Saxena SK. Global Trends in Epidemiology of Coronavirus Disease 2019 (COVID-19) Coronavirus Disease 2019 (COVID-19). Epidemiology, Pathogenesis, Diagnosis, and Therapeutics 2020; pp. 9-21.

[6]   Drosten C, Günther S, Preiser W, *et al.* Identification of a novel coronavirus in patients with severe acute respiratory syndrome. N Engl J Med 2003; 348(20): 1967-76.
[http://dx.doi.org/10.1056/NEJMoa030747] [PMID: 12690091]

[7]   Ksiazek TG, Erdman D, Goldsmith CS, *et al.* SARS Working Group. A novel coronavirus associated with severe acute respiratory syndrome. N Engl J Med 2003; 348(20): 1953-66.
[http://dx.doi.org/10.1056/NEJMoa030781] [PMID: 12690092]

[8]   Kahn JS, McIntosh K. History and recent advances in coronavirus discovery. Pediatr Infect Dis J

2005; 24(11) (Suppl.): S223-7.
[http://dx.doi.org/10.1097/01.inf.0000188166.17324.60] [PMID: 16378050]

[9]   Fehr AR, Perlman S. Coronaviruses: an overview of their replication and pathogenesis. Methods Mol Biol 2015; 2438-2437_2431.
[http://dx.doi.org/10.1007/978-1-4939-2438-7_1]

[10]   Paules CI, Marston HD, Fauci AS. Coronavirus infections-more than just the common cold. JAMA 2020; 323(8): 707-8.
[http://dx.doi.org/10.1001/jama.2020.0757] [PMID: 31971553]

[11]   Guan Y, Zheng BJ, He YQ, *et al.* Isolation and characterization of viruses related to the SARS coronavirus from animals in southern China. Science 2003; 302(5643): 276-8.
[http://dx.doi.org/10.1126/science.1087139] [PMID: 12958366]

[12]   Lau SK, Woo PC, Li KS, *et al.* Severe acute respiratory syndrome coronavirus-like virus in Chinese horseshoe bats. Proc Natl Acad Sci USA 2005; 102(39): 14040-5.
[http://dx.doi.org/10.1073/pnas.0506735102] [PMID: 16169905]

[13]   Kaplan RN, Riba RD, Zacharoulis S, *et al.* VEGFR1-positive haematopoietic bone marrow progenitors initiate the pre-metastatic niche. Nature 2005; 438(7069): 820-7.
[http://dx.doi.org/10.1038/nature04186] [PMID: 16341007]

[14]   Cui J, Li F, Shi ZL. Origin and evolution of pathogenic coronaviruses. Nat Rev Microbiol 2019; 17(3): 181-92.
[http://dx.doi.org/10.1038/s41579-018-0118-9] [PMID: 30531947]

[15]   Zaki AM, van Boheemen S, Bestebroer TM, Osterhaus AD, Fouchier RA. Isolation of a novel coronavirus from a man with pneumonia in Saudi Arabia. N Engl J Med 2012; 367(19): 1814-20.
[http://dx.doi.org/10.1056/NEJMoa1211721] [PMID: 23075143]

[16]   Hajjar SA, Memish ZA, McIntosh K. Middle East Respiratory Syndrome Coronavirus (MERS-CoV): a perpetual challenge. Ann Saudi Med 2013; 33(5): 427-36.
[http://dx.doi.org/10.5144/0256-4947.2013.427] [PMID: 24188935]

[17]   Ithete NL, Stoffberg S, Corman VM, *et al.* Close relative of human Middle East respiratory syndrome coronavirus in bat, South Africa. Emerg Infect Dis 2013; 19(10): 1697-9.
[http://dx.doi.org/10.3201/eid1910.130946] [PMID: 24050621]

[18]   Yi Y, Fang Y, Wu K, Liu Y, Zhang W. Comprehensive gene and pathway analysis of cervical cancer progression. Oncol Lett 2020; 19(4): 3316-32.
[http://dx.doi.org/10.3892/ol.2020.11439] [PMID: 32256826]

[19]   Liu SY, Song JC, Mao HD, Zhao JB, Song Q. Expert consensus on the diagnosis and treatment of heat stroke in China. Mil Med Res 2020; 7: 019-0229.
[http://dx.doi.org/10.1186/s40779-019-0229-2]

[20]   Chu H, Chan JF, Wang Y, *et al.* Comparative replication and immune activation profiles of SARS-CoV-2 and SARS-CoV in human lungs: an *ex vivo* study with implications for the pathogenesis of COVID-19. Clin Infect Dis 2020; 71(6): 1400-9.
[http://dx.doi.org/10.1093/cid/ciaa410] [PMID: 32270184]

[21]   Zhu N, Zhang D, Wang W, *et al.* China Novel Coronavirus Investigating and Research Team. A novel coronavirus from patients with pneumonia in China, 2019. N Engl J Med 2020; 382(8): 727-33.
[http://dx.doi.org/10.1056/NEJMoa2001017] [PMID: 31978945]

[22]   Zhai SL, Wei WK, Lv DH, *et al.* Where did SARS-CoV-2 come from? Vet Rec 2020; 186(8): 254.
[http://dx.doi.org/10.1136/vr.m740] [PMID: 32108071]

[23]   Rabi FA, Al Zoubi MS, Kasasbeh GA, Salameh DM, Al-Nasser AD. SARS-CoV-2 and coronavirus disease 2019: what we know so far. Pathogens 2020; 9(3): 231.
[http://dx.doi.org/10.3390/pathogens9030231] [PMID: 32245083]

[24]   Liu S-L, Saif LJ, Weiss SR, Su L. No credible evidence supporting claims of the laboratory engineering of SARS-CoV-2. Emerg Microbes Infect 2020; 9(1): 505-7.
[http://dx.doi.org/10.1080/22221751.2020.1733440] [PMID: 32102621]

[25]   Bulletin of the Atomic Sciences Experts know the new coronavirus is not a bioweapon They disagree on whether it could have leaked from a research lab 2020. Available from: https://thebulletin.org/2020/03/experts-know-the-new-coronavirus-i-
-not-a-bioweapon-they-disagree-on-whether-it-could-have-leaked-from-a-research-lab/

[26]   labroots. Conspiracy Theories Surrounding the Origins of SARS-CoV-2 2020. Available from: https://www.labroots.com/trending/genetics-and-genomics/17521/conspiracy-theor-
es-surrounding-origins-sars-cov-2

[27]   Zhou P, Yang X-L, Wang X-G, *et al.* A pneumonia outbreak associated with a new coronavirus of probable bat origin. Nature 2020; 579(7798): 270-3.
[http://dx.doi.org/10.1038/s41586-020-2012-7] [PMID: 32015507]

[28]   Andersen KG, Rambaut A, Lipkin WI, Holmes EC, Garry RF. The proximal origin of SARS-CoV-2. Nat Med 2020; 26(4): 450-2.
[http://dx.doi.org/10.1038/s41591-020-0820-9] [PMID: 32284615]

[29]   Pagano JK, Xie J, Erickson KA, *et al.* Actinide 2-metallabiphenylenes that satisfy Hückel's rule. Nature 2020; 578(7796): 563-7.
[http://dx.doi.org/10.1038/s41586-020-2004-7] [PMID: 32103196]

[30]   Lan J, Ge J, Yu J, *et al.* Structure of the SARS-CoV-2 spike receptor-binding domain bound to the ACE2 receptor. Nature 2020; 581(7807): 215-20.
[http://dx.doi.org/10.1038/s41586-020-2180-5] [PMID: 32225176]

[31]   Zhang T, Wu Q, Zhang Z. Pangolin homology associated with 2019-nCoV. bioRxiv 2020.

[32]   Sun J, He W-T, Wang L, *et al.* COVID-19: Epidemiology, evolution, and cross-disciplinary perspectives. Trends Mol Med 2020; 26(5): 483-95.
[http://dx.doi.org/10.1016/j.molmed.2020.02.008] [PMID: 32359479]

[33]   Yamada Y, Liu DX. Proteolytic activation of the spike protein at a novel RRRR/S motif is implicated in furin-dependent entry, syncytium formation, and infectivity of coronavirus infectious bronchitis virus in cultured cells. J Virol 2009; 83(17): 8744-58.
[http://dx.doi.org/10.1128/JVI.00613-09] [PMID: 19553314]

[34]   S Dr Priyanka, M Ranabir, c sourabrata, KS Amit, M Mahitosh, S Siddik. Mutations in spike protein of SARS-CoV-2 modulate receptor binding Membrane Fusion and Immunogenicity: An Insight into Viral Tropism and Pathogenesis of COVID-192020

[35]   Huang C, Wang Y, Li X, *et al.* Clinical features of patients infected with 2019 novel coronavirus in Wuhan, China. Lancet 2020; 395(10223): 497-506.
[http://dx.doi.org/10.1016/S0140-6736(20)30183-5] [PMID: 31986264]

[36]   Wang N, Li SY, Yang XL, *et al.* Serological evidence of bat SARS-related coronavirus infection in humans, china. Virol Sin 2018; 33(1): 104-7.
[http://dx.doi.org/10.1007/s12250-018-0012-7] [PMID: 29500691]

[37]   Ge X-Y, Li J-L, Yang X-L, *et al.* Isolation and characterization of a bat SARS-like coronavirus that uses the ACE2 receptor. Nature 2013; 503(7477): 535-8.
[http://dx.doi.org/10.1038/nature12711] [PMID: 24172901]

[38]   Wong MC, Javornik Cregeen SJ, Ajami NJ, Petrosino JF. Evidence of recombination in coronaviruses implicating pangolin origins of nCoV-2019. bioRxiv 2020.
[http://dx.doi.org/10.1101/2020.02.07.939207]

[39]   Sheahan T, Rockx B, Donaldson E, *et al.* Mechanisms of zoonotic severe acute respiratory syndrome coronavirus host range expansion in human airway epithelium. J Virol 2008; 82(5): 2274-85.

[http://dx.doi.org/10.1128/JVI.02041-07] [PMID: 18094188]

[40]   Ito T, Goto H, Yamamoto E, *et al.* Generation of a highly pathogenic avian influenza A virus from an avirulent field isolate by passaging in chickens. J Virol 2001; 75(9): 4439-43.
[http://dx.doi.org/10.1128/JVI.75.9.4439-4443.2001] [PMID: 11287597]

[41]   Li Q, Guan X, Wu P, *et al.* Early transmission dynamics in wuhan, china, of novel coronavirus-infected pneumonia. N Engl J Med 2020; 382(13): 1199-207.
[http://dx.doi.org/10.1056/NEJMoa2001316] [PMID: 31995857]

[42]   Li W, Zhang C, Sui J, *et al.* Receptor and viral determinants of SARS-coronavirus adaptation to human ACE2. EMBO J 2005; 24(8): 1634-43.
[http://dx.doi.org/10.1038/sj.emboj.7600640] [PMID: 15791205]

[43]   Xu X, Chen P, Wang J, *et al.* Evolution of the novel coronavirus from the ongoing Wuhan outbreak and modeling of its spike protein for risk of human transmission. Sci China Life Sci 2020; 63(3): 457-60.
[http://dx.doi.org/10.1007/s11427-020-1637-5] [PMID: 32009228]

[44]   Lan J, Ge J, Yu J, *et al.* Structure of the SARS-CoV-2 spike receptor-binding domain bound to the ACE2 receptor. Nature 2020; 581(7807): 215-20.
[http://dx.doi.org/10.1038/s41586-020-2180-5] [PMID: 32225176]

[45]   Walls AC, Park Y-J, Tortorici MA, Wall A, McGuire AT, Veesler D. Structure, Function, and Antigenicity of the SARS-CoV-2 Spike Glycoprotein. Cell 2020; 181(2): 281-292.e6.
[http://dx.doi.org/10.1016/j.cell.2020.02.058] [PMID: 32155444]

[46]   Mangar PP, Rai S, Lepcha S. Ranjan, VK, Rai, A. Comparative analysis based on the spike glycoproteins of SARS-CoV2 isolated from COVID 19 patients of different countries Preprints 2020.

[47]   Zhou P, Yang X-L, Wang X-G, Hu B, Zhang L, Zhang W, *et al.* Discovery of a novel coronavirus associated with the recent pneumonia outbreak in humans and its potential bat origin 2020.

[48]   Jaimes JA, André NM, Chappie JS, Millet JK, Whittaker GR. Phylogenetic analysis and structural modeling of SARS-CoV-2 spike protein reveals an evolutionary distinct and proteolytically sensitive activation loop. J Mol Biol 2020; 432(10): 3309-25.
[http://dx.doi.org/10.1016/j.jmb.2020.04.009] [PMID: 32320687]

[49]   virological.org. nCoV's relationship to bat coronaviruses & recombination signals (no snakes) - no evidence the 2019-nCoV lineage is recombinant 2020. Available from: http://virological.org/t/ncovs-relationship-to-bat-coronaviruses-recombination-signals-no-snakes-no-ev idence-the-2019-ncov-lineage -is-recombinant/331

[50]   Ji W, Wang W, Zhao X, Zai J, Li X. Homologous recombination within the spike glycoprotein of the newly identified coronavirus may boost cross species transmission from snake to human. J Med Virol 2020; 92.

[51]   Magiorkinis G, Magiorkinis E, Paraskevis D, *et al.* Phylogenetic analysis of the full-length SARS-CoV sequences: evidence for phylogenetic discordance in three genomic regions. J Med Virol 2004; 74(3): 369-72.
[http://dx.doi.org/10.1002/jmv.20187] [PMID: 15368527]

[52]   Paraskevis D, Kostaki EG, Magiorkinis G, Panayiotakopoulos G, Sourvinos G, Tsiodras S. Full-genome evolutionary analysis of the novel corona virus (2019-nCoV) rejects the hypothesis of emergence as a result of a recent recombination event. Infect Genet Evol 2020; 79: 104212-2.

[53]   Babcock GJ, Esshaki DJ, Thomas WD Jr, Ambrosino DM. Amino acids 270 to 510 of the severe acute respiratory syndrome coronavirus spike protein are required for interaction with receptor. J Virol 2004; 78(9): 4552-60.
[http://dx.doi.org/10.1128/JVI.78.9.4552-4560.2004] [PMID: 15078936]

[54]   Schoeman D, Fielding BC. Coronavirus envelope protein: current knowledge. Virol J 2019; 16: 19-1182.

[http://dx.doi.org/10.1186/s12985-019-1182-0]

[55]   Zhou P, Yang X, Wang X-G, Hu B, Zhang L, Zhang W, *et al.* A pneumonia outbreak associated with a new coronavirus of probable bat origin. Nature 2020; 579.
[http://dx.doi.org/10.1038/s41586-020-2012-7]

[56]   Zhao C, Zhang P, Zhou J, *et al.* Layered nanocomposites by shear-flow-induced alignment of nanosheets. Nature 2020; 580(7802): 210-5.
[http://dx.doi.org/10.1038/s41586-020-2161-8] [PMID: 32269352]

[57]   Imai Y, Meyer KJ, Iinishi A, Favre-Godal Q, Green R, Manuse S, *et al.* Author Correction: A new antibiotic selectively kills Gram-negative pathogens. Nature 2020; 580: 020-2063.
[http://dx.doi.org/10.1038/s41586-020-2063-9]

[58]   Wrapp D, Wang N, Corbett KS, *et al.* Cryo-EM structure of the 2019-nCoV spike in the prefusion conformation. Science 2020; 367(6483): 1260-3.
[http://dx.doi.org/10.1126/science.abb2507] [PMID: 32075877]

[59]   Letko M, Marzi A, Munster V. Functional assessment of cell entry and receptor usage for SARS-Co--2 and other lineage B betacoronaviruses. Nat Microbiol 2020; 5(4): 562-9.
[http://dx.doi.org/10.1038/s41564-020-0688-y] [PMID: 32094589]

[60]   Nao N, Yamagishi J, Miyamoto H, *et al.* Genetic predisposition to acquire a polybasic cleavage site for highly pathogenic avian influenza virus hemagglutinin. MBio 2017; 8(1): e02298-16.
[http://dx.doi.org/10.1128/mBio.02298-16] [PMID: 28196963]

[61]   Bagdonaite I, Wandall HH. Global aspects of viral glycosylation. Glycobiology 2018; 28(7): 443-67.
[http://dx.doi.org/10.1093/glycob/cwy021] [PMID: 29579213]

[62]   Follis KE, York J, Nunberg JH. Furin cleavage of the SARS coronavirus spike glycoprotein enhances cell-cell fusion but does not affect virion entry. Virology 2006; 350(2): 358-69.
[http://dx.doi.org/10.1016/j.virol.2006.02.003] [PMID: 16519916]

[63]   Menachery VD, Dinnon KH III, Yount BL Jr, *et al.* Trypsin treatment unlocks barrier for zoonotic bat coronavirus infection. J Virol 2020; 94(5): e01774-19.
[http://dx.doi.org/10.1128/JVI.01774-19] [PMID: 31801868]

[64]   Alexander DJ, Brown IH. History of highly pathogenic avian influenza. Rev Sci Tech 2009; 28(1): 19-38.
[http://dx.doi.org/10.20506/rst.28.1.1856] [PMID: 19618616]

[65]   Zhang H, Penninger JM, Li Y, Zhong N, Slutsky AS. Angiotensin-converting enzyme 2 (ACE2) as a SARS-CoV-2 receptor: molecular mechanisms and potential therapeutic target. Intensive Care Med 2020; 46(4): 586-90.
[http://dx.doi.org/10.1007/s00134-020-05985-9] [PMID: 32125455]

[66]   Kumar S, Nyodu R, Maurya VK, Saxena SK. Morphology, Genome Organization, Replication, and Pathogenesis of Severe Acute Respiratory Syndrome Coronavirus 2 (SARS-CoV-2) Coronavirus Disease 2019 (COVID-19). Springer 2020; pp. 23-31.

[67]   Mousavizadeh L, Ghasemi S. Genotype and phenotype of COVID-19: Their roles in pathogenesis. J Microbiol Immunol Infect 2020.
[http://dx.doi.org/10.1016/j.jmii.2020.03.022] [PMID: 32265180]

[68]   Zhang H, Penninger JM, Li Y, Zhong N, Slutsky AS. Angiotensin-converting enzyme 2 (ACE2) as a SARS-CoV-2 receptor: molecular mechanisms and potential therapeutic target. Intensive Care Med 2020; 46(4): 586-90.
[http://dx.doi.org/10.1007/s00134-020-05985-9] [PMID: 32125455]

[69]   Pal M, Berhanu G, Desalegn C, Kandi V. Severe acute respiratory syndrome coronavirus-2 (SARS-CoV-2): an update. Cureus 2020; 12(3): e7423-3.
[http://dx.doi.org/10.7759/cureus.7423] [PMID: 32337143]

[70]   Gorbalenya AE, Baker SC, Baric RS, de Groot RJ, Drosten C, Gulyaeva AA, *et al.* Coronaviridae Study Group of the International Committee on Taxonomy of Viruses. The species Severe acute respiratory syndrome-related coronavirus: classifying 2019-nCoV and naming it SARS-CoV-2. Nat Microbiol 2020; 5(4): 536-44.
[http://dx.doi.org/10.1038/s41564-020-0695-z] [PMID: 32123347]

[71]   Snijder EJ, Bredenbeek PJ, Dobbe JC, *et al.* Unique and conserved features of genome and proteome of SARS-coronavirus, an early split-off from the coronavirus group 2 lineage. J Mol Biol 2003; 331(5): 991-1004.
[http://dx.doi.org/10.1016/S0022-2836(03)00865-9] [PMID: 12927536]

[72]   van Boheemen S, de Graaf M, Lauber C, *et al.* Genomic characterization of a newly discovered coronavirus associated with acute respiratory distress syndrome in humans. MBio 2012; 3(6): 3.
[http://dx.doi.org/10.1128/mBio.00473-12] [PMID: 23170002]

[73]   Siddell SG, Walker PJ. Additional changes to taxonomy ratified in a special vote by the International Committee on Taxonomy of Viruses 2019; 164(October 2018): 943-6.

[74]   Li X, Zai J, Zhao Q, *et al.* Evolutionary history, potential intermediate animal host, and cross-species analyses of SARS-CoV-2. J Med Virol 2020; 92(6): 602-11.
[http://dx.doi.org/10.1002/jmv.25731] [PMID: 32104911]

[75]   Zhou P, Yang X-L, Wang X-G, Hu B, Zhang L, Zhang W, *et al.* Discovery of a novel coronavirus associated with the recent pneumonia outbreak in humans and its potential bat origin. bioRxiv 2022.

[76]   Black S. The jury is still out for SARS-CoV-2 intermediate host. The Science Advisory Board staff writer 2020.

[77]   Tang X, Wu C, Li X, Song Y, Yao X, Wu X, *et al.* On the origin and continuing evolution of SARS-CoV-2. Natl Sci Rev 2020.
[http://dx.doi.org/10.1093/nsr/nwaa036]

[78]   Lu R, Zhao X, Li J, *et al.* Genomic characterisation and epidemiology of 2019 novel coronavirus: implications for virus origins and receptor binding. Lancet 2020; 395(10224): 565-74.
[http://dx.doi.org/10.1016/S0140-6736(20)30251-8] [PMID: 32007145]

[79]   Zhu N, Zhang D, Wang W, *et al.* China Novel Coronavirus Investigating and Research Team. A novel coronavirus from patients with pneumonia in china, 2019. N Engl J Med 2020; 382(8): 727-33.
[http://dx.doi.org/10.1056/NEJMoa2001017] [PMID: 31978945]

[80]   Saitou N, Nei M. The neighbor-joining method: a new method for reconstructing phylogenetic trees. Mol Biol Evol 1987; 4(4): 406-25.
[PMID: 3447015]

[81]   Tamura K, Nei M, Kumar S. Prospects for inferring very large phylogenies by using the neighbor-joining method. Proc Natl Acad Sci USA 2004; 101(30): 11030-5.
[http://dx.doi.org/10.1073/pnas.0404206101] [PMID: 15258291]

[82]   Kumar S, Stecher G, Li M, Knyaz C, Tamura K. MEGA X: Molecular evolutionary genetics analysis across computing platforms. Mol Biol Evol 2018; 35(6): 1547-9.
[http://dx.doi.org/10.1093/molbev/msy096] [PMID: 29722887]

[83]   Xu J, Zhao S, Teng T, *et al.* Systematic comparison of two animal-to-human transmitted human coronaviruses: SARS-CoV-2 and SARS-CoV. Viruses 2020; 12(2): 244.
[http://dx.doi.org/10.3390/v12020244] [PMID: 32098422]

[84]   Chan JF, Kok KH. Genomic characterization of the 2019 novel human-pathogenic coronavirus isolated from a patient with atypical pneumonia after visiting Wuhan 2020.
[http://dx.doi.org/10.1080/22221751.2020.1719902]

[85]   Hu B, Zeng L-P, Yang X-L, *et al.* Discovery of a rich gene pool of bat SARS-related coronaviruses provides new insights into the origin of SARS coronavirus. PLoS Pathog 2017; 13(11)e1006698

[http://dx.doi.org/10.1371/journal.ppat.1006698] [PMID: 29190287]

[86]   Hoffmann M, Kleine-Weber H, Schroeder S, *et al.* SARS-CoV-2 cell entry depends on ACE2 and TMPRSS2 and is blocked by a clinically proven protease inhibitor. Cell 2020; 181(2): 271-280.e8.
[http://dx.doi.org/10.1016/j.cell.2020.02.052] [PMID: 32142651]

[87]   Shang J, Ye G, Shi K, *et al.* Structural basis of receptor recognition by SARS-CoV-2. Nature 2020; 581(7807): 221-4.
[http://dx.doi.org/10.1038/s41586-020-2179-y] [PMID: 32225175]

[88]   de Haan CA, Haijema BJ, Schellen P, *et al.* Cleavage of group 1 coronavirus spike proteins: how furin cleavage is traded off against heparan sulfate binding upon cell culture adaptation. J Virol 2008; 82(12): 6078-83.
[http://dx.doi.org/10.1128/JVI.00074-08] [PMID: 18400867]

[89]   Rehman SU, Shafique L, Ihsan A, Liu Q. Evolutionary trajectory for the emergence of novel coronavirus SARS-CoV-2. Pathogens 2020; 9(3): 240.
[http://dx.doi.org/10.3390/pathogens9030240] [PMID: 32210130]

[90]   Cui J, Li F, Shi Z-L. Origin and evolution of pathogenic coronaviruses. Nat Rev Microbiol 2019; 17(3): 181-92.
[http://dx.doi.org/10.1038/s41579-018-0118-9] [PMID: 30531947]

[91]   Tai W, He L, Zhang X, *et al.* Characterization of the receptor-binding domain (RBD) of 2019 novel coronavirus: implication for development of RBD protein as a viral attachment inhibitor and vaccine. Cell Mol Immunol 2020; 17(6): 613-20.
[http://dx.doi.org/10.1038/s41423-020-0400-4] [PMID: 32203189]

[92]   Cho SY, Kang J-M, Ha YE, *et al.* MERS-CoV outbreak following a single patient exposure in an emergency room in South Korea: an epidemiological outbreak study. Lancet 2016; 388(10048): 994-1001.
[http://dx.doi.org/10.1016/S0140-6736(16)30623-7] [PMID: 27402381]

[93]   Paules CI, Marston HD, Fauci AS. Coronavirus infections—more than just the common cold. JAMA 2020; 323(8): 707-8.
[http://dx.doi.org/10.1001/jama.2020.0757] [PMID: 31971553]

[94]   Yuen K-S, Ye Z-W, Fung S-Y, Chan C-P, Jin D-Y. SARS-CoV-2 and COVID-19: The most important research questions. Cell Biosci 2020; 10: 40.
[http://dx.doi.org/10.1186/s13578-020-00404-4] [PMID: 32190290]

[95]   Hoehl S, Rabenau H, Berger A, *et al.* Evidence of SARS-CoV-2 infection in returning travelers from Wuhan, China. N Engl J Med 2020; 382(13): 1278-80.
[http://dx.doi.org/10.1056/NEJMc2001899] [PMID: 32069388]

[96]   Moore M, Gelfeld B, Okunogbe A, Paul C. Identifying future disease hot spots: infectious disease vulnerability index. Rand Health Q 2017; 6(3): 5.
[PMID: 28845357]

[97]   Wilson ME, Chen LH. Travellers give wings to novel coronavirus (2019-nCoV). Oxford University Press 2020.
[http://dx.doi.org/10.1093/jtm/taaa015]

[98]   Bogoch II, Watts A, Thomas-Bachli A, Huber C, Kraemer MU, Khan K. Potential for global spread of a novel coronavirus from China. J of travel med 2020; 27: 0-11.

CHAPTER 3

Evaluating SARS-CoV-2 Entry Pathways SARS-CoV-2 Entry Pathways

Muhammad Kalim[1,*], Firasat Hussain[2,*], Hayat Khan[3], Kashif Rahim[2], Muhammad Shuaib[4], Amjad Islam Aqib[5] and Jinbiao Zhan[1]

[1] Department of Biochemistry, and Cancer Institute of the Second Affiliated Hospital, Zhejiang University, School of Medicine, Hangzhou 310058, China

[2] Department of Microbiology, Cholistan University of Veterinary & Animal Sciences, Bahawalpur-63100, Pakistan

[3] Department of Microbiology, University of Swabi, Khyber Pakhtunkhwa 23561, Pakistan

[4] School of Ecology and Environmental Science, Yunnan University, Kunming, China

[5] Department of Medicine Cholistan University of Veterinary and Animal Sciences Bahawalpur-63100, Pakistan

Abstract: Coronaviruses (CoVs) are members of the *Coronaviridae* family that possess positive-sense RNA. These are enveloped viruses causing severe acute respiratory syndrome (SARS), the Middle East respiratory syndrome (MERS), and currently coronavirus disease-19 (COVID-19) in humans. Still, there is less information available about the biology of Severe Acute Respiratory Syndrome-Coronavirus-2 (SARS-CoV-2). Recently, it was suggested that endocytosis mechanism studies and autophagy implicate importance in the viral entrance and an infection. These suggestions ascertain that endocytosis and intracellular trafficking studies have become essential target sites for developing therapeutic approaches. Initially, it was thought that coronaviruses possibly enter the host cell through direct diffusion, evading the membrane barriers. Laterally, it was found that the virus may enter the cell through the mechanism of endocytosis. Entry pathways and endocytosis of other viruses and especially SARS-CoV discussed here may expand the cellular range of viral endocytosis studies, pathogenesis, and infection. It may provide new information for pharmacokinetic studies and vaccine development. This chapter discussed some current advances in our understanding of cellular pathways of SARS-CoV-2 attachment, molecular signaling during virus entry, and trafficking mechanism studies.

Keywords: Coronaviruses, COVID-19, Clathrin, Endocytosis, SARS-CoV.

* Corresponding authors Firasat Hussain and Muhammad Kalim: Department of Microbiology, Cholistan University of Veterinary & Animal Sciences, Bahawalpur 63100, Pakistan. E-mail:firasathussain@cuvas.edu.pk and Department of Biochemistry, and Cancer Institute of the Second Affiliated Hospital, Zhejiang University, School of Medicine, Hangzhou 310058, China, E-mail:kalimutman@yahoo.com

Kamal Niaz & Muhammad Farrukh Nisar (Eds.)

INTRODUCTION

Coronavirus has startled people in the entire world after the complete lockdown started in Wuhan city in China on February 23, 2020, which posed the leading public health issue and governance challenge worldwide. Previously, it was named 2019-nCoV-2 (2019-novel coronavirus type 2), and at present, it was called SARS-CoV-2 (Severe Acute Respiratory Syndrome Coronavirus-2). The coronavirus (CoVs) has its place in the *Coronaviridae* family, which possesses 26-32 kb extraordinary large ssRNA genome [1]. CoVs are enveloped viruses found in avian hosts and several mammals like bats, camels, dogs, and masked palm civets. After the entry of SARS-CoV-2, individuals having weak immune systems are more prone to disease [2 - 4]. The coronavirus family is consequently titled to looks like crown-shaped projections arranged on the membrane surface under the microscope. COVID-19 is a member of *Betacoronaviruses* that also comprises the previously reported SARS and MERS human CoVs. Seven different strains of human CoVs (HCoVs) and this novel COVID-19 strain were reported so far. These strains are named *Alpha corona viruses* that include 229E and NL63 strains and *Betacoronaviruses* that comprise of HKU1, OC43, SARS, MERS, and COVID-19 HCoVs [5, 6]. The schematic diagram of the coronavirus is shown in Fig. (**1**).

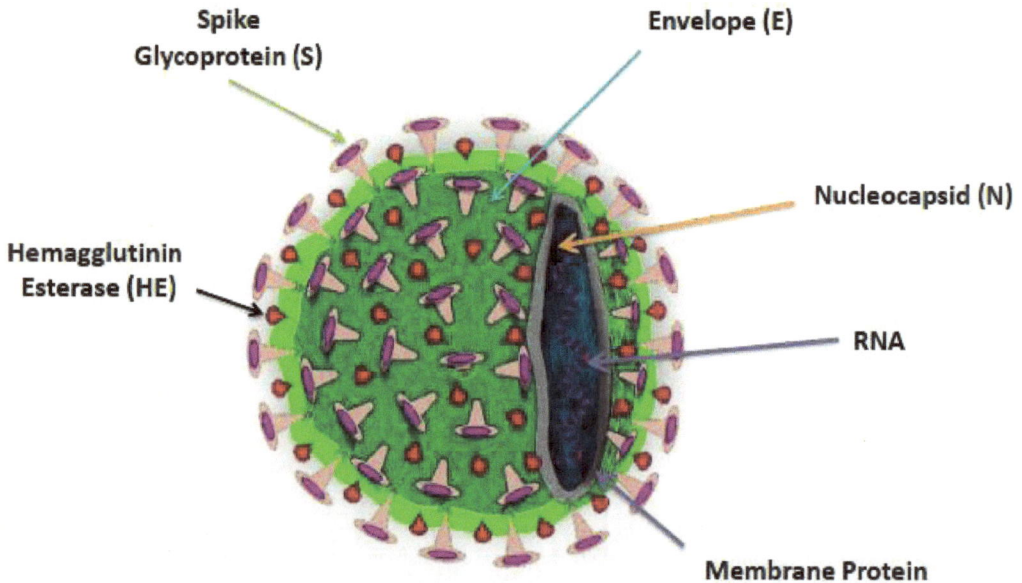

Fig. (1). Schematic representation of coronavirus structure.

Currently, vaccine development is underway, and researchers are developing potent therapeutic drugs and vaccines for COVID-19 to reduce the threat. Various international organizations, industrial researchers, and academic research groups are working on vaccine development. Former works to utilize angiotensin-converting-enzyme-2 (ACE2) binding receptor for vaccine development as it represents potent attachment site for endocytosis reported previously for SARS-CoV-2 and SARS CoV. Researchers investigated three different vaccination strategies. The first aim was to develop a whole virus vaccine. The whole vaccine provokes a quick and sharp immune response to the newly developed COVID-19 infection. Secondly, to develop a subunit vaccine to sensitize the immune system to certain viral subunits as reported S-spike proteins in SARS-CoV-2. The S-spike protein helps in the attachment and endocytosis of the virus. The third strategy was to developed nucleic acid, DNA, or RNA vaccines [7, 8].

The first COVID-19 clinical trial of vaccine development was started on March 16, 2020, in Seattle that included four volunteers. Several clinical trials evaluated different repurposing antiviral agents such as corticosteroid, vasodilators, bevacizumab, lipoic acid, and recombinant ACE2 development against SARS-CoV-2 before April 2020. Current antiviral medications such as chloroquine, hydroxychloroquine, Remdesivir, Ritonavir, and Lopinavir are being assessed to treat COVID-19 infection. It was found that spike protein arrangement initially is membrane protease plays an essential role in SARS-CoV-2 entry through binding with the ACE2 receptor molecule. These outcomes intend that the spike protein inhibitions by antibodies can halt the viral entry and further multiplications in the host environment. The spike proteins are considered intensely by scientists to develop potent SARS-CoV-2 vaccines. The possible entry of the virus to human cells through spike proteins helps in viral replication and pathogenesis. The complete topology of spike proteins comprised of the extracellular domain, transmembrane, and intracellular domain and their amino acid positions are shown in Fig.(2).

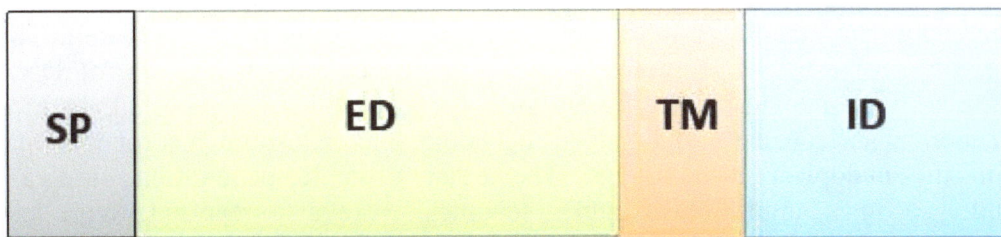

Fig. (2). Complete topology of spike protein presents the position of amino acids. Entry ID: (P59594). SP: Signal Peptides (1-13); ED: Extracellular Domain (14-1195); TM: Trans-membrane (1196-1216); ID: Intracellular Domain (1217-1255).

The spike glycoproteins (14-1255) comprise three sub-regions that play an essential role in attachment, fusion, and endocytosis. These are spike proteins S1 possess amino acid sequence alignment from 14 to 667, which helps in the attachment of virion to the membrane surface by interconnecting with the receptor molecule. The S2 subunit protein acting as a class I fusion protein ranges from 668 to 1255 amino acid sequences that help the fusion of the virion and membranes. The third sub-region S2' comprised 798 to 1255 amino acid sequences that play a vital role in S2 cleavage occurring upon endocytosis of virus (Fig. **3**).

S1 (14-667)

SDLDRCTTFDDVQAP.............AGICASYHTVSLLR

S2 (668-1255)

STSQKSIVAYTMLSGAD.............SEPVLKGVKLHYT

S2' (798-1255)

SFIEDLLFNKVTLA.............SEPVLKGVKLHYT

Fig. (3). Amino acid sequence analysis of spike protein.

Previously, it was discussed that spike protein plays an essential role in eliciting an immune response. The major achievement of the virus endocytosis mechanism is to carry its genomic DNA/RNA from an infected cell to the healthy one. Most viruses consume the endocytosis approach to enter the cell cytoplasm and lead to the endocytic vacuole or other inner cell compartments of the host cell. The uncoating of RNA viruses mostly occurs in the cytoplasm and that of DNA viruses in the nucleus. Six different sites for virus diffusion reported, such as membrane surface, early and mature endosome, late endosome, macropinosome, and the endoplasmic reticulum. The other possible penetration sites are endolysosomes, amphisomes, and lysosomes, were also reported. With less evidence, other viruses can consume additional pathways by engaging different receptor sites. The study focuses on attachment and endocytosis of SARS-CoV-2 and the molecular mechanism of intracellular trafficking studies.

Virus Attachment

The specificity of viral attachment and infection depends on the structural composition and receptor molecules on the membrane surface of the host cell that allows viral particles to enter inside. The specificity and choice of receptors contribute to endocytosis and eventually to disease development. Most probably, the enveloped viruses as COVID-19 attach through spike glycoprotein molecules, whereas the non-enveloped viruses utilize the fusion strategies, spike proteins, fibers, and surface depressions for their attachment and entrance. Generally, the cellular receptor molecules for virus attachment are highly comprehensive, extending from proteoglycans to glycoproteins and lipids [9]. These molecules assist simply for binding and absorption of viruses to the cell surface, whereas others have additional roles in signal stimulation, endocytosis, and the alteration of the bound virus. Most viruses utilize carbohydrates to enter into cells. The transferrin and LDL receptors utilize well-known binding receptors. Proteins in body fluids, antibodies, and complement factors also play bridging functions between the virus and binding receptors [10]. Essentially, virus interfaces with receptors can result in modifications in viral protein structures partially or in the whole virus particles.

Recently, a new class of attachment partners was found that mainly required stimulating the signaling pathways to assist the entry of viruses. These were called accessory factors. The accessory factors include tyrosine kinases, phosphatidyl-serine receptors (TAM and TIM), and integrins receptors [11 - 13]. A solution protein can mediate these interactions, Gas6 that interacts with phosphatidyl-serine receptors in the virus surface and tyrosine kinases, Axl, during viral uptake activation by using Macropinocytosis. Viruses often utilize more than one type of receptors, either similar, in the arrangement or interrelating with other cells. HCV, coxsackie B virus, HIV-1, and rotavirus are few examples of viruses that interact sequentially with diverse surface receptor molecules [14]. It was reported that herpes viruses might carry multiple receptor binding glycoproteins with different specificity and therefore can enter into different cell types [15]. It is predictable that the available studies are confusing and untrustworthy to elaborate the endocytosis of many viruses, including COVID-19, due to the fundamental complexity and severity of virus binding to the host cell. It is worth noticing that receptor molecules might be escorted by an additional co-receptor that stimulates a defined entry pathway or steadies the viral particles at the cell membrane surface. In addition to direct fusion with the membrane, it was also reported that the SARS-CoV could assume the endocytic routes that lead to the viral nucleotide multiplications and expressions. The entrance can increase the cellular assortment of SARS-CoV in ACE2 negative colonic enterocytes and live tissues. It doesn't involve as macropinocytosis-dependent entrance particular binding receptor molecules [16]. Studies revealed that SARS-CoV entry might also implicate receptor-mediated clathrin/caveolin dependent endocytosis, clathrin/caveolin-independent endocytosis. It also involve a pathway containing lipid rafts mechanism as shown in Fig. (**4**).

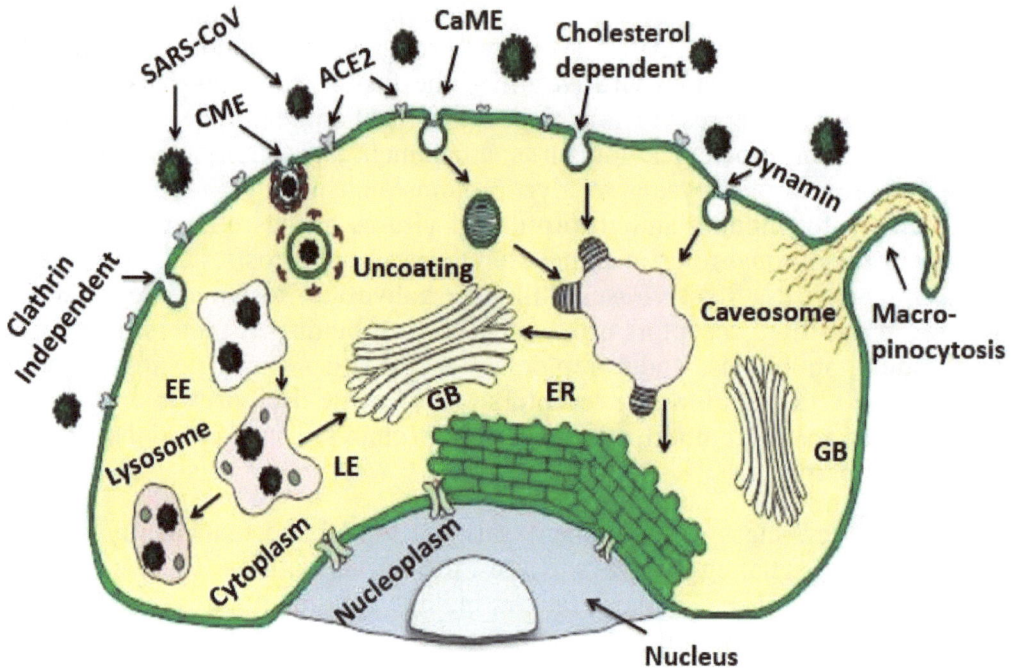

Fig. (4).   Endocytosis of viruses. Viruses are internalized through various endocytic mechanisms after attachment to the cell surface. These mechanisms of endocytosis mostly occur in five different locations as CME (Clathrin Mediated Endocytosis), CaME (Caveolin mediated endocytosis), clathrin independent mechanism, Cholesterol dependent, and dynamin-dependent. CME that carries viruses to EE (Early endosome), LE (Late endosome), and finally to lysosome. CaME, mostly related to the cholesterol-dependent mechanism in function, triggers viruses like Coxsackie B, SV40, Echo 1, and mouse polyomaviruses to Cavesome. Many viruses in further steps move to GB (Golgi bodies) and ER (Endoplasmic reticulum) while in the early step towards EE. Clathrin-independent pathways exist for arenaviruses and influenza viruses. The dynamin-dependent pathway is used by Echovirus 1 for the endocytosis mechanism. Similarly, the adenoviruses utilize the macropinocytosis mechanism of entry. SARS-CoV (Severe acute respiratory syndrome coronavirus) binds with ACE2 receptor proteins to enter the cell.

Membrane Fusion and SARS-CoV-2 Induced Signaling

Viruses essentially come in two different types *i.e.,* envelop viruses that carry lipid envelopes decorated with viral proteins and spikes as designed in COVID-19, and without lipid envelop naked viruses. The envelop viruses developed well-organized penetration machinery to enter the viral particle into cell cytosol through membrane fusion. The endocytosis mechanism is often triggered by low pH environment ranging (5.0-6.0) in the endocytic vesicles during late endosome formation [17]. Similarly, the HIV and herpes simplex virus acquire neutral pH to fuse there. Moreover, the structural changes of surface protein result in previously concealed amino acid residues (amphipathic/hydrophobic of fusion peptide molecules). During protein maturation, the metastable state is often achieved that elicits membrane arrangement potency for the entry of viruses in a low pH environment. The changes result in close contact of the viral and cellular membrane, finally provokes complete fusion of membrane surfaces. These contacts also result in mixing of lipids and ultimately delivering the viral nucleocapsid into the cell cytosol.

The viral fusion with the membrane is relatively well understood, but the endocytosis of naked viruses still needs to explore. Mostly, endocytosis might occur through the disruption of the virus-carrying vesicles or pores in the endosomal chamber. These openings are lined by virus proteins that make a network connecting through a gap in the viral layer. Low pH helps in the switching of the capsid holes most prominently [18].

The precise endocytosis pathways of virus that mostly depends on the physiognomies of the virus and the host. The actin barrier in the plasma membrane does not have contended endocytosis and can depend on endosome environmental acidic pH to pledge the fusion and penetration reactions [19]. The endocytosis also depends on the shape and size of the virus. The larger size usually utilizes actin-dependent phagocytosis, and long tubules like viruses utilize macropinocytosisas found in mimivirus, and *Ebola virus,* respectively [20].

The entry of SARS-CoV into cells was initially recognized by direct fusion with the plasma membrane. Latterly, it was found that it may depend on pH and protease cathepsin L of the endosome [21 - 23]. The binding receptor ACE2 was recognized as a prominent receptor molecule for CoVs in humans and bats, additionally for SARS-CoV-2 [24]. On the other hand, the virus can infect different target cells by binding with ACE2 receptors or integrin to access the host cells.

Endocytosis of SARS-CoV-2

Endocytosis involves the budding off of cellular vesicles from the cell membrane and releases its contents into the ' 'cell's cytosol modulating several essential cellular functions of the cell. These functions comprised internalization of extracellular load, receptor regulations on the membrane surface, lipid control on the surface membrane and inside compartments, cell to cell signaling, and chemical neurotransmission channel functions [25 - 27]. The above discussed essential functions of endocytosis demonstrate its application widely in drug delivery and endocytosis of viral particles. Various forms of endocytosis, including clathrin-mediated endocytosis (CME), caveolin mediated endocytosis (CaME), macropinocytosis, and phagocytosis, present vital routes in cellular transport [28].

CME represents the prominent route in endocytosis constitutes a large proportion of endocytic events. It involves the assembly of coated pits that induces well-defined vesicles of 50 nm that internalize up to 200 nm particles in size. Various CoVs, including SARS and MERS and murine hepatitis virus (MHV) constantly revealed the contribution of the endocytic pathway for viral entry and infection into numerous types of cells. Amongst them, clathrin-mediated and cathepsin-mediated S protein cleavage is found two vital steps for the entry of viruses and infections. The appliance is similarly appropriate to numerous other CoVs like IBV [29]. The CaME originates from small lipid rafts of 50 nm in size blebs. The penetration usually involves the fusion as reported in COVID-19 enveloped virus, whereas the non-enveloped viruses involved pore formation or membrane break. It was also reported that enveloped viruses such as the Sendai virus, HSV-1, and retroviruses could penetrate directly into the cell due to pH-independent fusion protein. These viruses do not require low pH for endocytosis. Most probably, the few RNA viruses also replicate inside the cytosol when getting through specific organelles [30]. The DNA viruses and their capsids, except for poxviruses and iridoviruses, subsequently get into the nucleus for replication.

The cell entry mechanism is an important step of viral transmission, especially for the Betacoronaviruses. It was reported that all CoVs represent surface glycoproteins or spikes that attach with the receptors on host cells mediating the endocytosis mechanism studies [31]. The single spike region called receptor-binding domain (RBD) facilitates the interface with the host cell receptors converting RBD with spike fusion peptide by nearby host proteases [32 - 34]. ACE2 was reported well-known host receptor for SARS-CoV and dipeptidyl peptidase-4 (DPP-4) for MERS-CoV [35, 36]. The studies revealed that spike RBD is proficient in independent folding in spike proteins that hold all the structural evidence for the virus-host receptors attachment. Previously, it was found that substituting RBD of lineage B bat virus, Rp3 permitted the virus to enter the ACE2 positive cells [8]. As discussed before, initially, it was reported that the entry of SARS-CoV into cells was a direct fusion of viruses at the membrane surface. Later, it was revealed that SARS-CoV enters the cell *via* a pH-dependent manner utilizing endosomal cathepsin L involvement in endocytosis. One study showed that SARS-CoV could enter the cells through receptor-mediated and pH-sensitive endocytosis. Also, the specific routes of entry are clathrin and caveolin independent pathway where lipid raft performs an essential function in endocytosis [37].

Clathrin-Mediated Endocytosis

CME typically originates with the formation of clathrin-coated pits that occupy 2% of the total membrane. Its lifetime is short and formed in a minute, invaginates inward, and form coated vesicles. It was found that about 2500 vesicles leave the membrane in a minute of cultured fibroblast. The coated vesicles can shed their coverings followed by fusion with early endosomes. Any foreign substance dissolved in the fluid is internalized or recycled back to the surface and this process of endocytosis is called fluid-phase endocytosis. Moreover, the scaffolding proteins clathrin, additional significant elements involved in CME comprised epsin, ampiphisin, Eps15, dynamin, adaptor protein 2 (AP2), actin, and PIP2 (Phospholipid phosphatidylinositol 4, 5- bisphosphate) [38, 39]. These factors make a composite on the plasma membrane inner sides to originate depths at endocytosis sites. The most prominent factor in localizing the internalization sites is PIP2 which marks less than 1% of all lipids. PIP2 makes a connection with various membrane proteins. CME is comprised of different steps. These are the formation of clathrin coated pits (CCP), capturing cargo in coated pits, induction of membrane invagination, and un-coating and breaking vesicles [40]. All these processes occur in a concise time *in vivo*. At the same time, the blueprint of endocytosis has been recognized. The major factors are being identified biophysical comprehension into the energetics of making and supporting high membrane curvature leftovers mainly mysterious. It was recently reported that SARS-CoV might utilize the CME in hepatocellular carcinoma cell lines HepG2 and COS7 [41]. CME is a significant and primary receptor-mediated source of entry. Previously, the live tissues showed less abundance or mimicked the expression of ACE2 proteins [16]. The entry mechanism found in MHV was also clathrin-dependent same as HCoV-NL63 which are transported to the lysosome to fuse [42, 43].

Clathrin Coated Pits (CCP) Formation

It has been found that the development of CCP requires proteins complex that comprised Eps15, FCHo1/2, and intersectin 1 [44]. The coat assembly initiation occurs by employing AP-2 proteins to the surface membrane through the FCHo complex by Eps15 factors. The PIP2 concentrations must be highly measured through the endocytosis process. The conversion of PIP3 to PIP2 and PIP occurs due to phosphoinositide phosphatase and synaptojanin, which is recruited by endophilin during endocytosis. Endophillin regulates the level of PIP [45]. The curvature is also mediated by PIP2 that coordinates with Epsin N- terminal homology (ENTH) and Bin amphiphysin Rvs homology (BAR) membrane domains. The role of Eps15 and Epsin in curvature generation and curvature recruitment in the nascent coat is still unclear. The Epsin15 coordinates with lipid

PIP2 and induces the curve in the membrane through lipid area asymmetry. Both epsin and Eps15 have similar functions. These have AP-2 binding domains that can connect multiple AP-2 molecules. The AP-2 adaptor protein, along with AP180 molecules, gathers the clathrin matrix, a triskelion scaffolding protein that possesses three-branch chains to attach with AP-2 and other clathrin molecules. AP-2 helps recruit clathrin that can further polymerize to form a basket-like framework on the membrane surface [46].

Cargo Capturing in Coated Pits

The functional activity of adaptin-associated kinase-1 (AAK1) is subsequently increased by the generation of the clathrin lattice structure. It phosphorylates AP-2 further to make enormous conformational changes. These changes create high-affinity attachment sites for transmembrane cargo and PIP2 [47]. The cargo binding occurs with AP-2 directly *via* the binding domain or indirectly *via* specific adaptor proteins forming cargo AP-2 complex that initiates PIPK1 activation. The reaction elevates PIP2 membrane activation, extending the clathrin coat in cargo availability [48, 49]. It was also reported that the CCP and cargo size could be compared due to the activation of PIPK1. If there is no availability of cargo, the CCP can be terminated at a critical coat size. This is due to the twisting firmness of the membrane that resists further developing the coat size to stabilize the membrane deformation [50].

Induction of Membrane Invagination and Clathrin Coat Growth

Epsin and activated AAK1 recruited more AP-2 to the developing coat during polymerization of clathrin that spreads the coat along the membrane. The association also disrupts the AP-2 attachment sites for Eps15 and epsin that push these proteins to the periphery slowing more AP-2 proteins near the coat. It was also reported that the growth of CCP and membrane invagination increases in CME [51]. It was also reported that curvature development is mediated by the clathrin coat itself, along with a combination of amphiphysin and epsin [52, 53]. The epsin induces more substantial curvature in the bilayer by introducing the N-terminal amphipathic helix. The developing clathrin designs the curvature and polymerizes to form a curved basket shape structure. Thus clathrin is supposed to play a more crucial role in endocytosis that stabilizes the reaction. A tubular neck region is formed after emerging from the membrane surface that is left uncovered by clathrin coat comprises excessive amounts of PIP2. Finally, the sensing domain of N-BAR recruits the endophilin and amphiphysin membrane proteins to the vesicle neck [54].

Uncoating of Vesicles

Dynamin recruitment to the neck of budding vesicles occurs due to amphiphysin that polymerizes in GTP dependent manner [55]. The dynamin collar pinching and PIP2 concentration result in the vesicle session from the cell membrane. Once, vesicle becomes free from the membrane, and the Rab5 is recruited by coated vesicles that dislocate both AP-2 and PIP2 binding [56]. The uncoating of AP-2 and PIP2 results in endosomal sorting or degradation of vesicles that depend on accessory and adaptor proteins found on the surface of vesicles [57]. It was found that viruses and capsids find their way after reached the cytosol towards the nucleus and/or to the particular site in the cytoplasm. Mostly, dynein and dynactin, microtubule-based motors play a vital role and moves along microtubules to the nucleus [58 - 60].

Viruses with large capsids, such as adenoviruses and herpes viruses, have developed mechanisms to release their genetic materials to the nucleus through nuclear pores. Small virus capsids, such as polyomaviruses and HBV, can enter the genetic material directly or through a modified manner into the nucleus by using nuclear pores [61 - 63]. Similarly, the influenza viruses divide their genome into eight different fragments due to excessive large size to pass through the nuclear pore. These fragments are assembled separately into viral ribonucleoproteins (vRNPs) that are small enough to overcome nuclear membrane barriers. Each individual possesses the nuclear localization signals necessary for importin-a and importin-b mediated nuclear transport [64, 65].

Viruses eventually discharge their genomic DNA/RNA into the cytosol to allow the endocytosis, transcription, and replication program. Uncoating of viruses is usually a stepwise procedure that involves different phases of entry. Sometimes it occurs before penetration into the cytosol, as in polyoma and adenoviruses. At the same time, in other cases, it penetrates the viral genome into the cytosol leaving behind the capsid as in picornaviruses [66, 67]. Some viruses use their enzymatic activity to enter the host cells, while others consume host-cell dynamics like ribosomes, proteasomes, and molecular motors [68]. Dynein, kinesin, and nucleoporins help in unwinding the capsid in adenoviruses to release the genetic materials. In HIV1, the uncoating is determined by the host factors due to the constancy of the capsid molecule and reverse transcription of viral RNA into DNA. The factors involved in uncoating are cyclophilin A and TRIM5a and are also stimulated through TNPO3 nuclear import receptors [62, 69, 70].

The entrance of CoVs can take place after encountering viral spike glycoprotein (S) with surface receptors that initiate the endocytosis of viruses. These viruses are carried in cargo through specific transport routes to the membrane fusion sites

[71]. Different CoVs possess various fusion sites as the site found in MERS-CoV in the early endosome. Whereas, the lysosomes were reported for MHV and FIPV (feline infectious peritonitis virus).

Caveolae/Lipid-Raft Dependent Endocytosis

Caveolae is a subgroup of lipid rafts that comprise unifying centers, caveolin, for the transduction of cellular signals. Caveolin is protein hairpin molecules of amino and carboxyl cytoplasmic termini. Caveolae (20kDa) organize lipid and protein molecules, expressed in different levels in different types of cells. These are also expressed in various other parts of cells [72, 73]. The inactive state of caveolin signaling molecules binds with CSD (caveolin scaffolding domain), activating and releasing the signal proteins [74, 75]. The CSD peptide sequence contains various binding motifs organizing the signaling molecules such as protein kinase A, protein kinase C, adenylyl cyclase (AC), Src, endothelial nitric oxide synthase, phosphatidylinositol-3-kinase (PI3K), mitogen-activated protein kinase, and heterotrimeric G complex proteins. The lipid rafts provide stages for the trafficking of proteins and transduction of signals containing glycosphingolipids and cholesterol on the membrane surface. The exceeding cholesterol level also delays the access of viruses to cells reported in dengue virus 2 (DEN2) and Japanese encephalitis virus (JEV) [76]. Caveolae/lipid raft-dependent endocytosis route shares specific mechanisms like clathrin-mediated but vary in their molecular dynamics.

Various reports were found that the activation of the p38 mitogen-activated protein kinase (MAPK) signaling pathway enhances viral replication. The uptake may involve caveolae and dynamin 2 lipid raft micro-domains [77, 78]. Simian virus 40 (SV40) had shown ligand-triggered caveolae-dependent endocytosis that recruits dynamin and assembles the cytoskeleton during the internalization process [79]. Similar results were found in avian reovirus (ARV) to trigger p38 MAPK, Ras, and Src signaling downstream pathways trailed through caveolin-1 mediated dynamin-dependent endocytosis [80]. These inductions and activation of the vial cycle in the early stages of ARV entry showed the combined effect of Src and p38 MAPK related to caveolin-1 and dynamin-2 cellular proteins.

Additionally, it was also shown that p38 MAPK activation also facilitates the replication of avian reovirus [81]. Although in most cases of endocytosis, integrins were reported essential in lipid rafts. However, in vest vile virus entry, cholesterol-rich microdomains membrane instead of integrins play vital roles. The uncoating of viruses and penetration in the endosome pathway from early endosome to late endosome requires a longer time as compared to CME by dynamin and caveolin regulations [82 - 84]. Viruses like KSHV do not require lipid rafts for their efficient attachment but utilize these pathways for additional functions during their infection [85].

Currently, two of seven CoVs in humans, namely, HCoV-229E and HCoV-OC43, utilize caveolae-mediated endocytosis. CD13 aggregates act as a binding receptor molecule for the HCoV-229E virus. It localizes with caveolin-1 in human fibroblasts that generate the cross-linking of the CD13 receptor, which got access to caveolae microdomain for successful endocytosis [86]. The entry mechanism was reported in HCT-8 cells for HCoV-OC43. It engages with caveolin-1 for internalization, and subsequent endocytosis through dynamin and actin-dependent manner [87]. Moreover, the caveolin-1 functions during entry of SARS-CoV remain contentious. Bioinformatics studies revealed the tens of caveolin-1 binding domains (CBD) in SARS-CoV proteins that showed the importance of caveolin-1 and lipid raft in SARS coronavirus infection [88]. However, it was found that key amino acid residue is gathered inside CBD that may not interact directly with caveolin-1. These interactions remind us that CBD is not a sufficient interaction mechanism and may undergo CMS [89].

Clathrin/caveolin independent endocytosis

Clathrin/caveolin independent pathway was initially reported for viral endocytosis in polyomavirus, mouse polyoma, and SV40 virus [84]. Numerous endocytic pathways were reported for different types of hCoVs. Although, viral fusion at the cell surface was studied in MHV that revealed an alternate entry pathway. Various studies showed that endocytosis of the A59 strain of MHV could be interrupted by lysosomotropic agents, not similar to others [42, 43]. Similarly, proteolysis of coronavirus S proteins shows the important feature in cell-cell interactions and viral host access. Numerous cleavage sites were recognized in CoVs that affect the entry of viruses through fusion or cell-cell interaction manner. During the assembly of new virions, the S protein of MHV strain sliced at the S1/S2 site through furin proteases by the secretory pathway of producer cell [90, 91]. It was shown that inhibition of S protein cleavage does not mark the entry of A59 strain but interrupt cell-cell fusion [90]. The same inhibition was found by low pH activated cathepsin protease inhibitors in feline CoVs and SARS-CoV while treating cell-bound particles that enhance cell to cell interactions and virus entry [92, 93]. In SARS-CoV, the proteolytic cleavage of the more downstream side than the S1 or S2 boundary was found important for cell entry [94].

Non-clathrin non-caveolin endocytosis

Several viruses like lymphocytic choriomeningitis virus (LCMV) exist cholesterol-dependent entry pathways instead of clathrin, dynamin, caveolin, lipid rafts actin dynamin, Arf6, and flotillin-1 dependent pathways. These viruses enter through non-coated pits and transfer directly to late endosomes without following the Rab5/EEA1 positive early endosome (EE) routes [95, 96]. Previously, in HSV-1, it was found that the virus can get into the cell through macro-pinocytosis. However, recently it was reported that the uptake could be phagocytoses facilitated by dynamin, nectin-1, and cholesterol [97 - 99]. Similarly, the influenza virus enters cells mainly through CME additionally other routes independent of clathrin and Caveolae dependent [100].

It is assumed that there may occur other new routes of endocytosis that need to be discovered and might serve as an important entry route for clathrin/caveolae-independent viruses. One experimental study conducted in HeLa and HaCaT cells showed that human papillomavirus type-16 (HPV-16) utilizes a similar entry mechanism to macropinocytosis. It occurs without activating Rho GTPases with small vesicles and no elevation of fluid uptake [101]. Similar features are in common with the human rhinovirus-14 and influenza virus [102, 103]. In LCMV, neuraminidase viruses and *Lassa viruses* utilize multi-vascular bodies avoiding early endosomes and internalize through clathrin/caveolin-dynamin-independent manners [95, 104]. *Acanthamoeba polyphagia* mimivirus, a 750 nm enveloped virus, uses amoeba as a host, using a phagocytosis-like mechanism to enter the human macrophages. However, viral endocytosis studies still need further elaborations.

Macropinocytosis

Macropinocytosis allows the drinking of extracellular soluble materials such as nutrients and antigens in response to cell stimuli to enter non-specifically into the cells. The process of taking a substance is so-called cell-drinking mechanism of endocytosis. Warren Lewis first observed in 1931 during his works on macrophages describing macropinocytosis as the inner folding using certain cell surface regions perturbs to fuse with the basal membrane, developing vesicular structures called macropinosomes. Structurally macropinosomes are large uncoated vesicles that significantly differ in size. Its diameters ranges from 0.2 to 5.0 μm [105]. The entry mechanism in macropinocytosis depends on actin that triggers a multifaceted signaling pathway that briefly alters the actin cytoskeleton's dynamics. It is a prominent entry pathway for predominant large viruses like filoviruses, poxviruses, adenoviruses, IAV, and HIV1 [20, 103, 106]. The virus-carrying macropinosomes endure the acidification process, maturation, and synthesis with LE or lysosome deeper in the cytoplasm. Various virus particles require to cover themselves in the form of cell debris or apoptotic inclusions to provoke the process of macropinocytosis as reported in the vaccinia virus (VACV), dengue virus, and lentiviral vectors [13, 107].

Viruses depending on macropinocytosis will be engulfed, similar to phagocytosis by inward invagination of membranes. This mechanism requires reorganization of the actin cytoskeleton to activate the Rho GTPases, PI3K, Cdc42, and other cellular kinases of actin modulatory factors. The binding of HIV1 glycoproteins envelope with primary CD4 receptors and one of the two co-receptors molecules (CXCR4 and CCR5) were found to generate signal cascades that cause actin cytoskeleton reorganization and Rac activation. These cascade mechanisms further provoke HIV-1 mediated membrane fusion [108, 109]. It was demonstrated that epidermal growth factor receptor molecules (EGFR) also play a vital role in the entrance of viruses as found in the hepatitis C virus that binds to CD81, inducing EGFR activation and internalization [110]. The binding activates multiple downstream signaling pathways. The entry mechanism reported in other viruses, including HCMV, influenza A virus, and adenoviruses, was facilitated by EGFR [111, 112].

The fusion of macropinosomes with EE and hind back to membrane surface takes place under different signaling regulations. The acidic environment of macropinosomes facilitates the entry of certain low pH-dependent viruses. Several viruses were found to utilize the macropinocytosis entry pathway as reported in HSV-1, vaccinia virus, coxsackievirus B (CVB), African swine fever virus (ASFV), HIV-1, KSHV, and HPV-16 [113 - 115]. The viral entry directly stimulates dextran uptake, polymerization of actin and EGFR, and activation of Rac1, Pak1, and PI3K/Akt signaling pathways [114]. Novel ligand-induced endocytic pathway different from classical macropinocytosis was found in HPV-16 concerning the size of vesicles, the sensitivity of cholesterol, and the necessity of GTPases [111, 115].

Some viruses do not enter macropinosomes but utilize macropinocytosis to trigger the infection as found in adenovirus type 2 [116]. Unlikely, macropinocytosis is not considered to be the main pathway of entrance mechanism in SARS-CoV pseudoviruses that influenced receptor-translocation from membrane surface to intracellular organelles. As macropinocytosis is not dependent on receptor-mediated endocytosis.

Integrins, Chemokines, and Heparin-Sulfate Receptors-Mediated Endocytosis

Various biological disciplines explain the significance of cell surface receptors organization with their signaling associates curiously. Current information has emphasized the significance of the co-localization of microdomain' ' receptors with their signal associates that assists cellular events during the endocytosis mechanism. Integrins play an essential role in signal transmission and interpretation from the external environment to inside cells through several signaling cascades. These are heterodimers comprised of α and β protein chains and abundant receptor molecules on cell surfaces in the extracellular matrix [117]. Several studies were found that report the regulation and trafficking of integrins.

Similarly, the role of small GTPases like Arf6 and members of the Rab family were highly appreciated in the trafficking of integrin molecules in cells [118]. The entry of the vaccinia virus with PI3K/Akt signals activation is mediated by integrins. Similarly, in KSHV, the αα3ββ integrin receptors help in binding with viral envelop glycoproteins molecules [119]. These interactions further induce FAK (focal adhesion kinase) activation, an essential step for consequent phosphorylation of other cellular kinase activities and cytoskeleton rearrangements. Similarly, in DENV-2, integrin αα5ββ3 was found in an endothelial structure that performs vital functions in endocytosis mechanism and infection [120].

Adenoviruses are reported as a significant source of acute infection. To understand the endocytosis and trafficking mechanism, the adenoviruses capsid proteins and penton initiate binding with integrins receptors that generate integrin-mediated endocytosis. These proteins organize stepwise events of the successful delivery of gene transfer, considerably causing an acute infection in humans [121]. In many cell types, the binding receptor CAR from Adenovirus forms a cell adhesion complex homodimer with neighboring cells that cooperate with surface integrins for an efficient viral entry [122]. Other viruses like poxvirus, HIV, and myxoma virus comprise the assumption of chemokine receptors that allow viruses to enter, and large, ake copies of them proliferate inside the host cell. Endocytosis of HIV generally involves the complex binding of the gp120/gp41 glycoprotein envelope to the CD4 receptor and G protein joined chemokine co-receptor CXCR4/ CCR5 that results in conformational alterations in protein' 's envelope [123]. Additionally, the HIV primary isolates consume the APJseven-transmembrane receptor molecules as a co-receptor molecule. The brief studies regarding HIV endocytosis show the contribution of actin polymerization, membrane- micro- domains, glycol- sphingolipids, chemokine, and CD4 signaling pathways to elucidate the entry mechanism [124].

Heparan sulfate typically exists as a proteoglycan form in the glycosaminoglycan family. It binds with extracellular matrix protein on the membrane surfaces. A similar mechanism of utilizing heparan-sulfate utilizing to bind with cell surface was also reported in herpesviruses, Rift valley fever virus (RVFV), and Aden-associated virus (AAV) [125 - 127]. The viral particles can initiate endocytosis after interaction with heparan sulfate that rapidly activates type I interferon by regulating heparan sulfate on the B cell membrane surface. However, the essential signaling pathways still need to be discovered.

CONCLUSION

The current worldwide ongoing epidemic of COVID-19 has arisen as a substantial global public health danger. Scientists and researchers worldwide have been sharply involved in the current situation to control the rapid spread of the virus through deep studying the molecular aspects and therapeutic studies. Presently, the exact endocytosis mechanism studies are still a topic of discussion that is considered an essential mechanism of viral entrance, specially SARS-CoV-2 endocytosis. For cell infection, viruses must attach to the membrane trailed by diffusion through downstream signaling. The cell membrane possesses a potential barrier for coming viruses. These viruses can get through these barriers by direct fusion with the membrane to release their capsid/nucleic acid to the cytosol or by endocytosis. The viral entry is mostly specific with their types or by using multiple pathways for entry mechanism. On the other side, the membrane components' diversity of host cells often limits the entry of viruses. The clarification of endocytosis will significantly benefit specific antiviral drug development.

The main theme of the viral particle is to carry its genetic material inside the cell then further to the uninfected cell. Mostly the viruses have gain advantages of the site-specific binding through receptor molecules to internalize inside the endocytic vacuoles or other compartments. Most RNA viruses achieved the benefits of the membrane transport system and reached the cytosol for replication. Similarly, the DNA viruses get access to the nucleus and finally uncoated their genome. Few viruses seem to penetrate directly through the membrane by fusion. Endocytosis of SARS-CoV involves receptor-mediated endocytosis, clathrin, and caveolin-independent endocytosis, and lipid-rafts mechanism. The endocytic mechanism still needs further elaboration to find out the exact entry route of coronavirus for potent drug and vaccine production.

CONSENT FOR PUBLICATION

Not Applicable.

CONFLICT OF INTEREST

The author confirms that this chapter contents have no conflict of interest.

ACKNOWLEDGEMENT

Declared none.

REFERENCES

[1]   Su S, Wong G, Shi W, *et al.* Epidemiology, genetic recombination, and pathogenesis of coronaviruses. Trends Microbiol 2016; 24(6): 490-502.
[http://dx.doi.org/10.1016/j.tim.2016.03.003] [PMID: 27012512]

[2]   Zhong NS, Zheng BJ, Li YM, *et al.* Epidemiology and cause of severe acute respiratory syndrome (SARS) in Guangdong, People's Republic of China, in February, 2003. Lancet 2003; 362(9393): 1353-8.
[http://dx.doi.org/10.1016/S0140-6736(03)14630-2] [PMID: 14585636]

[3]   Drosten C, Günther S, Preiser W, *et al.* Identification of a novel coronavirus in patients with severe acute respiratory syndrome. N Engl J Med 2003; 348(20): 1967-76.
[http://dx.doi.org/10.1056/NEJMoa030747] [PMID: 12690091]

[4]   Fouchier RA, Kuiken T, Schutten M, *et al.* Aetiology: Koch's postulates fulfilled for SARS virus. Nature 2003; 423(6937): 240.
[http://dx.doi.org/10.1038/423240a] [PMID: 12748632]

[5]   Zaki AM, van Boheemen S, Bestebroer TM, Osterhaus AD, Fouchier RA. Isolation of a novel coronavirus from a man with pneumonia in Saudi Arabia. N Engl J Med 2012; 367(19): 1814-20.
[http://dx.doi.org/10.1056/NEJMoa1211721] [PMID: 23075143]

[6]   Zhu N, Zhang D, Wang W, *et al.* A Novel Coronavirus from Patients with Pneumonia in China, 2019. N Engl J Med 2020; 382(8): 727-33.
[http://dx.doi.org/10.1056/NEJMoa2001017] [PMID: 31978945]

[7]   Li W, Moore MJ, Vasilieva N, *et al.* Angiotensin-converting enzyme 2 is a functional receptor for the SARS coronavirus. Nature 2003; 426(6965): 450-4.
[http://dx.doi.org/10.1038/nature02145] [PMID: 14647384]

[8]   Becker MM, Graham RL, Donaldson EF, *et al.* Synthetic recombinant bat SARS-like coronavirus is infectious in cultured cells and in mice. Proc Natl Acad Sci USA 2008; 105(50): 19944-9.
[http://dx.doi.org/10.1073/pnas.0808116105] [PMID: 19036930]

[9]   Helenius A. Virus Entry: Looking back and moving forward. J Mol Biol 2018; 430(13): 1853-62.
[http://dx.doi.org/10.1016/j.jmb.2018.03.034] [PMID: 29709571]

[10]   Flipse J, Wilschut J, Smit JM. Molecular mechanisms involved in antibody-dependent enhancement of dengue virus infection in humans. Traffic 2013; 14(1): 25-35.
[http://dx.doi.org/10.1111/tra.12012] [PMID: 22998156]

[11]   Mercer J, Helenius A. Apoptotic mimicry: phosphatidylserine-mediated macropinocytosis of vaccinia virus. Ann N Y Acad Sci 2010; 1209: 49-55.
[http://dx.doi.org/10.1111/j.1749-6632.2010.05772.x] [PMID: 20958316]

[12]   Morizono K, Xie Y, Olafsen T, *et al.* The soluble serum protein Gas6 bridges virion envelope phosphatidylserine to the TAM receptor tyrosine kinase Axl to mediate viral entry. Cell Host Microbe 2011; 9(4): 286-98.
[http://dx.doi.org/10.1016/j.chom.2011.03.012] [PMID: 21501828]

[13]   Meertens L, Carnec X, Lecoin MP, *et al.* The TIM and TAM families of phosphatidylserine receptors mediate dengue virus entry. Cell Host Microbe 2012; 12(4): 544-57.
[http://dx.doi.org/10.1016/j.chom.2012.08.009] [PMID: 23084921]

[14]   Coyne CB, Bergelson JM. Virus-induced Abl and Fyn kinase signals permit coxsackievirus entry through epithelial tight junctions. Cell 2006; 124(1): 119-31.
[http://dx.doi.org/10.1016/j.cell.2005.10.035] [PMID: 16413486]

[15]   Eisenberg RJ, Atanasiu D, Cairns TM, Gallagher JR, Krummenacher C, Cohen GH. Herpes virus fusion and entry: a story with many characters. Viruses 2012; 4(5): 800-32.
[http://dx.doi.org/10.3390/v4050800] [PMID: 22754650]

[16]   Hamming I, Timens W, Bulthuis ML, Lely AT, Navis G, van Goor H. Tissue distribution of ACE2 protein, the functional receptor for SARS coronavirus. A first step in understanding SARS pathogenesis. J Pathol 2004; 203(2): 631-7.
        [http://dx.doi.org/10.1002/path.1570] [PMID: 15141377]

[17]   Mellman I, Fuchs R, Helenius A. Acidification of the endocytic and exocytic pathways. Annu Rev Biochem 1986; 55: 663-700.
        [http://dx.doi.org/10.1146/annurev.bi.55.070186.003311] [PMID: 2874766]

[18]   Strauss M, Filman DJ, Belnap DM, Cheng N, Noel RT, Hogle JM. Nectin-like interactions between poliovirus and its receptor trigger conformational changes associated with cell entry. J Virol 2015; 89(8): 4143-57.
        [http://dx.doi.org/10.1128/JVI.03101-14] [PMID: 25631086]

[19]   Marsh M, Helenius A. Virus entry: open sesame. Cell 2006; 124(4): 729-40.
        [http://dx.doi.org/10.1016/j.cell.2006.02.007] [PMID: 16497584]

[20]   Saeed MF, Kolokoltsov AA, Albrecht T, Davey RA. Cellular entry of ebola virus involves uptake by a macropinocytosis-like mechanism and subsequent trafficking through early and late endosomes. PLoS Pathog 2010; 6(9)e1001110
        [http://dx.doi.org/10.1371/journal.ppat.1001110] [PMID: 20862315]

[21]   Ng ML, Tan SH, See EE, Ooi EE, Ling AE. Early events of SARS coronavirus infection in vero cells. J Med Virol 2003; 71(3): 323-31.
        [http://dx.doi.org/10.1002/jmv.10499] [PMID: 12966536]

[22]   Huang IC, Bosch BJ, Li F, *et al.* SARS coronavirus, but not human coronavirus NL63, utilizes cathepsin L to infect ACE2-expressing cells. J Biol Chem 2006; 281(6): 3198-203.
        [http://dx.doi.org/10.1074/jbc.M508381200] [PMID: 16339146]

[23]   Simmons G, Gosalia DN, Rennekamp AJ, Reeves JD, Diamond SL, Bates P. Inhibitors of cathepsin L prevent severe acute respiratory syndrome coronavirus entry. Proc Natl Acad Sci USA 2005; 102(33): 11876-81.
        [http://dx.doi.org/10.1073/pnas.0505577102] [PMID: 16081529]

[24]   Zhou P, Yang XL, Wang XG, *et al.* A pneumonia outbreak associated with a new coronavirus of probable bat origin. Nature 2020; 579(7798): 270-3.
        [http://dx.doi.org/10.1038/s41586-020-2012-7] [PMID: 32015507]

[25]   Schmidt AA. Membrane transport: the making of a vesicle. Nature 2002; 419(6905): 347-9.
        [http://dx.doi.org/10.1038/419347a] [PMID: 12353016]

[26]   Oved S, Yarden Y. Signal transduction: molecular ticket to enter cells. Nature 2002; 416(6877): 133-6.
        [http://dx.doi.org/10.1038/416133a] [PMID: 11894079]

[27]   Sorkin A, Von Zastrow M. Signal transduction and endocytosis: close encounters of many kinds. Nat Rev Mol Cell Biol 2002; 3(8): 600-14.
        [http://dx.doi.org/10.1038/nrm883] [PMID: 12154371]

[28]   Doherty GJ, McMahon HT. Mechanisms of endocytosis. Annu Rev Biochem 2009; 78: 857-902.
        [http://dx.doi.org/10.1146/annurev.biochem.78.081307.110540] [PMID: 19317650]

[29]   Wang H, Yuan X, Sun Y, *et al.* Infectious bronchitis virus entry mainly depends on clathrin mediated endocytosis and requires classical endosomal/lysosomal system. Virology 2019; 528: 118-36.
        [http://dx.doi.org/10.1016/j.virol.2018.12.012] [PMID: 30597347]

[30]   Salonen A, Ahola T, Kääriäinen L. Viral RNA replication in association with cellular membranes. Curr Top Microbiol Immunol 2005; 285: 139-73.
        [http://dx.doi.org/10.1007/3-540-26764-6_5] [PMID: 15609503]

[31]   Li F. Structure, function, and evolution of coronavirus spike proteins. Annu Rev Virol 2016; 3(1): 237-61.

[http://dx.doi.org/10.1146/annurev-virology-110615-042301] [PMID: 27578435]

[32] Simmons G, Zmora P, Gierer S, Heurich A, Pöhlmann S. Proteolytic activation of the SARS-coronavirus spike protein: cutting enzymes at the cutting edge of antiviral research. Antiviral Res 2013; 100(3): 605-14.
[http://dx.doi.org/10.1016/j.antiviral.2013.09.028] [PMID: 24121034]

[33] Matsuyama S, Nagata N, Shirato K, Kawase M, Takeda M, Taguchi F. Efficient activation of the severe acute respiratory syndrome coronavirus spike protein by the transmembrane protease TMPRSS2. J Virol 2010; 84(24): 12658-64.
[http://dx.doi.org/10.1128/JVI.01542-10] [PMID: 20926566]

[34] Bertram S, Glowacka I, Müller MA, *et al.* Cleavage and activation of the severe acute respiratory syndrome coronavirus spike protein by human airway trypsin-like protease. J Virol 2011; 85(24): 13363-72.
[http://dx.doi.org/10.1128/JVI.05300-11] [PMID: 21994442]

[35] Raj VS, Mou H, Smits SL, *et al.* Dipeptidyl peptidase 4 is a functional receptor for the emerging human coronavirus-EMC. Nature 2013; 495(7440): 251-4.
[http://dx.doi.org/10.1038/nature12005] [PMID: 23486063]

[36] Kuhn JH, Li W, Choe H, Farzan M. Angiotensin-converting enzyme 2: a functional receptor for SARS coronavirus. Cell Mol Life Sci 2004; 61(21): 2738-43.
[http://dx.doi.org/10.1007/s00018-004-4242-5] [PMID: 15549175]

[37] Wang H, Yang P, Liu K, *et al.* SARS coronavirus entry into host cells through a novel clathrin- and caveolae-independent endocytic pathway. Cell Res 2008; 18(2): 290-301.
[http://dx.doi.org/10.1038/cr.2008.15] [PMID: 18227861]

[38] Kirchhausen T. Three ways to make a vesicle. Nat Rev Mol Cell Biol 2000; 1(3): 187-98.
[http://dx.doi.org/10.1038/35043117] [PMID: 11252894]

[39] Czech MP. PIP2 and PIP3: complex roles at the cell surface. Cell 2000; 100(6): 603-6.
[http://dx.doi.org/10.1016/S0092-8674(00)80696-0] [PMID: 10761925]

[40] Ramanan V, Agrawal NJ, Liu J, Engles S, Toy R, Radhakrishnan R. Systems biology and physical biology of clathrin-mediated endocytosis 2011.
[http://dx.doi.org/10.1039/c1ib00036e]

[41] Inoue Y, Tanaka N, Tanaka Y, *et al.* Clathrin-dependent entry of severe acute respiratory syndrome coronavirus into target cells expressing ACE2 with the cytoplasmic tail deleted. J Virol 2007; 81(16): 8722-9.
[http://dx.doi.org/10.1128/JVI.00253-07] [PMID: 17522231]

[42] Eifart P, Ludwig K, Böttcher C, *et al.* Role of endocytosis and low pH in murine hepatitis virus strain A59 cell entry. J Virol 2007; 81(19): 10758-68.
[http://dx.doi.org/10.1128/JVI.00725-07] [PMID: 17626088]

[43] Qiu Z, Hingley ST, Simmons G, *et al.* Endosomal proteolysis by cathepsins is necessary for murine coronavirus mouse hepatitis virus type 2 spike-mediated entry. J Virol 2006; 80(12): 5768-76.
[http://dx.doi.org/10.1128/JVI.00442-06] [PMID: 16731916]

[44] Henne WM, Boucrot E, Meinecke M, *et al.* FCHo proteins are nucleators of clathrin-mediated endocytosis. Science 2010; 328(5983): 1281-4.
[http://dx.doi.org/10.1126/science.1188462] [PMID: 20448150]

[45] Song W, Zinsmaier KE. Endophilin and synaptojanin hook up to promote synaptic vesicle endocytosis. Neuron 2003; 40(4): 665-7.
[http://dx.doi.org/10.1016/S0896-6273(03)00726-8] [PMID: 14622570]

[46] Rappoport JZ, Kemal S, Benmerah A, Simon SM. Dynamics of clathrin and adaptor proteins during endocytosis. Am J Physiol Cell Physiol 2006; 291(5): C1072-81.
[http://dx.doi.org/10.1152/ajpcell.00160.2006] [PMID: 17035303]

[47] Collins BM, McCoy AJ, Kent HM, Evans PR, Owen DJ. Molecular architecture and functional model of the endocytic AP2 complex. Cell 2002; 109(4): 523-35.
[http://dx.doi.org/10.1016/S0092-8674(02)00735-3] [PMID: 12086608]

[48] Ungewickell EJ, Hinrichsen L. Endocytosis: clathrin-mediated membrane budding. Curr Opin Cell Biol 2007; 19(4): 417-25.
[http://dx.doi.org/10.1016/j.ceb.2007.05.003] [PMID: 17631994]

[49] Krauss M, Kinuta M, Wenk MR, De Camilli P, Takei K, Haucke V. ARF6 stimulates clathrin/AP-2 recruitment to synaptic membranes by activating phosphatidylinositol phosphate kinase type Igamma. J Cell Biol 2003; 162(1): 113-24.
[http://dx.doi.org/10.1083/jcb.200301006] [PMID: 12847086]

[50] Ehrlich M, Boll W, Van Oijen A, *et al.* Endocytosis by random initiation and stabilization of clathrin-coated pits. Cell 2004; 118(5): 591-605.
[http://dx.doi.org/10.1016/j.cell.2004.08.017] [PMID: 15339664]

[51] Lundmark R, Carlsson SR. Driving membrane curvature in clathrin-dependent and clathrin-independent endocytosis. Semin Cell Dev Biol 2010; 21(4): 363-70.
[http://dx.doi.org/10.1016/j.semcdb.2009.11.014] [PMID: 19931628]

[52] Yoon Y, Tong J, Lee PJ, *et al.* Molecular basis of the potent membrane-remodeling activity of the epsin 1 N-terminal homology domain. J Biol Chem 2010; 285(1): 531-40.
[http://dx.doi.org/10.1074/jbc.M109.068015] [PMID: 19880963]

[53] Rao Y, Ma Q, Vahedi-Faridi A, *et al.* Molecular basis for SH3 domain regulation of F-BAR-mediated membrane deformation. Proc Natl Acad Sci USA 2010; 107(18): 8213-8.
[http://dx.doi.org/10.1073/pnas.1003478107] [PMID: 20404169]

[54] Ringstad N, Gad H, Löw P, *et al.* Endophilin/SH3p4 is required for the transition from early to late stages in clathrin-mediated synaptic vesicle endocytosis. Neuron 1999; 24(1): 143-54.
[http://dx.doi.org/10.1016/S0896-6273(00)80828-4] [PMID: 10677033]

[55] Roux A, Uyhazi K, Frost A, De Camilli P. GTP-dependent twisting of dynamin implicates constriction and tension in membrane fission. Nature 2006; 441(7092): 528-31.
[http://dx.doi.org/10.1038/nature04718] [PMID: 16648839]

[56] Semerdjieva S, Shortt B, Maxwell E, *et al.* Coordinated regulation of AP2 uncoating from clathrin-coated vesicles by rab5 and hRME-6. J Cell Biol 2008; 183(3): 499-511.
[http://dx.doi.org/10.1083/jcb.200806016] [PMID: 18981233]

[57] Traub LM. Tickets to ride: selecting cargo for clathrin-regulated internalization. Nat Rev Mol Cell Biol 2009; 10(9): 583-96.
[http://dx.doi.org/10.1038/nrm2751] [PMID: 19696796]

[58] Yamauchi Y, Kiriyama K, Kubota N, Kimura H, Usukura J, Nishiyama Y. The UL14 tegument protein of herpes simplex virus type 1 is required for efficient nuclear transport of the alpha transinducing factor VP16 and viral capsids. J Virol 2008; 82(3): 1094-106.
[http://dx.doi.org/10.1128/JVI.01226-07] [PMID: 18032514]

[59] Bremner KH, Scherer J, Yi J, Vershinin M, Gross SP, Vallee RB. Adenovirus transport *via* direct interaction of cytoplasmic dynein with the viral capsid hexon subunit. Cell Host Microbe 2009; 6(6): 523-35.
[http://dx.doi.org/10.1016/j.chom.2009.11.006] [PMID: 20006841]

[60] Dodding MP, Way M. Coupling viruses to dynein and kinesin-1. EMBO J 2011; 30(17): 3527-39.
[http://dx.doi.org/10.1038/emboj.2011.283] [PMID: 21878994]

[61] Pasdeloup D, Blondel D, Isidro AL, Rixon FJ. Herpesvirus capsid association with the nuclear pore complex and viral DNA release involve the nucleoporin CAN/Nup214 and the capsid protein pUL25. J Virol 2009; 83(13): 6610-23.
[http://dx.doi.org/10.1128/JVI.02655-08] [PMID: 19386703]

[62] Strunze S, Engelke MF, Wang IH, *et al.* Kinesin-1-mediated capsid disassembly and disruption of the nuclear pore complex promote virus infection. Cell Host Microbe 2011; 10(3): 210-23.
[http://dx.doi.org/10.1016/j.chom.2011.08.010] [PMID: 21925109]

[63] Gallucci L, Kann M. Nuclear import of hepatitis B virus capsids and genome. Viruses 2017; 9(1)E21
[http://dx.doi.org/10.3390/v9010021] [PMID: 28117723]

[64] Wu WW, Sun YH, Panté N. Nuclear import of influenza A viral ribonucleoprotein complexes is mediated by two nuclear localization sequences on viral nucleoprotein. Virol J 2007; 4: 49.
[http://dx.doi.org/10.1186/1743-422X-4-49] [PMID: 17547769]

[65] Boulo S, Akarsu H, Ruigrok RW, Baudin F. Nuclear traffic of influenza virus proteins and ribonucleoprotein complexes. Virus Res 2007; 124(1-2): 12-21.
[http://dx.doi.org/10.1016/j.virusres.2006.09.013] [PMID: 17081640]

[66] Suomalainen M, Greber UF. Uncoating of non-enveloped viruses. Curr Opin Virol 2013; 3(1): 27-33.
[http://dx.doi.org/10.1016/j.coviro.2012.12.004] [PMID: 23332135]

[67] Fuchs R, Blaas D. Uncoating of human rhinoviruses. Rev Med Virol 2010; 20(5): 281-97.
[http://dx.doi.org/10.1002/rmv.654] [PMID: 20629045]

[68] Helenius A. Virus entry and uncoating. Fields virology 2007; 5: 99-118.

[69] Shah VB, Shi J, Hout DR, *et al.* The host proteins transportin SR2/TNPO3 and cyclophilin A exert opposing effects on HIV-1 uncoating. J Virol 2013; 87(1): 422-32.
[http://dx.doi.org/10.1128/JVI.07177-11] [PMID: 23097435]

[70] Arhel NJ, Souquere-Besse S, Munier S, *et al.* HIV-1 DNA Flap formation promotes uncoating of the pre-integration complex at the nuclear pore. EMBO J 2007; 26(12): 3025-37.
[http://dx.doi.org/10.1038/sj.emboj.7601740] [PMID: 17557080]

[71] Burkard C, Verheije MH, Wicht O, *et al.* Coronavirus cell entry occurs through the endo-/lysosomal pathway in a proteolysis-dependent manner. PLoS Pathog 2014; 10(11)e1004502
[http://dx.doi.org/10.1371/journal.ppat.1004502] [PMID: 25375324]

[72] Williams TM, Lisanti MP. The Caveolin genes: from cell biology to medicine. Ann Med 2004; 36(8): 584-95.
[http://dx.doi.org/10.1080/07853890410018899] [PMID: 15768830]

[73] Head BP, Insel PA. Do caveolins regulate cells by actions outside of caveolae? Trends Cell Biol 2007; 17(2): 51-7.
[http://dx.doi.org/10.1016/j.tcb.2006.11.008] [PMID: 17150359]

[74] Lisanti MP, Scherer PE, Tang Z, Sargiacomo M. Caveolae, caveolin and caveolin-rich membrane domains: a signalling hypothesis. Trends Cell Biol 1994; 4(7): 231-5.
[http://dx.doi.org/10.1016/0962-8924(94)90114-7] [PMID: 14731661]

[75] Okamoto T, Schlegel A, Scherer PE, Lisanti MP. Caveolins, a family of scaffolding proteins for organizing "preassembled signaling complexes" at the plasma membrane. J Biol Chem 1998; 273(10): 5419-22.
[http://dx.doi.org/10.1074/jbc.273.10.5419] [PMID: 9488658]

[76] Lee CJ, Lin HR, Liao CL, Lin YL. Cholesterol effectively blocks entry of flavivirus. J Virol 2008; 82(13): 6470-80.
[http://dx.doi.org/10.1128/JVI.00117-08] [PMID: 18448543]

[77] Banerjee S, Narayanan K, Mizutani T, Makino S. Murine coronavirus replication-induced p38 mitogen-activated protein kinase activation promotes interleukin-6 production and virus replication in cultured cells. J Virol 2002; 76(12): 5937-48.
[http://dx.doi.org/10.1128/JVI.76.12.5937-5948.2002] [PMID: 12021326]

[78] Rahaus M, Desloges N, Wolff MH. Replication of varicella-zoster virus is influenced by the levels of JNK/SAPK and p38/MAPK activation. J Gen Virol 2004; 85(Pt 12): 3529-40.

[http://dx.doi.org/10.1099/vir.0.80347-0] [PMID: 15557226]

[79]   Pelkmans L, Püntener D, Helenius A. Local actin polymerization and dynamin recruitment in SV40-induced internalization of caveolae. Science 2002; 296(5567): 535-9.
[http://dx.doi.org/10.1126/science.1069784] [PMID: 11964480]

[80]   Huang WR, Wang YC, Chi PI, *et al.* Cell entry of avian reovirus follows a caveolin-1-mediated and dynamin-2-dependent endocytic pathway that requires activation of p38 mitogen-activated protein kinase (MAPK) and Src signaling pathways as well as microtubules and small GTPase Rab5 protein. J Biol Chem 2011; 286(35): 30780-94.
[http://dx.doi.org/10.1074/jbc.M111.257154] [PMID: 21705803]

[81]   Ji WT, Lee LH, Lin FL, Wang L, Liu HJ. AMP-activated protein kinase facilitates avian reovirus to induce mitogen-activated protein kinase (MAPK) p38 and MAPK kinase 3/6 signalling that is beneficial for virus replication. J Gen Virol 2009; 90(Pt 12): 3002-9.
[http://dx.doi.org/10.1099/vir.0.013953-0] [PMID: 19656961]

[82]   Mercer J, Schelhaas M, Helenius A. Virus entry by endocytosis. Annu Rev Biochem 2010; 79: 803-33.
[http://dx.doi.org/10.1146/annurev-biochem-060208-104626] [PMID: 20196649]

[83]   Engel S, Heger T, Mancini R, *et al.* Role of endosomes in simian virus 40 entry and infection. J Virol 2011; 85(9): 4198-211.
[http://dx.doi.org/10.1128/JVI.02179-10] [PMID: 21345959]

[84]   Damm EM, Pelkmans L, Kartenbeck J, Mezzacasa A, Kurzchalia T, Helenius A. Clathrin- and caveolin-1-independent endocytosis: entry of simian virus 40 into cells devoid of caveolae. J Cell Biol 2005; 168(3): 477-88.
[http://dx.doi.org/10.1083/jcb.200407113] [PMID: 15668298]

[85]   Raghu H, Sharma-Walia N, Veettil MV, *et al.* Lipid rafts of primary endothelial cells are essential for Kaposi's sarcoma-associated herpesvirus/human herpesvirus 8-induced phosphatidylinositol 3-kinase and RhoA-GTPases critical for microtubule dynamics and nuclear delivery of viral DNA but dispensable for binding and entry. J Virol 2007; 81(15): 7941-59.
[http://dx.doi.org/10.1128/JVI.02848-06] [PMID: 17507466]

[86]   Schelhaas M. Come in and take your coat off - how host cells provide endocytosis for virus entry. Cell Microbiol 2010; 12(10): 1378-88.
[http://dx.doi.org/10.1111/j.1462-5822.2010.01510.x] [PMID: 20678171]

[87]   Owczarek K, Szczepanski A, Milewska A, *et al.* Early events during human coronavirus OC43 entry to the cell. Sci Rep 2018; 8(1): 7124.
[http://dx.doi.org/10.1038/s41598-018-25640-0] [PMID: 29740099]

[88]   Cai QC, Jiang QW, Zhao GM, Guo Q, Cao GW, Chen T. Putative caveolin-binding sites in SARS-CoV proteins. Acta Pharmacol Sin 2003; 24(10): 1051-9.
[PMID: 14531951]

[89]   Byrne DP, Dart C, Rigden DJ. Evaluating caveolin interactions: do proteins interact with the caveolin scaffolding domain through a widespread aromatic residue-rich motif? PLoS One 2012; 7(9)e44879
[http://dx.doi.org/10.1371/journal.pone.0044879] [PMID: 23028656]

[90]   de Haan CA, Stadler K, Godeke GJ, Bosch BJ, Rottier PJ. Cleavage inhibition of the murine coronavirus spike protein by a furin-like enzyme affects cell-cell but not virus-cell fusion. J Virol 2004; 78(11): 6048-54.
[http://dx.doi.org/10.1128/JVI.78.11.6048-6054.2004] [PMID: 15141003]

[91]   Luytjes W, Sturman LS, Bredenbeek PJ, *et al.* Primary structure of the glycoprotein E2 of coronavirus MHV-A59 and identification of the trypsin cleavage site. Virology 1987; 161(2): 479-87.
[http://dx.doi.org/10.1016/0042-6822(87)90142-5] [PMID: 2825419]

[92]   Matsuyama S, Taguchi F. Two-step conformational changes in a coronavirus envelope glycoprotein mediated by receptor binding and proteolysis. J Virol 2009; 83(21): 11133-41.

[http://dx.doi.org/10.1128/JVI.00959-09] [PMID: 19706706]

[93]   Regan AD, Shraybman R, Cohen RD, Whittaker GR. Differential role for low pH and cathepsin-mediated cleavage of the viral spike protein during entry of serotype II feline coronaviruses. Vet Microbiol 2008; 132(3-4): 235-48.
       [http://dx.doi.org/10.1016/j.vetmic.2008.05.019] [PMID: 18606506]

[94]   Ou X, Liu Y, Lei X, *et al.* Characterization of spike glycoprotein of SARS-CoV-2 on virus entry and its immune cross-reactivity with SARS-CoV. Nat Commun 2020; 11(1): 1620.
       [http://dx.doi.org/10.1038/s41467-020-15562-9] [PMID: 32221306]

[95]   Quirin K, Eschli B, Scheu I, Poort L, Kartenbeck J, Helenius A. Lymphocytic choriomeningitis virus uses a novel endocytic pathway for infectious entry *via* late endosomes. Virology 2008; 378(1): 21-33.
       [http://dx.doi.org/10.1016/j.virol.2008.04.046] [PMID: 18554681]

[96]   Borrow P, Oldstone MB. Mechanism of lymphocytic choriomeningitis virus entry into cells. Virology 1994; 198(1): 1-9.
       [http://dx.doi.org/10.1006/viro.1994.1001] [PMID: 8259643]

[97]   Nicola AV, Hou J, Major EO, Straus SE. Herpes simplex virus type 1 enters human epidermal keratinocytes, but not neurons, *via* a pH-dependent endocytic pathway. J Virol 2005; 79(12): 7609-16.
       [http://dx.doi.org/10.1128/JVI.79.12.7609-7616.2005] [PMID: 15919913]

[98]   Clement C, Tiwari V, Scanlan PM, Valyi-Nagy T, Yue BY, Shukla D. A novel role for phagocytosis-like uptake in herpes simplex virus entry. J Cell Biol 2006; 174(7): 1009-21.
       [http://dx.doi.org/10.1083/jcb.200509155] [PMID: 17000878]

[99]   Rahn E, Petermann P, Hsu MJ, Rixon FJ, Knebel-Mörsdorf D. Entry pathways of herpes simplex virus type 1 into human keratinocytes are dynamin- and cholesterol-dependent. PLoS One 2011; 6(10)e25464
       [http://dx.doi.org/10.1371/journal.pone.0025464] [PMID: 22022400]

[100] Sieczkarski SB, Whittaker GR. Influenza virus can enter and infect cells in the absence of clathrin-mediated endocytosis. J Virol 2002; 76(20): 10455-64.
       [http://dx.doi.org/10.1128/JVI.76.20.10455-10464.2002] [PMID: 12239322]

[101] Schelhaas M, Ewers H, Rajamäki ML, Day PM, Schiller JT, Helenius A. Human papillomavirus type 16 entry: retrograde cell surface transport along actin-rich protrusions. PLoS Pathog 2008; 4(9)e1000148
       [http://dx.doi.org/10.1371/journal.ppat.1000148] [PMID: 18773072]

[102] Khan AG, Pickl-Herk A, Gajdzik L, Marlovits TC, Fuchs R, Blaas D. Human rhinovirus 14 enters rhabdomyosarcoma cells expressing icam-1 by a clathrin-, caveolin-, and flotillin-independent pathway. J Virol 2010; 84(8): 3984-92.
       [http://dx.doi.org/10.1128/JVI.01693-09] [PMID: 20130060]

[103] de Vries E, Tscherne DM, Wienholts MJ, *et al.* Dissection of the influenza A virus endocytic routes reveals macropinocytosis as an alternative entry pathway. PLoS Pathog 2011; 7(3)e1001329
       [http://dx.doi.org/10.1371/journal.ppat.1001329] [PMID: 21483486]

[104] Kunz S. Receptor binding and cell entry of Old World arenaviruses reveal novel aspects of virus-host interaction. Virology 2009; 387(2): 245-9.
       [http://dx.doi.org/10.1016/j.virol.2009.02.042] [PMID: 19324387]

[105] Lim JP, Gleeson PA. Macropinocytosis: an endocytic pathway for internalising large gulps. Immunol Cell Biol 2011; 89(8): 836-43.
       [http://dx.doi.org/10.1038/icb.2011.20] [PMID: 21423264]

[106] Brindley MA, Hunt CL, Kondratowicz AS, *et al.* Tyrosine kinase receptor Axl enhances entry of Zaire ebolavirus without direct interactions with the viral glycoprotein. Virology 2011; 415(2): 83-94.
       [http://dx.doi.org/10.1016/j.virol.2011.04.002] [PMID: 21529875]

[107] Mercer J, Helenius A. Vaccinia virus uses macropinocytosis and apoptotic mimicry to enter host cells.

Science 2008; 320(5875): 531-5.
[http://dx.doi.org/10.1126/science.1155164] [PMID: 18436786]

[108]   Sieczkarski SB, Whittaker GR. Dissecting virus entry *via* endocytosis. J Gen Virol 2002; 83(Pt 7): 1535-45.
[http://dx.doi.org/10.1099/0022-1317-83-7-1535] [PMID: 12075072]

[109]   Harmon B, Ratner L. Induction of the Galpha(q) signaling cascade by the human immunodeficiency virus envelope is required for virus entry. J Virol 2008; 82(18): 9191-205.
[http://dx.doi.org/10.1128/JVI.00424-08] [PMID: 18632858]

[110]   Diao J, Pantua H, Ngu H, *et al.* Hepatitis C virus induces epidermal growth factor receptor activation *via* CD81 binding for viral internalization and entry. J Virol 2012; 86(20): 10935-49.
[http://dx.doi.org/10.1128/JVI.00750-12] [PMID: 22855500]

[111]   Chan G, Nogalski MT, Yurochko AD. Activation of EGFR on monocytes is required for human cytomegalovirus entry and mediates cellular motility. Proc Natl Acad Sci USA 2009; 106(52): 22369-74.
[http://dx.doi.org/10.1073/pnas.0908787106] [PMID: 20018733]

[112]   Eierhoff T, Hrincius ER, Rescher U, Ludwig S, Ehrhardt C. The epidermal growth factor receptor (EGFR) promotes uptake of influenza A viruses (IAV) into host cells. PLoS Pathog 2010; 6(9)e1001099
[http://dx.doi.org/10.1371/journal.ppat.1001099] [PMID: 20844577]

[113]   Mercer J, Helenius A. Virus entry by macropinocytosis. Nat Cell Biol 2009; 11(5): 510-20.
[http://dx.doi.org/10.1038/ncb0509-510] [PMID: 19404330]

[114]   Sánchez EG, Quintas A, Pérez-Núñez D, *et al.* African swine fever virus uses macropinocytosis to enter host cells. PLoS Pathog 2012; 8(6)e1002754
[http://dx.doi.org/10.1371/journal.ppat.1002754] [PMID: 22719252]

[115]   Schelhaas M, Shah B, Holzer M, *et al.* Entry of human papillomavirus type 16 by actin-dependent, clathrin- and lipid raft-independent endocytosis. PLoS Pathog 2012; 8(4)e1002657
[http://dx.doi.org/10.1371/journal.ppat.1002657] [PMID: 22536154]

[116]   Meier O, Boucke K, Hammer SV, *et al.* Adenovirus triggers macropinocytosis and endosomal leakage together with its clathrin-mediated uptake. J Cell Biol 2002; 158(6): 1119-31.
[http://dx.doi.org/10.1083/jcb.200112067] [PMID: 12221069]

[117]   Hynes RO. Integrins: bidirectional, allosteric signaling machines. Cell 2002; 110(6): 673-87.
[http://dx.doi.org/10.1016/S0092-8674(02)00971-6] [PMID: 12297042]

[118]   De Franceschi N, Hamidi H, Alanko J, Sahgal P, Ivaska J. Integrin traffic - the update. J Cell Sci 2015; 128(5): 839-52.
[PMID: 25663697]

[119]   Wang FZ, Akula SM, Sharma-Walia N, Zeng L, Chandran B. Human herpesvirus 8 envelope glycoprotein B mediates cell adhesion *via* its RGD sequence. J Virol 2003; 77(5): 3131-47.
[http://dx.doi.org/10.1128/JVI.77.5.3131-3147.2003] [PMID: 12584338]

[120]   Zamudio-Meza H, Castillo-Alvarez A, González-Bonilla C, Meza I. Cross-talk between Rac1 and Cdc42 GTPases regulates formation of filopodia required for dengue virus type-2 entry into HMEC-1 cells. J Gen Virol 2009; 90(Pt 12): 2902-11.
[http://dx.doi.org/10.1099/vir.0.014159-0] [PMID: 19710257]

[121]   Medina-Kauwe LK. Endocytosis of adenovirus and adenovirus capsid proteins. Adv Drug Deliv Rev 2003; 55(11): 1485-96.
[http://dx.doi.org/10.1016/j.addr.2003.07.010] [PMID: 14597142]

[122]   Farmer C, Morton PE, Snippe M, Santis G, Parsons M. Coxsackie adenovirus receptor (CAR) regulates integrin function through activation of p44/42 MAPK. Exp Cell Res 2009; 315(15): 2637-47.
[http://dx.doi.org/10.1016/j.yexcr.2009.06.008] [PMID: 19527712]

[123] Antonsson L, Boketoft A, Garzino-Demo A, Olde B, Owman C. Molecular mapping of epitopes for interaction of HIV-1 as well as natural ligands with the chemokine receptors, CCR5 and CXCR4. AIDS 2003; 17(18): 2571-9.
[http://dx.doi.org/10.1097/00002030-200312050-00004] [PMID: 14685051]

[124] Zhou N, Zhang X, Fan X, *et al.* The N-terminal domain of APJ, a CNS-based coreceptor for HIV-1, is essential for its receptor function and coreceptor activity. Virology 2003; 317(1): 84-94.
[http://dx.doi.org/10.1016/j.virol.2003.08.026] [PMID: 14675627]

[125] de Boer SM, Kortekaas J, de Haan CA, Rottier PJ, Moormann RJ, Bosch BJ. Heparan sulfate facilitates Rift Valley fever virus entry into the cell. J Virol 2012; 86(24): 13767-71.
[http://dx.doi.org/10.1128/JVI.01364-12] [PMID: 23015725]

[126] Shukla D, Spear PG. Herpesviruses and heparan sulfate: an intimate relationship in aid of viral entry. J Clin Invest 2001; 108(4): 503-10.
[http://dx.doi.org/10.1172/JCI200113799] [PMID: 11518721]

[127] Summerford C, Samulski RJ. Membrane-associated heparan sulfate proteoglycan is a receptor for adeno-associated virus type 2 virions. J Virol 1998; 72(2): 1438-45.
[http://dx.doi.org/10.1128/JVI.72.2.1438-1445.1998] [PMID: 9445046]

Part II: Genetic Alteration and Structural Determination of SARS-CoV-2 Proteins

CHAPTER 4

Genomic Characterization of SARS-CoV-2

Faisal Siddique[1,*], Muhammad Farrukh Nisar[2], Maida Manzoor[3], Firasat Hussain[1], Muhammad Saeed[4], Kashif Rahim[1] and Asif Javaid[5]

[1] *Department of Microbiology, Cholistan University of Veterinary & Animal Sciences, Bahawalpur, Pakistan*

[2] *Department of Physiology and Biochemistry, Cholistan University of Veterinary and Animal Sciences, Bahawalpur, Pakistan*

[3] *Institute of Microbiology, University of Agriculture, Faisalabad, Pakistan*

[4] *Department of Poultry Sciences, Cholistan University of Veterinary and Animal Sciences, Bahawalpur, Pakistan*

[5] *Department of Animal Nutrition, Cholistan University of Veterinary and Animal Sciences, Bahawalpur, Pakistan*

Abstract: Coronaviruses is associated with three big public health nightmares in the 21st century globally, such as acute respiratory syndrome coronavirus (SARS-CoV, in 2002), Middle East respiratory syndrome coronavirus (MERS-CoV, in 2012), and severe acute respiratory syndrome coronavirus type 2 (SARS-CoV-2, in 2020). They have caused respiratory diseases in humans, particularly in the elderly, children, and pre-existing comorbidities and immunocompromised patients. SARS-CoV-2 was first recorded in Wuhan city, Hubei Province, Chinathat severely affecting the world economy by more than $1 trillion. It consists of an enveloped lipid bilayer and a positive-sense RNA genome. The genome size is approximately 30 kb. The SARS-CoV-2 structure consists of many essential proteins such as spike glycoprotein (S), membrane (M), envelope (E), and nucleocapsid (NC). This chapter highlights the updated knowledge of SARS-CoV-2 infections such as current and background history, phylogenetic tree analysis of SARS-CoV-2, expression of ACE2 genes in human tissues, phylogenic of S surface glycoprotein gene, M protein, E protein, NC protein, evolutionary resemblance/comparison with SARS-CoV-2 and MERS gene, the role of replication of novel strain lead to COVID-19, factors involve in COVID-19 pathogenesis and conserved and non-conserved gene of SARS-CoV-2. This study may be a little supportive of the battle against COVID-19 infection worldwide.

Keywords: ACE2, Evolution, Genome, Replication, SARS-CoV-2, Spike protein.

*) **Corresponding author Faisal Siddique:** Department of Microbiology, Cholistan University of Veterinary & Animal Sciences, Bahawalpur 63100, Pakistan. E-mail:faisalsiddique@cuvas.edu.pk

Kamal Niaz & Muhammad Farrukh Nisar (Eds.)
All rights reserved-© 2021 Bentham Science Publishers

INTRODUCTION

The outbreak of severe acute respiratory syndrome-coronavirus (SARS-CoV), Middle East respiratory syndrome-coronavirus (MERS-CoV), and severe acute respiratory syndrome-coronavirus-2 (SARS-CoV-2) has shocked the world in 2003, 2012, and 2019 respectively. They were thought to be non-pathogenic or low pathogenic to humans two decades ago. The first epidemic of coronaviruses in a human was recorded in 2003 named SARS-CoV in Guangdong, China, and spread to more than twenty countries worldwide through worldwide journeying [1].

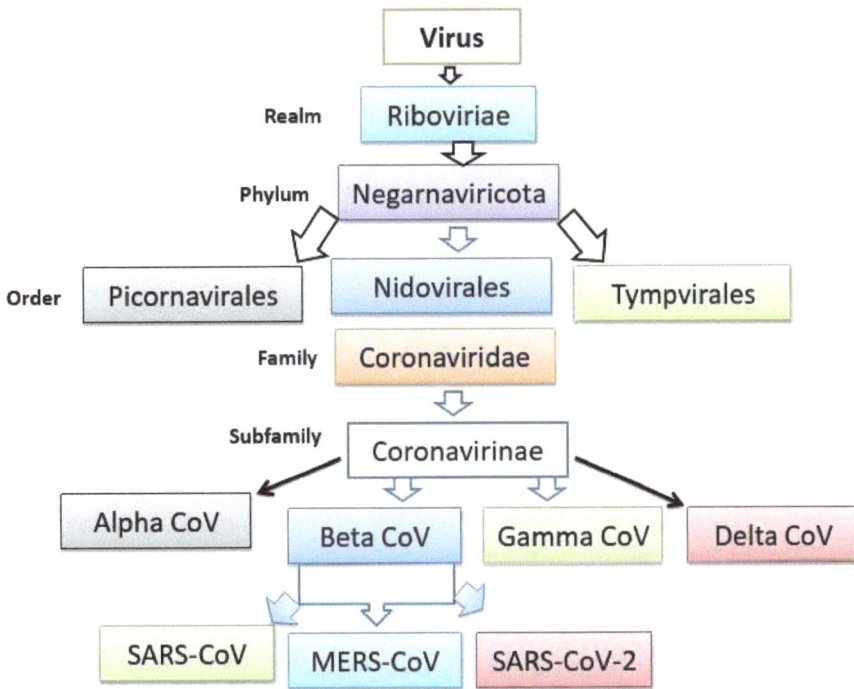

Fig. (1). Taxonomy of coronaviruses.

Coronaviruses have the aptitude to cause disease in humans, livestock, and birds. It belongs to *Nidovirale* order, *Coronaviridae* family and *Orthocoronavirinae* subfamily and beta-CoV genus [2]. They consist of an enveloped membrane, the largest RNA genome *i.e.* 34 kb in size [3]. The electron micrographs of coronaviruses indicated S or club-formed surface proteins looking like a crown. The corona is a Latin word that means crown [4].

Coronaviruses have been classified into genera *Alpha*, *beta*, *gamma*, and *delta* coronaviruses based on protein sequences presented in Fig. (**1**). Most human coronaviruses belong to beta-coronavirus genera, which further sub-categorized into A, B, C, and D lineages [5]. Most human coronaviruses belong to beta-coronavirus genera, which further sub-categorized into A, B, C, and D lineages [5].

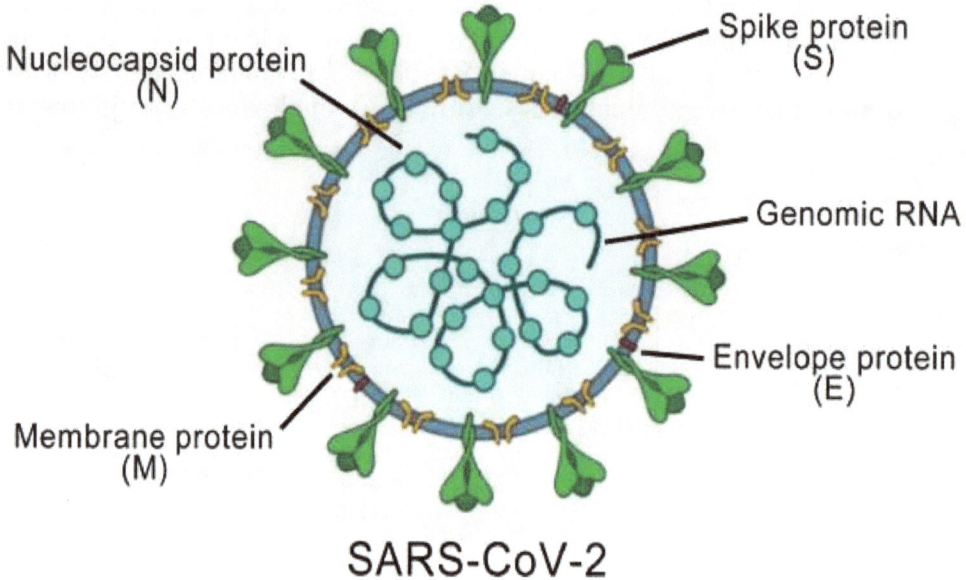

Fig. (2). Diagrammatical picture of a coronavirus [12].

Bats and rodents are the intermediate hosts of *alpha* and *beta* coronaviruses, while birds are the intermediate hosts of *gamma* and *delta* coronaviruses [6]. They can cross the species barrier and appear as new human pathogens, such as SARS-CoV-2 [7]. So far, various human-infected coronaviruses, such as HCoV-OC43, SARS-CoV, MERS, SARS-CoV-2, *etc.*, have been isolated and identified globally [8, 9]. The gene sequence of SARS-CoV-2 belongs to the β-coronavirus B line, which is more than 90% similar to bat and pangolin coronavirus genes.

The bat is believed to be the natural host of the new coronavirus SARS-CoV-2 based on the whole genome and phylogenetic sequence and to be infected by humans *via* an unknown intermediate host.

It has been reported that SARS-CoV-2 and SARS-CoV use the same enzyme converting receptors, *i.e.*, angiotensin 2, during human infection [10].

The SARS-CoV-2 genetic material acts as an infectious agent containing a 5'-methyl cap and a 3'-polyadenyl acid tail. SARS-CoV-2 has a total genome sequence of 29,811 nucleotides, including 8,903 5,482, 5,852, and 9,574 nitrogen base pairs, which are adenosine cytosine, guanine, and thymine, respectively [11]. The structure of SARS-CoV-2 is composed of a variety of structural proteins, including S glycoprotein, membrane (M), envelope (E), and core protein (N) presented in Fig. (**2**).

The petal or club-shaped S protein is densely packed M glycoproteins that help the virus attachment or fusion to host cells [13]. The pentameric small integral E protein is involved in the assembly and pathogenesis of the virus [14]. The type III integral type M associates with matrix formation. The nucleocapsid protein (NC) helps in genome encapsidation, protein, and RNA synthesis. All these structural proteins (S, M, E, and NC) of SARS-CoV-2 may act as an antigen towards human cells. They may stimulate antibody production and increase the immune response of T-cells [15].

Phylogenetic Tree Analysis of SARS-CoV-2

The phylogenetic or evolutionary analysis is a diagrammatic presentation that helps research how biological organisms, *e.g.,* bacteria, viruses, *etc.*, have evolved from their common ancestors. This phylogenetic tree is based on a comparative study of variations and similarities between genetic, geographical, and physical properties. Chinese scientists published the genomic sequence of Wuhan origin novel strain SARS-CoV-2 obtained from infected patients [7]. Phylogenetic analysis confirmed that this novel strain of the coronavirus is closely associated with MERS-CoV and SARS-CoV [16].

There are three main variants: A, B and C, that have been found based on amino acid changes during the phylogenetic analysis of one hundred and sixty SARS-CoV-2 genomes globally. Among them, variant A resembles bat coronaviruses. Variant A and C found in European and American countries as well as B genome in East Asian countries as depicted in Fig. (**3**) [17]. They used recently reported 96.2% similar human origin bat coronavirus genome [7] and labeled A. Generally, the phylogenetic network showed ancestral viral genomes prevailing together with their recently transformed daughter genomes during epidemics.

Another phylogenetic analysis of the SARS CoV 2 complete genome was done in Lombardy, Italy. Samples were obtained from infected SARS CoV 2 patients. Vero cells have been used for the growth of SARS CoV 2. The entire genome sequence was amplified by available specific primers and aligned with globally published genomes of SARS CoV 2 (a total of 157 genomes) publically available at GISAID. The phylogenetic study was done using a Bayesian Markov Chain Monte Carlo method achieved by software Beast version V.1.8.4 [18]. The evolutionary tree confirms that the genomic sequence of SARS CoV 2 strains produced in Italy was identical to the genomic sequence of Wuhan isolated first cases of typical pneumonia caused by SARS-CoV-2. Italy sequence is also closely related to Finnish, Brazilian, German, and Mexican one [19 - 21].

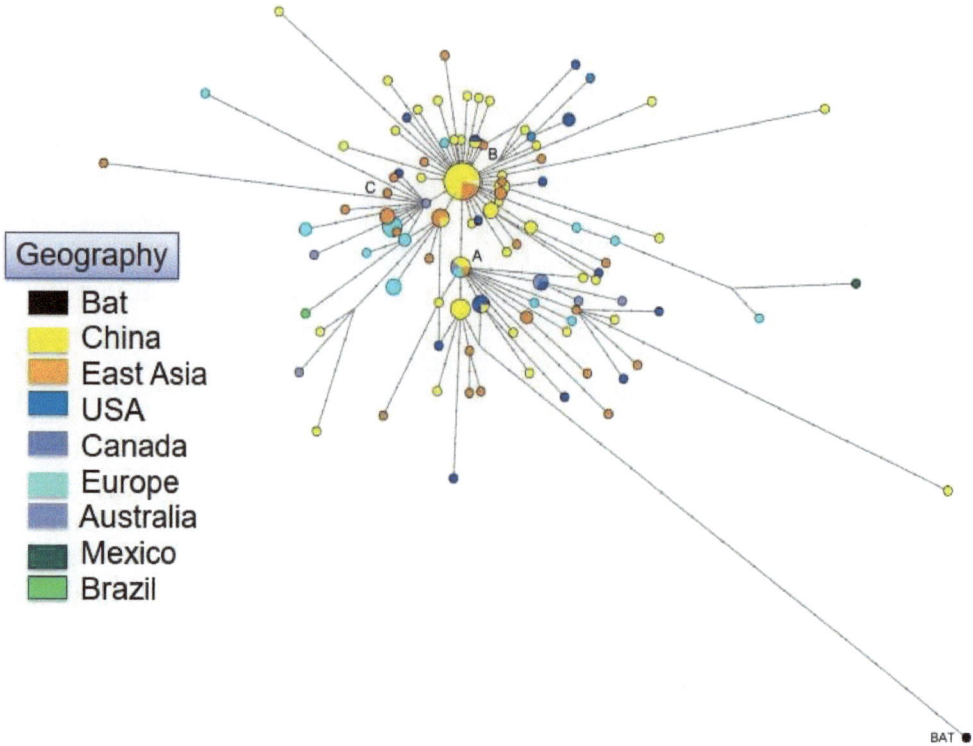

Fig. (3). Phylogenetic analysis of one hundred and sixty genomes of SARS-CoV-2 isolated globally. Bat coronavirus is represented in root cluster form. Various colored circles denoted taxa. Mutation in nucleotides represents the notch [7].

Zhang *et al.* [22] studied one hundred and sixty-nine samples for genomic analysis. They can be classified into two major genotypic clusters, such as Type I and Type II. The phylogenetic relationship between the SARS-CoV-2 genome and the BatCoV RaTG13 genome was investigated using FastTree software [23]. Phylogenetic examination revealed that the genome sequences of Type IA and IB similar to the genome sequence of bat viruses such as bat-SL-CoVZXC21, BatCoV RaTG13, and bat-SL-CoVZC45. This study recommended that Type I be an ancestral strain of human lineage B coronavirus and no direct connection with the Huanan seafood market [24]. Type II strain was transformed into Type I, *i.e.*, outbreak strain in Wuhan, China. These interpretations speculate that the Type II strain,, was caused by the outbreak in the seafood market in Huanan. Earlier reports also support this theory that outbreaks have no connection to Hunan's seafood market [25, 26]. Ogün *et al.* [27] collected samples from different patients hospitalized in Turkey. They isolated and identified the SARS-CoV-2 virus with the aid of RT-PCR. They further sequenced the isolated genomic material and comparison with already published SARS-CoV-2 sequenced globally. The results of the studies indicate that the virus was present earlier in Turkey, but the first case was identified late. Sub-cluster 4 and 8 lines have been extensively isolated and consist of approximately 80% of the SARS-CoV-2 genome isolated in the region.

Saif *et al.* [28] studied the adapted phylogenetic relationship of SARS-CoV-2. The genomic sequence of SARS-CoV-2 and the evolutionary relationship between SARS-CoV-2 and bat-CoVs was examined. They confirmed that bat was a natural reservoir host. They also verified the genetic modification in the S protein, E protein, and NC protein in a different region. The mutation had an impact on the replication, growth, and pathogenesis of SARS-CoV-2. Putative genetic alteration, *e.g.,* ORF3a, RdRp, *etc.*, have been identified. In the S gene, several recombination regions have been identified, which have demonstrated the adaptability strategy of the human host. Joseph *et al.* [29] studied the relationship between travel patterns and genomic epidemiology of SARS-CoV-2 infection in the USA. Up to March 2020, three hundred and fifty genomes of SARS-CoV-2 have been sequenced in the USA. They stated that the epidemic of novel strain could be caused by excessive domestic travel between one region, especially in the US state of Connecticut. They reported that the Connecticut epidemic was closely related to the Washington outbreak.

Expression of ACE2 Genes in Human Tissues

Researchers have been isolated, identified, and characterized COVID-19 from human epithelial and endothelial respiratory cells [30]. Lu *et al.* [25] reported that this novel coronavirus is similar to bat origin coronaviruses such as bat coronaviruses (bat-SL-CoVZC45 and bat-SL-CoVZXC21) based on complete genomic and proteomic sequencing and receptor-binding domain (RBD). Angiotensin-converting enzyme 2 (ACE2) is a binding receptor of SARS-CoV-2, MERS-CoV, HCoV-NL63, and SARS-CoV [10, 31]. However, SARS-CoV-2 did not use dipeptidyl peptidase 4 and aminopeptidase N receptors like other coronaviruses [10]. The RBD of the virus has a strong binding ability with ACE2 molecules [32].

ACE2is a metalloenzyme present in endothelial layers of arteries, kidneys, lungs, intestine, and heart [33]. ACE2 plays a significant role in the virulence of SARS-CoV-2 infection. ACE2 is also present in the brain mainly, the brain stem, striatum, hypothalamus, and cerebral cortex [34]. Anosmia and dysgeusia were also observed in patients during COVID-19 epidemics [35]. ACE2 is a class type 1 transmembrane protein, serves as the entry point of human coronaviruses, including SARS-CoV, SARS-CoV-2, MERS-CoV, and HCoV-NL63 by attachment of S proteins to the surface of the host cells [36, 37]. The genomic expression and spread of the ACE2 in human tissues may show the possible means of SARS-CoV-2 infection. Unfortunately, the pathogenesis and routes of SARS-CoV-2 infection are not well understood, yet host cell receptor studies' expression could help to understand better the global control of the COVID-19 infection [38].

The expression analysis of the ACE2 genome of SARS-CoV-2 was analyzed concerning human host cell receptors. The results of the research showed that SARS-CoV-2 mainly affects lung tissue. However, the lungs showed moderate ACE2 expression compared to the heart, small intestine, thyroid, and adipose tissue [39]. A similar study about the expression of ACE2 genes was conducted in the mouse. RT-PCR analysis with specific ACE2 primers indicated that cornea, testis, and liver tissue found strong expression of ACE2 genes as compared to lung, brain, kidney, and heart showed moderate expression. We found the ACE2 gene present in the cornea tissue but not in the optic nerve, iris, retina, and lens. Therefore, corneal tissue could be further affected by COVID-19 infection [40].

A current research investigated that the expression of ACE2 gene in humans found in the lung, esophagus keratinocytes, proximal tubules in kidney, cholangiocyte in the liver, colonocytes in the colon, enterocytes in ilium, rectum, epithelial cells in the stomach, and oral mucosa, pericytes in the eye tissue, pneumocytes (type II), brain and heart [33, 41, 42]. These outcomes have shown that high genomic expression of ACE2 cells is considered a major threat to SARS-CoV-2 infection [43].

Xu *et al.* [44] explored the genomic expression of the ACE2 receptor in epithelial cells of the buccal cavity based on public bulk-sequence RNA datasets such as Functional Annotation of The Mammalian Genome Cap Analysis of Gene Expression database and The Cancer Genome Atlas database. The findings of this research suggested that the epithelial cells of the tongue is enriched by the ACE2 receptor relative to the mouth floor, the oral tissue, the base of the tongue, and the gingival tissue of the oral cavity. The tongue in the oral cavity showed a high expression of the ACE2 receptor. These preliminary verdicts designated that the oral route could be considered vulnerable routes of entry to SARS-CoV-2 infection.

Phylogenic of Spike Surface Glycoprotein Gene (S)

The whole-genome sequencing technique identified and characterized a novel strain of coronavirus originated from Hubei, Wuhan province China has shown that this is a positive-sense RNA enveloped virus comprising a size of genome approximately29.9kb [45]. The genomic study of coronaviruses also identified different numbers of open reading frames (ORFs) [46]. The first open reading frame encrypts sixteen non-structural proteins and encodes two polyproteins (pp1ab and pp1a). Though, four essential components containing S, M, NC, and E, determined the remaining ORFs [47, 48]. Among them, S protein recognizes and binds with host cell receptor ACE2 for further pathogenesis. It may also help to develop the vaccine, antibodies, and antiviral [49, 50].

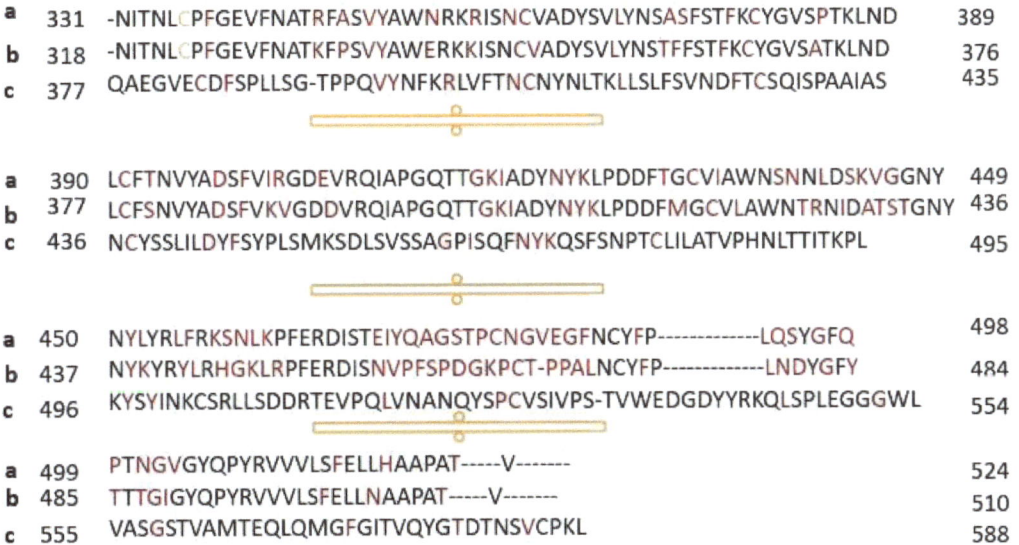

```
a   331  -NITNLCPFGEVFNATRFASVYAWNRKRISNCVADYSVLYNSASFSTFKCYGVSPTKLND      389
b   318  -NITNLCPFGEVFNATKFPSVYAWERKKISNCVADYSVLYNSTFFSTFKCYGVSATKLND      376
c   377  QAEGVECDFSPLLSG-TPPQVYNFKRLVFTNCNYNLTKLLSLFSVNDFTCSQISPAAIAS      435

a   390  LCFTNVYADSFVIRGDEVRQIAPGQTTGKIADYNYKLPDDFTGCVIAWNSNNLDSKVGGNY     449
b   377  LCFSNVYADSFVKVGDDVRQIAPGQTTGKIADYNYKLPDDFMGCVLAWNTRNIDATSTGNY     436
c   436  NCYSSLILDYFSYPLSMKSDLSVSSAGPISQFNYKQSFSNPTCLILATVPHNLTTITKPL      495

a   450  NYLYRLFRKSNLKPFERDISTEIYQAGSTPCNGVEGFNCYFP-------------LQSYGFQ     498
b   437  NYKYRYLRHGKLRPFERDISNVPFSPDGKPCT-PPALNCYFP-------------LNDYGFY     484
c   496  KYSYINKCSRLLSDDRTEVPQLVNANQYSPCVSIVPS-TVWEDGDYYRKQLSPLEGGGWL     554

a   499  PTNGVGYQPYRVVVLSFELLHAAPAT-----V-------                           524
b   485  TTTGIGYQPYRVVVLSFELLNAAPAT-----V-------                           510
c   555  VASGSTVAMTEQLQMGFGITVQYGTDTNSVCPKL                               588
```

Legends: a: SARS-CoV-2, b: SARS-CoV, and c: MERS-CoV

Fig. (4). Diagrammatic demonstration of the S glycoprotein of COVID-19. Previous characterized SARS-CoV and MERS domains were used in this picture, *i.e.*, internal fusion peptide (IFP), receptor-binding domain (RBD), heptad repeat 1/2 (HR1/2), N-terminal domain (NTD), SP (signal peptide), FP (fusion peptide), and the transmembrane domain (TM). Arrows designate the divisions of Spike protein into S1&S2 cleavage positions. Black and red frame indicated cleavage sites of furin and canonical furin-like motif at the S1 &S2 location, respectively [53].

The SARS-CoV-2 S protein is a large glycoprotein, approximately 180kDa, found on the surface of virions as a trimeric form. It is split into two S1 and S2 subunits. The RBD contains the receptor-binding motif in the loop region, which helps widespread attachment with the ACE2 receptor [31, 51]. The SI subunit of S protein is further categorized in two sub-domains *i.e.,* C & N terminal sub-domain, presented in Fig. (**4**). N terminal binding domain can bind the sialic acid receptor, and the C terminal domain bind with the proteinaceous receptor [52]. SARS-CoV-2 S1 C-domain recognizes host ACE2 receptors from humans, bats, and civets [10, 48].

Computer modeling of S glycoprotein showed that 77% and 80% amino acid sequence similarity in SARS-CoV-2 and SARS-CoV and CoV ZXC21 respectively presented in Fig. (**4**) [5, 54, 55]. The amino acid residue (394) of glutamine in the RBD of COVID-19 can be recognized on the ACE2 receptor [39].

A recent cryo-EM structure study has proved that the ACE2 binding mechanism SARS-CoV-2 and SARS-CoV S protein are similar [56]. The comparative analysis of SARS-CoV-2 and SARS-CoV S protein was performed based on bioinformatics methods. Both of them developed adjacent RGD motif and present in large quantities on the attachment surfaces, *i.e.,* extracellular matrix and cell surface proteins of the host cell. RGD motif includes arginine, glycine, and aspartic acid amino acids and is recognized and binds proteins integrins to the surface of host cells. The recognition of the evolutionary RGD motif may play a significant role in the early spread of person to person during SARS-CoV-2 infection [56].

An immunogenic effect of S glycoproteins of SARS-CoV-2 has been found and stimulates IFN-γ-specific T-cell response. The tropism of the virus could be changed due to the mutations in the S protein, which resulted in increasing viral pathogenesis and infecting new hosts [15]. SARS-CoV keeps some amino acid residues such as L472, D480, N479, T487, and Y442 in the RBD that permits the interspecies infection [24]. The mutation was observed in K479Nand S487T amino acid residues from civet to human. SARS-CoV2 contains amino acid residues like F486, N501, Q493, and L455, increasing interaction with the human ACE2 receptor. The two capping loops in the RBD of SARS-CoV-2 have solid binding ability with the ACE2 receptor [57].

Phylogenic of Nucleocapsid Protein Gene (NC)

NC is the leading viral protein found in the SARS-CoV-2 genome. It can form NC on its own, particularly in coronaviruses. It helps in genome packaging during replication. It protects the virus from a harsh environment, *e.g.,* poliovirus, yet, in

SARS-CoV-2, it provides an additional coat around genomic material. It is equipped with signature sequences, comprising structural motifs to play significant role pathogenesis of the virus to the host cells. Moreover, it is also known as the key immunogenic properties of antiserum. It is therefore used as a screening tool and as a vaccine candidate [58, 59].

NC is the most significant protein in SARS-CoV-2. The molecular weight of the NC protein is 50 KDa. It is consists of 422 amino acids. NC protein is highly antigenic and usually preserves its amino acid sequence by constructing this protein to prepare vaccine and diagnostic methods [22, 60]. The NC protein of COVID-19 is encrypted by the 9 open reading frames (ORF). It is used in transcription, replication, and genomic encapsidation [61]. It formed a complex of ribonucleoproteins during the packing of the positive-sense RNA genome and governing RNA synthesis and metabolism of the host cell [62, 63].

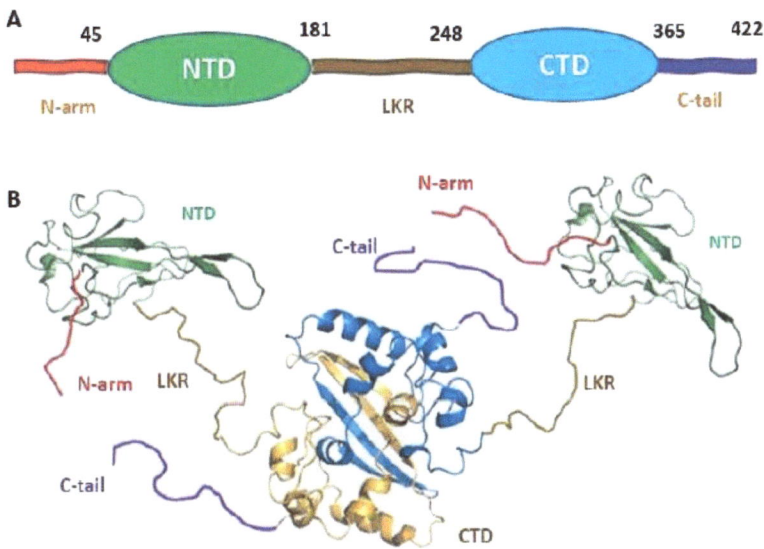

Fig. (5). Detailed structure of NC protein of COVID-19 (A) NTD and CTD structure of NC protein showed red and blue color respectively. (B) The assumed 3-D structure of the NC protein [66].

The conserved parts of NC protein comprise three domains as an N-terminal RNA-binding domain (NTD), a C-terminal dimerization domain (CTD), and an intrinsically disordered (SR)-rich linker for direct phosphorylation. The NTD binds with the 3′ end of the viral RNA genome while the C-terminal domain linkage the ribonucleoprotein complex to the viral membrane through its attachment with the matrix protein [64, 65]. The N-terminal domain region of NC comprises a positively charged sequence of amino acids utilized for a binding method of RNA. The C-terminal domain contains a lysine-rich amino acid region (between 373-390 amino acids) which activates nuclear localization signals. Middle of NC has an SR-rich motif that includes 177-207 amino acids.

Zheng *et al.* [66] detailed studied the correlation between NC and COVID-19 based on structure and function. To achieve their objectives, complete protein sequences were obtained containing 419 amino acids presented in Fig. (5a). The C and N terminal sub-domain of NC protein rich in β-strands are denoted in Fig. (5b).

Tilocca *et al.* [67] studied the taxonomical relationship of SARS-CoV-2 NC and other coronaviruses NC. The whole genomic sequence of NC proteins was done and phylogenetic classification of SARS-CoV-2 and other coronaviruses based on origin of nucleoprotein protein depicted in Fig. (6). NC protein structure of SARS-CoV-2 is similar to bat coronavirus RaTG13 and pangolin coronaviruses sequence. However, the low similarity was found in camels, canine, bovine, human enteric coronaviruses, and avian coronaviruses. This evolutionary taxonomy of SARS-CoV-2 and other coronaviruses was further protected with whole protein sequence by the multiple sequence alignment methods. It is revealed that SARS-CoV-2 shared 99% and 88% similarity with bat coronavirus RaTG13 and pangolin coronaviruses. The evolutionary phylogenetic analysis of the NC proteins revealed that SARS-CoV-2 NC similar to SARS-CoV and bat coronaviruses [10].

Phylogenic of Membrane Protein Gene (M)

The Membrane protein gene has been documented as a structural protein gene recently among different proteins in coronaviruses. M protein was first identified in the infectious bronchitis virus in 1990 [68]. Godet *et al.* [69] named this protein, *i.e.*, a small M protein. M is an abundant structural glycoprotein present in coronaviruses. M protein has unique features that help with intracellular budding. The small M protein is composed of 230 amino acids. It is divided into parts, such as the carboxy-terminal domain, N-terminal domain, and transmembrane domains [70]. Conserved amphipathic region present in the transmembrane domain in nearly all Coronaviridae [71]. The M protein genes present in the 3' one 3rd of the SARS-CoV-2 genome following S protein gene and nucleoprotein gene. M protein also carries additional genetic information at the 3' end containing the nucleoprotein sequence. The molecular weight of M protein is 20 to 38kDa [72]. M protein comprises small and large domains. The N-terminal glycosylated ectodomain is a small domain. C-terminal endo-domain is a large domain that spreads 7-8 nm into the viral particle [73]. M proteins present in dimer form and help in membrane curvature and binding in NC proteins [74]. M protein and N and E protein help stabilize the viral envelope and contribute to the formation of viral assembly [75].

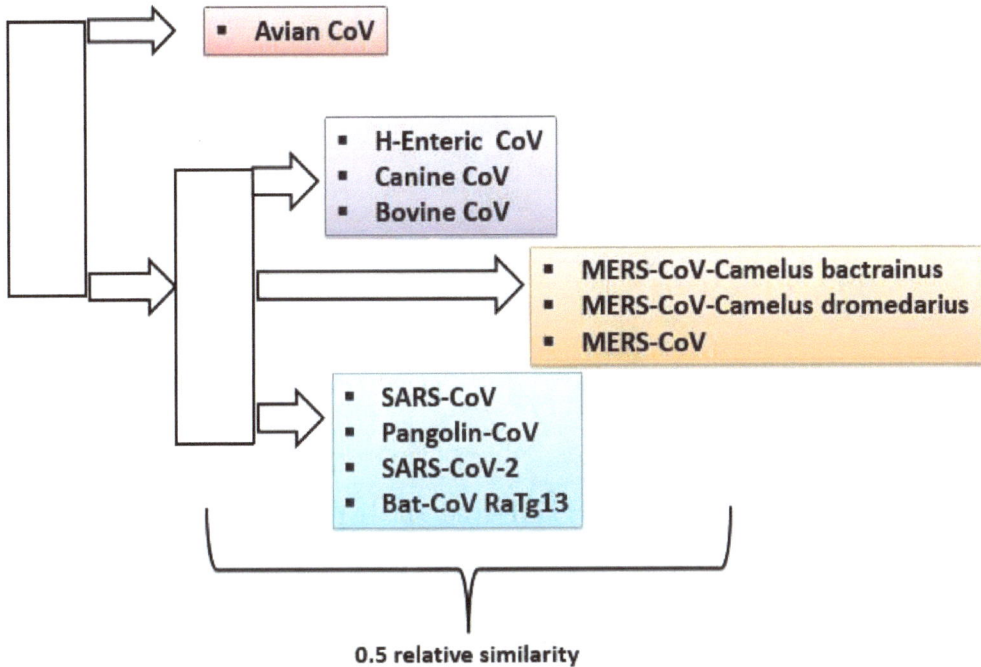

Fig. (6). Phylogenetic taxonomy of the SARS-CoV-2 and other animal coronaviruses based on whole-genome nucleoprotein sequence homology [67].

GenBank studies authorize that, alike to E and M proteins are generally conserved across SARS Coronaviruses. Multiple genetic sequences of bat coronavirus, pangolin coronavirus, and human SARS-CoV-2 in M protein showed that a similar pattern of the sequence was obtained. Yet, there is a difference present in the N-terminal position. Serine and asparagine amino acids residue present at 4 position in SARS-CoV-2 and bat and pangolin coronavirus genome respectively. Mutation of SARS-CoV-2 isolates has been reported at positions 70 and 89, *i.e.*, WA9-UW6 isolate, GenBank code MT163721, NIHE isolate, accession code MT127115, respectively. Due to mutation, Gly replaces the transmembrane with Arg at position 89. The mutation is predicted to have a significant effect on the protein properties of the membrane. We obtained a three-dimensional model of an M protein from the I-Tasser server (code QHD43419) presented in Fig. (7) [76].

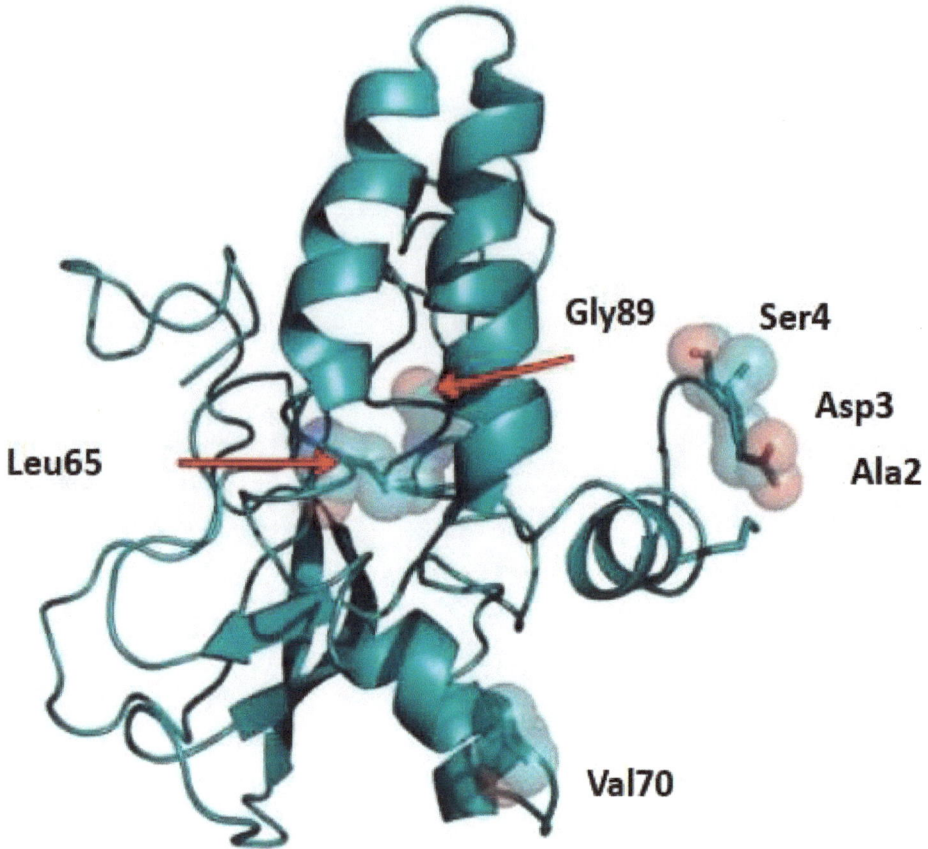

Fig. (7). Three-dimensional model of the M glycoprotein. Relevant residues are displayed as transparent space-filling spheres and labeled [76].

Phylogenic of Envelop Protein Gene (E)

The SARS-CoV-2 envelop E protein is unique which formed homotypic interaction and produced viroporins, *i.e.*, ion channel protein [77]. The ability of the enveloped protein to make homotypic interaction is the dependent transmembrane domain (TMD). Dimers, trimers, and pentamers were formed during homotypic interaction [78]. The E protein of SARS-CoV-2 is the smallest structural protein. It consists of 76-109 amino acids and is approximately 12 kDa [79, 80]. E protein is synthesized in large amounts during the replication cycle. However, a small amount is used for envelop formation [81]. A large portion of the E protein is present in the endoplasmic reticulum and Golgi complex, where it takes apart for assembly and budding formation [82]. The structure of E protein showed that it has two domains; a short hydrophilic domain contains 7-12 amino acids, and a large transmembrane hydrophobic domain comprises 25 amino acids presented in Fig. (**8**). Both domains end with carboxyl-terminal, *i.e.*, hydrophilic [83, 84]. The amphipathic α-helix present in the hydrophobic area of the E protein's transmembrane domain, which is formed an ion-conductive pore [82, 85]. The growth and replication of the virus require the host cell machinery. Many viruses like SARS-CoV-2 have utilized the host cell replication machinery to initiate infection by host-viral protein-protein interactions methods (PPIs) [86]. The first anti-apoptotic protein, such as Bcl-xL (B-cell lymphoma-extra-large), has been reported to interrelate with SARS-CoV-2 E protein during infection [87]. The SARS-CoVs E protein can associate with PALS1 (*Caenorhabditiselegans* lin-7 protein 1) through PDZ binding motif domain (PBM) *via* protein-protein interactions [88]. These different signaling techniques of SARS-CoVs are used for replication, growth, and pathogenesis during host cell interaction [89, 90]. The PBM is present in the last four amino acids of the SARS-CoV E C-terminal domain. The E protein binds different host proteins, including ATPase α-1 subunit, Bcl-xL, sodium/potassium (Na^+/K^+), stomatin, and PALS1. Enveloped proteins with Bcl-xl, PALS1, Na+/K+ ATPase α-1 subunit lead to lymphopenia, systemic infection, and decreased and imbalanced sodium channel in epithelial cells, respectively [14, 82, 87, 88]. Chromosomal investigation of SARS-CoV-2 E protein showed that the strong hydrophobicity is due to two neutral and non-polar amino acids, *i.e.*, valine and leucine, in the transmembrane domain region [45]. Two binding motifs, *i.e.*, postsynaptic density protein 95 and PBM binding motif recently discovered in E protein of SARS-CoVs [86, 91]. These binding motifs may be involved in the virulence of SARS-CoVs infection [88, 92]. The significance of the PBM motif domain has been studied in SARS-CoV-infected Vero cells. This PBM domain was investigated by deleting 9 amino acid residues but returned to virulence [14].

Evolutionary Resemblance/Comparison with SARS-CoV-2 and MERS-CoV Gene

Two major coronaviruses epidemics, namely SARS-CoV and MERS, have been reported in the last two decades [35]. On December 31, 2019, a new variant of coronavirus originated in Wuhan city, China, and has spread to more than two hundred countries worldwide. The virus termed SARS-CoV-2 and a disease called COVID-19 [48]. The origins of SARS-CoV-2, MERS-CoV, and SARS-CoV are primarily animals. Traveling and immunocompromised conditions of the human being are the most imminent threats to the transfer of COVID-19 worldwide. SARS-CoV, MERS-CoV, and SARS-CoV-2 have shared a variety of properties in terms of distribution and virulence. They cause respiratory problems in human beings. Human to human spread is possible among them. The SARS-CoV-2 is less virulent than that associated with SARS-CoV and MER-CoV in terms of mortality percentage [20].

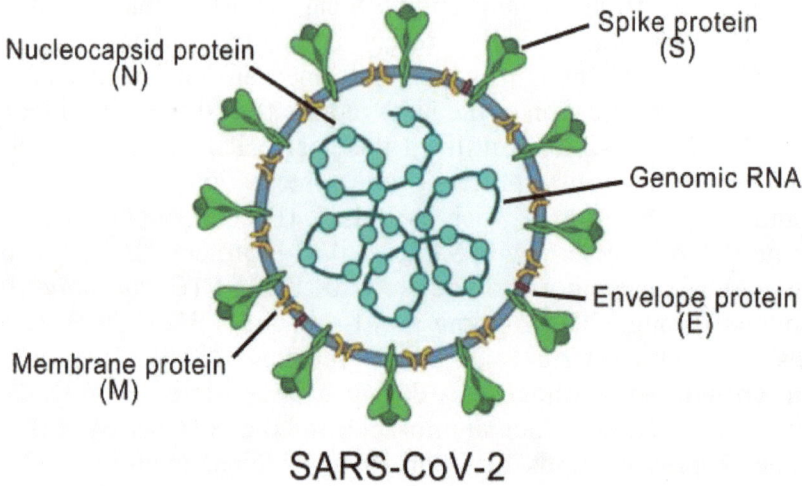

Fig. (8). The structural representation of the SARS-CoV E Protein. It comprises three domains, *i.e.*, N-terminal, T-terminal, and the C-terminal domain. The red color showed hydrophobic amino acid, and the blue color showed hydrophilic amino acids [14].

The genomic structure of SARS-CoV-2 is similar to MERS and SARS-CoV depicted in Fig. (**9**). It encloses ten open reading frames (ORFs). ORFs encode enzymes, *i.e.*, replicase, and four essential proteins, including E, S, M, and NC [20].

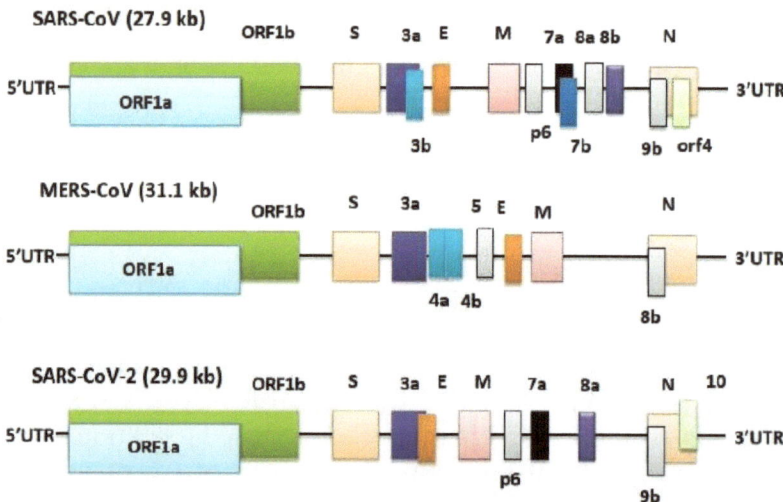

Fig. (9). Genomes comparison of SARS-CoV-2, MERS-CoV, and SARS-CoV [75].

Broncho-alveolar lavage fluid samples were collected from different viral pneumonia patients in china. They have all diagnosed COVID-19 with the help of the RT-PCR test and the next-generation sequencing method. Multiple sequence analysis of the COVID-19 genome showed that it is closely linked 87.99% and 87.23% to bat coronaviruses, *i.e.*, bat-SL-CoVZC45 bat-SL-CoVZXC21, respectively. E protein gene showed the highest similarities, *i.e.*, 98.7%, as followed by the S protein gene, *e.g.*, 75%. The SARS-CoV-2 genome shows less genetic likeness, *i.e.*, 79% and 50% of SARS-CoV and MERS-CoV, respectively. The S glycoprotein genome of SARS-CoV-2 is longer as compared to SARS-CoV and MERS-CoV S protein genes. The evolutionary analysis of RNA-dependent RNA polymerase and S protein genes has shown that these genes are far from SARS-CoV Spike and RNA-dependent RNA polymerase genes, indicating that it is a novel beta-coronavirus strain belonging to subgenus Sarbecovirus. The similarity between the S protein sub-domain S1 and S2 of SARS-CoV-2, and bat SARS-like coronavirus (bat-SL-CoVZC45 and bat-SL-CoVZXC21) have been reported 93% and 68%, respectively [30]. SARS-CoV-2 RBD of S1 was identical to the SARS-CoV S1 domain. Therefore, SARS-CoV and SARS-CoV-2 used similar ACE2 receptors to bind to the host cells. The gene sequence similarity of bat coronaviruses is less than 90% to SARS-CoV-2 which means that bats are not the direct descendants of COVID-19. Bat is the natural host of SARS-CoV, MERS-CoV, and SARS-CoV-2 [16, 75, 93].

Codon usage bias is another technique used for genomic evolutionary comparison of SARS-CoV-2 to SARS, MERS [59]. The virus structural and non-structural genes have been studied by the codon usage method [94]. Virus structural predominant S protein analysis showed that the number of thymine nucleotides was more, *i.e.*, 34%, followed by Adenine nucleotides, *e.g.*, 25%. The highest adenine-thymine (63%) ratio and lowest cytosine-guanine ratio (37%) have been observed in SARS-CoV-2 as compared with SARS-CoV and MERS-CoV [95]. Adenine and thymine are the predominant nucleotide in SARS-CoV-2 and are found in the 3rd position of the codon region [95]. Jiabao *et al.* [96] investigated the genetic homology of SARS-CoV-2 and SARS-CoV. The nucleotides sequence of both showed close homology. However, different regions of variation, *e.g.*, RD1-6, have been identified between them.

Replication of COVID-19 Lead to Pathogenesis

ORF1 is a specific gene present in all coronaviruses' downstream region.It encoded S and NC protein synthesis and helps in the replication process [97]. The S of glycoprotein is responsible for the binding of the SARS-CoV-2 virus to host cells. SARS-CoV-2 can use the same ACE2 receptors for cellular as MERS and SARS-CoV. These receptors are found in the lungs and alveoli of human beings. The cross-species and spread from person to person should be regulated by ACE2 receptors. The S glycoprotein of SARS-CoV-2 attaches with the ACE2 receptor on the surface of human cells. The binding efficacy of the glyco-Spike protein of SARS-CoV-2 with ACE2 is >20 times higher than the MERS and SARS-CoV [13]. Host cell proteases, *e.g.,* cell surface-associated transmembrane protease serine 2 (TMPRSS2), help cleavage or priming S protein after attachment presented in Fig. (**10**) [98].

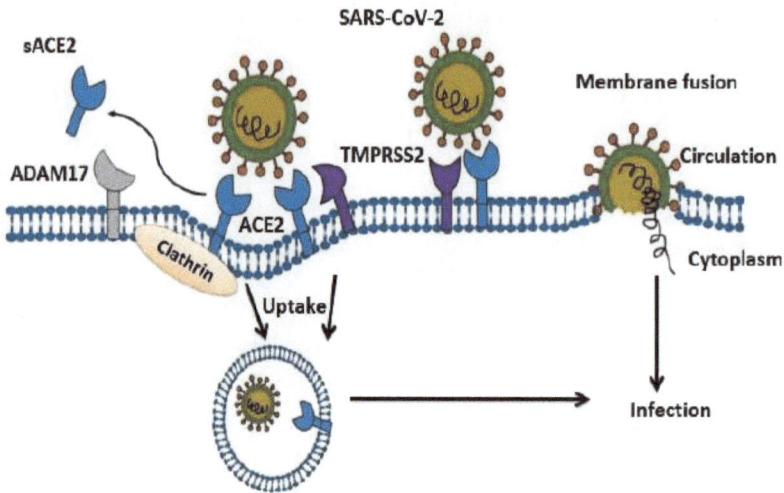

Fig. (10). ACE2 and TMPRSS2 receptor-mediated endocytosis [96].

Dipeptidyl peptidase four is a key receptor of MERS-CoV, while SARS-CoV-2 and HCoV-NL63 require ACE2 [99]. ACE2 receptor also presents other than the respiratory system, *e.g.,* brain, endothelial, and smooth cells in arteries. SARS-CoV-2 primarily attacks the lower respiratory tract, *e.g.,* alveoli and lungs, leading to alveolar damage and finally worsening respiratory misery presented in Fig.11 [44]. Therefore, SARS-CoV-2 spread other than the respiratory system. A similar pattern was seen in MERS-CoV and SARS-CoV infection [13].

S protein is further divided into two the S1 and S2 subunits. The primary function of the S1 subunit is to attach the virus through RBD and ACE2. S2 subunit helps envelop membrane fusion with the host cell membrane through the endosomal pathway [53]. After that, SARS-CoV-2 RNA is released into the host cytoplasm. The SARS-CoV-2 genomic RNA comprises approximately 28000 to 30000 nucleotides. These nucleotides encode several structural and non-structural proteins. Viral RNA synthesis or replicase-transcriptase proteins have a major role in the replication process. NC protein and nonstructural protein 2 (nsp2) are necessary for viral RNA synthesis. This encodes the open reading frame (ORF) 1a & 1b and contains produced two polyproteinsppla and pp1ab. Polyproteins, *e.g.,* pp1ab with ORF1a control ribosomal frame-shifting during the translation process. These polyproteins further produced different proteinases into small proteins. ORF 1a encodes non-structural proteins from NSP1-NSP11, and ORF1b translates non-structural proteins from NSP12-NSP16.Despite S protein fusion into host cells, other significant endocytic pathways like clathrin-dependent and independent help in virus entrance. The virus was assembled in the cytoplasm with the aid of viral RNA and proteins present at Golgi complex and endoplasmic reticulum. Finally, virions are released from host cells *via* vesicles presented in Fig. (**12**) [98].

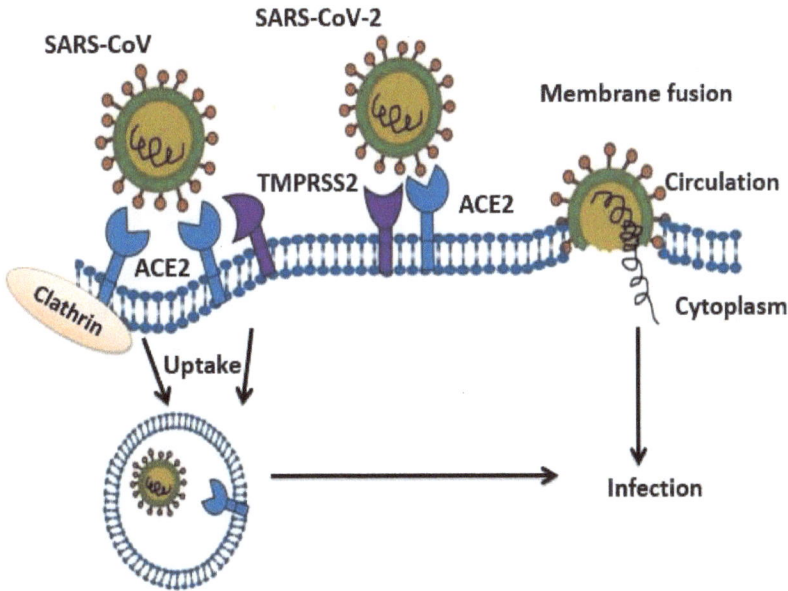

Fig. (11). The S protein of SARS-CoV-2 and SARS-CoV can attach the same receptors, *i.e.*, ACE2 and host cell protease TMPRSS2 [100].

Factors Involve in COVID-19 Pathogenesis

Host factors such as receptors, immune status, unusual habits *e.g.* smoking, *etc.* are significant values regarding pathogenesis [102]. Among them, the ACE2 receptor has a higher value. It belongs to the zinc metalloprotease of the angiotensin-converting enzyme family. The human ACE2 comprises 805 amino acids containing the catalytic domain in the N-terminal side and cytoplasmic tail from the C-terminal side of peptides [33]. Carboxypeptidase is broken down into ACE2 into I and II. Human ACE2 present in the different regions such as in nasal mucosa, tongue, oral mucosa, nasopharynx, smooth muscles in the arterial system, endothelial cells in the venous system, epithelial cells in trachea and alveoli, stratified epithelial cells in the esophagus, ileum, and colon. It is also present in myocardial cells, brain, urothelial cells in the bladder and renal proximal tubular cells [103]. The extensiveexpression of ACE2 in various tissue or organs has been associated with pathogenesis leading to pulmonary inflammation, loss of taste, neuritis, arthritis, pneumonitis, immune system dysfunction, and may cause multi-organ dysfunction during the advanced stage of SARS-CoV-2 infection [26, 42]. Blood coagulation has been found in all patients infected with COVID-19. However, there is no relationship between COVID-19 and disseminated intravascular coagulation (DIC). During a hypoxic state, vasoconstriction of alveolar capillaries can reduce blood pressure and activate the hypoxia-inducible factors. It inhibits the tissue factor and plasminogen activator inhibitor-1 (PAI-1) [104].

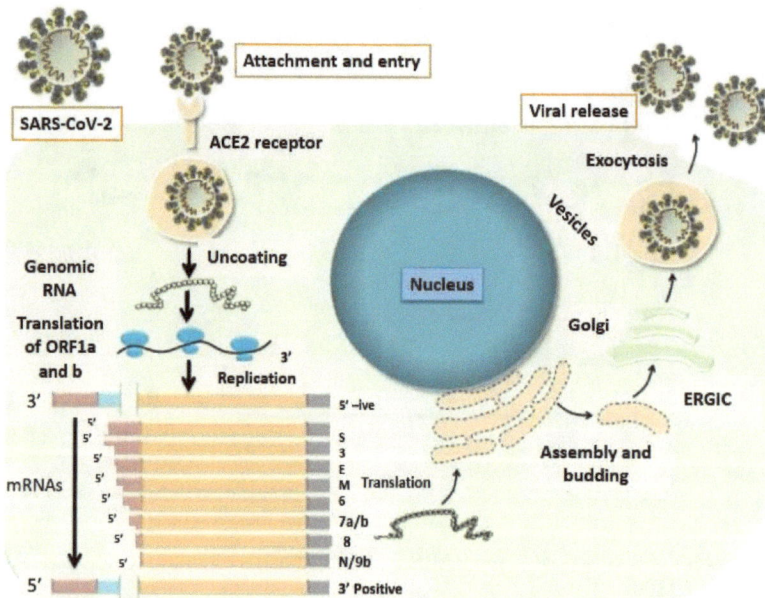

Fig. (12). Replication strategy of COVID-19 in host cells. Biosynthesis of different structural proteins and transcription of the RNA genome. Spike protein of SARS-CoV-2 binds with the ACE2 receptor of host cells. Then uncoating is done into the cytoplasm of the host cell. Translation of ORF1a and ORF1b encodes a non-structural protein (NSP1-NSP12). Finally, assembly of virion takes place and releases virions *via*vesicles by exocytosis [101].

ACE2 is an important regulator of the renin-angiotensin system (RAS). Angiotensin I, having no direct biological activity, exists as a precursor to angiotensin II and is transformed to the latter by removing two C-terminal residues fromACE2 primarily in the lung, kidneys, endothelial cells, and brain. Angiotensin II acts on venous and arterial smooth muscles to induce vasoconstriction and increase the CNS development. It also stimulates the secretion of aldosterone. It appears that apart from gaining its entry through the ACE2, the SARS-CoV-2 subsequently down-regulates the ACE2 expression leading to loss of its protective effects in various organs, which may have a significant impact on the pathogenesis of the disease. ACE2 expression is decreased in both males and females during aging. However, numerous animal research showed no gender-linked change of ACE2 expression, particularly in adult mice [105]. Yet, epidemiological data of new variants of coronavirus, *i.e.*, SARS-CoV-2, reported that sex and age have a significant value of susceptibility to SARS-CoV-2 infection. There is a strong relationship with various host determinants, *e.g.*, male sex, elderly age group, the existence of other chronic heart and lung diseases that are the most affected during the COVID-19 pandemic. In addition, data also showed that mortality was observed in those over 60 years of age with diabetes, heart, and pulmonary disease [106]. Raza *et al.* [107] reflect prevalence and genotypic analysis of SARS-CoV-2 patterns in Faisalabad, Pakistan, in which 37-47-year-old patients found high prevalence, *i.e.*, 17.18% however, no case was reported in children. The genome SARS-CoV-2 was isolated and characterized by clustering analysis. Genomic analysis of local isolate confirmed the similarity, *i.e.*, 79% towards SARS-CoVs.

The RBD of S protein initiated the attachment of SARS-CoV-2 with host cell ACE2 receptor. A similar pattern of attachment was reported during SARS-CoV and MERS-CoV infection. The host protease converts S protein into two subunits S1 and S2. The ACE2 receptor is mainly found in the bronchiolar epithelial cells, endothelial and smooth muscle cells of pulmonary vessels, *e.g.*, nerves and arteries, and epithelium of type II alveolar cells in the lungs. ACE2 is rich in differentiated cells as compared to poorly expressed in undifferentiated cells. These findings of the different studies help to explain the virulence of COVID-19 [54]. Due to its large surface area and high expressed ACE2 receptors, the lung is the most predominant target organ for SARS-CoV-2 infection. The alveolar type II cells act as a reservoir for the SARS-CoV-2 invasion due to the large-scale expression of ACE2 [108]. The relationship between human ACE2 with SARS-CoVs leads to the spread of the individual and severity of the disease [48]. The mutation of S proteins affects the binding ability to hACE2 [109]. To understand this mechanism or the binding ability of the S protein of SARS-CoV-2 used the biolayer interferometry method. We studied binding affinity and kinetics with hACE2 with SARS-CoV and SARS-CoV. The fourteen binding sites, *e.g.*, R426, Y475, Y440, T402, T487, Y491, Y484, Y442, Y436, G488, N473, Y491, Y472, and L472, of SARS-CoV with hACE2 had been reported previously [31]. Eight positions out of fourteen are conserved in SARS-CoV-2, although six sites are semi-conserved [1].

Animals and humans are the natural hosts of coronaviruses. They can cause mild to severe diseases in both animals and humans. The first epidemic of SARS-CoV infection was identified in 2002, China Province Guangdong leading to 774 deaths out of 8089 cases. SARS-CoV belongs to the genus beta coronavirus. The mortality rate of SARS-CoV infection may be as high as 50%, especially in patients over 60 years of age., The horseshoe bat is the natural reservoir host of SARS-CoV [110]. SARS-CoV was transmitted with the infected person only by direct or indirect methods after the onset of the disease. Strict quarantine measurements minimized this outbreak. The new variant of human coronavirus, *i.e.*, MERS-CoV, was identified and characterized in 2012. It caused severe respiratory system infection in human beings, and there was 29% case fatality rate worldwide. However, the plague did not exist after 2013. This information helps to understand the origination, replication, and pathogenesis of human coronaviruses [48].

The immune system of the host cell is another significant factor of SARS-CoV-2 infection leading to pathogenesis. The innate and adaptive immune system responded to viral infection and cleared the virus into the body of an infected individual. The Rig-1-like receptor family of an innate immune system has an essential role during initial infection. This family contains retinoic acid-inducible gene-1 (RIG-1), melanoma differentiation-associated protein-5 (MDA-5), and stimulator of interferon genes (STING), which recognized the viral ligands in the cytosol and also stimulated the IFN-β and inflammatory response [111]. MDA-5 is considered a more powerful cytosolic sensor for the recognition of SARS-CoV. Toll-like receptors also could recognize human coronaviruses. These sensors stimulate NF-κB, IRF3, and IRF7 (interferon regulatory factors 3 and 7), leading to activation of INF genes and pro-inflammatory cytokines.

The endoplasmic reticulum stress is closely linked with SARS-CoV infection and replication. The endoplasmic reticulum can maintain the protein synthesis of the host cell. During infection, the ER's capacity is overwhelmed, misfolded, and unfolded protein aggregated in the lumen, which initiates the ER stress [112]. The ER stress stimulates the unfolded protein response pathways (UPR) with the help of protein kinase RNA-like endoplasmic reticulum kinase (PERK). The stimulation of UPR has two main functions: first, increase the level of eIF2α (Eukaryotic Initiation Factor 2 alpha) and, secondly, stop protein synthesis production.

MERS-CoV generated ORF4a protein that inhibits endoplasmic reticulum induces stress granules. Moreover, pro-apoptotic genes are activated; inhibit the production of anti-apoptotic Bcl-2 proteins, and escape calcium to the cytoplasm during prolonged ER stress. These adoptive steps of the host cells are utilized to kill the replication process of the virus. On the other hand, CoV used multiple t escape mechanisms to destroy the immune system, increasing the magnitudes and length of the disease [112]. The S protein of SARS-CoV-2 inhibits or reduced the production of eIF3F, which modified the host translation process by decreasing the production of the pro-inflammatory cytokines, *e.g.,* IL-6, and IL-8 at an advanced phase of infection. These modulations play an essential role in SARS-CoV-2 the virulency, the severity, duration, and prognosis of the disease [112].

The epidemic, severity, and duration of diseases depend upon the route of transmission of SARS-CoV-2 infection. This virus mainly transfers infected individuals to healthy individuals by tiny respiratory droplets during coughing or sneezing [113]. On average, 3000 respiratory droplets should be produced during a single cough. These droplets contaminate land on different types of surfaces. These infected surfaces often transmit the virus to healthy individuals. The virus can withstand up to 3 days, 4 hours, and 24 hours in plastic and stainless steel, copper, and cardboard, respectively [[114]]. The SARS-CoV-2 will stay in the air for at least 3 hours. Indirect or fomites spread is not known to be the root cause of SARS-CoV-2 infection spread. This transmission method is minimized by using hand sanitizer, soap washing, and sterilization of the contaminated surfaces [115].

When SARS-CoV-2 entered the respiratory tract during the coughing of infected individuals and traveled through the respiratory tract, particularly through the mucosal membrane of the lung alveoli. S protein of the virus attaches with the help of surface receptors on the type II pneumocyte cells [113]. After binding, the virus entered the cytoplasm by receptors mediated endocytosis. Lysosomal enzymes break down the lipid layer of the virus. SARS-CoV-2 virus produced polyproteins in the host cell that will start replication with the help of the host RNA-dependent RNA polymerase. These polyproteins also synthesize structural proteins, *e.g.,* S, E, M, and NC of the virus [111]. The alveolar cells are damaged after releasing SARS-CoV-2 during budding. This destruction of pneumocytes activates pro-inflammatory mediators, *e.g.,* TNF-α, IL-1 &IL-6 [112]. Acute inflammation is seen in fever due to the release of IL-1 &IL-6 [116].

Moreover, these inflammatory mediators dilate and contract the blood vessel smooth muscles, leading to an increase in the permeability of the blood vessels. This can result in the leakage of plasma from the bloodstream, causing edema in type II pneumocyte cells. After the breakdown of the alveolar type II pneumocyte cells, it may stop the production of surfactant, hypoxia, dyspnea, shortness of breath, and developed severe condition, *i.e.,* acute respiratory distress syndrome (ARDS). The incubation period of COVID-19 ranges from 6-41 days. However, the average period is 5-7 days, primarily depends upon the age and immune status of the patients [105, 116]. Many other factors, *e.g.,* existing asthma, heart diseases, lung diseases, diabetes, smoking, use of ACE2 inhibitors, increased or greater the risk of COVID-19. ACE2 inhibitors increased 3-5 times of ACE2 upregulation, which exponentially amplified the replication of SARS-CoV-2, causing the development of the severe disease. Therefore, pre-existing hypertension condition patients are at more risk of SARS-CoV2 infection [117, 118].

The expression and secretion of ACE2 are more in chronic vascular diseases. Yet, severe COVID-19 has been documented in those who already have the chronic vascular disease [66]. Elderly-aged peoples with pre-existing medical conditions are more susceptible to COVID-19 than a healthy 30-year-old individual. In elder age, lung anatomic structure changes and atrophy of muscles lead to alteration of the respiratory tract's physiological function, *e.g.,* decreased lung reserve, immune barriers, and airway clearance mechanism. The ACE2 receptor also increased in the elderly. This manifestation results in a severe form of COVID-19 in aged people. Cardiovascular patients are more susceptible to infection with COVID-19 [66]. During SRAS-CoV-2 infection, cytokine storm produced which destruct the myocardial cells [24]. Numerous signs and symptoms, *e.g.,* fever, fatigue, anxiety, headache, cough, and dyspnea, were reported at the commencement of COVID-19. As stated earlier, the average incubation period is 5-7 days. Non-specific symptoms, just like the common cold, were present during the start of infection, yet, severe respiratory symptoms, *e.g.,* dyspnea, coughing, sneezing, *etc.*, are directly proportional to the replication of the virus [116]. The duration and severity of COVID-19 are directly proportional to the immune system of an individual [119].

Asymptomatic or milder symptoms have been observed if a person has a robust immune system. The strong immunity from individual control cytokine storm and inflammation during infection. The weak immune system with pre-existing medical illness leading to the more severe complications of COVID-19 [113]. Healthcare practitioners, for example, doctors, will manage symptomatic treatment. They placed the patient on a ventilator in the advanced stages of infection. The lethal complication of COVID-19, *i.e.*, ARDS was initiated 8 days after infection. ACE2 receptors are not only present in alveolar lung cells but also in the gastrointestinal tract enterocytes cells. Therefore, fatal pneumonia with diarrheal symptoms has been documented in older patients [25]. Opportunistic bacteria, *e.g., Streptococcus pneumonia, Haemophilus influenza,* and *Klebsiella pneumonia* may cause secondary bacterial pneumonia after 2nd week of infection [120].

Conserved genes of SARS-CoV-2

The RNA genome of SARS-CoV-2 consists of an open reading frame used for the replication process, accessory, and structural proteins. It is the most giant size positive-sense RNA virus and has a genome size of approximately 30 kb.

Moreover, it also contains *cis*-acting RNA in the untranslated region in 5 and 3 prime positions. *Cis*-acting RNA helps with replication, protein synthesis, and the packaging process [121]. A conserved region of SARS-CoV-2 RNA elements supports the diagnosis and antiviral targeting to cure the infection. Conserved structures play a significant role in the replication cycles of coronaviruses. Four stemloops are present in the 5th position of the UTR region and help in the replication process [122].

SARS-CoV-2 sequences contain conserved sequences, *i.e.*, the '3' and '5' untranslated region and the frame-shifting element. Fig. (**13**) represents the overlapping between SARS-CoV-2-conserved structured and SARS-CoV-2-conserved-unstructured sets [123].

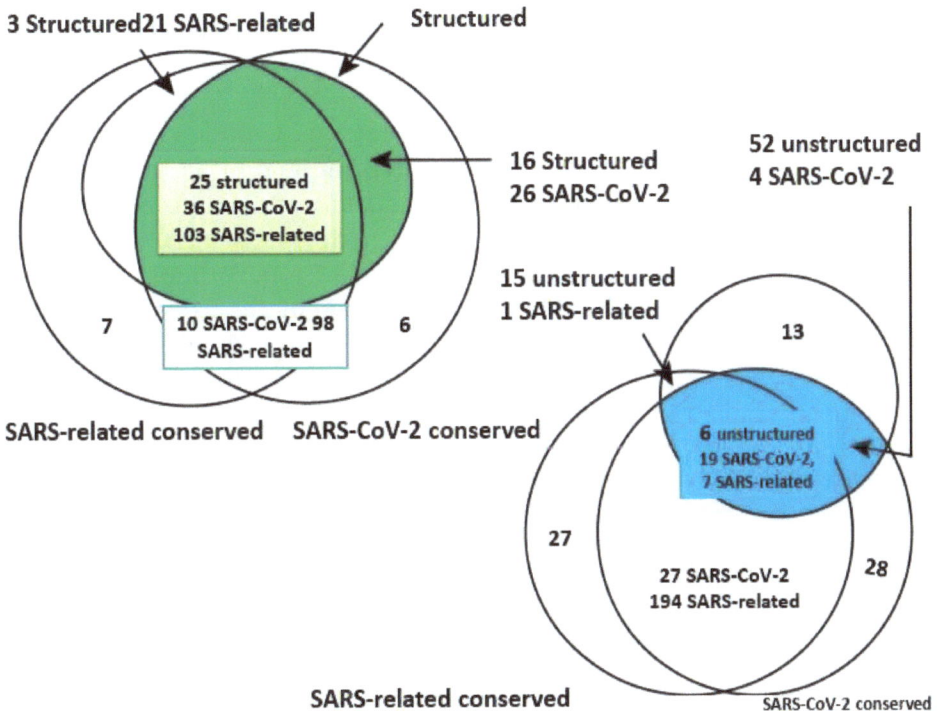

Fig. (13). Comparison between SARS-CoV-2 structured and SARS-CoV-2 unstructured region [123].

The RNA of coronavirus is infectious due to quick transcription and translation. The polymerase coding area is located at the 5' end of the SARS-CoV-2 genome and is composed of two open reading frames, *i.e.*, ORF1a and ORF1b. The S protein of SARS-CoV-2 has been shown in some conserved regions. It is further subdivided into S1 and S2 subunits. The S protein subunit S2 showed nucleotide sequence similarity towards about bat-SL-CoVZC45 coronavirus up to 94%. However, the S1 subunit had nucleotide sequence similarity towards bat-S--CoVZXC21 coronavirus of just68%. S1 domain is further categorized into N-terminal and C-terminal domains. Both of them can bind ACE2 host cell receptors [10, 124].

Roujian *et al.* [16] studied variation between amino acid sequences of SARS-CoV-2 S protein. Fifty preserved amino acid sequences have been identified between the SI subunit of the S protein of SARS-CoV-2 and SARS-CoV. Mutational variation was also observed in Bat coronaviruses in the S1 subunit. Deletion mutations were found in the C-terminal domain of the S1 subunit, particularly in bat-derived coronaviruses. Significant preserved immunogenic epitopes, *i.e.*, AO, havee been identified in the SARS-CoV-2 S protein subunit S2. AO4 is also present in SARS-CoV. 64% of amino acid homology of S1 subunits SARS-CoV-2 and SARS-CoV has been detected [125].

NC of SAR-CoV-2 contains three conserved regions include NTD (N-terminal RNA-binding domain), CTD (C-terminal dimerization domain), and SR (Ser/Arg linker). These are responsible for RNA attachment, oligomerization, and phosphorylation, respectively [126]. The detailed crystal structure of the NC protein of infectious bronchitis virus, SARS-CoV, mouse hepatitis virus, and HCoV-OC43 has been reported [127, 128]. Though, the novel nucleoprotein structure of SARS-CoV-2 remainsmostly unknown. The encoding region of the NC protein is conserved. Yet minor deviations between the virus strain Foshan and the Wuhan viral strain were observed. The SARS-CoV-2 encoding region of N protein amino acid sequences similarity of SARS-CoV-2, SARS-CoV, HCoV-OC43, and MERS-CoV were 90, 49, 48, and 36%, respectively [126, 129].

The E protein of the variant SARS-CoV-2 showed two conserved region features, *i.e.*, PBM (PDZ-binding Motif) and ion-channel. These stimulate cytokine storm and inflammation leading to the development of severe ARDS, *i.e.*, the main cause of mortality in COVID-19 [26]. Intikhab *et al.* [130] compared SARS-Co--2 E protein sequences for all known sequences present in the NCBI database to validate the conserved encoding region. This investigation showed that the homology of E protein of SARS-CoV-2 encoding conserved region in SARS and two bat-coronaviruses is 95% and 100%, respectively.

Non-conserved or Noncoding Genes of SARS-CoV-2

Non-conserved sequences have significant effects on controlling gene regulation during transcription. Tong *et al.* [131] investigated S and nucleoprotein non-conserved sequences in patients infected with SARS-CoV. Ten samples were collected and sequenced. The results of all samples showed that the S protein comprised the same 3768 nucleotides at the open reading frame that encoded 1255 amino acids. The nucleoprotein encoded the 422 amino acids and observed deletion, frameshift, and insertion in an open reading frame position. There was variation of three nucleotides sequences in S4, S7, and S8 patients. The arginine changes into glycine position at 29347 positions in the nucleoprotein gene obtained from the S4 patient. This result predicted that asparagine would change into aspartic acid due to the presence of non-conserved amino acids. The phenylalanine changes into serine at 22570 position of nucleotide in the S protein gene from S8 patient also due to non-conserved sequence.

Khailany *et al.* [132] studied the 95 genome sequences of SARS-CoV-2 available in GenBank. The sequence showed a strong relationship between the time and location of sample collection and genetic diversity. There were 116 mutations investigated. Among them, maximum mutations were observed in the ORF1ab gene, ORF8 gene in the N gene. The genomic variant of SARS-CoV-2 comprises 14 non-coding alleles, 46 missense, 2 insertions, and 1 deletion. All non-conservation genomic alterations were at 5' UTR or 3' UTR regions. The changes in amino acid sequences affect the rigorousness and transfer of the SARS-CoV-2 globally. The detailed knowledge about non-conserved genes in SARS-CoV-2 is still unknown.

CONCLUSION

The origin of the pandemic of SARS-CoV-2 in Wuhan, China, has spread worldwide. It will become a global threat towards the general public, specifically the elderly, immunocompromised, and healthcare staff. So, the zoonotic spread of this virus is not confirmed, but the phylogenetic analysis has shown that the bat is the primary reservoir host. SARS-CoV-2 is a novel strain comprised of a positive-sense RNA genome, enveloped lipid bilayer, and 30kb size approximately. The genetic sequence of SARS-CoV-2 belongs to lineage B *betacoronaviruses*, whichare more than 90% identical to bat and pangolin coronavirus genomes. The structure of SARS-CoV-2 consists of different structural proteins, including S (S), M, E, and NC. Phylogenetic analysis confirmed that this novel strain of the coronavirus is closely linked to MERS-CoV and SARS-CoV. Angiotensin-converting enzyme 2 is a primary receptor forSARS-CoV-2. The S protein of SARS-CoV-2 binds with the ACE2 receptor on the surface of human cells. The binding efficacy of the S protein of SARS-CoV-2 with ACE2 is > 20 fold higher as compared to the MERS-CoV and SARS-CoV. There is a strong relationship with several host determinants, *e.g.,* male sex, elderly age group, existence of other chronic heart and lung diseases that are the most affected during the COVID-19 pandemic. In addition, data also showed that mortality with diabetes, heart disease, and pulmonary disease was observed at over 60 years of age.

CONSENT FOR PUBLICATION

Not Applicable.

CONFLICT OF INTEREST

The author confirms that this chapter contents have no conflict of interest.

ACKNOWLEDGEMENT

Declared none.

REFERENCES

[1]   Walls AC, Park Y-J, Tortorici MA, Wall A, McGuire AT, Veesler D. Structure, function, and antigenicity of the SARS-CoV-2 spike glycoprotein. Cell 2020.
        [http://dx.doi.org/10.1016/j.cell.2020.11.032]

[2]   King AM, Adams MJ, Carstens EB, Lefkowitz EJ. Virus taxonomy. Ninth report of the International Committee on Taxonomy of Viruses 2012; 486-7.

[3]   Sexton NR, Smith EC, Blanc H, Vignuzzi M, Peersen OB, Denison MR. Homology-based identification of a mutation in the coronavirus RNA-dependent RNA polymerase that confers resistance to multiple mutagens. J Virol 2016; 90(16): 7415-28.
        [http://dx.doi.org/10.1128/JVI.00080-16] [PMID: 27279608]

[4]   Ye Z-W, Yuan S, Yuen K-S, Fung S-Y, Chan C-P, Jin D-Y. Zoonotic origins of human coronaviruses. Int J Biol Sci 2020; 16(10): 1686-97.
        [http://dx.doi.org/10.7150/ijbs.45472] [PMID: 32226286]

[5]   Chan JF-W, Kok K-H, Zhu Z, *et al.* Genomic characterization of the 2019 novel human-pathogenic coronavirus isolated from a patient with atypical pneumonia after visiting Wuhan. Emerg Microbes Infect 2020; 9(1): 221-36.
        [http://dx.doi.org/10.1080/22221751.2020.1719902] [PMID: 31987001]

[6]   Su S, Wong G, Shi W, *et al.* Epidemiology, genetic recombination, and pathogenesis of coronaviruses. Trends Microbiol 2016; 24(6): 490-502.
        [http://dx.doi.org/10.1016/j.tim.2016.03.003] [PMID: 27012512]

[7]   Zhou P, Yang X-L, Wang X-G, *et al.* A pneumonia outbreak associated with a new coronavirus of probable bat origin. nature 2020; 579(7798): 270-3.

[8]   Alshukairi AN, Zheng J, Zhao J, *et al.* High prevalence of MERS-CoV infection in camel workers in Saudi Arabia. MBio 2018; 9(5): e01985-18.
        [http://dx.doi.org/10.1128/mBio.01985-18] [PMID: 30377284]

[9]   Yin Y, Wunderink RG. MERS, SARS and other coronaviruses as causes of pneumonia. Respirology 2018; 23(2): 130-7.
        [http://dx.doi.org/10.1111/resp.13196] [PMID: 29052924]

[10]   Zhou P, Yang X-L, Wang X-G, *et al.* Discovery of a novel coronavirus associated with the recent pneumonia outbreak in humans and its potential bat origin. BioRxiv 2020.
        [http://dx.doi.org/10.1101/2020.01.22.914952]

[11]   Sah R, Rodriguez-Morales AJ, Jha R, *et al.* Complete genome sequence of a 2019 novel coronavirus (SARS-CoV-2) strain isolated in Nepal. Microbiol Resour Announc 2020; 9(11): e00169-20.

[http://dx.doi.org/10.1128/MRA.00169-20] [PMID: 32165386]

[12]   Shereen MA, Khan S, Kazmi A, Bashir N, Siddique R. COVID-19 infection: Origin, transmission, and characteristics of human coronaviruses. J Adv Res 2020; 24: 91-8.
[http://dx.doi.org/10.1016/j.jare.2020.03.005] [PMID: 32257431]

[13]   Wrapp D, Wang N, Corbett KS, *et al.* Cryo-EM structure of the 2019-nCoV spike in the prefusion conformation. Science 2020; 367(6483): 1260-3.
[http://dx.doi.org/10.1126/science.abb2507] [PMID: 32075877]

[14]   Schoeman D, Fielding BC. Coronavirus envelope protein: current knowledge. Virol J 2019; 16(1): 69.
[http://dx.doi.org/10.1186/s12985-019-1182-0] [PMID: 31133031]

[15]   Shang W, Yang Y, Rao Y, Rao X. The outbreak of SARS-CoV-2 pneumonia calls for viral vaccines. *npj.* Vaccines (Basel) 2020; 5(1): 1-3.
[PMID: 33375151]

[16]   Lu R, Zhao X, Li J, *et al.* Genomic characterisation and epidemiology of 2019 novel coronavirus: implications for virus origins and receptor binding. Lancet 2020; 395(10224): 565-74.
[http://dx.doi.org/10.1016/S0140-6736(20)30251-8] [PMID: 32007145]

[17]   Forster P, Forster L, Renfrew C, Forster M. Phylogenetic network analysis of SARS-CoV-2 genomes. Proc Natl Acad Sci USA 2020; 117(17): 9241-3.
[http://dx.doi.org/10.1073/pnas.2004999117] [PMID: 32269081]

[18]   Drummond AJ, Suchard MA, Xie D, Rambaut A. Bayesian phylogenetics with BEAUti and the BEAST 1.7. Mol Biol Evol 2012; 29(8): 1969-73.
[http://dx.doi.org/10.1093/molbev/mss075] [PMID: 22367748]

[19]   Hu D, Zhu C, Ai L, *et al.* Genomic characterization and infectivity of a novel SARS-like coronavirus in Chinese bats. Emerg Microbes Infect 2018; 7(1): 154.
[http://dx.doi.org/10.1038/s41426-018-0155-5] [PMID: 30209269]

[20]   Li Q, Guan X, Wu P, *et al.* Early transmission dynamics in Wuhan, China, of novel coronavirus–infected pneumonia. N Engl J Med 2020; 382(13): 1199-207.
[http://dx.doi.org/10.1056/NEJMoa2001316] [PMID: 31995857]

[21]   Zehender G, Lai A, Bergna A, *et al.* Genomic characterization and phylogenetic analysis of SARS-COV-2 in Italy. J Med Virol 2020; 92(9): 1637-40.
[http://dx.doi.org/10.1002/jmv.25794] [PMID: 32222993]

[22]   Zhang T, Wu Q, Zhang Z. Probable pangolin origin of SARS-CoV-2 associated with the COVID-19 outbreak. Curr Biol 2020.
[http://dx.doi.org/10.1016/j.cub.2020.03.063]

[23]   Price MN, Dehal PS, Arkin AP. FastTree 2--approximately maximum-likelihood trees for large alignments. PLoS One 2010; 5(3): e9490.
[http://dx.doi.org/10.1371/journal.pone.0009490] [PMID: 20224823]

[24]   Liu K, Chen Y, Lin R, Han K. Clinical features of COVID-19 in elderly patients: A comparison with young and middle-aged patients. J Infect 2020; 80(6): e14-8.
[http://dx.doi.org/10.1016/j.jinf.2020.03.005] [PMID: 32171866]

[25]   Lu H, Stratton CW, Tang YW. Outbreak of pneumonia of unknown etiology in Wuhan, China: The mystery and the miracle. J Med Virol 2020; 92(4): 401-2.
[http://dx.doi.org/10.1002/jmv.25678] [PMID: 31950516]

[26]   Huang C, Wang Y, Li X, *et al.* Clinical features of patients infected with 2019 novel coronavirus in Wuhan, China. Lancet 2020; 395(10223): 497-506.
[http://dx.doi.org/10.1016/S0140-6736(20)30183-5] [PMID: 31986264]

[27]   Adebali O, Bircan A, Circi D, *et al.* Phylogenetic Analysis of SARS-CoV-2 Genomes in Turkey. bioRxiv 2020.

[28]   Rehman SU, Shafique L, Ihsan A, Liu Q. Evolutionary trajectory for the emergence of novel coronavirus SARS-CoV-2. Pathogens 2020; 9(3): 240.
[http://dx.doi.org/10.3390/pathogens9030240] [PMID: 32210130]

[29]   Fauver JR, Petrone ME, Hodcroft EB, *et al.* Coast-to-coast spread of SARS-CoV-2 during the early epidemic in the United States. Cell 2020; 181(5): 990-996.e5.
[http://dx.doi.org/10.1016/j.cell.2020.04.021] [PMID: 32386545]

[30]   Zhu N, Zhang D, Wang W, *et al.* A novel coronavirus from patients with pneumonia in China, 2019. N Engl J Med 2020; 382(8): 727-33.
[http://dx.doi.org/10.1056/NEJMoa2001017] [PMID: 31978945]

[31]   Li F, Li W, Farzan M, Harrison SC. Structure of SARS coronavirus spike receptor-binding domain complexed with receptor. Science 2005; 309(5742): 1864-8.
[http://dx.doi.org/10.1126/science.1116480] [PMID: 16166518]

[32]   Xu J, Zhao S, Teng T, *et al.* Systematic comparison of two animal-to-human transmitted human coronaviruses: SARS-CoV-2 and SARS-CoV. Viruses 2020; 12(2): 244.
[http://dx.doi.org/10.3390/v12020244] [PMID: 32098422]

[33]   Hamming I, Timens W, Bulthuis M, Lely A, Navis Gv, van Goor H. Tissue distribution of ACE2 protein, the functional receptor for SARS coronavirus. A first step in understanding SARS pathogenesis. The Journal of Pathology: A Journal of the Pathological Society of Great Britain and Ireland 2004; 203(2): 631-7.

[34]   Kabbani N, Olds JL. Does COVID19 infect the brain? If so, smokers might be at a higher risk. Mol Pharmacol 2020; 97(5): 351-3.
[http://dx.doi.org/10.1124/molpharm.120.000014] [PMID: 32238438]

[35]   Cui J, Li F, Shi Z-L. Origin and evolution of pathogenic coronaviruses. Nat Rev Microbiol 2019; 17(3): 181-92.
[http://dx.doi.org/10.1038/s41579-018-0118-9] [PMID: 30531947]

[36]   Fehr AR. Perlman, S.Coronaviruses. Springer 2015; pp. 1-23.
[http://dx.doi.org/10.1007/978-1-4939-2438-7_1]

[37]   Hofmann H, Pyrc K, van der Hoek L, Geier M, Berkhout B, Pöhlmann S. Human coronavirus NL63 employs the severe acute respiratory syndrome coronavirus receptor for cellular entry. Proc Natl Acad Sci USA 2005; 102(22): 7988-93.
[http://dx.doi.org/10.1073/pnas.0409465102] [PMID: 15897467]

[38]   Qi F, Qian S, Zhang S, Zhang Z. Single cell RNA sequencing of 13 human tissues identify cell types and receptors of human coronaviruses. Biochem Biophys Res Commun 2020; 526(1): 135-40.
[http://dx.doi.org/10.1016/j.bbrc.2020.03.044] [PMID: 32199615]

[39]   Li M-Y, Li L, Zhang Y, Wang X-S. Expression of the SARS-CoV-2 cell receptor gene ACE2 in a wide variety of human tissues. Infect Dis Poverty 2020; 9(1): 45.
[http://dx.doi.org/10.1186/s40249-020-00662-x] [PMID: 32345362]

[40]   Ma D, Chen C-B, Jhanji V, *et al.* Expression of SARS-CoV-2 receptor ACE2 and TMPRSS2 in human primary conjunctival and pterygium cell lines and in mouse cornea. Eye (Lond) 2020; 34(7): 1212-9.
[http://dx.doi.org/10.1038/s41433-020-0939-4] [PMID: 32382146]

[41]   Baig AM, Khaleeq A, Ali U, Syeda H. Evidence of the COVID-19 virus targeting the CNS: tissue distribution, host–virus interaction, and proposed neurotropic mechanisms. ACS Chem Neurosci 2020; 11(7): 995-8.
[http://dx.doi.org/10.1021/acschemneuro.0c00122] [PMID: 32167747]

[42]   Xu X, Chen P, Wang J, *et al.* Evolution of the novel coronavirus from the ongoing Wuhan outbreak and modeling of its spike protein for risk of human transmission. Sci China Life Sci 2020; 63(3): 457-60.

[http://dx.doi.org/10.1007/s11427-020-1637-5] [PMID: 32009228]

[43]   Zou X, Chen K, Zou J, Han P, Hao J, Han Z. Single-cell RNA-seq data analysis on the receptor ACE2 expression reveals the potential risk of different human organs vulnerable to 2019-nCoV infection. Front Med 2020; 14(2): 185-92.
[http://dx.doi.org/10.1007/s11684-020-0754-0] [PMID: 32170560]

[44]   Xu H, Zhong L, Deng J, *et al.* High expression of ACE2 receptor of 2019-nCoV on the epithelial cells of oral mucosa. Int J Oral Sci 2020; 12(1): 8.
[http://dx.doi.org/10.1038/s41368-020-0074-x] [PMID: 32094336]

[45]   Wu Q, Zhang Y, Lü H, *et al.* The E protein is a multifunctional membrane protein of SARS-CoV. Genomics Proteomics Bioinformatics 2003; 1(2): 131-44.
[http://dx.doi.org/10.1016/S1672-0229(03)01017-9] [PMID: 15626343]

[46]   Song W, Gui M, Wang X, Xiang Y. Cryo-EM structure of the SARS coronavirus spike glycoprotein in complex with its host cell receptor ACE2. PLoS Pathog 2018; 14(8): e1007236.
[http://dx.doi.org/10.1371/journal.ppat.1007236] [PMID: 30102747]

[47]   Li Y, Surya W, Claudine S, Torres J. Structure of a conserved Golgi complex-targeting signal in coronavirus envelope proteins. J Biol Chem 2014; 289(18): 12535-49.
[http://dx.doi.org/10.1074/jbc.M114.560094] [PMID: 24668816]

[48]   Wan Y, Shang J, Graham R, Baric RS, Li F. Receptor recognition by the novel coronavirus from Wuhan: an analysis based on decade-long structural studies of SARS coronavirus. J Virol 2020; 94(7): e00127-20.
[http://dx.doi.org/10.1128/JVI.00127-20] [PMID: 31996437]

[49]   Du L, Tai W, Yang Y, *et al.* Introduction of neutralizing immunogenicity index to the rational design of MERS coronavirus subunit vaccines. Nat Commun 2016; 7(1): 13473.
[http://dx.doi.org/10.1038/ncomms13473] [PMID: 27874853]

[50]   He Y, Li J, Heck S, Lustigman S, Jiang S. Antigenic and immunogenic characterization of recombinant baculovirus-expressed severe acute respiratory syndrome coronavirus spike protein: implication for vaccine design. J Virol 2006; 80(12): 5757-67.
[http://dx.doi.org/10.1128/JVI.00083-06] [PMID: 16731915]

[51]   Zhu X, Liu Q, Du L, Lu L, Jiang S. Receptor-binding domain as a target for developing SARS vaccines. J Thorac Dis 2013; 5 (Suppl. 2): S142-8.
[PMID: 23977435]

[52]   Hulswit R. De Haan, C.; Bosch, B.-J.Advances in virus research. Elsevier 2016; Vol. 96: pp. 29-57.

[53]   Coutard B, Valle C, de Lamballerie X, Canard B, Seidah NG, Decroly E. The spike glycoprotein of the new coronavirus 2019-nCoV contains a furin-like cleavage site absent in CoV of the same clade. Antiviral Res 2020; 176: 104742.
[http://dx.doi.org/10.1016/j.antiviral.2020.104742] [PMID: 32057769]

[54]   Chan JF-W, Yuan S, Kok K-H, *et al.* A familial cluster of pneumonia associated with the 2019 novel coronavirus indicating person-to-person transmission: a study of a family cluster. Lancet 2020; 395(10223): 514-23.
[http://dx.doi.org/10.1016/S0140-6736(20)30154-9] [PMID: 31986261]

[55]   Xu Z, Shi L, Wang Y, *et al.* Pathological findings of COVID-19 associated with acute respiratory distress syndrome. Lancet Respir Med 2020; 8(4): 420-2.
[http://dx.doi.org/10.1016/S2213-2600(20)30076-X] [PMID: 32085846]

[56]   Yan R, Zhang Y, Guo Y, Xia L, Zhou Q. Structural basis for the recognition of the 2019-nCoV by human ACE2. BioRxiv 2020.
[http://dx.doi.org/10.1101/2020.02.19.956946]

[57]   Ortega JT, Serrano ML, Pujol FH, Rangel HR. Role of changes in SARS-CoV-2 spike protein in the interaction with the human ACE2 receptor: An *in silico* analysis. EXCLI J 2020; 19: 410-7.

[PMID: 32210742]

[58] Dinesh DC, Chalupska D, Silhan J, Veverka V, Boura E. Structural basis of RNA recognition by the SARS-CoV-2 nucleocapsid phosphoprotein. bioRxiv 2020.
[http://dx.doi.org/10.1101/2020.04.02.022194]

[59] Kandeel M, Elshazly K, El-Deeb W, Fayez M, Ghonim I. Species specificity and host affinity rather than tissue tropism controls codon usage pattern in respiratory mycoplasmosis. J Camel Pract Res 2019; 26(1): 29-40.
[http://dx.doi.org/10.5958/2277-8934.2019.00005.5]

[60] Guo L, Ren L, Yang S, *et al.* Profiling early humoral response to diagnose novel coronavirus disease (COVID-19). Clin Infect Dis 2020; 71(15): 778-85.
[http://dx.doi.org/10.1093/cid/ciaa310] [PMID: 32198501]

[61] Chang CK, Chen C-MM, Chiang MH, Hsu YL, Huang TH. Transient oligomerization of the SARS-CoV N protein--implication for virus ribonucleoprotein packaging. PLoS One 2013; 8(5): e65045.
[http://dx.doi.org/10.1371/journal.pone.0065045] [PMID: 23717688]

[62] Cong Y, Ulasli M, Schepers H, *et al.* Nucleocapsid protein recruitment to replication-transcription complexes plays a crucial role in coronaviral life cycle. J Virol 2020; 94(4): e01925-19.
[http://dx.doi.org/10.1128/JVI.01925-19] [PMID: 31776274]

[63] Sawicki S. Sawicki, D.Coronavirus replication and reverse genetics. Springer 2005; pp. 31-55.
[http://dx.doi.org/10.1007/3-540-26765-4_2]

[64] Chang M-S, Lu Y-T, Ho S-T, *et al.* Antibody detection of SARS-CoV spike and nucleocapsid protein. Biochem Biophys Res Commun 2004; 314(4): 931-6.
[http://dx.doi.org/10.1016/j.bbrc.2003.12.195] [PMID: 14751221]

[65] Keane SC, Liu P, Leibowitz JL, Giedroc DP. Functional transcriptional regulatory sequence (TRS) RNA binding and helix destabilizing determinants of murine hepatitis virus (MHV) nucleocapsid (N) protein. J Biol Chem 2012; 287(10): 7063-73.
[http://dx.doi.org/10.1074/jbc.M111.287763] [PMID: 22241479]

[66] Zheng Y-Y, Ma Y-T, Zhang J-Y, Xie X. COVID-19 and the cardiovascular system. Nat Rev Cardiol 2020; 17(5): 259-60.
[http://dx.doi.org/10.1038/s41569-020-0360-5] [PMID: 32139904]

[67] Tilocca B, Soggiu A, Sanguinetti M, *et al.* Comparative computational analysis of SARS-CoV-2 nucleocapsid protein epitopes in taxonomically related coronaviruses. Microbes Infect 2020; 22(4-5): 188-94.
[http://dx.doi.org/10.1016/j.micinf.2020.04.002] [PMID: 32302675]

[68] Smith AR, Boursnell ME, Binns MM, Brown TD, Inglis SC. Identification of a new membrane-associated polypeptide specified by the coronavirus infectious bronchitis virus. J Gen Virol 1990; 71(Pt 1): 3-11.
[http://dx.doi.org/10.1099/0022-1317-71-1-3] [PMID: 2154538]

[69] Godet M, L'Haridon R, Vautherot J-F, Laude H. TGEV corona virus ORF4 encodes a membrane protein that is incorporated into virions. Virology 1992; 188(2): 666-75.
[http://dx.doi.org/10.1016/0042-6822(92)90521-P] [PMID: 1316677]

[70] Ujike M, Taguchi F. Incorporation of spike and membrane glycoproteins into coronavirus virions. Viruses 2015; 7(4): 1700-25.
[http://dx.doi.org/10.3390/v7041700] [PMID: 25855243]

[71] Arndt AL, Larson BJ, Hogue BG. A conserved domain in the coronavirus membrane protein tail is important for virus assembly. J Virol 2010; 84(21): 11418-28.
[http://dx.doi.org/10.1128/JVI.01131-10] [PMID: 20719948]

[72] Armstrong J, Niemann H, Smeekens S, Rottier P, Warren G. Sequence and topology of a model intracellular membrane protein, E1 glycoprotein, from a coronavirus. Nature 1984; 308(5961): 751-2.

[http://dx.doi.org/10.1038/308751a0] [PMID: 6325918]

[73] Nal B, Chan C, Kien F, *et al.* Differential maturation and subcellular localization of severe acute respiratory syndrome coronavirus surface proteins S, M and E. J Gen Virol 2005; 86(Pt 5): 1423-34.
[http://dx.doi.org/10.1099/vir.0.80671-0] [PMID: 15831954]

[74] Neuman BW, Kiss G, Kunding AH, *et al.* A structural analysis of M protein in coronavirus assembly and morphology. J Struct Biol 2011; 174(1): 11-22.
[http://dx.doi.org/10.1016/j.jsb.2010.11.021] [PMID: 21130884]

[75] Malik YA. Properties of Coronavirus and SARS-CoV-2. Malays J Pathol 2020; 42(1): 3-11.
[PMID: 32342926]

[76] Bianchi M, Benvenuto D, Giovanetti M, Angeletti S, Ciccozzi M, Pascarella S. Sars-CoV-2 Envelope and Membrane Proteins: Structural Differences Linked to Virus Characteristics? BioMed Research International 2020; 2020

[77] Parthasarathy K, Ng L, Lin X, *et al.* Structural flexibility of the pentameric SARS coronavirus envelope protein ion channel. Biophys J 2008; 95(6): L39-41.
[http://dx.doi.org/10.1529/biophysj.108.133041] [PMID: 18658207]

[78] Torres J, Wang J, Parthasarathy K, Liu DX. The transmembrane oligomers of coronavirus protein E. Biophys J 2005; 88(2): 1283-90.
[http://dx.doi.org/10.1529/biophysj.104.051730] [PMID: 15713601]

[79] Arbely E, Khattari Z, Brotons G, Akkawi M, Salditt T, Arkin IT. A highly unusual palindromic transmembrane helical hairpin formed by SARS coronavirus E protein. J Mol Biol 2004; 341(3): 769-79.
[http://dx.doi.org/10.1016/j.jmb.2004.06.044] [PMID: 15288785]

[80] Kuo L, Hurst KR, Masters PS. Exceptional flexibility in the sequence requirements for coronavirus small envelope protein function. J Virol 2007; 81(5): 2249-62.
[http://dx.doi.org/10.1128/JVI.01577-06] [PMID: 17182690]

[81] Venkatagopalan P, Daskalova SM, Lopez LA, Dolezal KA, Hogue BG. Coronavirus envelope (E) protein remains at the site of assembly. Virology 2015; 478: 75-85.
[http://dx.doi.org/10.1016/j.virol.2015.02.005] [PMID: 25726972]

[82] Nieto-Torres JL, Dediego ML, Álvarez E, *et al.* Subcellular location and topology of severe acute respiratory syndrome coronavirus envelope protein. Virology 2011; 415(2): 69-82.
[http://dx.doi.org/10.1016/j.virol.2011.03.029] [PMID: 21524776]

[83] Liao Y, Yuan Q, Torres J, Tam JP, Liu DX. Biochemical and functional characterization of the membrane association and membrane permeabilizing activity of the severe acute respiratory syndrome coronavirus envelope protein. Virology 2006; 349(2): 264-75.
[http://dx.doi.org/10.1016/j.virol.2006.01.028] [PMID: 16507314]

[84] Surya W, Samsó M, Torres J. Structural and functional aspects of viroporins in human respiratory viruses: respiratory syncytial virus and coronaviruses. Respiratory Disease and Infection-A New Insight. 2013; pp. 47-76.
[http://dx.doi.org/10.5772/53957]

[85] Verdiá-Báguena C, Nieto-Torres JL, Alcaraz A, Dediego ML, Enjuanes L, Aguilella VM. Analysis of SARS-CoV E protein ion channel activity by tuning the protein and lipid charge. Biochim Biophys Acta 2013; 1828(9): 2026-31.
[http://dx.doi.org/10.1016/j.bbamem.2013.05.008] [PMID: 23688394]

[86] Javier RT, Rice AP. Emerging theme: cellular PDZ proteins as common targets of pathogenic viruses. J Virol 2011; 85(22): 11544-56.
[http://dx.doi.org/10.1128/JVI.05410-11] [PMID: 21775458]

[87] Yang Y, Peng F, Wang R, *et al.* The deadly coronaviruses: The 2003 SARS pandemic and the 2020 novel coronavirus epidemic in China. J Autoimmun 2020; 109: 102434.

[http://dx.doi.org/10.1016/j.jaut.2020.102434] [PMID: 32143990]

[88]   Teoh K-T, Siu Y-L, Chan W-L, *et al*. The SARS coronavirus E protein interacts with PALS1 and alters tight junction formation and epithelial morphogenesis. Mol Biol Cell 2010; 21(22): 3838-52.
[http://dx.doi.org/10.1091/mbc.e10-04-0338] [PMID: 20861307]

[89]   Subramani C, Nair VP, Anang S, *et al*. Host-Virus Protein Interaction Network Reveals the Involvement of Multiple Host Processes in the Life Cycle of Hepatitis E Virus. mSystems 2018; 3(1): e00135-17.
[http://dx.doi.org/10.1128/mSystems.00135-17] [PMID: 29404423]

[90]   Beale R, Wise H, Stuart A, Ravenhill BJ, Digard P, Randow F. A LC3-interacting motif in the influenza A virus M2 protein is required to subvert autophagy and maintain virion stability. Cell Host Microbe 2014; 15(2): 239-47.
[http://dx.doi.org/10.1016/j.chom.2014.01.006] [PMID: 24528869]

[91]   Münz M, Hein J, Biggin PC. The role of flexibility and conformational selection in the binding promiscuity of PDZ domains. PLOS Comput Biol 2012; 8(11): e1002749.
[http://dx.doi.org/10.1371/journal.pcbi.1002749] [PMID: 23133356]

[92]   Jimenez-Guardeño JM, Nieto-Torres JL, DeDiego ML, *et al*. The PDZ-binding motif of severe acute respiratory syndrome coronavirus envelope protein is a determinant of viral pathogenesis. PLoS Pathog 2014; 10(8): e1004320.
[http://dx.doi.org/10.1371/journal.ppat.1004320] [PMID: 25122212]

[93]   Perlman S. Another Decade, Another Coronavirus. N Engl J Med 2020; 382: 760-2.

[94]   Sheikh A, Al-Taher A, Al-Nazawi M, Al-Mubarak AI, Kandeel M. Analysis of preferred codon usage in the coronavirus N genes and their implications for genome evolution and vaccine design. J Virol Methods 2020; 277: 113806.
[http://dx.doi.org/10.1016/j.jviromet.2019.113806] [PMID: 31911390]

[95]   Kandeel M, Ibrahim A, Fayez M, Al-Nazawi M. From SARS and MERS CoVs to SARS-CoV-2: Moving toward more biased codon usage in viral structural and nonstructural genes. J Med Virol 2020; 92(6): 660-6.
[http://dx.doi.org/10.1002/jmv.25754] [PMID: 32159237]

[96]   Guzik TJ, Mohiddin SA, Dimarco A, *et al*. COVID-19 and the cardiovascular system: implications for risk assessment, diagnosis, and treatment options. Cardiovasc Res 2020; 116(10): 1666-87.
[http://dx.doi.org/10.1093/cvr/cvaa106] [PMID: 32352535]

[97]   van Boheemen S, de Graaf M, Lauber C, *et al*. Genomic characterization of a newly discovered coronavirus associated with acute respiratory distress syndrome in humans. MBio 2012; 3(6): e00473-12.
[http://dx.doi.org/10.1128/mBio.00473-12] [PMID: 23170002]

[98]   Hoffmann M, Kleine-Weber H, Schroeder S, *et al*. SARS-CoV-2 cell entry depends on ACE2 and TMPRSS2 and is blocked by a clinically proven protease inhibitor. Cell 2020; 181(2): 271-280.e8.
[http://dx.doi.org/10.1016/j.cell.2020.02.052] [PMID: 32142651]

[99]   Raj VS, Mou H, Smits SL, *et al*. Dipeptidyl peptidase 4 is a functional receptor for the emerging human coronavirus-EMC. Nature 2013; 495(7440): 251-4.
[http://dx.doi.org/10.1038/nature12005] [PMID: 23486063]

[100]   Mousavizadeh L, Ghasemi S. Genotype and phenotype of COVID-19: Their roles in pathogenesis. J Microbiol Immunol Infect 2020.
[http://dx.doi.org/10.1016/j.jmii.2020.03.022] [PMID: 32265180]

[101]   Kumar S. Nyodu, R.; Maurya, V.K.; Saxena, S.K.Coronavirus Disease 2019 (COVID-19). Springer 2020; pp. 23-31.
[http://dx.doi.org/10.1007/978-981-15-4814-7_3]

[102]   Nikhra V. The Agent and Host Factors in Covid-19: Exploring Pathogenesis and Therapeutic

Implications.

[103] Jiawei C, Quanlong J, Xian X, *et al.* Individual variation of the sars-cov-2 receptor ace2 gene expression and regulation. Biomed J Sci & Tech Res 2020; 27(2): 2020.

[104] Helms J, Tacquard C, Severac F, *et al.* High risk of thrombosis in patients with severe SARS-CoV-2 infection: a multicenter prospective cohort study. Intensive Care Med 2020; 46(6): 1089-98.
[http://dx.doi.org/10.1007/s00134-020-06062-x] [PMID: 32367170]

[105] Xie X, Chen J, Wang X, Zhang F, Liu Y. Age- and gender-related difference of ACE2 expression in rat lung. Life Sci 2006; 78(19): 2166-71.
[http://dx.doi.org/10.1016/j.lfs.2005.09.038] [PMID: 16303146]

[106] Chen J, Jiang Q, Xia X, *et al.* Individual variation of the SARS-CoV2 receptor ACE2 gene expression and regulation Aging Cell 2020; 19(7): e13168.

[107] Raza H, Wahid B, Rubi G, Gulzar A. Molecular epidemiology of SARS-CoV-2 in Faisalabad, Pakistan: A real-world clinical experience. Infect Genet Evol 2020; 84: 104374.
[http://dx.doi.org/10.1016/j.meegid.2020.104374] [PMID: 32450246]

[108] Zhang H, Penninger JM, Li Y, Zhong N, Slutsky AS. Angiotensin-converting enzyme 2 (ACE2) as a SARS-CoV-2 receptor: molecular mechanisms and potential therapeutic target. Intensive Care Med 2020; 46(4): 586-90.
[http://dx.doi.org/10.1007/s00134-020-05985-9] [PMID: 32125455]

[109] Kan B, Wang M, Jing H, *et al.* Molecular evolution analysis and geographic investigation of severe acute respiratory syndrome coronavirus-like virus in palm civets at an animal market and on farms. J Virol 2005; 79(18): 11892-900.
[http://dx.doi.org/10.1128/JVI.79.18.11892-11900.2005] [PMID: 16140765]

[110] de Wit E, van Doremalen N, Falzarano D, Munster VJ. SARS and MERS: recent insights into emerging coronaviruses. Nat Rev Microbiol 2016; 14(8): 523-34.
[http://dx.doi.org/10.1038/nrmicro.2016.81] [PMID: 27344959]

[111] Perrier A, Bonnin A, Desmarets L, *et al.* The C-terminal domain of the MERS coronavirus M protein contains a *trans*-Golgi network localization signal. J Biol Chem 2019; 294(39): 14406-21.
[http://dx.doi.org/10.1074/jbc.RA119.008964] [PMID: 31399512]

[112] Jin Y, Yang H, Ji W, *et al.* Virology, epidemiology, pathogenesis, and control of COVID-19. Viruses 2020; 12(4): 372.
[http://dx.doi.org/10.3390/v12040372] [PMID: 32230900]

[113] Wang C, Horby PW, Hayden FG, Gao GF. A novel coronavirus outbreak of global health concern. Lancet 2020; 395(10223): 470-3.
[http://dx.doi.org/10.1016/S0140-6736(20)30185-9] [PMID: 31986257]

[114] Boulos MNK, Geraghty EM. Geographical tracking and mapping of coronavirus disease COVID-19/severe acute respiratory syndrome coronavirus 2 (SARS-CoV-2) epidemic and associated events around the world: how 21st century GIS technologies are supporting the global fight against outbreaks and epidemics. Int J Health Geogr 2020; 19(1): 1-12.
[http://dx.doi.org/10.1186/s12942-020-00202-8]

[115] Fiorillo L, Cervino G, Matarese M, *et al.* COVID-19 Surface Persistence: A recent data summary and its importance for medical and dental settings. Int J Environ Res Public Health 2020; 17(9): 3132.
[http://dx.doi.org/10.3390/ijerph17093132] [PMID: 32365891]

[116] Rothan HA, Byrareddy SN. The epidemiology and pathogenesis of coronavirus disease (COVID-19) outbreak. J Autoimmun 2020; 109: 102433.
[http://dx.doi.org/10.1016/j.jaut.2020.102433] [PMID: 32113704]

[117] Yagil Y, Yagil C. Angiotensin converting enzyme-2 (ACE2) and its possible roles in hypertension, diabetes and cardiac function. Letters in Peptide Science 2003; 10(5): 377-85.
[http://dx.doi.org/10.1007/s10989-004-2387-6]

[118] Hussain A, Kaler J, Tabrez E, Tabrez S, Tabrez SSM. Novel COVID-19: A comprehensive review of transmission, manifestation, and pathogenesis. Cureus 2020; 12(5): e8184.
[PMID: 32566425]

[119] Lei J, Li J, Li X, Qi X. CT imaging of the 2019 novel coronavirus (2019-nCoV) pneumonia. Radiology 2020; 295(1): 18-8.
[http://dx.doi.org/10.1148/radiol.2020200236] [PMID: 32003646]

[120] Kannan S, Shaik Syed Ali P, Sheeza A, Hemalatha K. COVID-19 (Novel Coronavirus 2019) - recent trends. Eur Rev Med Pharmacol Sci 2020; 24(4): 2006-11.
[PMID: 32141569]

[121] Rangan R, Zheludev IN, Das R. RNA genome conservation and secondary structure in SARS-CoV-2 and SARS-related viruses BioRxiv 2020.
[http://dx.doi.org/10.1101/2020.03.27.012906]

[122] Bennett CF, Krainer AR, Cleveland DW. Antisense oligonucleotide therapies for neurodegenerative diseases. Annu Rev Neurosci 2019; 42: 385-406.
[http://dx.doi.org/10.1146/annurev-neuro-070918-050501] [PMID: 31283897]

[123] Rangan R, Zheludev IN, Hagey RJ, *et al.* RNA genome conservation and secondary structure in SARS-CoV-2 and SARS-related viruses: a first look. RNA 2020; 26(8): 937-59.
[http://dx.doi.org/10.1261/rna.076141.120] [PMID: 32398273]

[124] Gibson WT, Evans DM, An J, Jones SJ. ACE 2 coding variants: a potential x-linked risk factor for COVID-19 disease. bioRxiv 2020.

[125] Ou X, Liu Y, Lei X, *et al.* Characterization of spike glycoprotein of SARS-CoV-2 on virus entry and its immune cross-reactivity with SARS-CoV. Nat Commun 2020; 11(1): 1620.
[http://dx.doi.org/10.1038/s41467-020-15562-9] [PMID: 32221306]

[126] Chen I-J, Yuann J-MP, Chang Y-M, *et al.* Crystal structure-based exploration of the important role of Arg106 in the RNA-binding domain of human coronavirus OC43 nucleocapsid protein. Biochim Biophys Acta 2013; 1834(6): 1054-62.
[http://dx.doi.org/10.1016/j.bbapap.2013.03.003] [PMID: 23501675]

[127] Fan H, Ooi A, Tan YW, *et al.* The nucleocapsid protein of coronavirus infectious bronchitis virus: crystal structure of its N-terminal domain and multimerization properties. Structure 2005; 13(12): 1859-68.
[http://dx.doi.org/10.1016/j.str.2005.08.021] [PMID: 16338414]

[128] Grossoehme NE, Li L, Keane SC, *et al.* Coronavirus N protein N-terminal domain (NTD) specifically binds the transcriptional regulatory sequence (TRS) and melts TRS-cTRS RNA duplexes. J Mol Biol 2009; 394(3): 544-57.
[http://dx.doi.org/10.1016/j.jmb.2009.09.040] [PMID: 19782089]

[129] Kang S, Yang M, Hong Z, *et al.* Crystal structure of SARS-CoV-2 nucleocapsid protein RNA binding domain reveals potential unique drug targeting sites. Acta Pharm Sin B 2020; 10(7): 1228-38.
[http://dx.doi.org/10.1016/j.apsb.2020.04.009] [PMID: 32363136]

[130] Alam I, Kamau AK, Kulmanov M, *et al.* Functional pangenome analysis suggests inhibition of the protein E as a readily available therapy for COVID-2019. bioRxiv 2020.
[http://dx.doi.org/10.1101/2020.02.17.952895]

[131] Tong S, Lingappa JR, Chen Q, *et al.* Direct sequencing of SARS-coronavirus S and N genes from clinical specimens shows limited variation. J Infect Dis 2004; 190(6): 1127-31.
[http://dx.doi.org/10.1086/422849] [PMID: 15319863]

[132] Khailany RA, Safdar M, Ozaslan M. Genomic characterization of a novel SARS-CoV-2. Gene Rep 2020; 19: 100682.
[http://dx.doi.org/10.1016/j.genrep.2020.100682] [PMID: 32300673]

CHAPTER 5

Mutation of SARS-CoV-2

Umair Younas[1,*] and **Kashif Prince**[2]

[1] *Department of Livestock Management, Faculty of Animal Production and Technology, Cholistan University of Veterinary and Animal Sciences, Bahawalpur-63100, Pakistan*

[2] *Department of Medicine, Faculty of Veterinary Science, Cholistan University of Veterinary and Animal Sciences, Bahawalpur-63100, Pakistan*

Abstract: Coronavirus undergoes more frequent mutations over time. It is well understood with previous outbreaks of the diseases, like the severe acute respiratory syndrome (SARS) and the Middle East respiratory syndrome-coronavirus (MERS-CoV). The behavior and pattern of diseases change with the mutation, and the virus becomes a new virus of its out kind regarding morbidity and mortality. Virus from different origins has been observed to have mutations at various places of their genome resulting in changed disease pattern resulting in the worldwide outbreak of the coronavirus disease-19 (COVID-19). Mutation in coronavirus is a slow and emerging process that may be responsible for the modulation of viral transmission, virulence, and replication efficiency in different regions of the globe. SARS-CoV-2 is going to spread around the world, and novel mutation hotspots are emerging in the genome. There has been increasing in the genetic diversity of coronavirus in human hosts. Random mutations cause the diversification of the virus leading to drug resistance, the changed pathogenicity and infectivity. This variation could remain in the virus, but it could be transferred to the next generation. The study was conducted to focus on viral evolution through mutation in various geographic regions of the world.

Keywords: Coronavirus, COVID-19, Genome, Mutation, SARS-CoV-2.

INTRODUCTION

Coronavirus disease-19 caused by severe acute respiratory syndrome-coronaviru--2 (SARS-CoV-2), a novel virus that was emerged in fishmarket Wuhan Hubei province, China in December 2019. It was initially called a novel coronavirus 2019-nCoV, and later it was renamed as SARS-COV-2 that spread quickly to other parts of China and other countries around the globe [1]. More than 190 countries and territories were known to affect the coronavirus disease-19 (COVID-19) pandemic by the 23rd March 2020, whereas the number of

* **Corresponding author Umair Younas:** Department of Livestock Management, Faculty of Animal Production and Technology, Cholistan University of Veterinary and Animal Sciences, Bahawalpur-63100, Pakistan. E-mail: umairyounas@cuvas.edu.pk

Kamal Niaz & Muhammad Farrukh Nisar (Eds.)

confirmed and death cases reported was 464,142 and 21,200, respectively [2]. It was reported that a large variety of species may get infected from the coronavirus and emerged as a highly pathogenic virus for humans. Severe acute respiratory syndrome-coronavirus (SARS-CoV) and the Middle East respiratory syndrome (MERS) were reported in China, 2003 and Saudi Arabia 2012 respectively [3, 4].

According to another study, COVID-19 is a positive sense, 30kb length of single-stranded RNA genome that code for 4 structural and multiple non-structural proteins (nsp) responsible for millions of infected patients and more than 0.2 million deaths [5]. In another study, Gorbalenya *et al.* [6] and Stenglein *et al.* [7] reported the length of the coronavirus in the range of 27 to 34 kb.

Different recent studies reported that SARS-CoV-2 diverged from the SARS-CoV [8, 9]. Similarly, another study reported that an evolutionary tree shows a resemblance between SARS-coronavirus and SARS-CoV-2 [10, 11]. With a 30 kb genomic structure of SARS-CoV-2, it follows the properties of known genes of the coronavirus. The open reading frame (ORF)1ab poly protein constitutes 2/3rd of total genome size, membrane protein, envelope protein, nucleocapsid protein, and spike protein that are structural protein. The ORF1ab is also known as polyprotein replicase. Six ORFs are considered hypothetical proteins without any associated function and include ORF10, ORF8, ORF7b, ORF7a, ORF6, ORF3a [12].

A large number of mutations may occur due to RNA virus replication and may range from 10^{-4} to 10^{-6} per site in each replication round [13 - 16]. It was observed that the capacity of RNA viruses to rapidly evolve resulted due to the low fidelity replication, and RNA viruses might quickly adapt to host species under changing environmental stress [17, 18]. Whereas RNA-dependent RNA polymerase (RdRp) is considered a key regulator of nucleotide selectivity, fidelity and is the central point of RNA 'viruses' replication [19, 20].

Mutations in the virus's structural proteins play a vital role in determining the pathological properties of the virus, like virulence, antibody escape variants, and cellular tropism. Mutation in coronavirus is reported to be a slow and emerging process that may be responsible for the modulation of viral transmission, virulence, and replication efficiency in different regions of the globe [21, 22]. It is observed that coronavirus undergoes more frequent mutations over time. It is apparent with previous outbreaks of the diseases associated with the coronavirus, like MERS-CoV and SARS. A study reported on 32 genomes from the USA, Thailand and China suggested that there has been an increase in the genetic diversity of coronavirus in human hosts [11, 23].

Another study reported that among all known positive-sense RNA viruses, the large Nidoviruses including the coronavirus, replicate with high fidelity [24, 25]. Smith *et al.* [26] stated that for the maintenance of a large genome the increased fidelity is required in CoVs. 16 nsp are encoded by coronavirus, *i.e.*, nsp-1 to nsp-16. Among many of which are considered to play a role in fidelity regulation [27]. The study was conducted to understand the mutation hotspots in various regions of the globe along with their characterization, next-generation sequencing, random and site-directed mutation aspects, and specific mutation in SARS-Cov2.

Mutations Hotspots in Different Geographic Areas

SARS-CoV-2, commonly known as the coronavirus, is an RNA virus considered a virus with a high mutation rate. The mutation rate is estimated to be more than a million times as compared to their hosts. The virus may quickly get released from host immunity due to evolutionary capability and genomic variability. Thereby, resistance to various drugs may be developed [22]. It was reported that of a total of 3067 genomes, 105 are wild-type and mainly present in China. As a result of mutation, other strains with different genotypes were spread across the borders and accounted for 2963 strains [28].

It is studied that the coronavirus is swiftly spreading across the borders, and hotspot mutations were getting visible over time. In this regard, thirteen variation sites in the coronavirus have been characterized, including N, ORF-8, ORF3a, ORF1ab, and S region. It was observed that the mutation rate was 29.47% and 30.53% at position 8782 in ORF1a and 28144 in ORF8, respectively [29].

In another study, the mutation that is particular to contentwas also observed. Two mutations were shared by the Asian genome, *i.e.*, at 28144 and 28117 positions. Similarly, the Australian and African genomes shared 4 positions for mutations, *i.e.*, 29742, 28674, 11083, 1397, and 25563, 23403, 14408, 1059. In most of the mutations, a high ratio of substituting A by G and thus considered as transition mutation. Compared to the rest of the globe, America, New Zealand, and Australia were observed for high genome variability. It was reported that an intergenic variant (241 positions), Dd614G (spike), L4715L, F924F (ORF1ab) expressed in all viral strains excluding Asia. Similarly, except for Australia and Africa, the S5932F (ORF1ab), L84S (ORF8), and G251V (ORF3a) were noticed on all continents of the globe. Mutations in the viral genome were quite similar for Europe and Australia, including the 2 recurrent mutations Q57H and T265I (ORF3a). Ten recurrent mutations were shared among Dutch and European countries [28].

The balance between genomic variability and the integrity of genetic information may happen due to RNA virus mutation that results in viral adaption [30 - 32]. To understand the vital information for understanding the mechanism dealing with viral pathogenesis, immune escape, and viral drug resistance, the biological characterization of viral mutation could be useful.

Similarly, the development of diagnostic assays, antiviral drugs, and designing of new vaccines, the studies on viral mutation are crucial. Some viral enzymes are important for the mutagenic process in the viral genome responsible for replicating the nucleic acid under the influence of post replicative nucleic acid repair and/or with few or without proofreading capability. Some other processes responsible for generating mutation in the genome include recombination events, host enzymes, chemical and physical mutagens that cause spontaneous nucleic acid damage, and specific genetic elements that may produce new variants.

Pachetti *et al.* [22] randomly collected the database on an isolated genome sequence from 220 SARS-COV-2 patients to identify the recurrence of mutation hotspots across the borders. Data was divided into 4 geographic areas, *i.e.*, North America (Canadian and US patients), Europe (Genome from patients of Italy, Portugal, Luxemburg, Belgium, Sweden, Denmark, Finland, UK, Spain, Netherlands, France, Switzerland), Oceania (Australia) and Asia (South-East Asia, China, India, Japan).

The prevalence of mutation was confirmed at 26143, 28144, 11083, 8782, and 3036 positions [33 - 36]. As a result of the study, 8 new mutation hotspots were characterized, located at 28881, 23403, 18060, 17857, 17746, 14408, 2891, and 1397 positions. The mutations at positions 18060, 17857, and 17746 were predominant in North America, whereas positions 28881, 23403, 14408, 3036, and 2891 were exclusively present in Europe.

Of all mutations present in geographic areas, the cumulative mutation frequency is presented (Fig. **1**). The legend and nsp of the viral gene are reported to carry the mutations. The genome of North American and European patients presented an increased frequency of mutation as compared to region Asia. Also, the disparity in the pattern of mutation was observed in North America and Europe.

Mutations in SARS-CoV-2 are emerging though at a slow rate; however, the viral gene may get the ability to modulate for transmission to the host. Similarly, virulence and replication efficiency may also get tempered in various world regions [21, 22]. It is observed that the evolution of 11 clades has resulted from the accumulating mutations in the SARS-CoV-2 genome whereas, the parental clade O was appeared in Wuhan (China) [28].

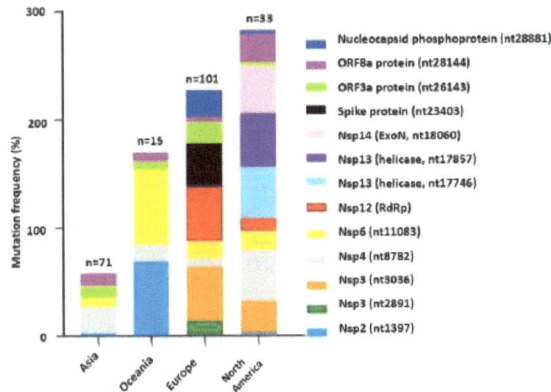

Fig. (1). Mutation frequency (SARS-CoV-2) in different geographic regions of the world. Hotspot mutations reported in literature (26143, 28144, 11083, 8782 and 3036) and Novel hotspot mutations (28881, 23403, 18060, 17857, 17746, 14408, 2891 and 1397) were categorized in to four geographic regions: North America (n=33), Europe (n=101), Oceania (n=15) and Asia (n=71) [22].

Characterization of Geographically Distinct Hotspots Overtime

Pachetti *et al.* [22] analyzed the genome to understand the expression of each mutation in different geographic regions over time. The genome was classified as per sample collection timing. Based on the analysis, 6 subgroups of the time were made, *i.e.*, Dec. 2019 for the genome examination taken from 5 patients; 1st to 15th Jan. 2020 (15 patients); 16th to 31st Jan.2020 (54 patients); 1st to 15th Feb.2020 (13 patients); 16th to 29th Feb.2020 (55 patients) and 1st to 13th Mar. 2020 (80 patient's genome analysis).

Over time, an increased rate of mutations was noted in Asia during viral spread. For the first time in December 2019, no mutation was observed in Asian genomes analysis. However, in Europe during January and February, the different SARS-CoV-2 mutations were recorded due to novel mutation at 14408 position that location was noticed in the RdRp gene. Further new mutations came to screen from the start of February 2020. The location of these mutations was 2891, 28881, and 23403. Whereas mutation at 2026 position was present (2.2%) in mid-January, for which an increase in frequency was noted [22].

Koyama *et al.* [37] analyzed the genome variants of SARS-Cov2 using four different databases and identified 6 major clades, *i.e.*, basal, D614G, L3606F, L84S, D448del, and G392D, along 14 sub-clades. The major clade D448del and G392D were first identified on February 8 and 20, 2020. Similarly, some sub-clades, including D614G/Q57H/T265I, D614G/203_204delinsKR/, D614G/Q57H, and L3606F/G251V/P765S were first observed in February 2020.

From the start of March 2020, a different set of hotspot mutations were observed in patients from North America. An outbreak was reported for positive cases of SARS-CoV-2 in Canada and USA hotspot mutations were distinctly featured in viral genomes. There was a report of three novel mutations at positions 18060, 17857, and 17746. European specific Corona mutations were absent from the viral genomes obtained from patients of North America as these viral genomes were possessing 14% RdRp mutations [22]. The unfortunate part of the naturally occurring mutation in RdRp may lead to drug resistance [38 - 40].

From the statistical point of view, the mutation is less likely to occur while considering the RNA replication and the significance of RdRp for viability. Correspond to that point mutation in the *Poliovirus* was observed to induce episodes of drug resistance [41]. On February 9, 2020, as per the available database, the RdRp mutation at position 14804 appeared for the first time in the UK. Thereafter, on February 20, 2020, a different mutation at position 14408 (AA; P to L) was first observed in Italy during a drastic increase in the number of SARS-CoV-2 infected patients reported by WHO. After February 9, 2020, the analysis of increase/decrease in each mutation frequency among various geographic regions was made. The results of our study that there was a significant increase (+61.7%) for genome possessing 3036 mutations followed by 60.5% increase in genome carrying the hotspot mutation at position 14408, 48.1% for mutation at position 23402, and 29.6% in 28881 mutations [22].

According to another study, the pool of mutations was monitored during the epidemic period along with their geographic location. At 716 site mutations were observed, of which 64% (457) were reported to have a non-synonymous effect. As a result of mutated alleles frequency, the 39 non-synonymous recurrent mutations were noted, including ten hotspot mutations and a prevalence of >0.10 in the population and distributed among 6 genes of SARS-CoV-2 [42].

Evolution of Mutation Overtime

In another study, SARS-CoV-2 genomes were collected after the virus's appearance during the first three months, *i.e.*, December 24, 2019 to March 25, 2020. The accumulation of mutations was noticed at a relatively constant rate. With the average value of 11.34 mutations/genome, the slight increase in accumulation of mutation was recorded for the strains selected at the end of March as compared to genomes that were collected in December, January, and February with average values as 10.59, 10.34, and 9.26, respectively which suggest the SNPs accumulation in SARS-CoV-2 genomes in the coming period. The various route of entries of the virus in different countries has been pointed out [42].

The genomic data of patients from four different database centers collected that encompassed 68 countries between February 1 and May 1 2020. They reported 5775 distinctive genome variants, including missense mutation (2969), synonymous mutations (1965), mutations in noncoding regions (484), non-coding deletion (142), and in-frame deletions (100), *etc*. The most common variants were the synonymous 3037C > T (6334 samples), P4715L in the ORF1ab (6319 samples), and D614G in the spike protein (6294 samples) [37].

A higher number of mutations were observed in the center of the outbreak period (end of January) when the mutation accumulations were studied. Similarly, at the start of April, an increased number of mutations was observed. The first mutation occurred that was appeared intergenic region related to ORF8 protein and nucleocapsid phosphoprotein. The Spike protein and ORF1ab expressed various hotspot mutations, including L84S and D614G, T265I, respectively [42].

Concurrent Prevalence of RdRp and Snp Mutations along with Other Mutations

The analysis of mutation frequency was made to observe the fact that RdRp (RNA dependent RNA polymerase) of RNA viruses is unable to carry out proofreading. There is an unequal distribution of mutations. The single nucleotide polymorphism mutations could be single or multiple mutations that may impact the pathogenicity and transmission pathway of SARS-CoV-2. It was noted that the more prevalent and significant types of co-mutations have occurred in European countries, *i.e.*, 23403, A>G; 3037, C>T; 241, C>T. The additional extended mutations were also found in the strain *i.e.* 23403, A>G; 14408, C>T; 3037, C>T, 241, C>T [43]. The WHO reported Italy with a major attack of SARS-CoV-2, which lead to 59,138 confirmed patients, and the death number was as high as 5476 till March 23, 2020 [44].

Studies were carried out to study the genome, and for this purpose, the genome was divided into 2 groups. The first group of genomes carrying a mutation at position 14408 (RdRp) affects patients from North America and Europe. Whereas the second group of genomes was without the mutation (RdRp). As compared to group-2, the first group showed an increased number of mutations. It noticed that the simultaneous occurrence of two, three, four, and five mutations present in 11.3%, 47.2%, 39.6%, and 1.9% genomes, respectively. The results of the group-2 analysis were the presence of one mutation in 29.8% of genomes. A simultaneous occurrence of two, three, four, five, and six was noted in 22.6%, 7.1%, 10.7%, 2.4%, and 3.6% genomes. Also, 23.8% of genomes showed no mutation at all. The locations of most reported mutations in group-2 were at 17857, 17746, 11083, 8782 regions. A significant difference was reported among group-1 and -2 for distribution of genome. However, it is insignificant when it came to the number of mutations, *i.e.*, 2, 5, and 5. A median of 3 point mutations was found in the viral strains of RdRp mutations with a range of 2-5 whereas a median of 1 mutation in viral strains with no RdRp mutation and a range of 0-3 (P<0.001). Regarding the frequency of mutation, it was stated that genome having mutations at position 28881, 23403, 3036 (Europe) and 18060, 17857, and 17746 (North America) showed a median of 3-4 mutations as compared to 1-2 mutations for the genomes that were not carrying any of these mutations (P<0.001). Statistically, the difference was significant that strongly implies that these mutations on the genome may be an indication for the presence of other mutations [22].

The RNA replication of SARS-CoV-2 is unique in terms of two RdRp. The first RNA polymerase is primer-dependent nsp12 compared to the second RNA polymerase, which is nsp8. The primase capacity for initiation of RNA replication without primers may be expressed through nsp8 [45]. The results were found consistent with the previous findings in which SARS-CoV-2 is classified as S and L types by the 2 co-mutations, *i.e.*, 28144, T>C and 8782, C>T [46]. In SARS-CoV-2 isolates, the 28144, T>C mutation was regarded as the most abundant SNP mutation where amino acid serine (S) becomes the mutated form of Leucine (L).

It was estimated that mutation occur in one generation based on SNP profiles of the viral genome from different world countries at other times. In the USA, in the two successive infection cases, the virus increase mutation at position 28854 (C>Y) between two community members. In SARS-CoV-2, the mutations may get accumulated and found ranging from 1 mutation to 14 mutations over the length of 30kb genome observed in the period between December 2019 till March 2020. In this way, we may estimate that 14 generations have been affected by the transmission of SARS-CoV-2 since the first reported case in December 2019 [43]. The mutations in SARS-CoV-2 are due to the low fidelity of reverse transcriptase [47, 48].

Homological Study of Mutant RdRp Protein

The high number of mutations could be a result of RNA virus replication, and the number of these mutations may range from a large number of mutations may occur as a result of RNA virus replication and may vary from 10^{-4} to 10^{-6} per site in each replication round [13 - 16]. It was observed that the capacity of RNA viruses to evolve resulted due to the low fidelity replication rapidly, and RNA viruses might easily adapt to host species under changing environmental stress [17, 49]. Whereas RdRp is considered a key regulator of nucleotide selectivity, fidelity and is the central point of RNA 'viruses' replication [19, 20].

Due to the direct involvement of the enzyme in viral replication, the RdRp mutant is considered to be interesting among various enzyme sites that were analyzed. Also, the mutagenic capacity of SARS-CoV-2 may be determined due to RdRp fidelity. It was observed that there is high homology between RdRps of SARS-CoV-2 and SARS-CoV. Therefore, the RdRp reference sequence was aligned for SARS-CoV-2 with the catalytic site sequence of RdRp in SARS-CoV. It was stated that due to nucleotide mutation at position 14408, the amino acid 323 substitution (P>L) does not fall in the catalytic site. Instead, it falls in a region of SARS-CoV, which is a poorly characterized Interface Domain structure, and is supposed to have interaction with other proteins that are responsible for RdRp activity regulation [50].

It is observed that RdRp of SARS-CoV makes a super complex which is a cylindrical and hollow structure along nsp-7 and -8 lead to conferring the process action to RdRp [51]. There is an interaction between nsp14 and replication super-complex. This interaction is important from the mutation rate point of view and to control the fidelity during RNA replication. There is a need for the identification of important RdRp residues that are involved. Therefore further research may be carried out to understand the role of 14408 mutation concern with the fidelity of RdRp. From the recent studies, it was observed that there is a direct interaction of nsp14 with CoV RdRp that is encoded in nsp-12 [52]. However, the overall fidelity regulation and the resultant effect of such interaction on the selectivity of nucleotide is not known [27].

Sexston *et al.* [27] analyzed whether nucleotide fidelity and selectivity determinants could be identified by homology modeling in CoV RdRps. For this purpose, CoV MHV (murine hepatitis virus) nsp-12 RdRp structure was modeled and then overlaid on the explained RdRp structure of picornavirus. The mapping of fidelity altering mutation was done on nsp-12 RdRp previously recognized in CVB3 (coxsackievirus B3). Thereafter engineered into murine hepatitis virus genome with and without [nsp-14 ExoN(+)] and [nsp-14 ExoN(-)], respectively. In this way, two mutations were identified that conferred the resistance to the 5-FU (mutagen 5-fluorouracil): nsp-12-V5531 and nsp-12-M611F. For nsp-1--V5531, Sexton *et al.* [27] also reported the resistance to 5-AZC (mutagen 5-azacytidine).

The altered fidelity of RdRp lowered the fitness relative to WT (wild type) viruses in most cases, as a result of which small changes like a 1.2 fold difference happened in the mutation accumulation [26, 53 - 55]. Despite the identity of no AA (amino acid) outside conserved motifs [26, 53, 56 - 60], the polymerase structure, including RNA-dependent RNA polymerase, looks like a cupped right hand with palm, fingers, and thumb domain [61]. The coronavirus is known as the largest known RNA virus genome, the length of that structure may range from 27-34kb [6, 7], and for the maintenance of such a large genome structure, increased fidelity is required.

Next-Generation Sequencing Reveals Diverse Mutations

The evolutionary step to surviving under varying environments and stressful conditions through various scales is developing low-frequency mutations or variants as a self-protective approach of cells and organisms from mitochondria to viruses and tumor cells [62 - 67]. There is a great adaptation of viruses, particularly RNA viruses, to evolve and mutate against host immune selection pressure. As a result of which a large number of variables among the population are generated though these variables are closely related genomes, also known as quasispecies [67, 68].

Next-generation sequencing is a novel method for discovering the virus to ensure the unbiased sequencing in coronavirus through genetic diversity is high. Unbiased next-generation sequencing is a costlier method and may be subjected to low abundance CoV sequences as non-viral sequences are present in the surveillance field samples [69].

Error-prone replication may cause the generation of minority variants in RNA viruses [49]. Enhancing the specificity and sensitivity determination of minority variants is considered a major challenge in virology. These viruses have a superior ability to adapt to a new environment and stress condition. Therefore emerges as vaccine and drug-resistant mutants include coronavirus [11, 12, 70], human immunodeficiency virus (HIV) [71 - 73], *poliovirus* [74], and hepatitis C virus (HCV) [75], *etc.*

The NGS (next-generation sequencing) is a rapidly grown technique in basic and clinical virology in the last decade [76], particularly for discovering the viruses [77] and diagnosis [78 - 81]. More sequencing reads are available at a lower cost, and multiplexing of samples is possible in the next-generation sequencing (NGS) technique compared to the conventional gold-standard Sanger sequencing [82]. Though the error rate is high (0.1% to 15%), large sequencing data are needed for NGS technologies depending on the application and platforms that may hinder rare mutation detection [66]. However, various error-corrective approaches have been developed to improve NGS technology to identify the low-frequency viral variant and applied for the investigation of viral quasispecies.

Due to the exclusive ability of NGS regarding sub-clonal variant detection within the population carrying diverse genetic information. The successful application of NGS was done for analysis and quantification of genetically diverse viral quasispecies. Also, various low-frequency vaccine or drug-resistant mutations that are therapeutically important have been reported. There is limited current NGS technologies to detect and quantify the viral minority variants with full accuracy.

Spike Protein in COVID-19 and Mutation Hotspots

The virus is composed of two things Genetic material and protein. Protein depicts many physiological and pathological properties in the host body. Each virus has its own characteristically defined proteins [83]. It was observed that there are 4 types of structural proteins in COVID-19 are termed S (spike), E (envelope), M (membrane), and N (nucleocapsid). Of these four proteins, the S, M, and E proteins are present outside the surface and contact the host environment. S proteins are knobs like structure on the surface of the virus it assists in virus entering inside host cells after receptor binding. Apart from this property S protein is an important immunogen and most accessible part of the virus that could be studied to make future vaccines successfully. These knob-like structures protrude out from the surface if we see them in an electron microscope. Spike protein is made up of S1 and S2 protein subunits or monomers. These two combine to make the spike protein. There is a vital role of structural 'proteins' mutation as they help understand the virus's pathological properties, like virulence, antibody escape variants, and cellular tropism. It is observed that the coronavirus undergoes more frequent mutations over time. As, tt is evident with previous outbreaks of the diseases associated with the coronavirus, like SARS and MERS-CoV [84].

The behavior and pattern of diseases change with the mutation, and the virus becomes a new virus of its kind regarding morbidity and mortality. Virus from different origins has been observed to have mutations at various places of their genome resulting in changed disease pattern resulting in the worldwide outbreak of the COVID-19. Spike protein has 1273 amino acids in the form of two subunits or subdomains called S1 and S2. These proteins perform a different but very crucial part of viral pathogenesis. Subdomain S1 has the receptor-binding domain and is involved in its attachment to the angiotensin-converting enzyme 2 (ACE2) receptors. The fusion of the virus is associated with S2 of the spike protein [84].

Multiple sequence alignment of COVID-19 spike proteins has been confirmed from a different origin. There are many positions at which mutations are observed, but some positions are more frequent. In a study conducted in the USA, it was observed most of the mutations occurred at position 614, mutation D to G in 99 isolates of coronavirus. The receptor-binding domain (RBD) of the coronavirus falls between 331 aa to 524 aa [85]. In this region, three different mutations have been observed, which are A348T, G476S, and V483A, with the last one showing the highest number of mutations. In South American viral strains, the mutation was observed at position 614 from D to G, which was the same as the North American strain, but there was more mutation at positions 348, 476, and 483. These mutations were not observed in any Australian isolate. Less than 50% of European isolates have shown the same mutation at position 614 as observed in other isolates. No such mutation was observed in Chinese isolates. Phylogeny of 342 American samples showed that the virus diverged in at least 20 clusters. Out of these 20 clusters, 3 clusters were observed to be prominent. Cluster 1 was comprised of G476S and clusters 2 shown mutations V483A. All these mutations were on the RBD of the spike protein. This shows the virus is mutating to become more infective, which is also depicted by the outbreak. Mutation at 614 from Aspartic Acid to Glycine was the largest cluster from all isolates. Aspartic acid is prominent negatively charged acidic amino acid, but glycine is a small and neutral amino acid, and due to this, there is a behavior change. A few sites in spike protein have shown no mutation in any isolate and are conserved as such. These portions lie between 241-320, 641-880, 961-1040, and 1121-1200. Out of these major sequences, between 641 to 880, 961 to 1040, and 1121 to 1200 fall on the S2 domain of the spike protein. It shows that most non-changing regions fall on the S2 domain and could be used for future vaccines. The present outbreak also called COVID-19, originated from the bat where spike glycoprotein mutation resulted in its transfer tohumans [86].

Effect of Random and Site-Directed Mutation

Random mutations cause the diversification of the virus leading to drug resistance and the changed pathogenicity and infectivity. This variation could remain in the virus, but it could be transferred to the next generation. Site-directed and random substitution mutation could cause various effects on the ligand-binding region on coronavirus. Retroviral genomes can mutate randomly to develop evading power from the host immune system, which could reduce the chances of survival of the virus in the human body [87, 88]. Sites of mutation are very important to determine the viability of the virus. The proteins help in viral replication. These proteins are encoded in ORF1 and consist of almost half of the viral genome structure. There are two polyproteins translated from this region, *i.e.*, ORF1a and ORF1b. These are nsp, and they are processed through main protease and papain-like proteases. Various antiviral drugs have been tested for the treatment of coronaviruses like anti-influenza and anticancer agent. These drugs include lopinavir, ritonavir [89], indinavir [90], chloroquine, and hydroxychloroquine [91, 92] with variable results.

SARS virus protease has two protomers that combine to form a dimer. Each dimer has three domains. Six stranded beta barrels are antiparallel present in domains 1 and 2, and cleft between these two domains express the substrate-binding site.

The 3rd domain is 5 alpha-helix and is connected to both domains with a long loop. It was reported that hydroxychloroquine and indinavir contain a high affinity for protease. A more binding affinity between HIS163 and the indinavir complex is reported that may involve the hydrogen binding and LEU141, GLY170, GLU 166 in hydrophobic interactions. Hydroxychloroquine has an affinity with THR190 and GLU166 involved in hydrogen bonding and HIS41 in hydrophobic interaction [93].

Though the ligand-binding site largely remains conserved, a few studies have shown that the mutation disturbs the binding ability of the drugs. The THR190 and GLY170 are mainly responsible for the interaction with Hydroxytoluene and Indinavir, respectively. Changing the position of threonine and glycine with non-polar and polar residues presented the variation in binding affinity and binding energies. A study was conducted to see the effect of a random mutation on the binding affinity of the drug. These 100 genome regions from the proteases were selected from ORF1 a and b. Throughout the hundred samples, the ligand-binding site was conserved. The Uniform substitution algorithm was run and generated random mutations with produced 200 mutant proteases. Results showed binding affinity has a lower variation for the hydroxychloroquine despite the mutations. The binding affinity of hydroxychloroquine and indinavir was changed significantly [93].

Viral protease is the protein that catalyzes the breakdown of the peptide bonds specific to viral glycoprotein precursors. The basic role of viral proteases is to mediate assembly and disassembly that lead glycoprotein to capsid formation upon entry of virus to a new cell [94]. Protease is more likely to affect by coronavirus infection. The process of protease function is to identify the substrate and get bind to it. If protease has a difference in structure due to mutation, the resistance develops [95]. Hydrophobic interactions are more important than hydrogen bonding in binding molecular surfaces to the receptor binding affinities [96]. Indinavir has a higher binding affinity mainly due to the hydrophobic interaction. Only two mutations GLY170 and THR190, are responsible for affecting the ligand binding.

The Specific Mutations in RdRp Helicase and Polymerase in SARS-CoV-2

ORF 1ab of the SARS-CoV-2 is the region where those genes are encoded, which are non-structure and perform various vital functions, including replication and translation. Besides these, it also possesses the 3'-5'exonuclease, helicase, RdRp, nsp-1 to 4, nsp-6 to 10, and 3C like proteinase [31]. The sequence analysis of the ORF1ab shows its importance of mutation, especially RNA-dependent RNA polymerases and helicase enzymes. These are the most important enzymes in determining the virus multiplication and replication, resulting in infectivity and pathogenesis. Rigidity occurs in the structure due to mutation at position 4715 (in the context of polyprotein) and 323 on RdRp.

Similarly, there is disability and protein structure flexibility due to mutation in helicase at position 5828 of polyprotein or 504. Such protein dynamin alterations and structure medication might cause many changes in the RNA unwinding, which is a complex stem-loop structure. Similarly, the changes in the affinity of RdRp helicase turn the viral RNA replication. This structural analysis can help in the drug targeting and therapeutic interactions of SARS-CoV-2 [97].

The life cycle of this single-stranded RNA virus encompasses the attachment to the receptor and its penetration, translation, replication, assembly, and egress. If we see all these steps individually, each step has two parts to perform these uniformly. These two parts are host, and the viral factors are compulsory to perform all these steps, and any change in these factors at any stage causes the modification of the process positively or negatively. Viral proteins have two categories, like all other organisms, which are structural and nonstructural proteins. Structural protein is those proteins that make the body of the virus. The capsid portion of the protein is mainly made up of protein portion. It provides strength and support to the virus and protects the more vulnerable parts of the virus, which are genetic material, from the harms of the environment, and it also makes a structure to aid in penetration to host cells by any means. The nonstructural proteins are also called the functional proteins; these are the major portion of the enzymes involved in all functions of the virus, including the RNA translation and replication [12, 98]. RNA-dependent RNA polymerase is a crucial protein called nonstructural protein 12 (nsp12), present in SARS-CoV-2. This enzyme helps in viral RNA replication. Helicase is the enzyme that helps in an essential step to RNA multiplication that is unwinding of the complex RNA structure RNA polymerase cannot excess each component to the RNA. To work properly, RNA should be in a straight form which is obtained by the helicase enzyme. Proteins are three-dimensional structures that have to perform various functions and are very dynamic. Their biological properties and functions are affected by the dynamics and conformations. These proteins' structure is coded on the ORF1ab portion of the coronavirus. So, any change or mutation at that part should affect the conformation and dynamic of these most important proteins, so the modulation of the proteins depends on the mutation of genes that are encoding these proteins.

Mutations in RNA viruses are more frequent and easier. Most of the RNA viruses mutate widely over time, and this mutation leads to change in many viral properties making viruses more potent, more infective, and lethal over time. The fidelity of RNA polymerase determines the mutation rate. The mutation determines the evolution of the virus, its properties to protect itself from the host immune system, and overall, various changes observed in the viral genome [30, 31]. In population, RNA polymerase, in turn, is also prone to mutation. This affects the fidelity of the virus. There are increased chances of the viral mutation leading to the emergence of the drug-resistant phenotypes of the virus. These mutations could change from area to area. There could be geographically region-specific virulence of the virus variant, which needs careful targeting the protein for designing the antiviral drug or vaccine candidate. Due to high mutation frequency, it is difficult to develop the vaccine or drug from RNA viruses. After S protein of coronavirus, the RdRp is also a significant target for therapeutic interventions and vaccine development.

Mutation in the ORF1ab caused enzyme's protein structure, leading to a change in functional processes. Most of the mutations in the ORF1ab region are RdRp and helicase enzyme regions. Both of these enzymes play a very important role in the RNA replication of the virus. Any mutation leads to change in stability, conformation, and flexibility of the virus. In the case of RdRp, the mutation was observed from Proline to Leucine that leads to the damage to two turn structures (positions 323 and 324). Proline amino acid is ubiquitous in the turns, and it is termed a helix breaker. Leucine is the amino acid that provides stability in the alpha-helix of the enzyme structure [99]. It is expected that the replacement of the proline results in a more stabilized form of the enzyme. Vibrational entropy energy is one of the important Parmenter that determine the stability of the protein. This amino acid shift leads to a decrease the molecular flexibility and increasing the stability of the protein. Determination of enzyme stability, deformation energy, and atomic fluctuation are vital parameters. The amount of local flexibility in a protein may be determined through deformation energy, and the absolute atomic motion amplitude may be described through atomic fluctuation. These parameters confirmed that proline to leucine mutation resulted in the more rigid and less flexible RNA-dependent RNA polymerase molecule.

On the other hand, proline to leucine mutation in the helicase leads to a decrease in rigidity and a rise in molecular flexibility, making the helicase less stable. Leucine has an aliphatic R group and non-polar whereas, proline is an uncharged R group and polar. Secondary structure prediction of proline to leucine mutation in helicase depicted many significant changes. Two turn structures were lost at the position of 503 and 504 due to this mutation. Three sheets were observed to be added at positions 504, 503, and 502 of the protein. From positions, 500 to 504 five helices got added in the mutated strain compared to the wild type. The stability of the decreased and flexibility was observed to increased due to this mutation. Both of these proteins are determinant for RNA replication, so any change in these enzymes leads to modification. The replication of viral RNA is influenced by these mutations. With the increase in the rate of mutation, the new variants may escape from the host's immune mechanism and make it possible to dodge the humoral immune responses establishing the antibody escape mutants, which may result in the expansion of viral tissue tropism. This mutation can make either a very virulent form of the virus or an attenuated form [97].

Specific Mutation Pattern of Whole-Genome in SARS-CoV-2 and Bat-SAR--CoV

Coronavirus is a small-sized virus ranging in size from 65nm to 125nm in diameter. The genetic material in the coronavirus is single-stranded RNA, and the size of nucleic material is 26 kbs to 32kbs in length. There are four subgroups of the coronavirus alpha, beta, gamma, and delta. It was considered that these viruses do not affect human beings until the infection of a human being with the SARS and SARS-CoV in 2002 in China [100]. After almost a decade, MERS-CoV caused an epidemic in Middle Eastern countries [101]. Many people were recently infected and died in the major population of Wuhan, China in the 2019 virus outbreak. This was named as novel coronavirus and, more specifically, COVID-19.

Genomics of the SARS CoV-2 is 80% identical to the previous human coronavirus (SARS-like bat Coronavirus [12]. Structural proteins are encoded by 4 genes (S, E, M, and N genes) that determine the structure. The ORF1ab is the largest gene in SARS-CoV-2, which encodes pp1ab proteins and 15 nsps. The ORF1a gene encodes for pp1a protein which contains 10 nsps [12, 69, 102]. The evolutionary tree shows that the SARS-CoV-2 is very close to the SARS-coronavirus [10, 11]. Still, there are many notable variations among the SARS-CoV-2 and SARS-coronavirus. It includes the absence of the 8a protein, fluctuation in numbers of amino acids 8b and 3c proteins in SARS-CoV-2 [12]. It is also observed that the spike glycoprotein of COVID-19 is modified *via* homologous recombination. The spike protein in SARS-CoV-2 is a mixture of bat SARS-CoV and an unknown beta coronavirus [23]. Cell receptors and the mechanism of cell entry are the same for both SARS-CoV and SARS-CoV-2. Both use ACE2 cell receptors [103, 104]. A single mutation in the SARS-CoV-2 has significantly increased the binding affinity with ACE2 receptors.

SARS-CoV-2 More Pathogenic than Other SARS and MERS

There are other coronaviruses apart from *beta* coronavirus, which causes diseases in human beings such as cold and croup. Such viruses are the underclass of alpha coronavirus, and their example is 229E and NL63. To understand the severity of the COVID-19, we should generally learn the coronavirus's pathophysiology

(SARS and MERS). The life cycle of the virus consists of attachment, penetration, biosynthesis, mutation, and release. These are five stages similar to all other mammalian viruses and they follow the same procedure until the release of the newly formed virus from the cell. SARS-CoV-2 invades into the after binding to the receptor site. The virus binds on the host cell on the proper site, which is called receptor. The infectivity of the virus depends on the receptors. If some cell does not have receptors for the virus, there will be no attachment or penetration of the virus to the host cells. The proper receptor is must for virus attachment. If there is no attachment in the process of the virus, will be hindered. After attachment, the next step is the entry of the virus into the host cell. The entry of the virus to the host cell takes place by endocytosis or membrane fusion. When the viral content reaches the host cell, they find their way directly to the host cell nucleus to take up the host machinery to produce viral protein and genetic material. This step is called biosynthesis of RNA. In the end, viral particles are made and released from the host cell. This is called maturation [105].

As we discussed earlier, there are 4 types of structural proteins in COVID-19 termed S, E, M, and N proteins [83]. Outside the viral surface, the S protein consists of glycoprotein, transmembrane trimetric and protruding out of the viral surfaces. The spike proteins determine the type of coronavirus, its diversity and host tropism, and receptor recognition. There are two functional units of the S protein S1 fit to the receptors of host cells and S2 involved in the union of the cellular and viral membrane. ACE-2 is the functional receptor for SARS-CoV. And SARS-CoV-2 [102, 106]. This receptor expression is higher in the lungs, heart, ileum, kidney, and bladder [107]. And most of the symptoms associated with the coronavirus are also associated with these organs. Lung epithelial cells have the highest expression of ACE2, and the most obvious symptoms are associated with lungs and lung failure and respiratory issues leading the death.

The protease cleavage is reported in spike protein to alter the binding of SARS-CoV-2 to host protein. A model was proposed to explain S protein activation in SARS CoV and MERS CoV. It is a two-step procedure in which cleavage of S1/S2 cleave site occurs for priming and cleavage for activation occurs at the S2 site, a position adjacent to the fusion peptide with the S2 subunit [108 - 110]. At cleavage sites of S1/S2, both subunits of S protein remain in the state of the non-covalent bond after the cleavage. The stabilization is done at the profusion state between the distal S1 and the membrane-anchored S2 subunit [111]. Cleavage at the S2 site activated the spike for membrane fusion by the irreversible conformational change. A range of different proteases can cleave and trigger the coronavirus spike in this way. It is unique among the other viruses [112]. The unique characteristic associated with the SARS-CoV-2 among other coronaviruses is the furin cleavage site at the S1/S2 site. During the biosynthesis, the S1/S2 Covid-19 is completely cleaved though different from SARS-CoV, where it is incorporated into the assembly without cleavage [111].

The ACE2 is highly expressed on the apical side of the lung epithelial cells in the alveolar [113, 114]. And the virus has needed these receptors to enter the cells, so these areas are at more risk of viral attack. This is also observed that most of the patients have early lung injury in the distal airway. Airways are protected by three ways from the infectious agents, *i.e.*, dendritic cells, alveolar macrophages, and epithelial cells. These are the most important sections of innate immunity [115]. Dendritic Cells are permanent residents beneath the epithelium. On the apical side of the epithelium, the Macrophages are present. These macrophages and dendritic cells are the first line of defense against the invader, which is nonspecific. This response fights back until the body's proper and specific response is formed in the form of T and b cell Responses. T cell response starts with presenting the antigen *via* DC and macrophages to the T cells [116]. Macrophages and DC phagocytose the apoptotic cells infected by the virus and take viral antigen and present them to the cells for a more adaptive immune response [117]. The virus can also be presented from the primary infected cells, but it is mainly the viral antigen presentation from the apoptotic cells. In addition to ACE2, the SARS-CoV may also bind to DC-SIGN and its related proteins whereas, DC-SIGN is dendritic cell-specific intercellular adhesion molecule 3 grabbing non-integrin and DC-SIGN-related proteins in addition to the ACE2 [118 - 120]. DC-SIGN is highly expressed on these to APCs, *i.e.*, dendritic cells and macrophages. This could be one target for the direct attack to the SARS-CoV-2 and can help infect these cells and direct the antigen presentation.

After that, APCs move to the draining lymph nodes to present the viral antigens to the T cells. CD4+ and CD8+ both play a vital role in this regard. CD4+ cells activate the B cells for the production of antigen-specific antibodies. In contrast, the CD8+ activates the T cells to activate the T cell-mediated immune response, which will kill the virally infected cells. The patients with severe COVID-19 showed that there was lymphopenia, particularly in reducing the peripheral blood T cells [121 - 123]. Proinflammatory cytokines are observed to have a higher concentration in the patients. These cytokines include granulocyte colony-stimulating factor, monocyte chemoattractant protein 1, IL-10, IL6, TNF-α, and macrophage inflammatory protein 1 α [123, 124]. The level of IL6 was higher in those patients whose conditions were worse. CD4+ and CD8+ T cells were activated in the patient who have higher expression of CD69, CD38, and CD44 [125]. If the T cells get exhausted or less in number, there is more progression of the disease. The patient with severe COVID-19 was observed to carry the pathogenic CD4+T cells along with IFN-γ expression and granulocyte-macrophage colony-stimulating factor [121].

Infected lung epithelial cells are observed to produce IL-8 along with IL-6 in SARS-CoV [115]. Interleukin 8 is a well-known chemical signal for neutrophil and T cells. Large numbers of inflammatory cells were observed in the lungs which were affected by COVID-19 [104, 126]. In such cells, there was a great activity of innate immune cells and adaptive immune cells. In the innate immune cells, most cells are neutrophils that can act in two ways, good and bad. It is bad because it can cause tissue injury in lungs [40, 122, 127, 128]. In the adaptive immune response, the T cells were observed to be more active than the B cells, and in the T cells, most of the cells were cytotoxic T cells [129]. These cells can kill the virus and kill the lung cells causing tissue injury [130]. The circulating monocytes are also increased in the patient of COVID-19.

Thrombosis and pulmonary embolism are other symptoms along with respiratory symptoms. The various activities performed by endothelium, like fibrinolysis, avoid the aggregation and promoting vasodilation. Thus, a vital role is played by endothelium in thrombotic regulation [127, 131]. The profile showing a higher level of chemicals to help coagulation is likely to indicate significant endothelial damage. Endothelial cells also express the ACE2 [131, 132], and more than half of the lung tissue is endothelial tissue [133]. Endothelial injury increases microvascular permeability, and this permeability leads to viral invasion.

Infants and young children have shown milder symptoms in the COVID-19 than the other respiratory issues in which young kids are more at risk [134]. At old age, the patient with COVID-19 is observed to have pathological T cells. It was reported that during the early age of life, the CD4+ T cells are reduced regarding Th1 cell production (associated proinflammatory cytokines) and thus skewed towards Th2 [135]. The T cells at a young age have less ability to kill the cells, which can explain the susceptibility of the infants to the SARS-CoV-2. A study was conducted in the macaques in which age and severity of the infection were compared of SARS-CoV infection. Results showed that lung injury was higher in old macaques due to robust cell inflammatory responses than the young age [136]. Similar results were obtained in the mice infected with SARS-CoV [137]. Severe disease of the COVID-19 is associated with the massive proinflammatory responses that cause ARDS and multiorgan failures. This response is also different at different ages [138]. With age, proinflammatory cytokines are increased, and their responses become more robust. This leads to more inflammation of the lungs, but this is not like that at a younger age. With the advancement of age, the number of other pathogens also increases in the respiratory passage compared to the young this could also contribute to the severity of the disease [139].

CONCLUSION AND FUTURE PERSPECTIVES

Keeping in view the studies around the globe, the SARS-Cov2 pandemic has massively caused a giant impact on the economy and health. It is concluded that the mutation accumulation and emergence of different major clades and sub-clades in various geographic regions played an active role in worsens the condition. The virus is evolving, and strains from different geographic regions might coexist whereas, different mutation patterns may characterize each strain. The emergence of mutations on the viral genome's structural part, including RdRp, Spikes, and nucleocapsid coding genes, leads to the new variants. Mutations have a direct and/or indirect role where virus transmission and disease severity might affect. The imperative consequence exists in response to the emergence of various subclones of SARS-Cov2 that can affect viral phenotype. Similarly, the comprehensive knowledge of RdRp contribution to the mutation phenomenon is vital so that the mutation pattern may be thoroughly investigated.

The complete understanding of genetic diversity and Covid-19 evolution has become a priority matter to combat disease. There is a need to perform the complete bioinformatic and genomic analysis in the future. Also, the maximum number of possible implications of mutation must be under observation so that important insights will be helpful to understand the molecular basis of disease severity.

CONSENT FOR PUBLICATION

Not Applicable.

CONFLICT OF INTEREST

The author confirms that this chapter contents have no conflict of interest.

ACKNOWLEDGEMENT

Declared none.

REFERENCES

[1]   Surveillances V. The epidemiological characteristics of an outbreak of 2019 novel coronavirus diseases (COVID-19)—China, 2020. China CDC Weekly 2020; 2(8): 113-22.
[http://dx.doi.org/10.46234/ccdcw2020.032]

[2]   Organization, W.H. Coronavirus disease 2019 (COVID-19): situation report 2020; 72.

[3]   Peiris JS, Lai ST, Poon LL, *et al.* Coronavirus as a possible cause of severe acute respiratory syndrome. Lancet 2003; 361(9366): 1319-25.
[http://dx.doi.org/10.1016/S0140-6736(03)13077-2] [PMID: 12711465]

[4]   Zaki AM, van Boheemen S, Bestebroer TM, Osterhaus AD, Fouchier RA. Isolation of a novel

coronavirus from a man with pneumonia in Saudi Arabia. N Engl J Med 2012; 367(19): 1814-20.
[http://dx.doi.org/10.1056/NEJMoa1211721] [PMID: 23075143]

[5]   Astuti I, Ysrafil . Severe Acute Respiratory Syndrome Coronavirus 2 (SARS-CoV-2): An overview of viral structure and host response. Diabetes Metab Syndr 2020; 14(4): 407-12.
[http://dx.doi.org/10.1016/j.dsx.2020.04.020] [PMID: 32335367]

[6]   Gorbalenya AE, Enjuanes L, Ziebuhr J, Snijder EJ. Nidovirales: evolving the largest RNA virus genome. Virus Res 2006; 117(1): 17-37.
[http://dx.doi.org/10.1016/j.virusres.2006.01.017] [PMID: 16503362]

[7]   Stenglein MD, Jacobson ER, Wozniak EJ, *et al.* Ball python nidovirus: a candidate etiologic agent for severe respiratory disease in Python regius. MBio 2014; 5(5): e01484-14.
[http://dx.doi.org/10.1128/mBio.01484-14] [PMID: 25205093]

[8]   Yeşilbağ K, Aytoğu G. Coronavirus host divergence and novel coronavirus (Sars-CoV-2) outbreak. Clinical and Experimental Ocular Trauma and Infection 2020; 2(1): 1-9.

[9]   Andersen KG, Rambaut A, Lipkin WI, Holmes EC, Garry RF. The proximal origin of SARS-CoV-2. Nat Med 2020; 26(4): 450-2.
[http://dx.doi.org/10.1038/s41591-020-0820-9] [PMID: 32284615]

[10]   Hui DS, I Azhar E, Madani TA, *et al.* The continuing 2019-nCoV epidemic threat of novel coronaviruses to global health - The latest 2019 novel coronavirus outbreak in Wuhan, China. Int J Infect Dis 2020; 91: 264-6.
[http://dx.doi.org/10.1016/j.ijid.2020.01.009] [PMID: 31953166]

[11]   Li B, Si H-R, Zhu Y, *et al.* Discovery of bat coronaviruses through surveillance and probe capture-based next-generation sequencing. MSphere 2020; 5: 1.: e00807-19.
[http://dx.doi.org/10.1128/mSphere.00807-19] [PMID: 31996413]

[12]   Wu A, Peng Y, Huang B, *et al.* Genome composition and divergence of the novel coronavirus (2019-nCoV) originating in China. Cell Host Microbe 2020; 27(3): 325-8.
[http://dx.doi.org/10.1016/j.chom.2020.02.001] [PMID: 32035028]

[13]   Sanjuán R, Nebot MR, Chirico N, Mansky LM, Belshaw R. Viral mutation rates. J Virol 2010; 84(19): 9733-48.
[http://dx.doi.org/10.1128/JVI.00694-10] [PMID: 20660197]

[14]   Crotty S, Cameron CE, Andino R. RNA virus error catastrophe: direct molecular test by using ribavirin. Proc Natl Acad Sci USA 2001; 98(12): 6895-900.
[http://dx.doi.org/10.1073/pnas.111085598] [PMID: 11371613]

[15]   Smith EC, Denison MR. Implications of altered replication fidelity on the evolution and pathogenesis of coronaviruses. Curr Opin Virol 2012; 2(5): 519-24.
[http://dx.doi.org/10.1016/j.coviro.2012.07.005] [PMID: 22857992]

[16]   Castro C, Arnold JJ, Cameron CE. Incorporation fidelity of the viral RNA-dependent RNA polymerase: a kinetic, thermodynamic and structural perspective. Virus Res 2005; 107(2): 141-9.
[http://dx.doi.org/10.1016/j.virusres.2004.11.004] [PMID: 15649560]

[17]   Sanjuán R. From molecular genetics to phylodynamics: evolutionary relevance of mutation rates across viruses. PLoS Pathog 2012; 8(5): e1002685.
[http://dx.doi.org/10.1371/journal.ppat.1002685] [PMID: 22570614]

[18]   Domingo E. Mechanisms of viral emergence. Vet Res 2010; 41(6): 38.
[http://dx.doi.org/10.1051/vetres/2010010] [PMID: 20167200]

[19]   Arnold JJ, Vignuzzi M, Stone JK, Andino R, Cameron CE. Remote site control of an active site fidelity checkpoint in a viral RNA-dependent RNA polymerase. J Biol Chem 2005; 280(27): 25706-16.
[http://dx.doi.org/10.1074/jbc.M503444200] [PMID: 15878882]

[20] Campagnola G, McDonald S, Beaucourt S, Vignuzzi M, Peersen OB. Structure-function relationships underlying the replication fidelity of viral RNA-dependent RNA polymerases. J Virol 2015; 89(1): 275-86.
[http://dx.doi.org/10.1128/JVI.01574-14] [PMID: 25320316]

[21] Jia Y, Shen G, Zhang Y, *et al.* Analysis of the mutation dynamics of SARS-CoV-2 reveals the spread history and emergence of RBD mutant with lower ACE2 binding affinity BioRxiv 2020.

[22] Pachetti M, Marini B, Benedetti F, *et al.* Emerging SARS-CoV-2 mutation hot spots include a novel RNA-dependent-RNA polymerase variant. J Transl Med 2020; 18(1): 179.
[http://dx.doi.org/10.1186/s12967-020-02344-6] [PMID: 32321524]

[23] Li LQ, Huang T, Wang YQ, *et al.* COVID-19 patients' clinical characteristics, discharge rate, and fatality rate of meta-analysis. J Med Virol 2020; 92(6): 577-83.
[http://dx.doi.org/10.1002/jmv.25757] [PMID: 32162702]

[24] Eckerle LD, Becker MM, Halpin RA, *et al.* Infidelity of SARS-CoV Nsp14-exonuclease mutant virus replication is revealed by complete genome sequencing. PLoS Pathog 2010; 6(5): e1000896.
[http://dx.doi.org/10.1371/journal.ppat.1000896] [PMID: 20463816]

[25] Smith EC, Blanc H, Surdel MC, Vignuzzi M, Denison MR. Coronaviruses lacking exoribonuclease activity are susceptible to lethal mutagenesis: evidence for proofreading and potential therapeutics. PLoS Pathog 2013; 9(8): e1003565.
[http://dx.doi.org/10.1371/journal.ppat.1003565] [PMID: 23966862]

[26] Smith EC, Sexton NR, Denison MR. Thinking outside the triangle: replication fidelity of the largest RNA viruses. Annu Rev Virol 2014; 1(1): 111-32.
[http://dx.doi.org/10.1146/annurev-virology-031413-085507] [PMID: 26958717]

[27] Sexton NR, Smith EC, Blanc H, Vignuzzi M, Peersen OB, Denison MR. Homology-based identification of a mutation in the coronavirus RNA-dependent RNA polymerase that confers resistance to multiple mutagens. J Virol 2016; 90(16): 7415-28.
[http://dx.doi.org/10.1128/JVI.00080-16] [PMID: 27279608]

[28] Maitra A, Sarkar MC, Raheja H, *et al.* Mutations in SARS-CoV-2 viral RNA identified in Eastern India: Possible implications for the ongoing outbreak in India and impact on viral structure and host susceptibility. J Biosci 2020; 45(1): 76.
[http://dx.doi.org/10.1007/s12038-020-00046-1] [PMID: 32515358]

[29] Wang C, Liu Z, Chen Z, *et al.* The establishment of reference sequence for SARS-CoV-2 and variation analysis. J Med Virol 2020; 92(6): 667-74.
[http://dx.doi.org/10.1002/jmv.25762] [PMID: 32167180]

[30] Domingo E, Holland JJ. RNA virus mutations and fitness for survival. Annu Rev Microbiol 1997; 51(1): 151-78.
[http://dx.doi.org/10.1146/annurev.micro.51.1.151] [PMID: 9343347]

[31] Domingo E. Viruses at the edge of adaptation. Virology 2000; 270(2): 251-3.
[http://dx.doi.org/10.1006/viro.2000.0320] [PMID: 10792982]

[32] Domingo E. Quasispecies theory in virology. J Virol 2002; 76(1): 463-5.
[http://dx.doi.org/10.1128/JVI.76.1.463-465.2002] [PMID: 33739796]

[33] Tang X, Wu C, Li X, *et al.* On the origin and continuing evolution of SARS-CoV-2. Natl Sci Rev 2020.
[http://dx.doi.org/10.1093/nsr/nwaa036]

[34] Shen Z, Xiao Y, Kang L, *et al.* Genomic diversity of SARS-CoV-2 in Coronavirus Disease 2019 patients. Clin Infect Dis 2020.
[http://dx.doi.org/10.1093/cid/ciaa203]

[35] Phan T. Genetic diversity and evolution of SARS-CoV-2. Infect Genet Evol 2020; 81: 104260.

[http://dx.doi.org/10.1016/j.meegid.2020.104260] [PMID: 32092483]

[36]   Najjar M, Suebsuwong C, Ray SS, *et al.* Structure guided design of potent and selective ponatinib-based hybrid inhibitors for RIPK1. Cell Rep 2015; 10(11): 1850-60.
[http://dx.doi.org/10.1016/j.celrep.2015.02.052] [PMID: 25801024]

[37]   Koyama T, Platt D, Parida L. Variant analysis of SARS-CoV-2 genomes. Bull World Health Organ 2020; 98(7): 495-504.
[http://dx.doi.org/10.2471/BLT.20.253591] [PMID: 32742035]

[38]   Agostini ML, Andres EL, Sims AC, *et al.* Coronavirus susceptibility to the antiviral remdesivir (GS-5734) is mediated by the viral polymerase and the proofreading exoribonuclease. MBio 2018; 9(2): e00221-18.
[http://dx.doi.org/10.1128/mBio.00221-18] [PMID: 29511076]

[39]   Goldhill DH, Te Velthuis AJW, Fletcher RA, *et al.* The mechanism of resistance to favipiravir in influenza. Proc Natl Acad Sci USA 2018; 115(45): 11613-8.
[http://dx.doi.org/10.1073/pnas.1811345115] [PMID: 30352857]

[40]   Young RE, Thompson RD, Larbi KY, *et al.* Neutrophil elastase (NE)-deficient mice demonstrate a nonredundant role for NE in neutrophil migration, generation of proinflammatory mediators, and phagocytosis in response to zymosan particles *in vivo.* J Immunol 2004; 172(7): 4493-502.
[http://dx.doi.org/10.4049/jimmunol.172.7.4493] [PMID: 15034066]

[41]   Pfeiffer JK, Kirkegaard K. A single mutation in poliovirus RNA-dependent RNA polymerase confers resistance to mutagenic nucleotide analogs *via* increased fidelity. Proc Natl Acad Sci USA 2003; 100(12): 7289-94.
[http://dx.doi.org/10.1073/pnas.1232294100] [PMID: 12754380]

[42]   Laamarti M, Alouane T, Kartti S, *et al.* Large scale genomic analysis of 3067 SARS-CoV-2 genomes reveals a clonal geodistribution and a rich genetic variations of hotspots mutations bioRxiv 2020.

[43]   Yin C. Genotyping coronavirus SARS-CoV-2: methods and implications. Genomics 2020; 112(5): 3588-96.
[http://dx.doi.org/10.1016/j.ygeno.2020.04.016] [PMID: 32353474]

[44]   Organization WH. Infection prevention and control during health care when COVID-19 is suspected: interim guidance, March 19 2020. World Health Organization 2020.

[45]   te Velthuis AJ, van den Worm SH, Snijder EJ. The SARS-coronavirus nsp7 I nsp8 complex is a unique multimeric RNA polymerase capable of both *de novo* initiation and primer extension. Nucleic Acids Res 2012; 40(4): 1737-47.
[http://dx.doi.org/10.1093/nar/gkr893] [PMID: 22039154]

[46]   Zhang L, Shen FM, Chen F, Lin Z. Origin and evolution of the 2019 novel coronavirus. Clin Infect Dis 2020; 71(15): 882-3.
[http://dx.doi.org/10.1093/cid/ciaa112] [PMID: 32011673]

[47]   Stern A, Te Yeh M, Zinger T, *et al.* The evolutionary pathway to virulence of an RNA virus. Cell 2017; 169(1): 35-46.
[http://dx.doi.org/10.1016/j.cell.2017.03.013]

[48]   Denison MR, Graham RL, Donaldson EF, Eckerle LD, Baric RS. Coronaviruses: an RNA proofreading machine regulates replication fidelity and diversity. RNA Biol 2011; 8(2): 270-9.
[http://dx.doi.org/10.4161/rna.8.2.15013] [PMID: 21593585]

[49]   Domingo E, Sheldon J, Perales C. Viral quasispecies evolution. Microbiol Mol Biol Rev 2012; 76(2): 159-216.
[http://dx.doi.org/10.1128/MMBR.05023-11] [PMID: 22688811]

[50]   Kirchdoerfer RN, Ward AB. Structure of the SARS-CoV nsp12 polymerase bound to nsp7 and nsp8 co-factors. Nat Commun 2019; 10(1): 2342.
[http://dx.doi.org/10.1038/s41467-019-10280-3] [PMID: 31138817]

[51]   Zhai Y, Sun F, Li X, *et al.* Insights into SARS-CoV transcription and replication from the structure of the nsp7-nsp8 hexadecamer. Nat Struct Mol Biol 2005; 12(11): 980-6.
[http://dx.doi.org/10.1038/nsmb999] [PMID: 16228002]

[52]   Subissi L, Posthuma CC, Collet A, *et al.* One severe acute respiratory syndrome coronavirus protein complex integrates processive RNA polymerase and exonuclease activities. Proc Natl Acad Sci USA 2014; 111(37): E3900-9.
[http://dx.doi.org/10.1073/pnas.1323705111] [PMID: 25197083]

[53]   Vignuzzi M, Stone JK, Andino R. Ribavirin and lethal mutagenesis of poliovirus: molecular mechanisms, resistance and biological implications. Virus Res 2005; 107(2): 173-81.
[http://dx.doi.org/10.1016/j.virusres.2004.11.007] [PMID: 15649563]

[54]   Pfeiffer JK, Kirkegaard K. Increased fidelity reduces poliovirus fitness and virulence under selective pressure in mice. PLoS Pathog 2005; 1(2): e11.
[http://dx.doi.org/10.1371/journal.ppat.0010011] [PMID: 16220146]

[55]   Severson WE, Schmaljohn CS, Javadian A, Jonsson CB. Ribavirin causes error catastrophe during Hantaan virus replication. J Virol 2003; 77(1): 481-8.
[http://dx.doi.org/10.1128/JVI.77.1.481-488.2003] [PMID: 12477853]

[56]   Gnädig NF, Beaucourt S, Campagnola G, *et al.* Coxsackievirus B3 mutator strains are attenuated *in vivo*. Proc Natl Acad Sci USA 2012; 109(34): E2294-303.
[http://dx.doi.org/10.1073/pnas.1204022109] [PMID: 22853955]

[57]   Dapp MJ, Heineman RH, Mansky LM. Interrelationship between HIV-1 fitness and mutation rate. J Mol Biol 2013; 425(1): 41-53.
[http://dx.doi.org/10.1016/j.jmb.2012.10.009] [PMID: 23084856]

[58]   Bruenn JA. A structural and primary sequence comparison of the viral RNA-dependent RNA polymerases. Nucleic Acids Res 2003; 31(7): 1821-9.
[http://dx.doi.org/10.1093/nar/gkg277] [PMID: 12654997]

[59]   Lang DM, Zemla AT, Zhou CL. Highly similar structural frames link the template tunnel and NTP entry tunnel to the exterior surface in RNA-dependent RNA polymerases. Nucleic Acids Res 2013; 41(3): 1464-82.
[http://dx.doi.org/10.1093/nar/gks1251] [PMID: 23275546]

[60]   Butcher SJ, Grimes JM, Makeyev EV, Bamford DH, Stuart DI. A mechanism for initiating RNA-dependent RNA polymerization. Nature 2001; 410(6825): 235-40.
[http://dx.doi.org/10.1038/35065653] [PMID: 11242087]

[61]   Ng KK-S, J.J. Arnold, C.E. Cameron. In RNA Interference. Springer 2008; pp. 137-56.

[62]   Barzon L, Lavezzo E, Militello V, Toppo S, Palù G. Applications of next-generation sequencing technologies to diagnostic virology. Int J Mol Sci 2011; 12(11): 7861-84.
[http://dx.doi.org/10.3390/ijms12117861] [PMID: 22174638]

[63]   He Y, Wu J, Dressman DC, *et al.* Heteroplasmic mitochondrial DNA mutations in normal and tumour cells. Nature 2010; 464(7288): 610-4.
[http://dx.doi.org/10.1038/nature08802] [PMID: 20200521]

[64]   Mwenifumbo JC, Marra MA. Cancer genome-sequencing study design. Nat Rev Genet 2013; 14(5): 321-32.
[http://dx.doi.org/10.1038/nrg3445] [PMID: 23594910]

[65]   Salehi F, Baronio R, Idrogo-Lam R, *et al.* CHOPER filters enable rare mutation detection in complex mutagenesis populations by next-generation sequencing. PLoS One 2015; 10(2): e0116877.
[http://dx.doi.org/10.1371/journal.pone.0116877] [PMID: 25692681]

[66]   Salk JJ, Schmitt MW, Loeb LA. Enhancing the accuracy of next-generation sequencing for detecting rare and subclonal mutations. Nat Rev Genet 2018; 19(5): 269-85.

[http://dx.doi.org/10.1038/nrg.2017.117] [PMID: 29576615]

[67]   Woo H-J, Reifman J. A quantitative quasispecies theory-based model of virus escape mutation under immune selection. Proc Natl Acad Sci USA 2012; 109(32): 12980-5.
[http://dx.doi.org/10.1073/pnas.1117201109] [PMID: 22826258]

[68]   Andino R, Domingo E. Viral quasispecies. Virology 2015; 479-480: 46-51.
[http://dx.doi.org/10.1016/j.virol.2015.03.022] [PMID: 25824477]

[69]   Lu I-N, Muller CP, He FQ. Applying next-generation sequencing to unravel the mutational landscape in viral quasispecies. Virus Res 2020; 283: 197963.
[http://dx.doi.org/10.1016/j.virusres.2020.197963] [PMID: 32278821]

[70]   Zhu N, Zhang D, Wang W, *et al.* A novel coronavirus from patients with pneumonia in China, 2019. N Engl J Med 2020; 382(8): 727-33.
[http://dx.doi.org/10.1056/NEJMoa2001017] [PMID: 31978945]

[71]   James KL, de Silva TI, Brown K, *et al.* Low-bias RNA sequencing of the HIV-2 genome from blood plasma. J Virol 2018; 93(1): e00677-18.
[http://dx.doi.org/10.1128/JVI.00677-18] [PMID: 30333167]

[72]   Kyeyune F, Gibson RM, Nankya I, *et al.* Low-frequency drug resistance in HIV-infected Ugandans on antiretroviral treatment is associated with regimen failure. Antimicrob Agents Chemother 2016; 60(6): 3380-97.
[http://dx.doi.org/10.1128/AAC.00038-16] [PMID: 27001818]

[73]   Rawson JMO, Gohl DM, Landman SR, *et al.* Single-strand consensus sequencing reveals that HIV type but not subtype significantly impacts viral mutation frequencies and spectra. J Mol Biol 2017; 429(15): 2290-307.
[http://dx.doi.org/10.1016/j.jmb.2017.05.010] [PMID: 28502791]

[74]   Acevedo A, Brodsky L, Andino R. Mutational and fitness landscapes of an RNA virus revealed through population sequencing. Nature 2014; 505(7485): 686-90.
[http://dx.doi.org/10.1038/nature12861] [PMID: 24284629]

[75]   Itakura J, Kurosaki M, Higuchi M, *et al.* Resistance-associated NS5A variants of hepatitis C virus are susceptible to interferon-based therapy. PLoS One 2015; 10(9): e0138060.
[http://dx.doi.org/10.1371/journal.pone.0138060] [PMID: 26368554]

[76]   Houldcroft CJ, Beale MA, Breuer J. Clinical and biological insights from viral genome sequencing. Nat Rev Microbiol 2017; 15(3): 183-92.
[http://dx.doi.org/10.1038/nrmicro.2016.182] [PMID: 28090077]

[77]   Datta S, Budhauliya R, Das B, Chatterjee S, Vanlalhmuaka , Veer V. Next-generation sequencing in clinical virology: Discovery of new viruses. World J Virol 2015; 4(3): 265-76.
[http://dx.doi.org/10.5501/wjv.v4.i3.265] [PMID: 26279987]

[78]   Barzon L, Lavezzo E, Costanzi G, Franchin E, Toppo S, Palù G. Next-generation sequencing technologies in diagnostic virology. J Clin Virol 2013; 58(2): 346-50.
[http://dx.doi.org/10.1016/j.jcv.2013.03.003] [PMID: 23523339]

[79]   Gardy JL, Loman NJ. Towards a genomics-informed, real-time, global pathogen surveillance system. Nat Rev Genet 2018; 19(1): 9-20.
[http://dx.doi.org/10.1038/nrg.2017.88] [PMID: 29129921]

[80]   Kuroda M, Katano H, Nakajima N, *et al.* Characterization of quasispecies of pandemic 2009 influenza A virus (A/H1N1/2009) by *de novo* sequencing using a next-generation DNA sequencer. PLoS One 2010; 5(4): e10256.
[http://dx.doi.org/10.1371/journal.pone.0010256] [PMID: 20428231]

[81]   Prachayangprecha S, Schapendonk CM, Koopmans MP, *et al.* Exploring the potential of next-generation sequencing in detection of respiratory viruses. J Clin Microbiol 2014; 52(10): 3722-30.
[http://dx.doi.org/10.1128/JCM.01641-14] [PMID: 25100822]

[82]   Shendure J, Balasubramanian S, Church GM, *et al.* DNA sequencing at 40: past, present and future. Nature 2017; 550(7676): 345-53.
[http://dx.doi.org/10.1038/nature24286] [PMID: 29019985]

[83]   Bosch BJ, van der Zee R, de Haan CA, Rottier PJ. The coronavirus spike protein is a class I virus fusion protein: structural and functional characterization of the fusion core complex. J Virol 2003; 77(16): 8801-11.
[http://dx.doi.org/10.1128/JVI.77.16.8801-8811.2003] [PMID: 12885899]

[84]   Banerjee AK, Begum F, Ray U. Mutation Hot Spots in Spike Protein of COVID-19 2020.

[85]   Tai W, He L, Zhang X, *et al.* Characterization of the receptor-binding domain (RBD) of 2019 novel coronavirus: implication for development of RBD protein as a viral attachment inhibitor and vaccine. Cell Mol Immunol 2020; 17(6): 613-20.
[http://dx.doi.org/10.1038/s41423-020-0400-4] [PMID: 32203189]

[86]   Angeletti S, Benvenuto D, Bianchi M, Giovanetti M, Pascarella S, Ciccozzi M. COVID-2019: The role of the nsp2 and nsp3 in its pathogenesis. J Med Virol 2020; 92(6): 584-8.
[http://dx.doi.org/10.1002/jmv.25719] [PMID: 32083328]

[87]   Woo HJ, Reifman J. Quantitative modeling of virus evolutionary dynamics and adaptation in serial passages using empirically inferred fitness landscapes. J Virol 2014; 88(2): 1039-50.
[http://dx.doi.org/10.1128/JVI.02958-13] [PMID: 24198414]

[88]   Eigen M. Selforganization of matter and the evolution of biological macromolecules. Naturwissenschaften 1971; 58(10): 465-523.
[http://dx.doi.org/10.1007/BF00623322] [PMID: 4942363]

[89]   Chang Y-C, Tung Y-A, Lee K-H, *et al.* Potential therapeutic agents for COVID-19 based on the analysis of protease and RNA polymerase docking 2020.

[90]   Contini A. Virtual screening of an FDA approved drugs database on two COVID-19 coronavirus proteins 2020.

[91]   Dayer MR. Old drugs for newly emerging viral disease, COVID-19: Bioinformatic Prospective 2020.

[92]   Molina JM, Delaugerre C, Le Goff J, *et al.* No evidence of rapid antiviral clearance or clinical benefit with the combination of hydroxychloroquine and azithromycin in patients with severe COVID-19 infection. Med Mal Infect 2020; 50(4): 384.
[http://dx.doi.org/10.1016/j.medmal.2020.03.006] [PMID: 32240719]

[93]   Sunny JS, Balachandran S, Solaipriya S, Saleena LM. Comparison of random and site directed mutation effects on the efficacy between lead SARS-CoV2 anti-protease drugs Indinavir and Hydroxychloroquine 2020.

[94]   Babé LM, Craik CS. Viral proteases: evolution of diverse structural motifs to optimize function. Cell 1997; 91(4): 427-30.
[http://dx.doi.org/10.1016/S0092-8674(00)80426-2] [PMID: 9390549]

[95]   Kurt Yilmaz N, Swanstrom R, Schiffer CA. Improving viral protease inhibitors to counter drug resistance. Trends Microbiol 2016; 24(7): 547-57.
[http://dx.doi.org/10.1016/j.tim.2016.03.010] [PMID: 27090931]

[96]   Patil R, Das S, Stanley A, Yadav L, Sudhakar A, Varma AK. Optimized hydrophobic interactions and hydrogen bonding at the target-ligand interface leads the pathways of drug-designing. PLoS One 2010; 5(8): e12029.
[http://dx.doi.org/10.1371/journal.pone.0012029] [PMID: 20808434]

[97]   Begum F, Mukherjee D, Das S, *et al.* Specific mutations in SARS-CoV2 RNA dependent RNA polymerase and helicase alter protein structure, dynamics and thus function: Effect on viral RNA replication bioRxiv 2020.
[http://dx.doi.org/10.1101/2020.04.26.063024]

[98]   Ziebuhr J. In Coronavirus replication and reverse genetics. Springer 2005; pp. 57-94.
[http://dx.doi.org/10.1007/3-540-26765-4_3]

[99]   Howland J. Structure and Mechanism in Protein Science. A guide to Enzyme Catalysis and Protein
Folding-Alan Fersht, WH Freeman and Company, New York, 1999, 631 pp, ISBN 0-7167-3268-8,
$53.00. Biochem Mol Biol Educ 2001; 1(29): 36.
[http://dx.doi.org/10.1016/S0307-4412(99)00114-4]

[100]   Zhong NS, Zheng BJ, Li YM, *et al.* Epidemiology and cause of severe acute respiratory syndrome
(SARS) in Guangdong, People's Republic of China, in February, 2003. Lancet 2003; 362(9393):
1353-8.
[http://dx.doi.org/10.1016/S0140-6736(03)14630-2] [PMID: 14585636]

[101]   Wang N, Shi X, Jiang L, *et al.* Structure of MERS-CoV spike receptor-binding domain complexed
with human receptor DPP4. Cell Res 2013; 23(8): 986-93.
[http://dx.doi.org/10.1038/cr.2013.92] [PMID: 23835475]

[102]   Chen Y, Liu Q, Guo D. Emerging coronaviruses: Genome structure, replication, and pathogenesis. J
Med Virol 2020; 92(4): 418-23.
[http://dx.doi.org/10.1002/jmv.25681] [PMID: 31967327]

[103]   Gralinski LE, Menachery VD. Return of the Coronavirus: 2019-nCoV. Viruses 2020; 12(2): 135.
[http://dx.doi.org/10.3390/v12020135] [PMID: 31991541]

[104]   Xu X, Chen P, Wang J, *et al.* Evolution of the novel coronavirus from the ongoing Wuhan outbreak
and modeling of its spike protein for risk of human transmission. Sci China Life Sci 2020; 63(3): 457-
60.
[http://dx.doi.org/10.1007/s11427-020-1637-5] [PMID: 32009228]

[105]   Yuki K, Fujiogi M, Koutsogiannaki S. COVID-19 pathophysiology: A review. Clin Immunol 2020;
215: 108427.
[http://dx.doi.org/10.1016/j.clim.2020.108427] [PMID: 32325252]

[106]   Li W, Moore MJ, Vasilieva N, *et al.* Angiotensin-converting enzyme 2 is a functional receptor for the
SARS coronavirus. Nature 2003; 426(6965): 450-4.
[http://dx.doi.org/10.1038/nature02145] [PMID: 14647384]

[107]   Ni L, Zhou L, Zhou M, Zhao J, Wang DW. Combination of western medicine and Chinese traditional
patent medicine in treating a family case of COVID-19. Front Med 2020; 14(2): 210-4.
[http://dx.doi.org/10.1007/s11684-020-0757-x] [PMID: 32170559]

[108]   Belouzard S, Chu VC, Whittaker GR. Activation of the SARS coronavirus spike protein *via* sequential
proteolytic cleavage at two distinct sites. Proc Natl Acad Sci USA 2009; 106(14): 5871-6.
[http://dx.doi.org/10.1073/pnas.0809524106] [PMID: 19321428]

[109]   Millet JK, Whittaker GR. Host cell entry of Middle East respiratory syndrome coronavirus after two-
step, furin-mediated activation of the spike protein. Proc Natl Acad Sci USA 2014; 111(42): 15214-9.
[http://dx.doi.org/10.1073/pnas.1407087111] [PMID: 25288733]

[110]   Ou X, Liu Y, Lei X, *et al.* Characterization of spike glycoprotein of SARS-CoV-2 on virus entry and
its immune cross-reactivity with SARS-CoV. Nat Commun 2020; 11(1): 1620.
[http://dx.doi.org/10.1038/s41467-020-15562-9] [PMID: 32221306]

[111]   Walls AC, Park Y-J, Tortorici MA, Wall A, McGuire AT, Veesler D. Structure, function, and
antigenicity of the SARS-CoV-2 spike glycoprotein. Cell 2020.
[http://dx.doi.org/10.1016/j.cell.2020.11.032]

[112]   Belouzard S, Millet JK, Licitra BN, Whittaker GR. Mechanisms of coronavirus cell entry mediated by
the viral spike protein. Viruses 2012; 4(6): 1011-33.
[http://dx.doi.org/10.3390/v4061011] [PMID: 22816037]

[113]   Hamming I, Timens W, Bulthuis M, Lely A, Navis Gv, van Goor H. Tissue distribution of ACE2

protein, the functional receptor for SARS coronavirus. A first step in understanding SARS pathogenesis. The Journal of Pathology: A Journal of the Pathological Society of Great Britain and Ireland 2004; 203(2): 631-7.

[114] Jia HP, Look DC, Shi L, *et al.* ACE2 receptor expression and severe acute respiratory syndrome coronavirus infection depend on differentiation of human airway epithelia. J Virol 2005; 79(23): 14614-21.
[http://dx.doi.org/10.1128/JVI.79.23.14614-14621.2005] [PMID: 16282461]

[115] Yoshikawa T, Hill T, Li K, Peters CJ, Tseng C-TK. Severe acute respiratory syndrome (SARS) coronavirus-induced lung epithelial cytokines exacerbate SARS pathogenesis by modulating intrinsic functions of monocyte-derived macrophages and dendritic cells. J Virol 2009; 83(7): 3039-48.
[http://dx.doi.org/10.1128/JVI.01792-08] [PMID: 19004938]

[116] Channappanavar R, Zhao J, Perlman S. T cell-mediated immune response to respiratory coronaviruses. Immunol Res 2014; 59(1-3): 118-28.
[http://dx.doi.org/10.1007/s12026-014-8534-z] [PMID: 24845462]

[117] Fujimoto I, Pan J, Takizawa T, Nakanishi Y. Virus clearance through apoptosis-dependent phagocytosis of influenza A virus-infected cells by macrophages. J Virol 2000; 74(7): 3399-403.
[http://dx.doi.org/10.1128/JVI.74.7.3399-3403.2000] [PMID: 10708457]

[118] Jeffers SA, Tusell SM, Gillim-Ross L, *et al.* CD209L (L-SIGN) is a receptor for severe acute respiratory syndrome coronavirus. Proc Natl Acad Sci USA 2004; 101(44): 15748-53.
[http://dx.doi.org/10.1073/pnas.0403812101] [PMID: 15496474]

[119] Marzi A, Gramberg T, Simmons G, *et al.* DC-SIGN and DC-SIGNR interact with the glycoprotein of Marburg virus and the S protein of severe acute respiratory syndrome coronavirus. J Virol 2004; 78(21): 12090-5.
[http://dx.doi.org/10.1128/JVI.78.21.12090-12095.2004] [PMID: 15479853]

[120] Yang Z-Y, Huang Y, Ganesh L, *et al.* pH-dependent entry of severe acute respiratory syndrome coronavirus is mediated by the spike glycoprotein and enhanced by dendritic cell transfer through DC-SIGN. J Virol 2004; 78(11): 5642-50.
[http://dx.doi.org/10.1128/JVI.78.11.5642-5650.2004] [PMID: 15140961]

[121] Zhou Y, Fu B, Zheng X, *et al.* Pathogenic T-cells and inflammatory monocytes incite inflammatory storms in severe COVID-19 patients. Natl Sci Rev 2020.
[http://dx.doi.org/10.1093/nsr/nwaa041]

[122] Liu S, Su X, Pan P, *et al.* Neutrophil extracellular traps are indirectly triggered by lipopolysaccharide and contribute to acute lung injury. Sci Rep 2016; 6: 37252.
[http://dx.doi.org/10.1038/srep37252] [PMID: 27849031]

[123] Liu Y, Du X, Chen J, *et al.* Neutrophil-to-lymphocyte ratio as an independent risk factor for mortality in hospitalized patients with COVID-19. J Infect 2020; 81(1): e6-e12.
[http://dx.doi.org/10.1016/j.jinf.2020.04.002] [PMID: 32283162]

[124] Huang C, Wang Y, Li X, *et al.* Clinical features of patients infected with 2019 novel coronavirus in Wuhan, China. Lancet 2020; 395(10223): 497-506.
[http://dx.doi.org/10.1016/S0140-6736(20)30183-5] [PMID: 31986264]

[125] Zheng M, Gao Y, Wang G, *et al.* Functional exhaustion of antiviral lymphocytes in COVID-19 patients. Cell Mol Immunol 2020; 17(5): 533-5.
[http://dx.doi.org/10.1038/s41423-020-0402-2] [PMID: 32203188]

[126] Tian S, Hu W, Niu L, Liu H, Xu H, Xiao S-Y. Pulmonary pathology of early phase 2019 novel coronavirus (COVID-19) pneumonia in two patients with lung cancer. J Thorac Oncol 2020; 15(5): 700-4.
[http://dx.doi.org/10.1016/j.jtho.2020.02.010] [PMID: 32114094]

[127] Wang M, Hao H, Leeper NJ, Zhu L. Thrombotic regulation from the endothelial cell perspectives.

Arterioscler Thromb Vasc Biol 2018; 38(6): e90-5.
[http://dx.doi.org/10.1161/ATVBAHA.118.310367] [PMID: 29793992]

[128] Koutsogiannaki S, Shimaoka M, Yuki K. The use of volatile anesthetics as sedatives for acute respiratory distress syndrome. Transl Perioper Pain Med 2019; 6(2): 27-38.
[PMID: 30923729]

[129] Fang M, Siciliano NA, Hersperger AR, *et al.* Perforin-dependent CD4+ T-cell cytotoxicity contributes to control a murine poxvirus infection. Proc Natl Acad Sci USA 2012; 109(25): 9983-8.
[http://dx.doi.org/10.1073/pnas.1202143109] [PMID: 22665800]

[130] Small BA, Dressel SA, Lawrence CW, *et al.* CD8(+) T cell-mediated injury *in vivo* progresses in the absence of effector T cells. J Exp Med 2001; 194(12): 1835-46.
[http://dx.doi.org/10.1084/jem.194.12.1835] [PMID: 11748284]

[131] Lovren F, Pan Y, Quan A, *et al.* Angiotensin converting enzyme-2 confers endothelial protection and attenuates atherosclerosis. Am J Physiol Heart Circ Physiol 2008; 295(4): H1377-84.
[http://dx.doi.org/10.1152/ajpheart.00331.2008] [PMID: 18660448]

[132] Thatcher SE, Zhang X, Howatt DA, *et al.* Angiotensin-converting enzyme 2 deficiency in whole body or bone marrow-derived cells increases atherosclerosis in low-density lipoprotein receptor-/- mice. Arterioscler Thromb Vasc Biol 2011; 31(4): 758-65.
[http://dx.doi.org/10.1161/ATVBAHA.110.221614] [PMID: 21252069]

[133] Zeng H, Pappas C, Belser JA, *et al.* Human pulmonary microvascular endothelial cells support productive replication of highly pathogenic avian influenza viruses: possible involvement in the pathogenesis of human H5N1 virus infection. J Virol 2012; 86(2): 667-78.
[http://dx.doi.org/10.1128/JVI.06348-11] [PMID: 22072765]

[134] Li M, Yao D, Zeng X, *et al.* Age related human T cell subset evolution and senescence. Immun Ageing 2019; 16(1): 24.
[http://dx.doi.org/10.1186/s12979-019-0165-8] [PMID: 31528179]

[135] Connors TJ, Ravindranath TM, Bickham KL, *et al.* Airway CD8+ T cells are associated with lung injury during infant viral respiratory tract infection. Am J Respir Cell Mol Biol 2016; 54(6): 822-30.
[http://dx.doi.org/10.1165/rcmb.2015-0297OC] [PMID: 26618559]

[136] Smits SL, de Lang A, van den Brand JM, *et al.* Exacerbated innate host response to SARS-CoV in aged non-human primates. PLoS Pathog 2010; 6(2): e1000756.
[http://dx.doi.org/10.1371/journal.ppat.1000756] [PMID: 20140198]

[137] Roberts A, Deming D, Paddock CD, *et al.* A mouse-adapted SARS-coronavirus causes disease and mortality in BALB/c mice. PLoS Pathog 2007; 3(1): e5.
[http://dx.doi.org/10.1371/journal.ppat.0030005] [PMID: 17222058]

[138] Wong HR, Freishtat RJ, Monaco M, Odoms K, Shanley TP. Leukocyte subset-derived genome-wide expression profiles in pediatric septic shock. Pediatric critical care medicine: a journal of the Society of Critical Care Medicine and the World Federation of Pediatric Intensive and Critical Care Societies 2010; 11(3): 349.

[139] Nickbakhsh S, Mair C, Matthews L, *et al.* Virus-virus interactions impact the population dynamics of influenza and the common cold. Proc Natl Acad Sci USA 2019; 116(52): 27142-50.
[http://dx.doi.org/10.1073/pnas.1911083116] [PMID: 31843887]

CHAPTER 6

Biochemical Characterization of SARS-CoV-2 Spike Protein Proteolytic Processing

Hayat Khan[1,*], Firasat Hussain[2,*], Muhammad Kalim[3], Shafi Ullah[4], Kashif Rahim[2] and Faisal Siddique[2]

[1] *Department of Microbiology, University of Swabi, Khyber Pakhtunkhwa 23561, Pakistan*

[2] *Department of Microbiology, Cholistan University of Veterinary & Animal Sciences, Bahawalpur-63100, Pakistan*

[3] *Department of Biochemistry, and Cancer Institute of the Second Affiliated Hospital, Zhejiang University, School of Medicine, Hangzhou 310058, China*

[4] *Cardiology Unit, Khyber Teaching Hospital (KTH), Peshawar, Pakistan*

Abstract: Coronavirus spike (S) glycoproteins belong to class I viral fusion protein. Spike protein has S1 and S2 domain that respectively are involved in receptor-binding and fusion of virus-host membrane. Spike protein of SARS-CoV-2 interacts with human angiotensin-converting enzyme-2 (hACE-2), expressing predominantly on the lungs and intestinal cells as a receptor. Although the receptor-binding motif of SARS-CoV-2 shares only 50% homology with that of SARS-CoV, its affinity towards hACE-2 are many folds higher. The host proteases mediate the membrane fusion reaction through the cleavage of S protein between S1 and S2. The S of SARS-CoV-2 harbors cleavage site for furin or furin-like protease, which sets the SARS-CoV-2 apart from SARS and SARS-like other coronaviruses. The S protein is cleaved either by one or several host proteases depending upon the infecting cells and virus strains. Based on the presence of a different type of host protease, the CoVs decides whether to enter cells *via* the cell membrane route or endocytosis. Unlike SARS-CoV, S of SARS-Co-2 causes typical syncytium formation (cell-cell fusion) among the infected cells. Besides receptor binding, S protein is a major target of neutralizing antibodies following infection. However, antibodies raised against SARS-CoV either weakly or fail to neutralize the SARS-CoV-2, suggesting no cross-protection between them. Being is a driver of viral entry, the spike protein of SARS-CoV-2 is a good candidate for vaccine development. Furthermore, the role of host proteases in the membrane is also very significant for the designing of entry inhibitors. The purpose of this chapter is to summarize the detailed structure, fusogenic potential, protease-driven activation, and cross-neutralization of spike protein with antibodies from SARS-CoV and sera of recovered patients.

---

* Corresponding authors Firasat Hussain and Hayat Khan: Department of Microbiology, Cholistan University of Veterinary & Animal Sciences, Bahawalpur 63100, Pakistan. E-mail:firasathussain@cuvas.edu.pk, Department of Microbiology, University of Swabi, Khyber Pakhtunkhwa 23561, Pakistan. E-mail:hayatkhan@uoswabi.edu.pk, hayatbiotech@ yahoo.com

Keywords: Angiotensin-converting enzyme-2, Furin, Host protease, SARS-CoV-2, Spike protein.

INTRODUCTION

Coronaviruses cause infection both in human and animals and causes a wide range of clinical manifestations such as respiratory, renal, and neurological diseases [1]. Coronaviruses are a group of ssRNA, positive sense enveloped viruses. The genome is in the form of a single linear RNA segment. They belong to the family Coronaviradae and are grouped into four genera; alpha, beta, gamma, and delta coronaviruses [1]. Genus beta has a further four; A, B, C, and D lineages. Beginning the 21st century, three *beta* coronaviruses has crossed the species barrier. It caused three severe zoonotic outbreaks of viral pneumonia; severe acute respiratory syndrome-coronavirus (SARS-CoV, 2002–2003), Middle East respiratory syndrome-coronavirus (MERS-CoV, 2012), and later emerged severe acute respiratory syndrome coronavirus-2 (SARS-CoV-2, December 2019) [1 - 3]. Lineage B of beta coronaviruses; SARS-CoV first emerged in China during 2002-2003 and quickly transmitted to other countries of the world that caused around 8000 infections and 800 deaths worldwide [4]. SARS-CoV is transmitted from bat to human, whereas civet cat is considered the intermediate animal reservoir [5, 6]. The second beta coronavirus of lineage C, called MERS-CoV was initially reported from Saudi Arabia [3] with 2494 confirmed infections and 858 deaths so far [4]. It is confined to the Middle East, and the dromedary camel is believed as an intermediate host of MERS-CoV. At the end of 2019 new coronavirus, SARS-CoV-2, surfaced in patients suffering from severe pneumonia in Wuhan city of China [7 - 9]. The virus spread across the globe very quickly. The World Health Organization (WHO) declared SARS-CoV-2 infection a global health emergency of international concern. The virus caused 4.32 million confirmed infections, and 0.30 million patients lost their lives until mid-May 2020 [10]. The virus was isolated from patients and sequenced. The SARS-CoV-2 was classified into lineage B of beta coronaviruses. Phylogenetically, SARS-CoV-2 is a close relative of RaTG13, a SARS-like (SL) coronavirus discovered in bat during 2013 in China [11]. SARS-CoV-2 shares about 96% and 82% nucleotide sequence identities with RaTG13 and SARS-CoV, respectively, speculating it might evolve from SARS-like bat coronavirus. Nevertheless, the intermediate animal reservoir, if any, is still unknown [12]. Besides these three highly pathogenic *beta* coronaviruses, four other known human coronaviruses; two *alpha* hCoV-NL63 and hCoV-229E, and two *beta* HCoV-OC43, HKU1 that cause mild respiratory infection [13 - 18].

All the coronaviruses infect the host cell *via* binding of viral spike (S) glycoprotein with a surface-exposed host receptor. The virus's cellular and tissue tropism is thus primarily determined by viral recognition of host receptors along with other cellular intrinsic factors [19]. Remarkably, excluding HCoV-OC43 and HKU1 binds to sugar moieties of the surface-exposed cellular receptor for attachment [20], whereas the rest of human coronaviruses recognize protein receptors. The HCoV-229E and MERS-CoV recognize respectively human aminopeptidase N [21] and human dipeptidyl peptidase 4 (hDPP4 or hCD26) [22, 23]. The SARS-CoV, SARS-CoV-2, and hCoV-NL63 bind to human angiotensin-converting enzyme 2 (hACE2) for cellular attachment [19, 24 - 28].

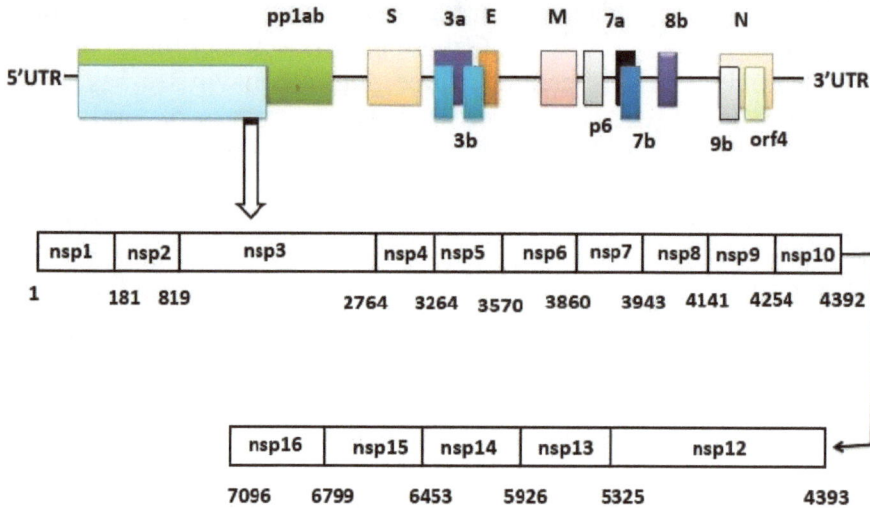

Fig. (1). Schematic diagram of the genomic organization of IVDC-HB-01/2019 (HB01) strain. The open reading frame encodes the largest protein pp1ab; orf1ab. The pp1ab is cleaved into 15 nsps (nsp1-nsp10 and nsp12-nsp16). The orf1a gene encodes pp1a protein that harbors 10 nsps (nsp1-nsp10). Besides these, four structural genes encode spike (S), envelope (E), membrane (M), and nucleocapsid (N) protein. The accessory genes are distributed among the structural genes.

The whole-genome sequencing of viral genomes isolated from different patients in Wuhan reveals that the genome of SARS-CoV-2 is 29844-29891 bases long, encoding around 9860 residues and missing haemagglutinin-esterase gene [13, 29]. The genome codes for a total of 27 proteins and harbors 14 open reading frames (ORFs) (Fig.1). The two-third of the genome at 5′ terminus contains orf1(ab/a) that encodes for 15 nonstructural proteins mutually implicated in viral replication and perhaps in escaping from the human immune system. Located at 3′ end, one-third of genomic codes structural and accessory proteins [30]. Hypervariable genomic hot spots lie in S and other non-structural genes [31].

Spike (S) protein is the glycosylated trimeric protein that protrudes out from coronaviruses' viral envelope. It gives them the characteristic shape of corona (A crown-like) [32]. Mostly, the S protein is cleaved by cellular proteases into S1 and

S2 segments. The S1 engages with receptor recognition, and S2 brings about viral and host membrane fusion [33]. In many coronaviruses, the S protein is chopped at the border of S1, and S2 subunits. It is non-covalently stays together in a prefusion manner [34 - 40]. The S1 is subdivided into the NTD and C-terminal domain (CTD). Either one is involved in engagement with host receptors in various CoVs. The SARS-CoV, MERS-CoV, and SARS-CoV-2 exploit CTD (also known as receptor binding domain) for receptor attachment [19, 20, 22], while mouse hepatitis coronavirus uses NTD for receptor binding [41]. The RBD of the SARS- CoV-2 also lies in the CTD of S1 and forms more atomic interaction with hACE2 than SARC-CoV speculating possible explanation for the rapid expansion of Coronavirus Disease-19 (COVID-19) [19]. SARS-CoV and MERS-CoV S activation is brought about by a two-step successive protease cleavage model [34, 38]. Initially, the cleavage is primed at the junction of S1 and S2, followed by cleavage activation at 'S2' position. The S protein is cleaved either by one or several host proteases depending upon the infecting cells and virus strains. The various types of host proteases discovered so far are trypsin, cathepsins, furin, human airway trypsin-like protease (HAT), transmembrane protease serine protease-2 (TMPRSS-2), and transmembrane protease serine protease-2 (TMPRSS-4) [38, 39, 42 - 47]. The coronavirusesCoVs decide whether to enter cells *via* cell membrane route or endocytosis based on these different types of host protease. Furthermore, SARS-CoV-2 S contains a cleavage site for furin at the border of S1/S2 processed as S is being synthesized. The furin cleavage site separates SARSCoV-2 from SARS-CoV and other SARS-like coronaviruses [48]. This chapter will discuss the structure, function, expression, and role of S protein in the membrane fusion during coronavirus entry. Furthermore, therapeutic aspects and future research perspectives of S protein had also been discussed in detail.

Expression of Spike Protein

As described before, the coronavirus S glycoprotein interacts with the host receptor for viral entry. It is a major target of host humoral response. It harbors antigenic determinants [35, 48, 49], which underscores the significance of spike glycoprotein in the entry of virus and interaction with the immune system. Anchored in the viral envelope, S glycoprotein performs two vital functions: receptor attachment and fusing viral and cell membranes [50]. The fusion of membrane leads to the release of viral genomic RNA in the target cells, followed by the initiation of viral replication [51].

After the release of genomic RNA, translation of orf1(ab/a) produces a complex of 15 non-structural proteins known as viral replicase-transcriptase complex (RTC) (Fig. **1**). The RTC mediates viral replication and subsequent transcription of subgenomic viral RNAs. Subgenomic RNAs are later translated into 4 structural (spike, envelope, membrane, and nucleocapsid) and several other accessory proteins. After synthesis, all the structural proteins except nucleocapsid anchor into the endoplasmic reticulum (ER) membrane. From the ER, these travel to the endoplasmic reticulum-Golgi apparatus intermediate compartment (ERGIC) *via* the secretory pathway. Coronavirus particles assemble in the ERGIC. Finally, the mature virus particles bud out the infected cell through exocytosis [52]. In the ERGIC, the monomeric form of S proteins undergoes extensive N-glycosylation followed by trimerization [53]. During biosynthesis, the S glycoprotein of some coronaviruses (MERS-CoV and SARS-CoV-2) is also processed partially by furin and/or furin-like proteases inside the Golgi Bodies [40, 54, 55]. Spike protein of some coronaviruses, which does not incorporate into viral envelope also transport to the cell surface [56].

Structure of Spike Protein

The type I transmembrane S glycoprotein is encoded by ORF downstream of RTC ORF and is well conserved across all coronaviruses. The S protein is 180-kDa that is involved in receptor engagement and viral entry. Spike protein is partitioned into amino (N) S1 and carboxyl (C) S2 terminal domains. The N-terminus S1 and C-terminus S2 harbor, respectively, receptor-binding motif and membrane fusion domain (Fig. **2**) [50, 53, 57].

The S1 subunit form the bulbous head, and the S2 subunit form the transmembrane stalk, as revealed from the structural modeling of the monomeric form of coronaviruses S protein (Fig. **2B**). The S1 subunit is further organized into an NTD and C-terminal domains (CTD) (Fig. **2**). Either one or both act as receptor-binding domains (RBD). A short stretch within the RBD directly interacts with the receptor is called receptor binding motif (RBM). The S1 is relatively more variable as opposed to S2 [58]. As a general rule of thumb, the NTD interacts with sugar-based receptors (such as NTD of HCoV-OC43 and HKU1 viruses), where CTD of S1 binds to protein-based receptors (such as CTD of MERS-CoV, SARS-CoV, SARS-CoV 2, and hCoV-NL63). Nevertheless, exceptions exist, *e.g.,* NTD of mouse hepatitis virus binds the proteinaceous receptor, CEACAM1 [7, 24 - 27, 59, 60]. Both SARS-CoV and SARS-CoV-2 exploit the CTD of S1 for binding to hACE2 [25, 27], found richly on pneumocytes and enterocytes [61]. The RBM of SARS-CoV and SARS-CoV-2 shares ~50% sequence homology, but little is known about whether these differences reinforce or reduce RBM-hACE2 engagement. However, it is uncertain if these variations contribute to a relatively stronger interaction between SARS-CoV-2 S and hACE2 [62]. Nevertheless, some *in vitro* analyses reveal greater interaction between spike protein of SARS-CoV-2 and hACE2 than that of

SARS-CoV [19, 62]. On the other hand, another study reports a comparable affinity of RBD of both SARS-CoV-2 and SARS-CoV for hACE2 [63], requiring further study to explore the impact of amino acid alteration in RBM on interaction with ACE2.

MERS-CoV also utilizes CTD for binding to proteinaceous dipeptidyl peptidase 4 (DPP4) [23], expressed on lung and kidney cells [64]. The highly conserved nature of DPP4 across a wide range of different species (*e.g.,* bats, dromedaries, humans) highlights the zoonotic potential of MERS-CoV. Besides DPP4, MERS-CoV S has also been shown to interact with sialic acid receptors that contribute further to the zoonotic competency of MERS-CoV [65].

Coronavirus S glycoprotein belongs to class I viral fusion protein owing to S2 architecture [66]. Within class I viral protein, S2 mostly consists of alpha-helices. The function of S is regulated by proteolytic priming or cleavage at the designated position to produce the fusion-competent form of S [67]. The S2 is subdivided into different types of motifs; the first is the fusion peptide (FP), a functional fusogenic component of the spike protein.

The FP is a small piece of 15-25 residues, which is well-conserved across the viral family. Primarily, the FP consists of nonpolar amino acid (*e.g.,* glycine or alanine) that anchors into the cellular membrane to induce the process of the membrane of fusion [68]. The FP is highly rendered to mutation, and single point mutation can abrogate the fusion event [69]. Nevertheless, FP is poorly understood because these requirements are just guidelines for identifying the FP region but not the absolute description of the FP.

Several regions of FP have been described for the SARS-CoV S2. Regions 770-788, 873-888, 1185-1202, and 798-835 implicated in membrane fusion events have been identified by different researchers for the SARS-CoV [69 - 72]. Research studies explicitly centering on the FP of MERS-CoV are relatively scarce. Mutational analysis with gigantic unilamellar vesicles reveals FP region 888-898 of MERS-CoV (RSARSAIEDLLFDKV) containing important nonpolar residues capable of forming syncytium [73]. Based on the pairwise alignment, the FP of SARS-CoV-2 is 93% homologous with SARS-CoV FP, demonstrating a high degree of conservation across two viruses.

Two heptad repeats, HR1 and HR2, are located after the fusion region in S2 (Fig. **3**). Heptad region 2 (HR2) is shorter than the heptad region 1 (HR1). The HR1 and HR2 are heptapeptides, HPPHCPC, repeats where H indicates hydrophobic or conventionally huge residues, P and C respectively show polar and other charged amino acids [74]. Because heptapeptide repeats, the HR assumes alpha-helices with an outward polar interface to drive fusogenic reaction [66]. Anchored in the viral membrane, the transmembrane domain lies next to the HR2 (Fig. **2c**). The last C-terminal part of S2 is the cytoplasmic tail located interior to the viral envelope.

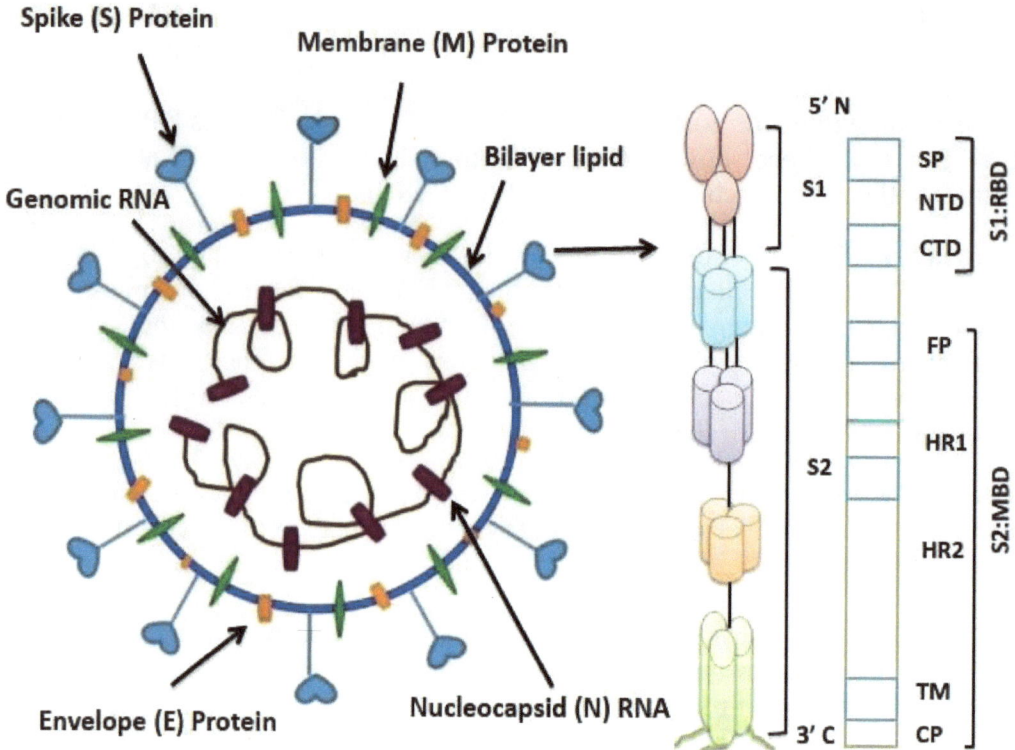

Fig. (2). Spike Protein of Coronavirus. A. Cartoon figure of Coronavirus particle. The particle has an outer layer of host-derived lipid membrane with three transmembrane structural proteins: spike (S), membrane (M), and envelope (E). The genomic RNA is encased the interior with nucleocapsid (N) protein. B. Cartoonic diagram of spike protein trimer. C. Functional components of the spike protein. The spike protein subunits: S1 and S2, along with their functional components, have been shown. SP (signal peptide, red); NTD (N-terminal domain; blue), CTD (C-terminal domain; orange), FP (fusion peptide; yellow), HR1 (heptad repeat 1; grey), HR2 (heptad repeat 2; light green), TM (transmembrane; pink), and CP (cytoplasmic; dark green).

Human ACE2 is a Receptor for SARS-CoV-2

Following the COVID-19 epidemic in China, great attention was paid to discover the cellular receptor and entry mechanism of SARS-CoV-2. Several studies reveal that like its closest friend, SARS-CoV, SARS-CoV-2 also uses hACE2 as a receptor for its entry [24, 27, 63, 75, 76]. Walls *et al* demonstrates that MLV based pseudo-type particle (pp) of SARS-CoV-2 S transduce the Vero E6 cells known to express ACE2 and support replication of SARS-CoV [2, 63, 77]. The experiment was carried out based on high homology (75%) between S proteins of both viruses. The hACE2 as primary receptor was re-confirmed by transfecting baby hamster kidney (BHK) cells with pp SARS-CoV-2 S transiently expressing hACE2. Before the hACE2 expression, the cells were resistant to ppSARS-CoV 2 S transfection. The crystallography analysis shows that the CTD of SARS-CoV2 S1 harbors RBD containing 14 residues interacting with hACE2 [76]. However, the site-directed mutagenesis demonstrates that only these residues are not sufficient for the entry of the virus, but the surrounding residues are also critical for the productive infection [76]. Relative affinity of both SARS-CoV and SARS-CoV-2 RBDs with hACE2 shows that despite the high level of homology among RBDs of both viruses, the substituted residues in CTD of SARS-CoV-2 somewhat firming receptor contacts as opposed to RBD of SARS-CoV [78]. Similarly, *in vitro* analysis demonstrates that receptor binding affinity of SARS-CoV-2 RBD is 10-20 folds higher than RBD of SARS-CoV [79], which might explain why SARS-CoV-2 has relatively higher virulence and transmission.

Furthermore, the cryoelectron microscopy (cryo-EM) analysis reveals that the hACE2 dimerizes upon interacting with the B0AT1 (an amino acid transporter) and CTD of SARS-CoV2 [62]. Each monomer of the ACE2 binds with one molecule of SARS-CoV 2 CTD [62]. The interacting residues among the RBD of SARS-CoV-2 and hACE2 have also been determined using crystallography [19]. ACE2 is found mainly on the cell surface of the lung, small intestine, endothelial cells of arteries and veins in the majority of organs. Various parts of the brain, such as the cerebral cortex, hypothalamus, brain stem, and striatum, also express ACE2 [80]. Expression of hACE2 in the various tissues of the nervous system might render them susceptible to the SARS-CoV-2 infection and suggest the probable cause of neurological manifestation and insomnia associated with COVID-19 [81]. The suffering of many patients with insomnia and parageusia (loss/change of taste) suggest early indication of COVID-19 infection [81], which was later identified as characteristic symptoms of COVID-19.

SARS-CoV-2 S-Mediated Cell-Cell Fusion

Unlike SARS-CoV, SARS-CoV-2 infected cells induce syncytia formation, proposing that SARS-CoV-2 might largely use cell surface fusion pathway for entry to target cells. In the cell-cell fusion system, the spike protein of SARS-CoV-2 may perhaps efficiently induce the syncytium formation among the effector and target cells even in the absence of trypsin (exogenous protease). At the same time, the SARS-CoV S is unable to do so. Most viruses enter the cell more efficiently through the plasma membrane fusion pathway because the endosomal membrane fusion pathway is more disposed to innate antiviral immunity of the infected host cell [82, 83]. However, most lineages B of the beta coronaviruses lack the S1/S2 furin site, and their spike glycoproteins are intact in native conformation. For example, SARS-CoV enters host cells mostly through the endosomal fusion pathway. The spike glycoprotein is cleaved and triggered by the endosomal proteolytic enzyme (cathepsin L) [34]. The SARS- CoV S prefers the cell membrane fusion pathway over the endosomal pathway if the S1/S2 furin cleavage site is introduced in the spike glycoprotein [84].

Interestingly, the S1/S2 cleavage site for furin is present in the spike glycoprotein of SARS-CoV-2. However, its role in membrane fusion and the life cycle of the virus is still obscure. Recent findings propose that SARS-CoV-2 primarily utilizes proteolytic enzyme, transmembrane protease/serine subfamily member 2 (TMPRSS2), to fuse plasma membrane, suggesting that the use of TMPRSS2 inhibitor may provide an opportunity for inhibiting SARS-CoV-2 S mediated fusion of viral entry [85]. Infected cells form syncytia naturally the following infection with live SARS-CoV-2, which is rarely described in the case of SARS-CoV infection [86]. SARS-CoV-2 form syncytia both in transient expressing ACE2 receptor cells (ACE2/293T cells) and naturally expressing ACE2 receptor cells (Huh-7 cells) [86].

Cross Reaction of T62 Antibodies and SARS-CoV-2 Spike Protein

The T62 are polyclonal antibodies (PAb) raised in rabbits against the spike S1 subunit of SARS-CoV. The T62 is also written as anti-SARS-CoV S1 rabbit PAb. The T62 is used for various purposes, including cross-neutralization of other coronaviruses. The antibody was produced in the rabbit and purified by the Sino Biological (SB) Beijing, China [60]. Although there is a high degree of homology between the spike protein of SARS-CoV-2 and SARS-CoV, polyclonal rabbit anti-SARS S1 antibodies (T62) do not bind well to spike protein SARS-CoV-2 and hence poorly neutralize SARS-CoV-2 entry to the target cell. The T62 antibody weakly interacts with the SARS-CoV 2 S in the western blot analysis. The T62 antibody also 'doesn't impede the transfection of HEK293T cells effectively with SARS-CoV-2 S pseudovirions. It speculates that the T62 is not effective in the neutralization of SARS-CoV-2. The NTDs and RBD harbor binding epitopes for the T62. Site direct mutagenesis suggests that residues of RBDs involved in the receptor binding do not interact directly with T62 [60].

Cross-Neutralization of COVID-19 Sera

S glycoproteins protrude out from the viral envelope and facilitate viral entry, so it is the major target of neutralizing immunoglobulins following infection. Being the entry mediator and target of neutralizing antibodies, S protein is also the main focus of designing therapeutics and prophylaxes. It is believed that recovery from one coronavirus infection might protect the other because the RBDs of the coronaviruses are highly sequenced conserved. Hoverer, different reports provide contradictory findings. One study finds that sera from the convalescent patients of COVID-19 and SARS weakly neutralize each other, suggesting that those who recovered from viral infection are not protected well from other viral infections [60].

Similarly, as described earlier, antibodies raised against the spike protein of SARS-CoV cannot hamper the entry of SARS-CoV-2. Likewise, the murine monoclonal and polyclonal antibodies raised against RBD of SARS-CoV cannot interact with the spike protein of SARS-CoV-2, indicating antigenic difference among the two [19]. However, another study demonstrates that the SARS-CoV spike protein provokes antibodies that potently neutralize the SARS-CoV-2 [63]. Based on not these contradictory findings, there is an urgent need for pan-CoVs vaccine development that can target highly conserved regions across coronaviruses.

Activation of SARS-CoV-2 Spike Protein

As described, the coronavirus S protein mediates both receptor binding and membrane fusion. For membrane fusion, the S protein is primed first by a suitable protease at the interface of S1 and S2, followed by induction just upstream of the FP of S2. The interesting thing is that this event can be triggered by different proteases that determine the virus's tissue tropism. Protease availability determines whether SARS-CoV and MERS-CoV fuse at the plasma membrane or endosomal membrane. The SARS-CoV-2 also uses plasma membrane and endocytic pathways for viral entry (Fig. **3**) [85]. If an appropriate protease is available on the plasma membrane, the virus will enter through the early pathway route; otherwise, the virus will use the endosomal membrane pathway.

Early Pathway

Cell-cell fusion studies provide an early clue that SARS-CoV uses the plasma membrane pathway for viral entry. It was found that HEK293T cells that express SARS-CoV S protein transiently induce cell-cell fusion with target E6 Vero cells in the presence of a low concentration of exogenous trypsin. However, a similar setup lacking trypsin but using a low pulse of pH cannot do so [87]. Likewise, exogenous trypsin also triggers MERS-CoV and SARS-CoV-2 S protein facilitated Vero E6 and 293T cell-cell fusion, respectively [46, 60]. Furthermore, trypsin treatment of retroviral-based pseudo particles of SARS-CoV (SARSpp) and MERS-CoV (MERSpp) S proteins following interacting with their corresponding receptors enhance the viral infection at the cell surface membrane [45, 88]. Before receptor binding, trypsin treatment abrogates infection, because trypsin treatment causes irreversible conformational changes in the S protein, making it unable to mediate membrane fusion [39, 88, 89]. However, this phenomenon needs to explore for SARS-CoV-2. It has also been shown that other exogenous proteases, thermolysin, and elastase also promote cellular entry. It occursin SARS-CoV, and MERS-CoV live viruses into Vero E6 cells after receptor binding [46, 89, 90]. As the elastin is expressed by the inflammatory cells of the lungs after the SAR-CoV infection, this is very important clinically because it might further progress the SARS-CoV infection.

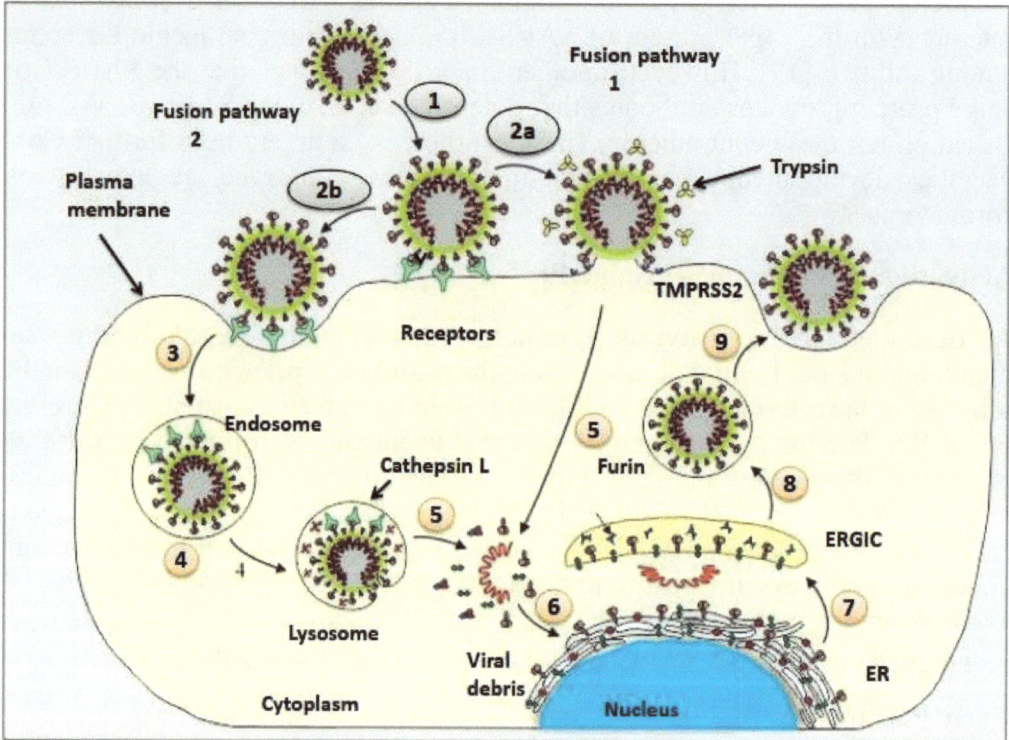

Fig. (3). Model of coronavirus dual entry pathway. This model describes two pathways of viral entry: early pathway and late pathway.

Even though the exogenous proteases can induce the fusion event, they are unable to describe the mechanistic approach of fusion in the respiratory tract of humans, which is the main target of coronaviruses. This is because the coronaviruses S glycoprotein needs to be cleaved only after binding to the receptor and not prior. However, the timely use of exogenous proteases in the *in vivo* environment is hard to regulate. Therefore, transmembrane proteases provide a great deal of interest because they are confined to the cell membrane where viruses encounter the receptor. Type II transmembrane serine proteases (TTSPs) are examples of membrane-localized proteases that play an important role in the viral infection of the influenza virus [91]. The TMPRSS2 and TMPRSS4 can induce and spread influenza viral infection even in the absence of extracellular trypsin [92 - 94].

Similarly, TMPRSS11a (TTSP protease) can induce exogenously SARS-CoV S mediated fusion [95]. Further studies inquired whether membrane-anchored TTSP can trigger the S glycoprotein of the SARS-CoV as well. In the absence of extracellular proteases, the SAR-CoV fuses at the surface of TMPRSS2 expressing cells [96 - 98]. Likewise, membrane-localized TMPRSS2 also induces the infection of MERS-CoV *in vitro* [44, 45]. The SARS-CoV-2 also uses membrane-bound TMPRSS2 for viral entry at the cell surface, similar to SARS-CoV and MERS-CoV [85, 99].

Additional membrane-localized proteases also activate CoVs infection at the cell surface at a different level. The TMPRSS11a and TMPRSS11e also promote the viral infection of MERS-CoV S [100]. Even if TMPRSS4 induces S protein-mediated syncytia formation in SARS-CoV and MERS-CoV, it is inefficient to prevent both viruses [45, 96]. Similarly, TMPRSS2, 4, 11a, 11d, and 11e improve S-mediated syncytium formation in SARS-CoV-2. However, it is yet to be discovered whether these protease trigger spike protein for viral infection [60]. This is because of the high in vitro expression of S protein and its interaction with broader surface areas in cell-cell fusion assay, which promotes high fusion compared to viral-cell fusion *in vivo* [96].

Furthermore, activation of transmembrane proteases differs among SARS-CoV and MERS-CoV. TMPRSS11d, a human airway trypsin-like protease (HAT), induces the S mediated infection in MARS-CoV but is incapable of doing so in the case of SARS-CoV [43, 100]. It is notable to say that the spike glycoprotein of CoVs evolved in a way that renders it to different types of proteases for cleavage and activation, providing a probable explanation for their animal-human transmission behavior.

Even if there is a high level of sequence homology between the S2 fusion domains of SARS-CoV and MERS-CoV, both practices required different fusion mechanisms at the cell surface for their entry into the host cell. The S glycoprotein of MERS-CoV S harbors S1/S2 cleavage site for the furin, whereas SARS-CoV S lacks such site [38]. During synthesis, the furin and/or furin –protease in the trans-Golgi network (TGN) process the S protein by acting upon the furin cleavage site [101]. The S of MERS-CoV is pre-cleaved during its biosynthesis at the S1/S2 site (Millet and Whittaker, 2014). Subsequently, the pre-cleavage promote further TMPRSS2 cleavage at 'S2' to triggers cell surface fusion of MARS-CoV. The TMPRSS2 mediated entry of MARS-CoV is inhibited in case there is no pre-cleavage [39]. It has been demonstrated that specific basic amino acids are believed to involve in inducing furin cleavage of MERS-CoV S at the 'S2' site for viral entry [38]. Still, the precise mechanism is yet to be explored role [102]. However, there is no evidence that the S protein of both SARS-CoV and SARS-CoV-2 S at 'S2' position is furin sensitive for the cleavage.

The S protein of SARS-CoV does not need to be pre-cleaved during biosynthesis for subsequent viral entry at the cell surface. Although it is assumed that the pre-cleavage causes the conformation changes in S protein in a way that uncovers the 'S2' for the subsequent cell-surface fusion event, however, prior binding of S to receptor creates changes in the conformation of S protein [39]. Furthermore, receptor binding of SARS-CoV S protein is 10-20 times greater than that of MERS-CoV, which might compensate for the pre-cleavage deficiency in SARS-CoV. The cleavage diversity of S at S1/S2 possibly suggests coronaviruses' transmission and subsequent infection to a new host with relatively weak receptor binding. Surprisingly, overexpression of TMPRSS2 causes infection of a cell with uncleaved S protein of MERS-CoV, thus circumventing the need for pre-cleavage for viral infection [54], once again underscores the flexibility of CoVs S protein.

Surprisingly, the S protein of SARS-CoV-2 possesses a potential cleavage site furin protease at the S1/S2 position, which is a unique characteristic of SARS-CoV-2 among SARS-like CoVs [63, 79, 103]. Western plot analysis shows that S is also cleaved during the biosynthesis at the position of S1/S2 like the pre-cleavage event of MERS-CoV S protein [63].

Late Pathway

Coronavirusescan enter through an alternative route of endocytosis if the extracellular or membrane-anchored proteases are absent [104, 105]. If there is no pre-cleavage of MERS-CoV S protein at S1/S2 position, then the virus will enter *via* endocytosis respective of cell surface proteases [39]. The pH of endosomes declines as the virus progresses to the interior of the cell *via* endocytosis. Low pH induces the fusion of viral and endosomal membranes in viruses like VSV and influenza. The infection of these viruses can be inhibited on treatment with lysosomotropic agents. Asit prevents acidification of endosomes [106]. The SARS-CoV can infect cells upon treatment with lysosomotropic agents. It speculates that SARS-CoV is a sensitive acidic condition of the endosome [87]. Additional factors may also contribute to the fusion of coronaviruses in endosomes because low pH treatment cannot decrease SARS-CoV infection.

The acidic environment of the endosome activates proteases. Cathepsin is a member of cysteine proteases. Cathepsin proteases are activated in a sequential event. Cathepsins B and L are activated respectively in early and late endosomes, which activate other proteases of the same family [107, 108]. Furthermore, the exogenous use of cathepsin inhibitor effectively reduces the viral entry of SARS-CoV [88, 109] and MERS-CoV [44].

Similarly, SARS-CoV-2 is also sensitive to cathepsin B and L inhibitors [60, 85]. The use of cathepsin B and or L inhibitors can provide sufficient proof. These coronaviruses fuse within the late endosome [45, 60, 88], together with observing the direct movement of SARS-CoV towards late endosomes [110]. Thus, rather than the direct effect of low pH on the S protein of SARS-CoV, MERS-CoV, and SARS-CoV-2, the acidic environment of the endosome turns on cathepsin L, which later on activates S proteins of all these viruses for further fusion events.

Cleavage Sites of Spike Protein

Even though the same set of proteases are required to activate SARS-CoV and MERS-CoV activation, their S protein is cleaved by proteases at different cleavage sites, which probably results in slightly different functions. For example, TMPRSS2 acts on the 'S2' site of SARS-CoV S protein for fusion at the cell surface [54, 111]. Nevertheless, this requires furin-mediated pre-cleavage of S protein at S1/S2 position during biosynthesis of the spike protein of MERS-CoV [38, 39, 54]. In contrast, SARS-CoV does not need to do so [111]. However, in the case of SARS-CoV-2, it is yet to be found whether the pre-cleavage of S protein at the S1/S2 site during biosynthesis is required for the subsequent cell surface fusion. Scientists are interested in the S1/S2 furin cleavage because of its association with the tropism and virulence of the virus. The cleavage site of a less pathogenic strain of influenza consists of single basic amino acids, while that of more pathogenic is furin polybasic site [112]. Most of the cell lines express furin and furin-like proteases, suggesting that strain of influenza that contains furin cleavage site in HA results in the expansion of viral tropism. Based on this phenomenon in influenza, it is believed that the presence of furin cleavage site allows the more efficient spread of SARS-CoV-2 as compared to other SARS-like-CoVs [63, 103], though it is still to be proved experimentally. Furthermore, it is also be determined where the SARS-CoV-2 retrieved the furin sites, *i.e.,* whether during transmission from animal to human or human to human [113]. This is very important to unravel the pathogenicity of emerging coronaviruses.

Unlike TMPRSS2, exogenous trypsin has different requirements for cleavage. In the case of SARS-CoV, trypsin activates the S protein in two steps sequential process; first, it causes cleavage of arginine (R) at position 667 of S1/S2 site and then cleaves R797 at 'S2' site (R797) for plasma membrane fusion [34]. However, TMPRSS2 does not cleave at S1/S2 site. This feature underscores the FP of coronaviruses' adaptability because it is prone to cleavage by various proteases leading to a bit different activity. Furthermore, the elastase and trypsin cleave the

S protein of SARS-CoV respectively at T795 and R797 of 'S2' site, which supports further the flexibility of coronaviruses FP [90]. This also reveals that S can also accommodate different cleavage sites. However, the elastase facilitates maximum fusion at the plasma membrane when the S is cleaved at the R797 site, revealing that although the S has different cleavage sites, there are preferred ones also. The precise cleavage positions of MERS-CoV and SARS-CoV-2 S protein for the extracellular proteases are still unknown. It would be interesting to know if there are slight changes in these viruses' cleavage sites for various proteases.

Endosomal protease, cathepsin L cleaves S protein of SARS-CoV at T678 slightly downstream of S1/S2 location; however, functional studies are required to determine this even [114]. For MERS-CoV, cathepsin L requires S1/S2 & 'S2' positions to activate S protein. However, the mutation in S2 results in a slight reduction of cathepsin L mediated fusion of MERS-CoV [54]. It reveals that cathepsin L might use a secondary cleavage site to activate the MERS-CoV S protein. Practically it is hard to determine these sites for the cathepsin, though it has been shown that cathepsin L prefers aromatic amino acids at the S2 cleavage site [115]. Although the endocytic pathway seems similar for the SARS-CoV, MERS-CoV, and SARS-CoV-2. However, the position and number of cleavage sites for cathepsin L may vary among the S proteins of these viruses. It can influence the entry proficiency of the MERS-CoV or SARS-CoV-2 endocytic pathway. In general, the vast array of proteases that activate SARS-CoV, MERS-CoV, and SARS- CoV-2 proves the capability of these viruses in infecting a wide range of different cell types that express this set of proteases and hence provide a possible explanation for the expanded tropism of these viruses.

Function of Spike Proteins

Receptor Binding of Spike Protein

As described, the S protein serves as both receptor recognition and fusogenic. It has been shown in multiple studies that hACE2 is the principal receptor of SARS-CoV-2 [27, 60, 63, 76, 85]. Structural modeling of SARS-CoV-2 S underscores receptor usage in similar passion as of SARS-CoV [116] despite genetic heterogeneity in the RBD among the two. At the interface of S1 and S2, the S of SARS-CoV-2 harbors an extended loop structure that contains basic amino acids and is believed to be proteolytically sensitive. Like other coronaviruses, this loop is considered to be involved in the interaction with the receptor and fusion of membrane fusion for viral entry. The cryo-EM structure of SARS-CoV-2 S reveals that one monomer of the trimer is in the up position possible for binding with the receptor [79]. The binding ridge in RBD of SARS-CoV-2 S forms a more compact conformation as compared to RBD of SARS-CoV [117]. Furthermore, the two receptor binding hotspots of the virus at the interface of hACE2/RBD are stabilized by the amino acid changes in the RBD of SARS-CoV-2 [117]. These structural features are responsible for the increased affinity of SARS-CoV-2 S with hACE2 [7, 117].

Moreover, interactive analysis of various residues in the biomolecular complex of SARS-CoV-2 S and hACE2 demonstrate polar contacts between ala475, asn487, glu484, tyr453 of RBD, respectively with ser19, gln24, lys31, his34 of hACE2. Similarly, lys417 residue makes ionic interaction with asp30 of hACE2. Spike protein residues gly446, tyr449, gly496, gln498, thr500, and gly502 contribute hydrogen bond interaction with residues asp38, tyr41, gln42, lys353, and asp355 of hACE2, respectively. Furthermore, hydrophobic interactions are also involved in the virus-receptor binding among the amino acids tyr489 and phe486 of RBD and receptor residues phe28, leu79, met82, and tyr83. However, above all, the polar interaction is the most effective one because mutation of single hydrophilic residue K353A abrogates these virus-receptor interface contacts [7].

Spike Protein-Driven Membrane Fusion

The process whereby the enveloped viruses fuse their envelope with the plasma membrane of the host is called viral membrane fusion. As a result of viral membrane fusion, the viruses deliver their genome within host cells and ultimately produce the progeny viruses within the cells [118, 119]. Following receptor binding, the coronaviruses fuse their membrane with the cell membrane of host cells such that both membranes become proximal. Nevertheless, membrane fusion does not spontaneously take place because it requires high energy to close the two membranes nearby [120, 121]. The fusion protein of the viruses provides the energy for membrane fusion, just like the catalyst.

Fusion proteins are grouped into three discrete classes (I, II, and III) due to their structural and functional characteristics [66, 67]. As described earlier, the coronaviruses S protein belongs to class I fusion protein because of its fusion domain structural characteristics, protease requirement for activation, and presence of heptapeptide repeats that assume a six-helix bundle structure during the fusion process [35]. Class I fusion proteins work in a sequence of states to drive the fusion of viral and host membrane. The first is the pre-fusion native state, and the second is the pre-fusion metastable state, the third is the pre-hairpin intermediate state, and the fourth and last one is a post-fusion stable state. The pre-fusion form is adopted during the synthesis of S protein. The proteolytic cleavage at S1/S2 turns the S protein into the pre-fusion metastable state. After cleavage, the S1 and S2 domains separate and adhere together non-covalently [122].

The metastable state of FP has to transition to the next state and passes through an energy transition barrier. Next, a trigger provides energy to cross the kinetic barrier. As a result, FP of the S is anchored into the host cell membrane and finally adopts the pre-hairpin intermediate state. The triggers are generally environmental signals that tell the virus about its microenvironment. For example, in the case of the influenza virus, when the virus moves along the endocytic route. The acidic environment of the endosome brings about conformational changes in the fusion protein. It inserts the FP in the endosomal membrane and thus began the membrane fusion of both virus and endosome fusion protein [123]. The triggering event is tightly regulated to ensure the fusion of the virus at an appropriate position. This regulation is particularly critical because the conformation changes in the class I viral fusion proteins are usually irreversible and should be triggered fuse at an optimal condition.

Moreover, the FP of influenza is exposed due to the triggering process because it is hidden inside the fusion domain to prevent its hydrophobic statefrom the surrounding hydrophilic environment. However, FP of both SARS-CoV and MERS-CoV are surface exposed partly [49]. This appears to be a characteristic of coronaviruses fusion because the FP of murine hepatitis virus is surface exposed in the prefusion state [48].

Following insertion in the host membrane, the three HR1 regions of fusion combine to form a coiled-coil trimer. In contrast, the three HR2 regions interact with hydrophobic furrows of HR1 trimer in an antiparallel fashion and eventually form a fusion core or six-helix bundle (6HB) [124]. The 6HB brings viral and host membrane inproximity for subsequent fusion. The membrane fusion itself is a two-step process: hemifusion and pore formation. Hemifusion is the fusion of outer layers of viral and host membrane. The merged outer layer and inner layer mix in pore formation, forming a tubular connection between the host's viral interior and cytoplasm, allowing the viral genome to release into the host cell cytoplasm [125].

The fusion of membrane depends on the lipid contents of viral &/or host cellular membranes [126]. Both sphingolipids and cholesterol tend to form microdomains together in the viral and host membranes. These microdomains are called lipid rafts which floats within the sea of phospholipids [127]. Lipid rafts perform two functions in the membrane fusion; first, it provides hotspots for the entry of virus as viral receptors may be concentrated within the lipid rafts, second cholesterol reduces the energy required for the membrane fusion [128]. It is believed that hACE2 is focused on the lipid raft; hence the cholesterol is required for the viral entry of SARS-CoV [129]. However, the exact mechanism is still unknown. Besides concentrating the viral receptor, cholesterol may directly affect the fusion reaction by promoting the formation of fusion intermediate, but this needs to prove experimentally for the coronaviruses. The DPP4, a receptor of MERS-CoV, associates with lipid raft in the human T cell line (Jurkat cell line) [130]. However, the DPP4 needs to be determined in the lipid raft of susceptible cell lines and hence the role of cholesterol upon the viral entry of MERS-CoV. It will be of great interest to know the role of cholesterol in the viral entry of SARS-CoV-2.

The microenvironment of the host cells highly influences the membrane fusion of coronaviruses. Exogenous proteases and pH of the microenvironment affect directly or indirectly the fusion of SARS-CoV and MERS-CoV. The presence of calcium ions enables FP to induce membrane ordering and hence subsequent fusion. Similarly, calcium ions have been shown to involve proper positioning and insertion of rubella and Ebola viruses [131 - 133]. Furthermore, calcium chelating agents reduce the infectivity of SARS and MERS pseudo-type particles [134]. It helps calcium in the endocytic pathway for the viral entry of both viruses. It has to be determined yet whether calcium ions influence the fusion of SARS-CoV-2.

Antigenicity of Spike Protein

Following infection, the spike glycoprotein of SARS-CoV-2 elicits the adaptive arm of the immune system, so the S protein harbors antigenic determinants for the adaptive immune system. At the moment, there are neither effective vaccines nor antivirals for the COVID-19. However, there some conventional therapeutic strategies for the SARS-CoV-2 but associated with many limitations, as many people develop asymptomatic infection suggesting that the immune system is the key player to clear the virus before symptoms appear. Immune-mediated clearance of the virus surely uses adaptive immunity, speculating that immunization will indeed protect against this deadly viral pandemic. For instance, the RBD of both SARS-CoV and MERS-CoV proved to raise effectively neutralizing antibodies [135, 136].

Nevertheless, due to antigenic and electrostatic distribution differences among the spike protein of SARS-CoV and SARS-CoV-2, it is uncertain whether the formerly designed RBD-based subunit vaccine of SARS-CoV will provide effective prophylaxis against SARS-CoV-2. Notably, there is a high level of homology (~90%) among S2 regions of SARS-CoV and SARS-CoV-2, which harbor neutralizing antigenic determinants [135, 136]. It has been observed that less than 40% of SARS-CoV-2 patients develop antibodies at the end of the first week of onset of the disease. It quickly increased to 100% at the end of the second week [137]. This suggests that the patient develops adaptive immunity by day-15 since the onset, which clears the virus by own.

Furthermore, cross-neutralization studies reveal that the murine antisera of SARS-CoV inhibit the entry of SARS-CoV-2 [63], suggesting the presence of antigenic determinants on spike glycoprotein SARS-CoV-2 and highlight the importance of the S in the development of the vaccine. Nevertheless, despite the same binding target (ACE2), three out of four monoclonal antibodies that bind effectively to RBD of SRAS-CoV failed to exhibit apparent binding to RBD of SARS-CoV-2 [138]. Limited cross-reactivity of antibodies provides the importance to explore further antigenic differences among the epitopes of both SARS-CoV and SARS-CoV-2 S protein. Antibody epitope bioinformatics tools suggest that the limited cross-reactivity stems from the presence of novel antigenic determinants in the non-conserved region of SARS-CoV-2 that cannot be recognized by antibodies raised against SARS-CoV [139]. These will offer favorable progress for SARS-CoV-2 vaccine research and development.

Moreover, the antigenic variation in S protein of both SARS-CoV-2 and SARS-CoV reveals that most cytotoxic T lymphocyte epitopes are novel in SARS-CoV-2, and only six epitopes are novel common among the two. This speculates that SARS-CoV-2 exhibits high antigenic variation with SARS-CoV [140]. The common identical epitopes may be used for the vaccine design for both viruses, whereas the navel epitopes can lead to developing the fresh, and potent vaccine.

FUTURE PERSPECTIVE

Spike protein drives the entry of coronaviruses, including the newly pandemic SARS-CoV-2. The S protein is a good target for designing pan-CoVs drugs because the fusion mechanism governed by the S protein and its protein sequence are well conserved. However, better knowledge of the fusion mechanism must unravel the potential target within the S protein.

Although surface fusion of coronavirus is supposed to clinically more significant because the pneumocytes of the lung express TMPRSS2 protease on its surface, however, *in vivo* setup required proving this. The available TMPRSS2 knockout mice model is ineffective for studying the viral infection and immunopathology of SARS-CoV or MERS-CoV. However, SARS-CoV can be detected in the alveoli of knockout mice [141]. This supposes that the virus may enter *via* the endosomal route rather than the cell surface and endosomal proteases (*e.g.,* cathepsin L) ways. It might trigger the fusion event supporting the clinical relevancy of the endosomal route. So, it is imperative to explore the role of endosomal protease. Determining the possible obscure site in the spike protein for the endosomal protease such as cathepsin L could explore other domains in the S protein for membrane fusion. Moreover, MERS-CoV and SARS-CoV-2 are believed to be cleaved at S1/S2 and S2' sites sequentially [38, 63, 79, 103]. MERS-CoV S is pre-cleaved by furin or furin-like proteases at the S/S2 site as it is being synthesized, but furin mediated pre-cleavage event of SARS-CoV-2 S protein is still obscure. However, the presence of the furin site would influence the viral entry of SARS-CoV-2. Therefore, *in vivo* investigations are required to discover the role of these proteases inactivation and subsequent S mediated fusion of SARS-CoV-2. As the *in vivo* system is clinically more significant, so it can progress in planning entry inhibitors. As described before, cholesterol and calcium ions play some role in one way or another in the viral entry of coronaviruses. Further studies are required to understand the role of these two in SARS-CoV-2 entry. The resultant outcomes would lead the drug designers for novel anti-CoVs therapeutics.

Currently, the HR2 region is a significant target of agents that interfere with the fusion of coronaviruses. Current studies on anti-coronavirus fusogenic have identified HR2 peptides as a promising countermeasure. The EK1 peptide has been potent against pseudo-type particles of SARS-CoV, MERS-CoV, and SARS-CoV-2 in micromolar concentration [86]. Moreover, the EK1 has also been studied in mice infected with MERS-CoV with profound therapeutic outcomes. However, the peptide has been injected half an hour after the viral challenge. It would be interesting if the effect is analyzed on the different time scales of post-infection to obtain comprehensive information about its efficacy.

Research should extend further on the mechanistic study of viral entry, leading the scientific community to develop novel entry inhibitors. Different features of vial-membrane fusion processes such as receptor bind domain, FP, lipid, and ionic contents may provide viral fusion reaction (S domains, proteases, lipid compositions, and ionic environments) proved as a significant target for various types of agents interfering with viral fusion. The scientists are dedicated to what they can do for the management of coronavirus infection.

Moreover, the ACE2 architecture is the same in other vertebrates [142]. Structural analysis reveals that ACE2 from other vertebrates binds effectively to the RBD of SARS-CoV-2 S protein, suggesting that these can host virus infection [143, 144]. Therefore, the interaction of RBD and hACE2 needs to be characterized to design antiviral strategies for intervening receptor-viral interaction [145, 146].

Besides viruses that infect humans, there are animal viruses with homologous fusion proteins, thus, demonstrating more similar features than their human counterparts. Isolating and culturing these animal viruses would provide important information about future outbreaks and crossing species barriers.

Currently, available therapeutics for coronaviruses treatment have limited potency in various populations and species. The development of novel therapeutics that intervene with different stages of the viral life cycle is crucial, especially in immunocompromised individuals. It happens due to the emerging of drug-resistant strains of coronaviruses [147 - 149]. The main focus is on designing therapeutic strategies to inhibit viral entry into host cells, impede viral replication, and interfere with virus-host interactions [150]. Antigenic variations for immune evasion and crossing species barriers require large-scale effective countermeasures [151].

Extensive mutations in the coronavirus genome are the main barrier to developing an effective vaccine for the COVID [152]. Genetic alterations in the antigenic determinants of spike proteins result in new strains [135, 153]. As a result of genetic alteration in the epitopes, the antibodies raised against the previous stains cannot recognize the newly emerging stains. Hence, immunity against one strain cannot provide protection [154]. The urgency of novel therapeutics in critical cases stems from the appearance of drug-resistant strains [155]. In the last few years, drugs interfering with various stages of the viral life cycle, such as entry, replication, and virus-host interaction, have been designed to treat viral diseases [156]. Recently, virus-immune system interaction has gained significant attention and is the main focus of antiviral targets [157]. Biomolecules such as immunomodulators and bacterial metabolites are being investigated for enhancing immunity.

Coronavirus infections are zoonotic, so understanding the mechanism of crossing species barriers would be greatly informative for disease prevention. Nevertheless, the primary, intermediate animal host of SARS-CoV-2, if there exists, is yet to be discovered. To provide insight into the future cross-species transmission of coronavirus, interactive analysis of hACE2 and S protein other strains are of prime importance. Different studies demonstrate that cross-reactive antibodies weakly interact with viruses of other strains, so there is an urgent need to identify the well-conserved antigenic determinant(s) within the spike protein for future development pan-coronaviruses vaccine. Moreover, diverse polyclonal antibodies respond to different strains of coronaviruses replicate in animal reservoirs. It may provide an immediate countermeasure for the neutralization of immune escape mutant strain.

CONCLUSION

Coronavirus spike (S) glycoprotein is a 180-kDa protein that drives receptor attachment and viral entry to the host cells. Spike protein is structured into amino (N) S1 and carboxyl (C) S terminal domains involved in the receptor attachment and membrane fusion. The RBD of SARS-CoV-2 is located within the C-terminal region of S1. Besides the high level of homology among the RBDs of SARS-CoV and SARS-CoV-2, the affinity of SARS-CoV-2 RBD is many folds higher for the hACE2 receptor. Unlike SARS-CoV spike protein, SARS-CoV-2 spike glycoprotein induces syncytia formation among the infected cells even in the lack of exogenous protease. Spike proteins drive fusion reaction between viral and host membrane for viral entry. A fusion reaction is triggered by the S2 domain and cellular proteases such as trypsin, cathepsins, furin, HAT, TMPRSS-2, and TMPRSS-4. The presence of this different type of host protease determines whether coronaviruses enter host cells *via* cell membrane route or endocytosis. Although the same set of proteases is required to activate spike protein, different coronaviruses harbor various cleavage sites. SARS-CoV-2 possesses a cleavage site for furin or furin-like protease, which sets apart SARS-CoV-2 from SARS-CoV and other SARS-like CoVs.

Furthermore, polyclonal rabbit anti-SARS S1 antibodies (T62) 'don't bind well to spike protein of SARS-CoV-2 and hence weakly neutralize SARS-CoV-2 entry to the target cell. Similarly, sera from the convalescent patients of COVID-19 and SARS weakly neutralize each other, suggesting that those who recovered from one viral infection do not provide against the other. Therefore, there is an urgent pan-coronaviruses vaccine development that can target highly conserved regions across coronaviruses. Moreover, membrane fusion is a sequential process that is driven by heptapeptide repeats (HR1 and HR2) of S2. The HR1 and HR2 assume 6HB which causes the fusion of viral and host cell membrane. Future perspective involves various aspects to be revealed such as interfering viral entry by targeting surface proteases and HR2 region, investigating the role of furin site, cholesterol and calcium in viral entry, interactive analysis of SARS-CoV-2 spike, and hACE2 from other vertebrates to prevent a future outbreak of coronaviruses and lastly developing of the pan-coronaviruses vaccine.

CONSENT FOR PUBLICATION

Not Applicable.

CONFLICT OF INTEREST

The author confirms that this chapter contents have no conflict of interest.

ACKNOWLEDGEMENT

Declared none.

REFERENCES

[1]   Malaviya P, Rathore VS. Bioremediation of pulp and paper mill effluent by a novel fungal consortium isolated from polluted soil. Bioresour Technol 2007; 98(18): 3647-51.
[http://dx.doi.org/10.1016/j.biortech.2006.11.021] [PMID: 17208440]

[2]   Drosten C, Günther S, Preiser W, *et al.* Identification of a novel coronavirus in patients with severe acute respiratory syndrome. N Engl J Med 2003; 348(20): 1967-76.
[http://dx.doi.org/10.1056/NEJMoa030747] [PMID: 12690091]

[3]   Zaki AM, van Boheemen S, Bestebroer TM, Osterhaus AD, Fouchier RA. Isolation of a novel coronavirus from a man with pneumonia in Saudi Arabia. N Engl J Med 2012; 367(19): 1814-20.
[http://dx.doi.org/10.1056/NEJMoa1211721] [PMID: 23075143]

[4]   Memish ZA, Perlman S, Van Kerkhove MD, Zumla A. Middle East respiratory syndrome. Lancet 2020; 395(10229): 1063-77.
[http://dx.doi.org/10.1016/S0140-6736(19)33221-0] [PMID: 32145185]

[5]   Guan Y, Zheng BJ, He YQ, *et al.* Isolation and characterization of viruses related to the SARS coronavirus from animals in southern China. Science 2003; 302(5643): 276-8.
[http://dx.doi.org/10.1126/science.1087139] [PMID: 12958366]

[6]   Li W, Shi Z, Yu M, *et al.* Bats are natural reservoirs of SARS-like coronaviruses. Science 2005; 310(5748): 676-9.
[http://dx.doi.org/10.1126/science.1118391] [PMID: 16195424]

[7]   Huang C, Wang Y, Li X, *et al.* Clinical features of patients infected with 2019 novel coronavirus in Wuhan, China. Lancet 2020; 395(10223): 497-506.
[http://dx.doi.org/10.1016/S0140-6736(20)30183-5] [PMID: 31986264]

[8]   Calisher C, Carroll D, Colwell R, *et al.* Statement in support of the scientists, public health professionals, and medical professionals of China combatting COVID-19. Lancet 2020; 395(10226): e42-3.
[http://dx.doi.org/10.1016/S0140-6736(20)30418-9] [PMID: 32087122]

[9]   Zhu N, Zhang D, Wang W. A novel coronavirus from patients with pneumonia in China, 2019 [published January 24. N Engl J Med 2020.
[http://dx.doi.org/10.1056/NEJMoa2001017]

[10]   Organization, W.H. Coronavirus disease 2019 (COVID-19): situation report 2020; 85.

[11]   Zhou D, Cai W, Zhang W. An adaptive wavelet method for nonlinear circuit simulation. IEEE Trans Circ Syst I Fundam Theory Appl 1999; 46(8): 931-8.
[http://dx.doi.org/10.1109/81.780374]

[12]   Wang D, Hu B, Hu C, *et al.* Clinical characteristics of 138 hospitalized patients with 2019 novel coronavirus–infected pneumonia in Wuhan, China. JAMA 2020; 17(11): 1061-1.
[http://dx.doi.org/10.1001/jama.2020.1585]

[13]   Lu R, Zhao X, Li J, *et al.* Genomic characterisation and epidemiology of 2019 novel coronavirus: implications for virus origins and receptor binding. Lancet 2020; 395(10224): 565-74.
[http://dx.doi.org/10.1016/S0140-6736(20)30251-8] [PMID: 32007145]

[14]   Wevers BA, van der Hoek L. Recently discovered human coronaviruses. Clin Lab Med 2009; 29(4): 715-24.
[http://dx.doi.org/10.1016/j.cll.2009.07.007] [PMID: 19892230]

[15]   Chiu SS, Chan KH, Chu KW, *et al.* Human coronavirus NL63 infection and other coronavirus infections in children hospitalized with acute respiratory disease in Hong Kong, China. Clin Infect Dis 2005; 40(12): 1721-9.
[http://dx.doi.org/10.1086/430301] [PMID: 15909257]

[16]   Gorse GJ, O'Connor TZ, Hall SL, Vitale JN, Nichol KL. Human coronavirus and acute respiratory illness in older adults with chronic obstructive pulmonary disease. J Infect Dis 2009; 199(6): 847-57.
[http://dx.doi.org/10.1086/597122] [PMID: 19239338]

[17]   Jean A, Quach C, Yung A, Semret M. Severity and outcome associated with human coronavirus OC43 infections among children. Pediatr Infect Dis J 2013; 32(4): 325-9.

[http://dx.doi.org/10.1097/INF.0b013e3182812787] [PMID: 23337903]

[18]   Jevšnik M, Uršič T, Žigon N, Lusa L, Krivec U, Petrovec M. Coronavirus infections in hospitalized pediatric patients with acute respiratory tract disease. BMC Infect Dis 2012; 12(1): 365.
[http://dx.doi.org/10.1186/1471-2334-12-365] [PMID: 23256846]

[19]   Wang C, Horby PW, Hayden FG, Gao GF. A novel coronavirus outbreak of global health concern. Lancet 2020; 395(10223): 470-3.
[http://dx.doi.org/10.1016/S0140-6736(20)30185-9] [PMID: 31986257]

[20]   Li F, Li W, Farzan M, Harrison SC. Structure of SARS coronavirus spike receptor-binding domain complexed with receptor. Science 2005; 309(5742): 1864-8.
[http://dx.doi.org/10.1126/science.1116480] [PMID: 16166518]

[21]   Li Z, Tomlinson AC, Wong AH, *et al.* The human coronavirus HCoV-229E S-protein structure and receptor binding. eLife 2019; 8: e51230.
[http://dx.doi.org/10.7554/eLife.51230] [PMID: 31650956]

[22]   Lu G, Hu Y, Wang Q, *et al.* Molecular basis of binding between novel human coronavirus MERS-CoV and its receptor CD26. Nature 2013; 500(7461): 227-31.
[http://dx.doi.org/10.1038/nature12328] [PMID: 23831647]

[23]   Raj VS, Mou H, Smits SL, *et al.* Dipeptidyl peptidase 4 is a functional receptor for the emerging human coronavirus-EMC. Nature 2013; 495(7440): 251-4.
[http://dx.doi.org/10.1038/nature12005] [PMID: 23486063]

[24]   Hofmann H, Pyrc K, van der Hoek L, Geier M, Berkhout B, Pöhlmann S. Human coronavirus NL63 employs the severe acute respiratory syndrome coronavirus receptor for cellular entry. Proc Natl Acad Sci USA 2005; 102(22): 7988-93.
[http://dx.doi.org/10.1073/pnas.0409465102] [PMID: 15897467]

[25]   Li W, Moore MJ, Vasilieva N, *et al.* Angiotensin-converting enzyme 2 is a functional receptor for the SARS coronavirus. Nature 2003; 426(6965): 450-4.
[http://dx.doi.org/10.1038/nature02145] [PMID: 14647384]

[26]   Wu K, Li W, Peng G, Li F. Crystal structure of NL63 respiratory coronavirus receptor-binding domain complexed with its human receptor. Proc Natl Acad Sci USA 2009; 106(47): 19970-4.
[http://dx.doi.org/10.1073/pnas.0908837106] [PMID: 19901337]

[27]   Zhou P, Yang X L, Wang X-G, *et al.* A pneumonia outbreak associated with a new coronavirus of probable bat origin. nature 2020; 579(7798): 270-3.

[28]   Guan WJ, Ni ZY, Hu Y, *et al.* Clinical characteristics of coronavirus disease 2019 in China. N Engl J Med 2020; 382(18): 1708-20.
[http://dx.doi.org/10.1056/NEJMoa2002032] [PMID: 32109013]

[29]   Chan JF-W, Kok K-H, Zhu Z, *et al.* Genomic characterization of the 2019 novel human-pathogenic coronavirus isolated from a patient with atypical pneumonia after visiting Wuhan. Emerg Microbes Infect 2020; 9(1): 221-36.
[http://dx.doi.org/10.1080/22221751.2020.1719902] [PMID: 31987001]

[30]   Wu A, Peng Y, Huang B, *et al.* Genome composition and divergence of the novel coronavirus (2019-nCoV) originating in China. Cell Host Microbe 2020; 27(3): 325-8.
[http://dx.doi.org/10.1016/j.chom.2020.02.001] [PMID: 32035028]

[31]   Wen F, Yu H, Guo J, Li Y, Luo K, Huang S. Identification of the hyper-variable genomic hotspot for the novel coronavirus SARS-CoV-2. J Infect 2020; 80(6): 671-93.
[http://dx.doi.org/10.1016/j.jinf.2020.02.027] [PMID: 32145215]

[32]   Lu G, Wang Q, Gao GF. Bat-to-human: spike features determining 'host jump' of coronaviruses SARS-CoV, MERS-CoV, and beyond. Trends Microbiol 2015; 23(8): 468-78.
[http://dx.doi.org/10.1016/j.tim.2015.06.003] [PMID: 26206723]

[33]   Lai M. Coronaviridae Fields virology 2007; 1305-18.

[34]   Belouzard S, Chu VC, Whittaker GR. Activation of the SARS coronavirus spike protein *via* sequential proteolytic cleavage at two distinct sites. Proceedings of the National Academy of Sciences, 2009; 106(14): 5871-6.
[http://dx.doi.org/10.1073/pnas.0809524106] [PMID: 19321428]

[35]   Bosch BJ, van der Zee R, de Haan CA, Rottier PJ. The coronavirus spike protein is a class I virus fusion protein: structural and functional characterization of the fusion core complex. J Virol 2003; 77(16): 8801-11.
[http://dx.doi.org/10.1128/JVI.77.16.8801-8811.2003] [PMID: 12885899]

[36]   Burkard C, Verheije MH, Wicht O, *et al.* Coronavirus cell entry occurs through the endo-/lysosomal pathway in a proteolysis-dependent manner. PLoS Pathog 2014; 10(11): e1004502.
[http://dx.doi.org/10.1371/journal.ppat.1004502] [PMID: 25375324]

[37]   Kirchdoerfer RN, Cottrell CA, Wang N, *et al.* Pre-fusion structure of a human coronavirus spike protein. Nature 2016; 531(7592): 118-21.
[http://dx.doi.org/10.1038/nature17200] [PMID: 26935699]

[38]   Millet JK, Whittaker GR. Host cell entry of Middle East respiratory syndrome coronavirus after two-step, furin-mediated activation of the spike protein. Proc Natl Acad Sci USA 2014; 111(42): 15214-9.
[http://dx.doi.org/10.1073/pnas.1407087111] [PMID: 25288733]

[39]   Park J-E, Li K, Barlan A, *et al.* Proteolytic processing of Middle East respiratory syndrome coronavirus spikes expands virus tropism. Proc Natl Acad Sci USA 2016; 113(43): 12262-7.
[http://dx.doi.org/10.1073/pnas.1608147113] [PMID: 27791014]

[40]   Walls A, Tortorici MA, Bosch BJ, *et al.* Crucial steps in the structure determination of a coronavirus spike glycoprotein using cryo-electron microscopy. Protein Sci 2017; 26(1): 113-21.
[http://dx.doi.org/10.1002/pro.3048] [PMID: 27667334]

[41]   Taguchi F, Hirai-Yuki A. Mouse hepatitis virus receptor as a determinant of the mouse susceptibility to MHV infection. Front Microbiol 2012; 3: 68.
[http://dx.doi.org/10.3389/fmicb.2012.00068] [PMID: 22375141]

[42]   Bertram S, Dijkman R, Habjan M, *et al.* TMPRSS2 activates the human coronavirus 229E for cathepsin-independent host cell entry and is expressed in viral target cells in the respiratory epithelium. J Virol 2013; 87(11): 6150-60.
[http://dx.doi.org/10.1128/JVI.03372-12] [PMID: 23536651]

[43]   Bertram S, Glowacka I, Müller MA, *et al.* Cleavage and activation of the severe acute respiratory syndrome coronavirus spike protein by human airway trypsin-like protease. J Virol 2011; 85(24): 13363-72.
[http://dx.doi.org/10.1128/JVI.05300-11] [PMID: 21994442]

[44]   Gierer S, Bertram S, Kaup F, *et al.* The spike protein of the emerging betacoronavirus EMC uses a novel coronavirus receptor for entry, can be activated by TMPRSS2, and is targeted by neutralizing antibodies. J Virol 2013; 87(10): 5502-11.
[http://dx.doi.org/10.1128/JVI.00128-13] [PMID: 23468491]

[45]   Qian Z, Dominguez SR, Holmes KV. Role of the spike glycoprotein of human Middle East respiratory syndrome coronavirus (MERS-CoV) in virus entry and syncytia formation. PLoS One 2013; 8(10): e76469.
[http://dx.doi.org/10.1371/journal.pone.0076469] [PMID: 24098509]

[46]   Shirato K, Kawase M, Matsuyama S. Middle East respiratory syndrome coronavirus infection mediated by the transmembrane serine protease TMPRSS2. J Virol 2013; 87(23): 12552-61.
[http://dx.doi.org/10.1128/JVI.01890-13] [PMID: 24027332]

[47]   Shirogane Y, Takeda M, Iwasaki M, *et al.* Efficient multiplication of human metapneumovirus in Vero cells expressing the transmembrane serine protease TMPRSS2. J Virol 2008; 82(17): 8942-6.

[http://dx.doi.org/10.1128/JVI.00676-08] [PMID: 18562527]

[48]   Walls AC, Tortorici MA, Bosch B-J, *et al.* Cryo-electron microscopy structure of a coronavirus spike glycoprotein trimer. Nature 2016; 531(7592): 114-7.
[http://dx.doi.org/10.1038/nature16988] [PMID: 26855426]

[49]   Yuan Y, Cao D, Zhang Y, *et al.* Cryo-EM structures of MERS-CoV and SARS-CoV spike glycoproteins reveal the dynamic receptor binding domains. Nat Commun 2017; 8: 15092.
[http://dx.doi.org/10.1038/ncomms15092] [PMID: 28393837]

[50]   Belouzard S, Millet JK, Licitra BN, Whittaker GR. Mechanisms of coronavirus cell entry mediated by the viral spike protein. Viruses 2012; 4(6): 1011-33.
[http://dx.doi.org/10.3390/v4061011] [PMID: 22816037]

[51]   Kuo L, Koetzner CA, Hurst KR, Masters PS. Recognition of the murine coronavirus genomic RNA packaging signal depends on the second RNA-binding domain of the nucleocapsid protein. J Virol 2014; 88(8): 4451-65.
[http://dx.doi.org/10.1128/JVI.03866-13] [PMID: 24501403]

[52]   de Haan CA, Rottier PJ. Molecular interactions in the assembly of coronaviruses. Adv Virus Res 2005; 64: 165-230.
[http://dx.doi.org/10.1016/S0065-3527(05)64006-7] [PMID: 16139595]

[53]   Heald-Sargent T, Gallagher T. Ready, set, fuse! The coronavirus spike protein and acquisition of fusion competence. Viruses 2012; 4(4): 557-80.
[http://dx.doi.org/10.3390/v4040557] [PMID: 22590686]

[54]   Kleine-Weber H, Elzayat MT, Hoffmann M, Pöhlmann S. Functional analysis of potential cleavage sites in the MERS-coronavirus spike protein. Sci Rep 2018; 8(1): 16597.
[http://dx.doi.org/10.1038/s41598-018-34859-w] [PMID: 30413791]

[55]   Yang Y, Du L, Liu C, *et al.* Receptor usage and cell entry of bat coronavirus HKU4 provide insight into bat-to-human transmission of MERS coronavirus. Proc Natl Acad Sci USA 2014; 111(34): 12516-21.
[http://dx.doi.org/10.1073/pnas.1405889111] [PMID: 25114257]

[56]   Fehr A, Perlman S. Coronaviruses: Methods and Protocols. The Pirbright Institute 2015.

[57]   Wu F, Zhao S, Yu B, *et al.* A new coronavirus associated with human respiratory disease in China. Nature 2020; 579(7798): 265-9.
[http://dx.doi.org/10.1038/s41586-020-2008-3] [PMID: 32015508]

[58]   Wong SK, Li W, Moore MJ, Choe H, Farzan M. A 193-amino acid fragment of the SARS coronavirus S protein efficiently binds angiotensin-converting enzyme 2. J Biol Chem 2004; 279(5): 3197-201.
[http://dx.doi.org/10.1074/jbc.C300520200] [PMID: 14670965]

[59]   Peng G, Sun D, Rajashankar KR, Qian Z, Holmes KV, Li F. Crystal structure of mouse coronavirus receptor-binding domain complexed with its murine receptor. Proc Natl Acad Sci USA 2011; 108(26): 10696-701.
[http://dx.doi.org/10.1073/pnas.1104306108] [PMID: 21670291]

[60]   Xu X, Chen P, Wang J, *et al.* Evolution of the novel coronavirus from the ongoing Wuhan outbreak and modeling of its spike protein for risk of human transmission. Sci China Life Sci 2020; 63(3): 457-60.
[http://dx.doi.org/10.1007/s11427-020-1637-5] [PMID: 32009228]

[61]   Hamming I, Timens W, Bulthuis M, Lely A, Navis Gv, van Goor H. Tissue distribution of ACE2 protein, the functional receptor for SARS coronavirus. A first step in understanding SARS pathogenesis. The Journal of Pathology: A Journal of the Pathological Society of Great Britain and Ireland 2004; 203(2): 631-7.

[62]   Yan R, Zhang Y, Li Y, Xia L, Guo YY, Zhou Q. Structural basis for the recognition of SARS-CoV-2 by full-length human ACE2. Science 2020; 27;367(6485): 1444-8.

[http://dx.doi.org/10.1001/jama.2020.1585]

[63]   Walls AC, Park Y-J, Tortorici MA, Wall A, McGuire AT, Veesler D. Structure, function, and antigenicity of the SARS-CoV-2 spike glycoprotein. Cell 2020.
[http://dx.doi.org/10.1016/j.cell.2020.11.032]

[64]   van Doremalen N, Miazgowicz KL, Milne-Price S, *et al.* Host species restriction of Middle East respiratory syndrome coronavirus through its receptor, dipeptidyl peptidase 4. J Virol 2014; 88(16): 9220-32.
[http://dx.doi.org/10.1128/JVI.00676-14] [PMID: 24899185]

[65]   Li W, Hulswit RJG, Widjaja I, *et al.* Identification of sialic acid-binding function for the Middle East respiratory syndrome coronavirus spike glycoprotein. Proc Natl Acad Sci USA 2017; 114(40): E8508-17.
[http://dx.doi.org/10.1073/pnas.1712592114] [PMID: 28923942]

[66]   White JM, Delos SE, Brecher M, Schornberg K. Structures and mechanisms of viral membrane fusion proteins: multiple variations on a common theme. Crit Rev Biochem Mol Biol 2008; 43(3): 189-219.
[http://dx.doi.org/10.1080/10409230802058320] [PMID: 18568847]

[67]   White JM, Whittaker GR. Fusion of enveloped viruses in endosomes. Traffic 2016; 17(6): 593-614.
[http://dx.doi.org/10.1111/tra.12389] [PMID: 26935856]

[68]   Teasdale JD. Emotional processing, three modes of mind and the prevention of relapse in depression. Behav Res Ther 1999; 37 (Suppl. 1): S53-77.
[http://dx.doi.org/10.1016/S0005-7967(99)00050-9] [PMID: 10402696]

[69]   Madu IG, Belouzard S, Whittaker GR. SARS-coronavirus spike S2 domain flanked by cysteine residues C822 and C833 is important for activation of membrane fusion. Virology 2009; 393(2): 265-71.
[http://dx.doi.org/10.1016/j.virol.2009.07.038] [PMID: 19717178]

[70]   Sainz B Jr, Rausch JM, Gallaher WR, Garry RF, Wimley WC. Identification and characterization of the putative fusion peptide of the severe acute respiratory syndrome-associated coronavirus spike protein. J Virol 2005; 79(11): 7195-206.
[http://dx.doi.org/10.1128/JVI.79.11.7195-7206.2005] [PMID: 15890958]

[71]   Guillén J, Kinnunen PK, Villalaín J. Membrane insertion of the three main membranotropic sequences from SARS-CoV S2 glycoprotein. Biochim Biophys Acta 2008; 1778(12): 2765-74.
[http://dx.doi.org/10.1016/j.bbamem.2008.07.021] [PMID: 18721794]

[72]   Guillén J, Pérez-Berná AJ, Moreno MR, Villalaín J. A second SARS-CoV S2 glycoprotein internal membrane-active peptide. Biophysical characterization and membrane interaction. Biochemistry 2008; 47(31): 8214-24.
[http://dx.doi.org/10.1021/bi800814q] [PMID: 18616295]

[73]   Alsaadi EAJ, Neuman BW, Jones IM. A fusion peptide in the spike protein of MERS coronavirus. Viruses 2019; 11(9): 825.
[http://dx.doi.org/10.3390/v11090825] [PMID: 31491938]

[74]   Chambers K, McCarthy P. Stellar absorption features in high-redshift radio galaxies. Astrophys J 1990; 354: L9-L12.
[http://dx.doi.org/10.1086/185710]

[75]   Ou X, Liu Y, Lei X, *et al.* Characterization of spike glycoprotein of SARS-CoV-2 on virus entry and its immune cross-reactivity with SARS-CoV. Nat Commun 2020; 11(1): 1620.
[http://dx.doi.org/10.1038/s41467-020-15562-9] [PMID: 32221306]

[76]   Letko M, Marzi A, Munster V. Functional assessment of cell entry and receptor usage for SARS-Co-2 and other lineage B betacoronaviruses. Nat Microbiol 2020; 5(4): 562-9.
[http://dx.doi.org/10.1038/s41564-020-0688-y] [PMID: 32094589]

[77]   Ksiazek TG, Erdman D, Goldsmith CS, *et al.* A novel coronavirus associated with severe acute

respiratory syndrome. N Engl J Med 2003; 348(20): 1953-66.
[http://dx.doi.org/10.1056/NEJMoa030781] [PMID: 12690092]

[78] Wang Q, Zhang Y, Wu L, *et al.* Structural and functional basis of SARS-CoV-2 entry by using human ACE2. Cell 2020; 181(4): 894-904.e9.
[http://dx.doi.org/10.1016/j.cell.2020.03.045] [PMID: 32275855]

[79] Wrapp D, Wang N, Corbett KS, *et al.* Cryo-EM structure of the 2019-nCoV spike in the prefusion conformation. Science 2020; 367(6483): 1260-3.
[http://dx.doi.org/10.1126/science.abb2507] [PMID: 32075877]

[80] Kabbani N, Olds JL. Does COVID19 infect the brain? If so, smokers might be at a higher risk. Mol Pharmacol 2020; 97(5): 351-3.
[http://dx.doi.org/10.1124/molpharm.120.000014] [PMID: 32238438]

[81] Baig AM, Khaleeq A, Ali U, Syeda H. Evidence of the COVID-19 virus targeting the CNS: tissue distribution, host–virus interaction, and proposed neurotropic mechanisms. ACS Chem Neurosci 2020; 11(7): 995-8.
[http://dx.doi.org/10.1021/acschemneuro.0c00122] [PMID: 32167747]

[82] Shirato K, Kanou K, Kawase M, Matsuyama S. Clinical isolates of human coronavirus 229E bypass the endosome for cell entry. J Virol 2016; 91(1): e01387-16.
[PMID: 27733646]

[83] Shirato K, Kawase M, Matsuyama S. Wild-type human coronaviruses prefer cell-surface TMPRSS2 to endosomal cathepsins for cell entry. Virology 2018; 517: 9-15.
[http://dx.doi.org/10.1016/j.virol.2017.11.012] [PMID: 29217279]

[84] Follis KE, York J, Nunberg JH. Furin cleavage of the SARS coronavirus spike glycoprotein enhances cell-cell fusion but does not affect virion entry. Virology 2006; 350(2): 358-69.
[http://dx.doi.org/10.1016/j.virol.2006.02.003] [PMID: 16519916]

[85] Hoffmann M, Kleine-Weber H, Schroeder S, *et al.* SARS-CoV-2 cell entry depends on ACE2 and TMPRSS2 and is blocked by a clinically proven protease inhibitor. Cell 2020; 181(2): 271-280.e8.
[http://dx.doi.org/10.1016/j.cell.2020.02.052] [PMID: 32142651]

[86] Xia S, Liu M, Wang C, *et al.* Inhibition of SARS-CoV-2 (previously 2019-nCoV) infection by a highly potent pan-coronavirus fusion inhibitor targeting its spike protein that harbors a high capacity to mediate membrane fusion. Cell Res 2020; 30(4): 343-55.
[http://dx.doi.org/10.1038/s41422-020-0305-x] [PMID: 32231345]

[87] Simmons G, Reeves JD, Rennekamp AJ, Amberg SM, Piefer AJ, Bates P. Characterization of severe acute respiratory syndrome-associated coronavirus (SARS-CoV) spike glycoprotein-mediated viral entry. Proc Natl Acad Sci USA 2004; 101(12): 4240-5.
[http://dx.doi.org/10.1073/pnas.0306446101] [PMID: 15010527]

[88] Simmons G, Gosalia DN, Rennekamp AJ, Reeves JD, Diamond SL, Bates P. Inhibitors of cathepsin L prevent severe acute respiratory syndrome coronavirus entry. Proc Natl Acad Sci USA 2005; 102(33): 11876-81.
[http://dx.doi.org/10.1073/pnas.0505577102] [PMID: 16081529]

[89] Matsuyama S, Ujike M, Morikawa S, Tashiro M, Taguchi F. Protease-mediated enhancement of severe acute respiratory syndrome coronavirus infection. Proc Natl Acad Sci USA 2005; 102(35): 12543-7.
[http://dx.doi.org/10.1073/pnas.0503203102] [PMID: 16116101]

[90] Belouzard S, Madu I, Whittaker GR. Elastase-mediated activation of the severe acute respiratory syndrome coronavirus spike protein at discrete sites within the S2 domain. J Biol Chem 2010; 285(30): 22758-63.
[http://dx.doi.org/10.1074/jbc.M110.103275] [PMID: 20507992]

[91] Choi S-Y, Bertram S, Glowacka I, Park YW, Pöhlmann S. Type II transmembrane serine proteases in

cancer and viral infections. Trends Mol Med 2009; 15(7): 303-12.
[http://dx.doi.org/10.1016/j.molmed.2009.05.003] [PMID: 19581128]

[92]   Bertram S, Glowacka I, Blazejewska P, *et al.* TMPRSS2 and TMPRSS4 facilitate trypsin-independent spread of influenza virus in Caco-2 cells. J Virol 2010; 84(19): 10016-25.
[http://dx.doi.org/10.1128/JVI.00239-10] [PMID: 20631123]

[93]   Böttcher E, Matrosovich T, Beyerle M, Klenk H-D, Garten W, Matrosovich M. Proteolytic activation of influenza viruses by serine proteases TMPRSS2 and HAT from human airway epithelium. J Virol 2006; 80(19): 9896-8.
[http://dx.doi.org/10.1128/JVI.01118-06] [PMID: 16973594]

[94]   Chaipan C, Kobasa D, Bertram S, *et al.* Proteolytic activation of the 1918 influenza virus hemagglutinin. J Virol 2009; 83(7): 3200-11.
[http://dx.doi.org/10.1128/JVI.02205-08] [PMID: 19158246]

[95]   Kam Y-W, Okumura Y, Kido H, Ng LF, Bruzzone R, Altmeyer R. Cleavage of the SARS coronavirus spike glycoprotein by airway proteases enhances virus entry into human bronchial epithelial cells *in vitro*. PLoS One 2009; 4(11): e7870.
[http://dx.doi.org/10.1371/journal.pone.0007870] [PMID: 19924243]

[96]   Glowacka I, Bertram S, Müller MA, *et al.* Evidence that TMPRSS2 activates the severe acute respiratory syndrome coronavirus spike protein for membrane fusion and reduces viral control by the humoral immune response. J Virol 2011; 85(9): 4122-34.
[http://dx.doi.org/10.1128/JVI.02232-10] [PMID: 21325420]

[97]   Matsuyama S, Nagata N, Shirato K, Kawase M, Takeda M, Taguchi F. Efficient activation of the severe acute respiratory syndrome coronavirus spike protein by the transmembrane protease TMPRSS2. J Virol 2010; 84(24): 12658-64.
[http://dx.doi.org/10.1128/JVI.01542-10] [PMID: 20926566]

[98]   Shulla A, Heald-Sargent T, Subramanya G, Zhao J, Perlman S, Gallagher T. A transmembrane serine protease is linked to the severe acute respiratory syndrome coronavirus receptor and activates virus entry. J Virol 2011; 85(2): 873-82.
[http://dx.doi.org/10.1128/JVI.02062-10] [PMID: 21068237]

[99]   Matsuyama S, Nao N, Shirato K, *et al.* Enhanced isolation of SARS-CoV-2 by TMPRSS2-expressing cells. Proc Natl Acad Sci USA 2020; 117(13): 7001-3.
[http://dx.doi.org/10.1073/pnas.2002589117] [PMID: 32165541]

[100] Zmora P, Hoffmann M, Kollmus H, *et al.* TMPRSS11A activates the influenza A virus hemagglutinin and the MERS coronavirus spike protein and is insensitive against blockade by HAI-1. J Biol Chem 2018; 293(36): 13863-73.
[http://dx.doi.org/10.1074/jbc.RA118.001273] [PMID: 29976755]

[101] Millet JK, Whittaker GR. Host cell proteases: Critical determinants of coronavirus tropism and pathogenesis. Virus Res 2015; 202: 120-34.
[http://dx.doi.org/10.1016/j.virusres.2014.11.021] [PMID: 25445340]

[102] Horvath S, Oshima J, Martin GM, *et al.* Epigenetic clock for skin and blood cells applied to Hutchinson Gilford Progeria Syndrome and *ex vivo* studies. Aging (Albany NY) 2018; 10(7): 1758-75.
[http://dx.doi.org/10.18632/aging.101508] [PMID: 30048243]

[103] Coutard B, Valle C, de Lamballerie X, Canard B, Seidah NG, Decroly E. The spike glycoprotein of the new coronavirus 2019-nCoV contains a furin-like cleavage site absent in CoV of the same clade. Antiviral Res 2020; 176: 104742.
[http://dx.doi.org/10.1016/j.antiviral.2020.104742] [PMID: 32057769]

[104] Inoue Y, Tanaka N, Tanaka Y, *et al.* Clathrin-dependent entry of severe acute respiratory syndrome coronavirus into target cells expressing ACE2 with the cytoplasmic tail deleted. J Virol 2007; 81(16): 8722-9.
[http://dx.doi.org/10.1128/JVI.00253-07] [PMID: 17522231]

[105] Wang H, Yang P, Liu K, *et al.* SARS coronavirus entry into host cells through a novel clathrin- and caveolae-independent endocytic pathway. Cell Res 2008; 18(2): 290-301.
[http://dx.doi.org/10.1038/cr.2008.15] [PMID: 18227861]

[106] Ochiai H, Sakai S, Hirabayashi T, Shimizu Y, Terasawa K. Inhibitory effect of bafilomycin A1, a specific inhibitor of vacuolar-type proton pump, on the growth of influenza A and B viruses in MDCK cells. Antiviral Res 1995; 27(4): 425-30.
[http://dx.doi.org/10.1016/0166-3542(95)00040-S] [PMID: 8540761]

[107] Qiu Z, Hingley ST, Simmons G, *et al.* Endosomal proteolysis by cathepsins is necessary for murine coronavirus mouse hepatitis virus type 2 spike-mediated entry. J Virol 2006; 80(12): 5768-76.
[http://dx.doi.org/10.1128/JVI.00442-06] [PMID: 16731916]

[108] Regan AD, Shraybman R, Cohen RD, Whittaker GR. Differential role for low pH and cathepsin-mediated cleavage of the viral spike protein during entry of serotype II feline coronaviruses. Vet Microbiol 2008; 132(3-4): 235-48.
[http://dx.doi.org/10.1016/j.vetmic.2008.05.019] [PMID: 18606506]

[109] Huang I-C, Bosch BJ, Li F, *et al.* SARS coronavirus, but not human coronavirus NL63, utilizes cathepsin L to infect ACE2-expressing cells. J Biol Chem 2006; 281(6): 3198-203.
[http://dx.doi.org/10.1074/jbc.M508381200] [PMID: 16339146]

[110] Mingo RM, Simmons JA, Shoemaker CJ, *et al.* Ebola virus and severe acute respiratory syndrome coronavirus display late cell entry kinetics: evidence that transport to NPC1+ endolysosomes is a rate-defining step. J Virol 2015; 89(5): 2931-43.
[http://dx.doi.org/10.1128/JVI.03398-14] [PMID: 25552710]

[111] Reinke LM, Spiegel M, Plegge T, *et al.* Different residues in the SARS-CoV spike protein determine cleavage and activation by the host cell protease TMPRSS2. PLoS One 2017; 12(6): e0179177.
[http://dx.doi.org/10.1371/journal.pone.0179177] [PMID: 28636671]

[112] Sun X, Tse LV, Ferguson AD, Whittaker GR. Modifications to the hemagglutinin cleavage site control the virulence of a neurotropic H1N1 influenza virus. J Virol 2010; 84(17): 8683-90.
[http://dx.doi.org/10.1128/JVI.00797-10] [PMID: 20554779]

[113] Andersen KG, Rambaut A, Lipkin WI, Holmes EC, Garry RF. The proximal origin of SARS-CoV-2. Nat Med 2020; 26(4): 450-2.
[http://dx.doi.org/10.1038/s41591-020-0820-9] [PMID: 32284615]

[114] Bosch BJ, Bartelink W, Rottier PJ. Cathepsin L functionally cleaves the severe acute respiratory syndrome coronavirus class I fusion protein upstream of rather than adjacent to the fusion peptide. J Virol 2008; 82(17): 8887-90.
[http://dx.doi.org/10.1128/JVI.00415-08] [PMID: 18562523]

[115] Biniossek ML, Nägler DK, Becker-Pauly C, Schilling O. Proteomic identification of protease cleavage sites characterizes prime and non-prime specificity of cysteine cathepsins B, L, and S. J Proteome Res 2011; 10(12): 5363-73.
[http://dx.doi.org/10.1021/pr200621z] [PMID: 21967108]

[116] Jaimes JA, André NM, Chappie JS, Millet JK, Whittaker GR. Phylogenetic analysis and structural modeling of SARS-CoV-2 spike protein reveals an evolutionary distinct and proteolytically-sensitive activation loop. J Mol Biol 2020; 432(10): 3309-25.
[http://dx.doi.org/10.1016/j.jmb.2020.04.009] [PMID: 32320687]

[117] Shang J, Ye G, Shi K, *et al.* Structural basis of receptor recognition by SARS-CoV-2. Nature 2020; 581(7807): 221-4.
[http://dx.doi.org/10.1038/s41586-020-2179-y] [PMID: 32225175]

[118] Harrison SC. Viral membrane fusion. Virology 2015; 479-480: 498-507.
[http://dx.doi.org/10.1016/j.virol.2015.03.043] [PMID: 25866377]

[119] Harrison SC. Viral membrane fusion. Nat Struct Mol Biol 2008; 15(7): 690-8.

[http://dx.doi.org/10.1038/nsmb.1456] [PMID: 18596815]

[120] Cohen FS, Melikyan GB. The energetics of membrane fusion from binding, through hemifusion, pore formation, and pore enlargement. J Membr Biol 2004; 199(1): 1-14.
[http://dx.doi.org/10.1007/s00232-004-0669-8] [PMID: 15366419]

[121] Martens S, McMahon HT. Mechanisms of membrane fusion: disparate players and common principles. Nat Rev Mol Cell Biol 2008; 9(7): 543-56.
[http://dx.doi.org/10.1038/nrm2417] [PMID: 18496517]

[122] Tripet B, Howard MW, Jobling M, Holmes RK, Holmes KV, Hodges RS. Structural characterization of the SARS-coronavirus spike S fusion protein core. J Biol Chem 2004; 279(20): 20836-49.
[http://dx.doi.org/10.1074/jbc.M400759200] [PMID: 14996844]

[123] Carr CM, Kim PS. A spring-loaded mechanism for the conformational change of influenza hemagglutinin. Cell 1993; 73(4): 823-32.
[http://dx.doi.org/10.1016/0092-8674(93)90260-W] [PMID: 8500173]

[124] Guillén J, Pérez-Berná AJ, Moreno MR, Villalaín J. Identification of the membrane-active regions of the severe acute respiratory syndrome coronavirus spike membrane glycoprotein using a 16/18-mer peptide scan: implications for the viral fusion mechanism. J Virol 2005; 79(3): 1743-52.
[http://dx.doi.org/10.1128/JVI.79.3.1743-1752.2005] [PMID: 15650199]

[125] Lentz BR, Malinin V, Haque ME, Evans K. Protein machines and lipid assemblies: current views of cell membrane fusion. Curr Opin Struct Biol 2000; 10(5): 607-15.
[http://dx.doi.org/10.1016/S0959-440X(00)00138-X] [PMID: 11042461]

[126] Chernomordik LV, Kozlov MM. Mechanics of membrane fusion. Nat Struct Mol Biol 2008; 15(7): 675-83.
[http://dx.doi.org/10.1038/nsmb.1455] [PMID: 18596814]

[127] Simons K, Ikonen E. Functional rafts in cell membranes. nature 1997; 387(6633): 569-72.

[128] Yang S-T, Kreutzberger AJB, Lee J, Kiessling V, Tamm LK. The role of cholesterol in membrane fusion. Chem Phys Lipids 2016; 199: 136-43.
[http://dx.doi.org/10.1016/j.chemphyslip.2016.05.003] [PMID: 27179407]

[129] Glende J, Schwegmann-Wessels C, Al-Falah M, *et al.* Importance of cholesterol-rich membrane microdomains in the interaction of the S protein of SARS-coronavirus with the cellular receptor angiotensin-converting enzyme 2. Virology 2008; 381(2): 215-21.
[http://dx.doi.org/10.1016/j.virol.2008.08.026] [PMID: 18814896]

[130] Ishii T, Ohnuma K, Murakami A, *et al.* CD26-mediated signaling for T cell activation occurs in lipid rafts through its association with CD45RO. Proc Natl Acad Sci USA 2001; 98(21): 12138-43.
[http://dx.doi.org/10.1073/pnas.211439098] [PMID: 11593028]

[131] Dubé M, Rey FA, Kielian M. Rubella virus: first calcium-requiring viral fusion protein. PLoS Pathog 2014; 10(12): e1004530.
[http://dx.doi.org/10.1371/journal.ppat.1004530] [PMID: 25474548]

[132] Nathan L, Lai AL, Millet JK, *et al.* Calcium ions directly interact with the ebola virus fusion peptide To promote structure–function changes that enhance infection. ACS Infect Dis 2019.
[PMID: 31746195]

[133] Das DK, Bulow U, Diehl WE, *et al.* Conformational changes in the Ebola virus membrane fusion machine induced by pH, Ca2+, and receptor binding. PLoS Biol 2020; 18(2): e3000626.
[http://dx.doi.org/10.1371/journal.pbio.3000626] [PMID: 32040508]

[134] Lai AL, Millet JK, Daniel S, Freed JH, Whittaker GR. The SARS-CoV fusion peptide forms an extended bipartite fusion platform that perturbs membrane order in a calcium-dependent manner. J

Mol Biol 2017; 429(24): 3875-92.
[http://dx.doi.org/10.1016/j.jmb.2017.10.017] [PMID: 29056462]

[135]   Du L, He Y, Zhou Y, Liu S, Zheng B-J, Jiang S. The spike protein of SARS-CoV--a target for vaccine and therapeutic development. Nat Rev Microbiol 2009; 7(3): 226-36.
[http://dx.doi.org/10.1038/nrmicro2090] [PMID: 19198616]

[136]   Wang L, Shi W, Joyce MG, *et al.* Evaluation of candidate vaccine approaches for MERS-CoV. Nat Commun 2015; 6(1): 7712.
[http://dx.doi.org/10.1038/ncomms8712] [PMID: 26218507]

[137]   Zhao J, Yuan Q, Wang H, *et al.* Antibody responses to SARS-CoV-2 in patients of novel coronavirus disease 2019. Clin Infect Dis 2020; 71(16): 2027-34.
[http://dx.doi.org/10.1093/cid/ciaa344] [PMID: 32221519]

[138]   Tian X, Li C, Huang A, *et al.* Potent binding of 2019 novel coronavirus spike protein by a SARS coronavirus-specific human monoclonal antibody. Emerg Microbes Infect 2020; 9(1): 382-5.
[http://dx.doi.org/10.1080/22221751.2020.1729069] [PMID: 32065055]

[139]   Zheng M, Song L. Novel antibody epitopes dominate the antigenicity of spike glycoprotein in SARS-CoV-2 compared to SARS-CoV. Cell Mol Immunol 2020; 17(5): 536-8.
[http://dx.doi.org/10.1038/s41423-020-0385-z] [PMID: 32132669]

[140]   Kumar K, Ranjan C, Davim JP. Antigenic variation of SARS☐CoV☐2 in response to immune pressure. Molecular Ecology 2021; 30(14): 3548-59.

[141]   Iwata-Yoshikawa N, Okamura T, Shimizu Y, Hasegawa H, Takeda M, Nagata N. TMPRSS2 contributes to virus spread and immunopathology in the airways of murine models after coronavirus infection. J Virol 2019; 93(6): e01815-18.
[http://dx.doi.org/10.1128/JVI.01815-18] [PMID: 30626688]

[142]   Imai Y, Kuba K, Rao S, *et al.* Angiotensin-converting enzyme 2 protects from severe acute lung failure. Nature 2005; 436(7047): 112-6.
[http://dx.doi.org/10.1038/nature03712] [PMID: 16001071]

[143]   Mathewson AC, Bishop A, Yao Y, *et al.* Interaction of severe acute respiratory syndrome-coronavirus and NL63 coronavirus spike proteins with angiotensin converting enzyme-2. J Gen Virol 2008; 89(Pt 11): 2741-5.
[http://dx.doi.org/10.1099/vir.0.2008/003962-0] [PMID: 18931070]

[144]   Poon LLM, Peiris M. Emergence of a novel human coronavirus threatening human health. Nat Med 2020; 26(3): 317-9.
[http://dx.doi.org/10.1038/s41591-020-0796-5] [PMID: 32108160]

[145]   Senathilake K, Samarakoon S, Tennekoon K. Virtual screening of inhibitors against spike glycoprotein of 2019 novel corona virus: A drug repurposing approach 2020.
[http://dx.doi.org/10.20944/preprints202003.0042.v1]

[146]   Chen Y, Guo Y, Pan Y, Zhao ZJ. Structure analysis of the receptor binding of 2019-nCoV. Biochem Biophys Res Commun 2020.: S0006-291X(20)30339-9.
[http://dx.doi.org/10.1016/j.bbrc.2020.02.071] [PMID: 32081428]

[147]   Prajapat M, Sarma P, Shekhar N, *et al.* Drug targets for corona virus: A systematic review. Indian J Pharmacol 2020; 52(1): 56-65.
[http://dx.doi.org/10.4103/ijp.IJP_115_20] [PMID: 32201449]

[148]   Yang Y, Islam MS, Wang J, Li Y, Chen X. Traditional Chinese medicine in the treatment of patients

infected with 2019-new coronavirus (SARS-CoV-2): a review and perspective. Int J Biol Sci 2020; 16(10): 1708-17.
[http://dx.doi.org/10.7150/ijbs.45538] [PMID: 32226288]

[149]   Zhou G, Zhao Q. Perspectives on therapeutic neutralizing antibodies against the Novel Coronavirus SARS-CoV-2. Int J Biol Sci 2020; 16(10): 1718-23.
[http://dx.doi.org/10.7150/ijbs.45123] [PMID: 32226289]

[150]   Schaack GA, Mehle A. Experimental approaches to identify host factors important for influenza virus. Cold Spring Harb Perspect Med 2020; 10(12): a038521.
[http://dx.doi.org/10.1101/cshperspect.a038521] [PMID: 31871241]

[151]   Ahmed SF, Quadeer AA, McKay MR. Preliminary identification of potential vaccine targets for the COVID-19 coronavirus (SARS-CoV-2) based on SARS-CoV immunological studies. Viruses 2020; 12(3): 254.
[http://dx.doi.org/10.3390/v12030254] [PMID: 32106567]

[152]   Kim Y, Cheon S, Min C-K, *et al.* Spread of mutant Middle East respiratory syndrome coronavirus with reduced affinity to human CD26 during the South Korean outbreak. MBio 2016; 7(2): e00019-6.
[http://dx.doi.org/10.1128/mBio.00019-16] [PMID: 26933050]

[153]   Kleine-Weber H, Elzayat MT, Wang L, *et al.* Mutations in the spike protein of Middle East respiratory syndrome coronavirus transmitted in Korea increase resistance to antibody-mediated neutralization. J Virol 2019; 93(2): e01381-18.
[http://dx.doi.org/10.1128/JVI.01381-18] [PMID: 30404801]

[154]   Stebbing J, Phelan A, Griffin I, *et al.* COVID-19: combining antiviral and anti-inflammatory treatments. Lancet Infect Dis 2020; 20(4): 400-2.
[http://dx.doi.org/10.1016/S1473-3099(20)30132-8] [PMID: 32113509]

[155]   Zu ZY, Jiang MD, Xu PP, *et al.* Coronavirus disease 2019 (COVID-19): a perspective from China. Radiology 2020; 296(2): E15-25.
[http://dx.doi.org/10.1148/radiol.2020200490] [PMID: 32083985]

[156]   Peeri NC, Shrestha N, Rahman MS, *et al.* The SARS, MERS and novel coronavirus (COVID-19) epidemics, the newest and biggest global health threats: what lessons have we learned? Int J Epidemiol 2020; 49(3): 717-26.
[http://dx.doi.org/10.1093/ije/dyaa033] [PMID: 32086938]

[157]   Zumla A, Chan JF, Azhar EI, Hui DS, Yuen K-Y. Coronaviruses - drug discovery and therapeutic options. Nat Rev Drug Discov 2016; 15(5): 327-47.
[http://dx.doi.org/10.1038/nrd.2015.37] [PMID: 26868298]

CHAPTER 7

Crystal Structure Determination and Receptor Recognition Basis of SARS-CoV-2 Spike Glycoprotein

Maher Darwish[1,*]

[1] *Department of Pharmaceutical Chemistry and Drug Control, Faculty of Pharmacy, Wadi International University, Homs, Syria*

Abstract: A new coronavirus outbreak has emerged in Wuhan, China, in 2019 and turned into a global pandemic posing a massive public health concern. Its genome has been sequenced and showed pairwise percent identities of approximately 79.5% and 50% compared to severe acute respiratory syndrome-coronavirus (SARS-CoV) and the Middle East respiratory syndrome-coronavirus (MERS-CoV), respectively. The coronavirus spike glycoprotein is the primary determinant of viral tropism and is responsible for receptor binding and membrane fusion. The receptor-binding domain of severe acute respiratory syndrome-coronavirus-2 (SARS-CoV-2) has been characterized and structurally identified through X-ray crystallography and cryo-electron microscopy. The variations in residual sequences, hidden receptor binding domain, and furin-like cleavage nature of the spike clarified the higher receptor affinity and efficient spread among humans compared to SARS-CoV. The spike glycoprotein is a vital target for vaccines and therapeutic antibodies. Correspondingly, the potential implication of its structure elucidation in developing new and cross-neutralizing antibodies targeting the spike epitopes has been briefly discussed. Here, it is expected that the elaborated details of the molecular structure may facilitate the opportunity of developing therapeutics against SARS-CoV-2.

Keywords: COVID19, Crystal structure, Neutralizing antibody, Receptor binding domain, SARS-CoV-2, Spike glycoprotein, Vaccine.

INTRODUCTION

Earlier in 2018, the World Health Organization (WHO) published blueprint priority diseases, including some coronaviruses-mediated diseases such as the Middle East respiratory syndrome (MERS) and severe acute respiratory syndrome (SARS). Ssome other diseases, such as Ebola and Marburg virus diseases, and

* **Corresponding author Maher Darwish:** Department of Pharmaceutical Chemistry and Drug Control, Faculty of Pharmacy, Wadi International University, Homs, Syria;
E-mails: darwish_maher@ymail.com and maherdarwish@wiu.edu.sy

Kamal Niaz & Muhammad Farrukh Nisar (Eds.)
All rights reserved-© 2021 Bentham Science Publishers

Disease X that are presumably caused by an unknown pathogen and can cause a human epidemic or pandemic disease [1]. Less than one year later, acute pneumonia cases reported in Wuhan, China was designated by WHO as the first-ever Disease X. Very soon afterward, a novel coronavirus was recognized as the causative pathogen agent behind the emerged disease denoted COVID-19 by WHO [2]. The novel virus was firstly designated as 2019-nCoV and then referred to as SARS-CoV-2 by the Coronaviridae Study Group (CSG) of the International Committee on Taxonomy of Viruses (ICTV) [3, 4].

The coronaviruses, named following the surficial crown-like spikes in their structure, belong to the *Coronaviridae* family and the *Orthocoronaviridae* subfamily. They are classified into four genera: α-, β-, δ-, and γ-coronaviruses. The β-coronaviruses are further classified into four lineages: A, B, C, and D. Among the different genera, seven coronaviruses have been reported as human pathogens including HCoV-229E and HCoV-NL63 (α-coronaviruses), HCoV-OC43, and HCoV-HKU1 (β-coronaviruses lineage A), MERS-CoV (β-coronaviruses lineage C), SARS-CoV, and most recently SARS-CoV-2 (β-coronaviruses lineage B), a species comprises several viruses that can infect humans, bats, and many other different animals [5]. δ-coronaviruses and γ-coronaviruses are of an avian source original but are, yet, able to infect mammals in addition to avian species [6]. The new wave of infectious pneumonia caused by COVID-19 has witnessed a rapid spread around the globe and, on March 11, 2020, more than 118000 cases were confirmed in 114 countries, and 4291 people had died from the disease.

The assessment of COVID-19 by WHO was characterized as a pandemic outbreak and global health emergency, when sudden deaths appeared worldwide [7]. SARS-CoV-2 infection's main complication is pneumonia accompanied by respiratory tract infection. Fever and cough are widely reported among the notable symptoms of the disease. In contrast, some others are represented by breathing difficulties, muscular ache, fatigue, confusion, headache, sore throat, and even acute respiratory distress syndrome, leading to respiratory or multiorgan failure. COVID-19 is especially life-threatening for those elderly patients who suffer from chronic diseases such as diabetes, hypertension, immunodeficiency, liver, or cardiovascular disease. At the same time, a minor impact has been witnessed on children. The virus transmission is mediated mainly by respirational droplets or direct contact with polluted surfaces or objects, and traces have been detected in many biological samples such as saliva, stool, and blood [8].

The disease is opposed solely by quarantine procedures, travel restrictions, patient isolation, and supportive medical care with no specific cure available yet. Scientists from all over the world tried to build on the previous experience with coronaviruses. They collaboratively attempted to identify and analyze the novel agent behind the disease painstakingly. The research shortly culminated in demonstrating the sequence of the new virus (SARS-CoV-2), and the phylogenetic analysis exhibited a 96.2% consistency with Bat SARS-like coronavirus (BatCoV-RaTG13) genome sequence, whereas 79.5% identity to SARS-CoV is shared. Various probable intermediate hosts have been proposed, including main pangolins, but not mice and rats [9, 10]. One of the major targets of SARS-CoV-2 research is to build on the atomic-level iterative framework of virus-receptor interactions, anticipate species-specific receptor usage, and classify probable animal hosts and animal models of viruses. Accordingly, the vital characteristics of the membrane glycoproteins (GPs) responsible for the virus-receptor interactions were determined. The establishment of angiotensin-converting enzyme 2 (ACE2) receptor recognition by SARS-CoV-2 presented a perception of viral tropism and pathogenesi. In contrast, functional mapping domains in the spike protein (S-glycoprotein) enables inhibitors to be generated. These S-glycoproteins are imperative targets for antiviral medications and vaccines. Hence, endeavors to cure SARS-CoV-2 have dedicated especially inhibit the S-glycoprotein from facilitating virus entry inside the target cells and encouraging results obtained so far.

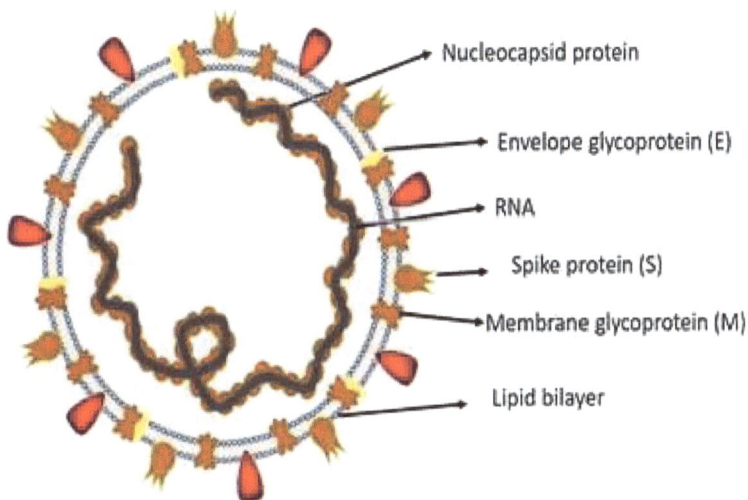

Fig. (1). The general structure of β-coronaviruses.

In this chapter, we throw the general structure of SARS-CoV-2 S and show that it uses ACE2 to enter the target cells. We also reveal the detailed atomic-level structure obtained by X-ray crystallography and cryo-electron microscopy of the virus-receptor interface identifying the key residues contributing to the interaction and cell entry. The overall similarities/differences with the original SARS-CoV as well as MERS-CoV are also well-manifested. Finally, we show the SARS-CoV-2 S-glycoprotein as a vital target for developing vaccines and virus-entry inhibitors.

Structure of SARS-CoV-2

In similitude to the other β-coronaviruses, SARS-CoV-2 is a spherical or moderately pleiomorphic virion in the nanoscale regimen (65-125 nm in diameter). It contains a non-segmented positive-sense RNA as a nucleic material that ranges from 26 to 32 kbs in length (Fig. **1**) [11].

The RNA genome of SARS-CoV-2, like MERS-CoV and SARS-CoV, has two regions; the first one is situated in the first open reading frame (ORF 1a/b) and comprises two-thirds of the genome. It decodes two polyproteins (pp1a and pp1ab). It expresses approximately 16 non-structural proteins (NSPs) such as papain-like protease, helicase, 3-chymotrypsin-like protease, and RNA-dependent RNA polymerase essential for the virus lifecycle [12]. The remaining third expresses five to eight auxiliary proteins and four vital structural proteins implanted in the surficial lipid bilayer hijacked from the host cell. The structural proteins comprise spike glycoprotein (S), membrane protein (M), a small envelope protein (E), and nucleocapsid protein (N) [13]. The coronavirus S-glycoprotein is the principal determining factor of viral tropism and is crucial for binding to the receptor and then fusion to the host cell membrane. It is a huge type I transmembrane glycoprotein (~ 180 kDa of ~1300 amino acids) assembled into a prominent trimer on the viral surface to produce the characteristic crown-like appearance. Its ectodomain is organized into two subunits, S1 and S2 (Fig. **2**). Both the amino-terminal domain (NTD) and receptor-binding domain (RBD) are parts of the S1 subunit and are responsible for binding to host receptors, while the S2 domain is in the S2 subunit mediates the viral fusion to the host membranes [6, 14]. The distances between the three interdomain are broadly distributed, ranging from 40 Å to 110 Å between S2 and NTD/RBD domains and 30 Å to 100 Å between NTD and RBD domains. These wide distributions designate improved structural flexibility in the domain planning of the four protomer arrangements [15]. The RBD domain spanning approximately 200 residues and contains two subdomains [16]. The first one is the core that is responsible for the construction of S trimer particles and is structurally composed of a twisted five-stranded antiparallel β sheet (β1, β2, β3, β4, and β7) with short connecting helices and loops. The second is external subdomain emerging between the β4 and β7 strands of the core, has a shape of extended insertion prevailed by a disulfide bond-stabilized flexible loop connecting short β5 and β6 strands, α4, and α5 helices. The small prolonged insertion forms the so-called receptor binding motif (RBM), which holds the majority of SARS-CoV-2 residues that contacts the receptor [17, 18]. The S2 subunit encompasses a hydrophobic looped fusion peptide (FP), two heptads repeat regions: heptad repeat 1 (HR1) and heptad repeat 2 (HR2), transmembrane domain (TM), and a cytoplasmic domain (CP), which suggests a coiled helix structure of the S2 subunit.

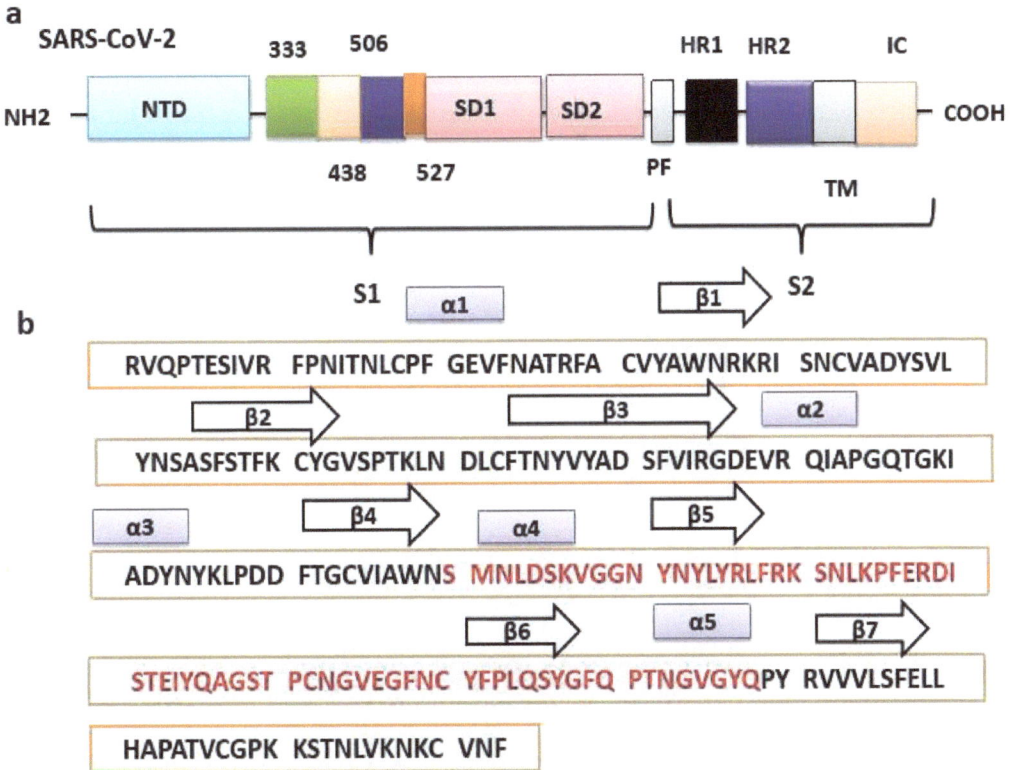

Fig. (2). The overall structure of SARS-CoV-2 S-glycoprotein.

ACE2 is the Cellular Receptor of SARS-CoV-2

The first step in virus infections is the interaction of viral units to host cell-surface receptors through the viral RBD on the spike protein. Receptor recognition is hence the determining factor of the viral tropism towards host cells and tissues. Furthermore, the variations at amino acid residues of a virus responsible for binding to the receptor in other species are also critical to modulate infection susceptibility across species [19, 20]. ACE2 is well-established as the host cell receptor for SARS-CoV. Consequently, scientists instantly following the outbreak of COVID-19 resolved that SARS-CoV-2 also utilizes human ACE2 (hACE2) as the target cellular receptor. This was achieved by carrying out virus contagion study using HeLa cells expressing or not the ACE2 proteins from humans and some other species, including bats, civets, pigs, and mice. The results implied that SARS-CoV-2 could benefit most of the ACE2 proteins, except for the mouse, to pass in ACE2-expressing cells while non-expressing HeLa cells failed to be beneficial. However, unlike some other human coronavirus receptors, SARS-CoV-2 did not bind with human aminopeptidase N (hAPN). However, it recognized the receptor of HCoV-229E or dipeptidyl peptidase 4 (DPP4 or CD26) of MERS-CoV [21, 22]. SARS-CoV-2 only could attach to ACE2 for virus entry (Fig. **3**) [23].

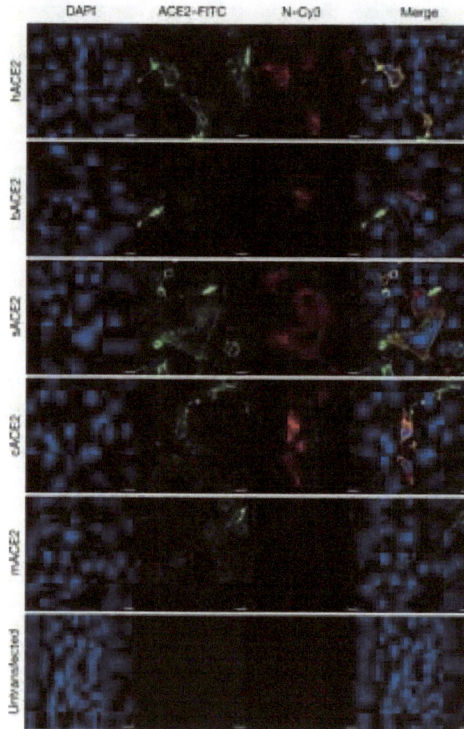

Fig. (3). Analysis of the receptor use of SARS-CoV-2.

ACE2 is a zinc-dependent membrane-bound peptidase of the M2-metalloprotease family widely expressed on the exterior surface of the endothelium of versatile tissues such as lungs, kidneys, small intestine, and renal tubes. ACE2 activates the splitting of angiotensin I peptide to produce vasodilator angiotensin 1-9. It also activates angiotensin II peptide to produce vasodilator angiotensin 1-7 and regulates blood pressure. Renin-angiotensin system blockers, including ACE inhibitors (ACEIs) and angiotensin receptor blockers (ARBs) are vastly benefited drugs for the medication of patients with cardiovascular diseases, including heart attack, hypertension, chronic kidney disease (nephropathy), and diabetes [24]. Nevertheless, the bodily role of ACE2 is entirely independent of its role as the viral receptor. Structurally, ACE2 comprises a large N-terminal peptidase ectodomain and a C-terminal collectrin-like domain (CLD). It ends with a single transmembrane helix and a ~40-residue intracellular segment. The peptidase domain (PD) is formed as a claw-like structure built of two α-helical lobes. The ACE2 activation position by enzymes is deeply hidden in a hole flanked by the two lobes [25, 26].

SARS-CoV-2 contact interaction with ACE2 is characterized as a strong one and is considered as a fundamental aspect in defining the host variety and cross-species transmissions of coronaviruses [27, 28]. SARS-CoV-2 entering process is established through the S-glycoprotein as forementioned. The S-glycoprotein exists in a metastable prefusion conformation subjected to a fundamental structural rearrangement to mediate the adhesion of the viral membrane and the host cell membrane [29]. The receptor binding is realized by the RBD of S1, which recognizes cell surface sugar molecules and directly engages, *via* its unique RBM, to the PD of ACE2. RBD is subjected to hinge-like conformational motions that rapidly cover or uncover the binding residues. The two situations are denoted as the "down" conformation and the "up" conformation, where the lying-down position agrees with the receptor-unreachable situation but effective for immune evasion and standing-up position coincides with the receptor reachable situation, which is considered to be unstable (Fig. 4) [30].

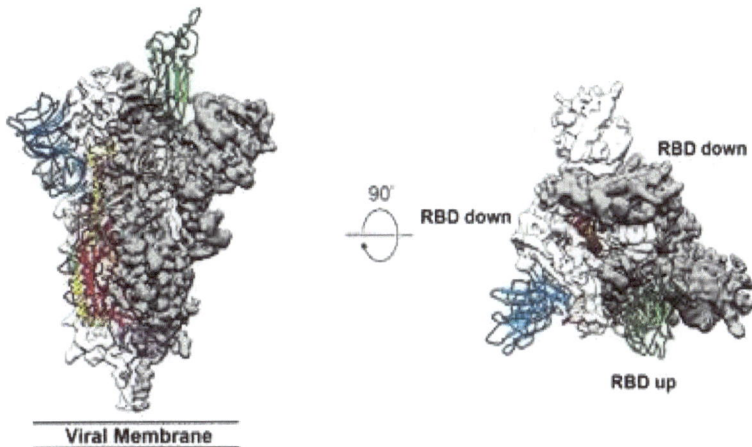

Fig. (4). Structure of SARS-CoV-2 S in the prefusion conformation.

The single-chain inactive precursor of S-glycoprotein undergoes a furin-like cleavage by the host cellular proteases. It comprises human airway trypsin-like protease (HAT), lysosomal proteases cathepsins, and transmembrane protease serine 2 (TMPRSS2) that cracks the S-glycoprotein and initiate more diffusion modifications. The splitting occurs at the interface between the S1 and S2 subunits to produce two noncovalently associated amino N-terminal S1 subunits and a carboxyl C-terminal S2 subunit [31, 32]. S1 can be further divided into

NTD and RBD, which both function as a receptor-adherence object, whereas SARS-CoV-2, SARS-CoV, and MERS-CoV employ the S1 RBD to identify the receptor, mouse hepatitis CoV binds the receptor with its S1 NTD [17]. Receptor binding also triggers conformational changes in the S2 subunit, HR1, and HR2 domains interact with each other to form a six-helix bundle (6-HB) fusion core, fetching viral and host cell membranes into juxtaposition to facilitate fusion through the exposure of fusion peptide [33 - 35]. Finally, SARS-CoV-2 S-glycoprotein enters the host cells mainly *via* endocytosis [36]. From receptor engagement to replication, the whole life cycle of the virus is fully illustrated in Fig.(**5**) [11].

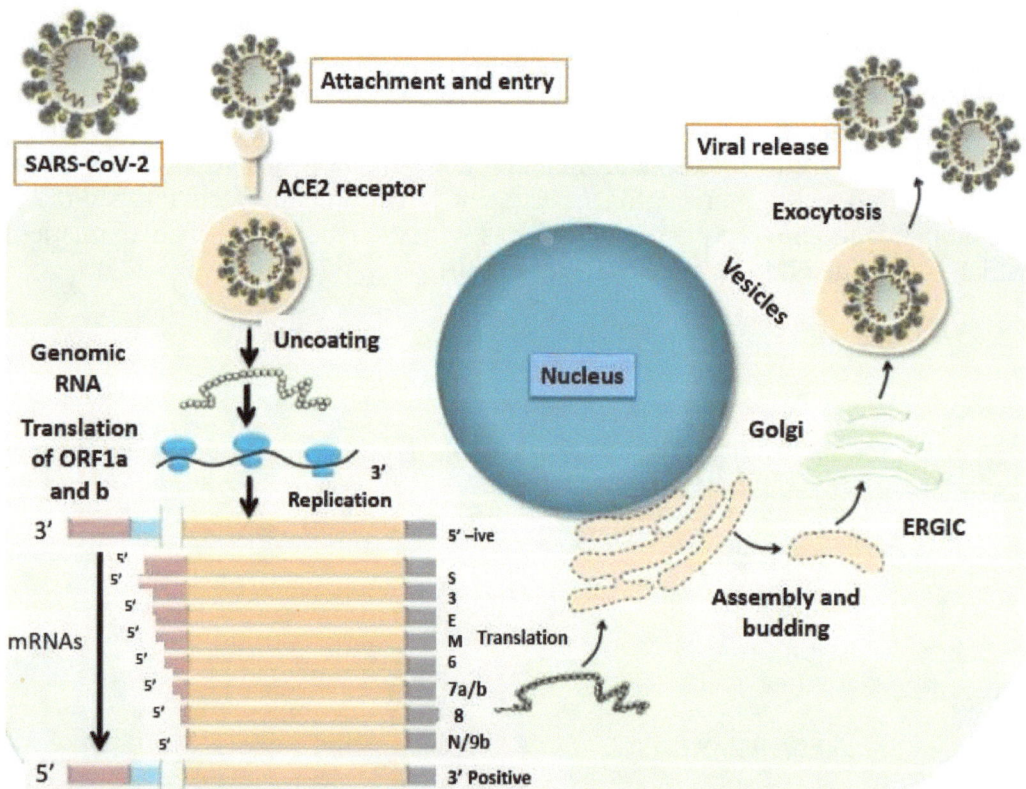

Fig. (5). The life cycle of SARS-CoV-2 in host cells.

Identification of Critical Binding Residues and Species-Specific ACE2–RBD Interactions

To establish a wider comprehension of the initial step in SARS-CoV-2 infection at the atomic-level, structural characterization of ACE2 key binding residues for the viral S-glycoprotein RBD has been identified using X-ray crystallography and cryo-electron microscopy (cryo-EM) structural analysis methods. The attained information was of great importance in elucidating the interface between SARS-CoV-2 and responsive cells. This would pave the way to target the connection area by neutralizing antibodies and would assist vaccine design to the SARS-CoV-2. The ACE2-RBD complexation is typical of protein-protein interactions (PPIs) that feature extended interfaces spanning many binding residues. Experimental and computational analyses of PPIs illustrated many contact residues that dominate the binding energy landscape [19].

X-ray Crystallography Method

The prolonged insertion in RBD, the RBM, bears the majority of SARS-CoV-2 linking residues that would facilitate binding to ACE2. The RBD contains nine cysteine residues in total, eight of which contribute to forming four pairs of disulfide bonds (Fig. **6**) [18]. Three of these four pairs are allocated in the core (C336-C361, C379-C432, and C391-C525) and assisting the stabilization of the β sheet structure. The last pair (C480-C488) attaches the loop in the terminal part of the RBM. On the other hand, the two α-helical lobes of ACE2 N-terminal PD contain a binding site between them to allow for the peptide substrate contact. The prolonged RBM in the SARS-CoV-2 RBD associates the lowest part of the ACE2 small lobe with the outer surface RBM in a concave shape to harbor the N-terminal helix of the ACE2.

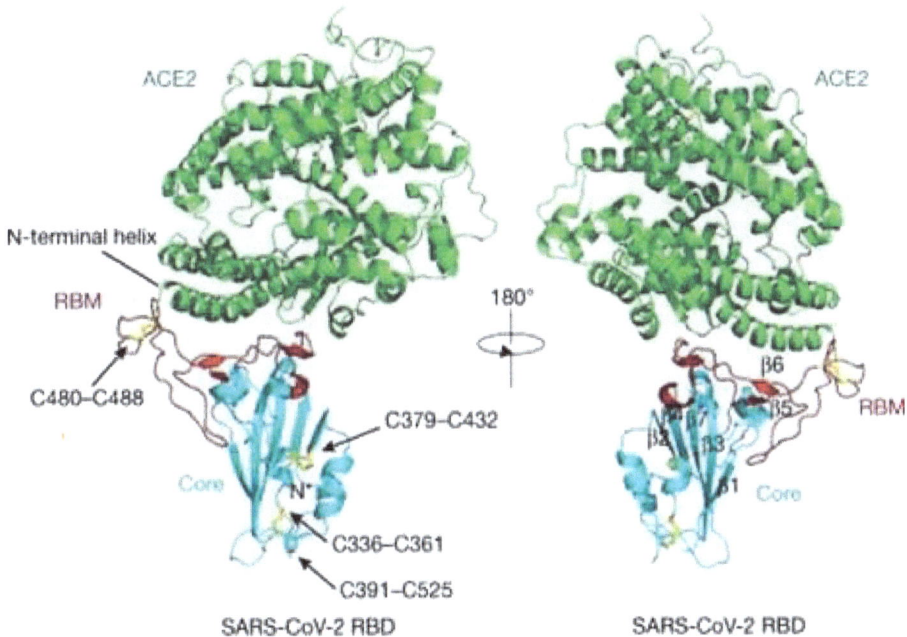

Fig. (6). The overall structure of the SARS-CoV-2 RBD bound to ACE2.

Both SARS-CoV-2 and SARS-CoV RBDs share a general mutual structure even in the RBM extended part that owns some sequence variations and one apparent conformational alteration in the distal end.

The total contact approach of the SARS-CoV-2 RBD to ACE2 is likewise closely undistinguishable from that detected in the formerly established structure of the SARS-CoV RBD/ACE2 complex. The cradling of the N-terminal helix of ACE2 by the outer surface of the RBM results in a large buried surface of 1,687 Å^2 (864 Å^2 on the RBD and 823 Å^2. Analysis of this interface demonstrated a total of 17 residues of the SARS-CoV-2 RBD in interaction with 20 residues of ACE2 [18]. A prominent feature presented between the viral ligand and receptor is the solid hydrophilic interactions with many hydrogen bonds and salt bridge ionic interactions (Table **1**) [18, 37]. Another noteworthy aspect is the participation of several tyrosine residues in forming hydrogen-bonding interactions with the polar hydroxyl group. Additional virus-receptor associates encompass SARS-CoV-2 RBD Y489 and F486 packing against hACE2 residues F28, L79, M82, and Y83, creating a small patch of hydrophobic contacts at the boundary [17]. In general, the virus-receptor attachment is governed by polar links intermediated by the hydrophilic residues.

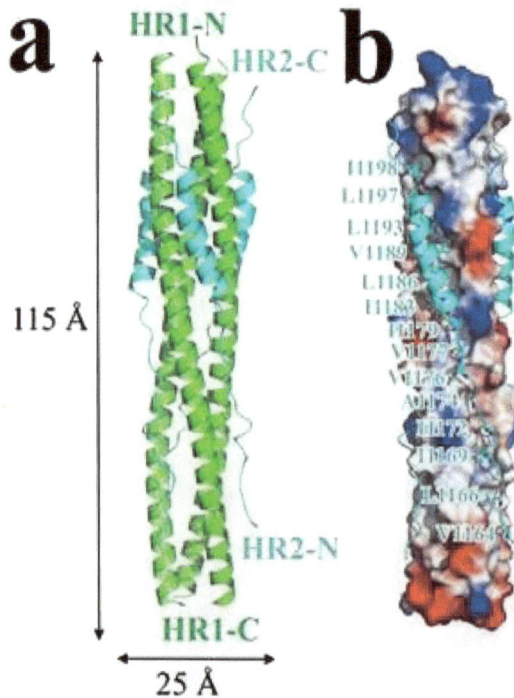

Fig. (7). The complete structure of post-fusion 6-HB in SARS-CoV-2.

In the S2 subunit structure, investigation of the 6-HB fusion core fashioned by HR1 and HR2 domains showed that it is arranged in a rod-like shape 115 Å in length and 25 Å in diameter (Fig. **7a**). The three HR1 domains create a parallel trimeric coiled-coil center, near which three HR2 domains are entwined in an antiparallel way. The two domains are bonded primarily by hydrophobic forces. Each pair of two neighboring HR1 helices creates a profound hydrophobic groove, accommodating the binding site for hydrophobic residues of the HR2 domain, including V1164, L1166, I1169, I1172, A1174, V1176, V1177, I1179, I1183, L1186, V1189, L1193, L1197 and I1198 (Fig. **7b**). The hydrophobic contacts amongst HR1 and HR2 are principally situated in the helical fusion core area [33].

Table 1. The polar links and salt bridges at the SARS-CoV-2 RBD/ACE2 interface.

	SARS-CoV-2 RBD	Distance(A)	ACE2 residues
Hydrogen Bonds	N487	2.4	Q24
	Q493	3.2	E35
	Y505	3.5	E37
	Y505	3.6	E37
	Y449	3.0	D38
	Y449	2.8	D38
	T500	2.7	Y41
	N501	3.7	Y41
	Q498	3.1	Q42
	G446	3.6	Q42
	Y449	3.2	Q42 Q42
	N487	2.5	Y83
	Y489	3.4	Y83 Q325 N330
	Y495	3.5	K353
	G496	3.1	K353
	G502	2.7	K353
	Y505	3.8	R393
Salt Bridges	K417	3.1	D30 E329 E329

Cryo-EM method

The cryo-EM structure alignment of SARS-CoV-2 RBD in the complex state with ACE2 is in analogy with the crystal structure obtained by *X-ray crystallography*. Extracellular PD of the ACE2 recognizes the RBD mainly through polar residues. The S-glycoprotein has its trimeric structure as one in "up conformation" and two in "down conformations". The connection of PD is established in S-glycoprotein when the ternary complex aligns with the RBD of the "up conformation". In contrast, attachment will not occur when the complex is overlaid on RDB in the "down conformation" [30]. The overall connection area between SARS-CoV-2 and ACE2 is also resolved primarily *via* polar contacts (Fig. **8a**). An extended loop region of the RBD spans the arch-shaped α1 helix of the ACE2-PD like a bridge. The α2 helix and a loop that connects the β3 and β4 antiparallel strands referred to as loop 3-4 of the PD. It also contributes to a small extent to the organization of the RBD. The connection may be divided into three clusters. The two ends of the bridge interact with the N and C termini of the α1 helix as well as small areas on the α2 helix and loop 3-4. The central segment of α1 promotes contact by accompanying two polar residues (Fig. **8a**). At the N terminus of α1, Q498, T500, and N501 of the RBD, develop a hydrogen-bonding network with Y41, Q42, K353, and R357 from ACE2 (Fig. **8b**). In the middle of the bridge, K417 and Y453 of the RBD interrelate with D30 and H34 of ACE2, respectively (Fig. **8c**). At the C terminus of α1, Q474 of the RBD is hydrogen attached to Q24 of ACE2. Meanwhile, F486 of the RBD networks with M82 of ACE2 through Van der Waals forces (Fig. **8d**) [38].

Comparison of SARS-CoV-2, SARS-CoV, and MERS-CoV

Phylogenetic analysis of the novel coronavirus exhibited that SARS-CoV-2, SARS-CoV, and bat-CoV-RaTG13 all belong to one clade that is different from MERS-CoV. The findings indicate an altered viral evolution from SARS and MERS, comprising bats as the animal reservoir (Table **1**) [38 - 40].

Table 2. Comparison of SARS-CoV-2, SARS-CoV, and MERS-CoV.

	Phylogenetic origin	Animal reservoir	Intermediate host	Receptor	Case fatality rate
SARS-CoV-2	Clade I, cluster IIa	Bats	Unknown	ACE2	2.3%
SARS-CoV	Clade I, cluster IIb	Bats	Palm civets	ACE2	9.5%
MERS-CoV	Clade II	Bats	Camels	DPP4	34.4%

On a genomic level, SARS-CoV-2 pairwise percent identities fall to approximately 79.5% and 50% compared to SARS-CoV and MERS-CoV, respectively. The S-glycoprotein of SARS-CoV-2 was revealed to be around 75%

analogous to the SARS-CoV spike. Significant variations between SARS-CoV and SARS-CoV-2 include the disappearance of 8a protein and dissimilarity in the total number of amino acids in 8b and 3c protein (Fig. **9**) [11].

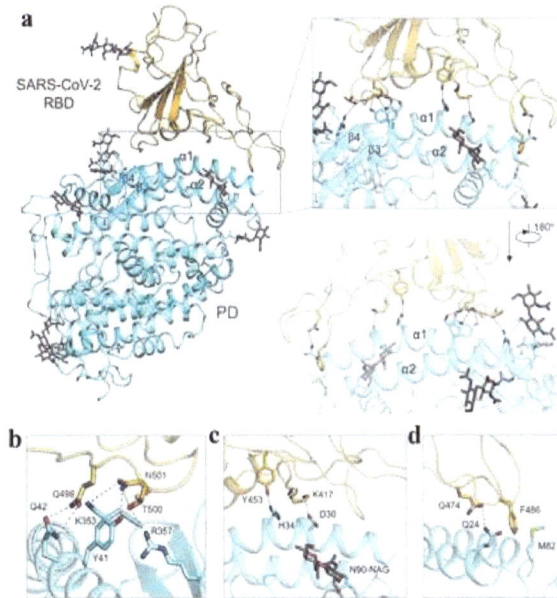

Fig. (8). Connections between RBD of SARS-CoV-2 and ACE2 (Cryo-EM).

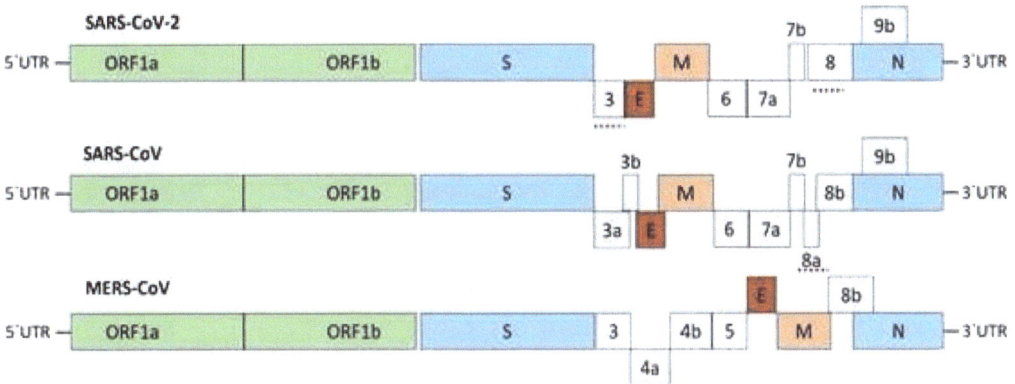

Fig. (9). β-coronaviruses genome organization.

SARS-CoV-2 and SARS-CoV seem to share identical clinical features. However, SARS-CoV-2 has a lower mortality rate than SARS-CoV and much lower than that of MERS (Table **2**).

SARS-CoV and MERS-CoV mutually target type II pneumocytes; while separately target ciliated bronchial epithelial cells and non-ciliated bronchial epithelial cells, respectively. On the other hand, SARS-CoV-2 can infect *ex vivo* with the same range of cell culture lines as SARS-CoV and MERS-CoV, *e.g.* Vero E6, Huh-7 cells, though primary human airway epithelial cells are its preferential cell type [6]. The pandemic feature of COVID 19 implies that the SARS-CoV-2 transmission rate is higher than that of SRAS-CoV and MERS-CoV. This is mainly attributed to the genetic recombination event at S-glycoprotein in the RBD area of SARS-CoV-2 that may have improved its spreading capacity and the higher binding affinity of SARS-CoV-2 RBD to hACE2 [11]. In detail, the S-glycoprotein of SARS-CoV-2 is modulated by homologous recombination. It is a mixture of BatCoV-RaTG13 (98%) and unknown β-coronavirus. The single N501T mutation in SARS-CoV-2 S-glycoprotein may have substantially boosted its binding affinity for ACE2 comparing with SARS-CoV [41]. The binding affinity between SARS-CoV-2 and ACE2 is evaluated between 4-fold and 10- to 20-fold greater [19, 30]. Accurately and to avoid literature controversy, SARS-CoV-2 RBD connects to hACE2 with considerably greater affinity than SARS-CoV RBD, supporting efficient cell entry. In contrast, paradoxically, the entire SARS-CoV-2 S-glycoprotein (RBD is mostly in the down conformation) has comparable to or lower hACE2 binding affinity than SARS-CoV S-glycoprotein (RBD is mostly in the up conformation). It is signifying that SARS-CoV-2 RBD, although more potent, is less exposed than SARS-CoV RBD. Moreover, it may be assumed that due to the lower severity in clinical implications of COVID-19, it can have a higher transmission among people than MERS and SARS [40].

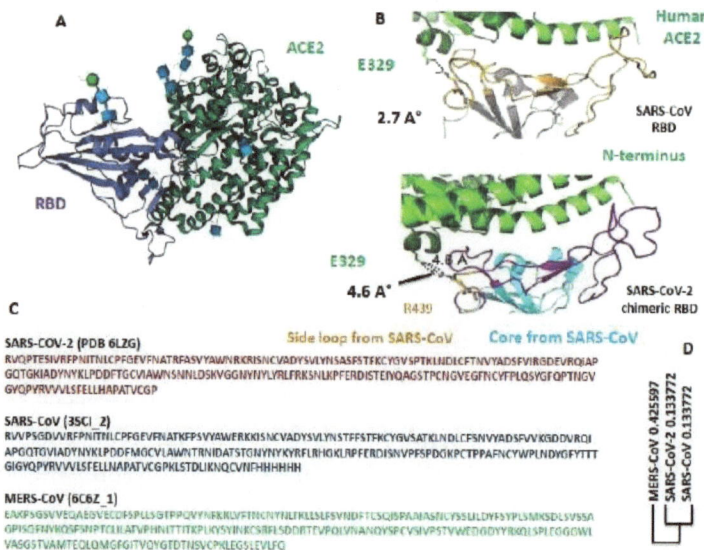

Fig. (10). Comparative structure and binding of SARS-CoV-2 and SARS-CoV to hACE2.

The receptor for SARS-CoV-2 is confirmed to be ACE2, similar to what has been identified with SARS-CoV. But it was not found to use dipeptidyl peptidase 4 (also known as CD26), the receptor for MERS-CoV. Although the two SARS viruses share the same human receptor [42], alignment of the three-dimensional structure and amino acid sequence of RBD of SARS-CoV-2 to those of SARS-CoV and MERS-CoV manifested a substantial topologic and sequence modification among the RBD of SARS-CoV-2 and those of the other two CoVs (Fig. **10b** and **10c**) [24]. SARS-CoV-2 RBD shares a 74.4% sequence identity of (166 amino acids) with SARS-CoV RBD, while only 17.9% (40 amino acids) is shared with MERS-CoV RBD (Fig. **10c**). This shows that SARS coronaviruses taxonomically dissent from MERS coronavirus (Fig. **10d**).

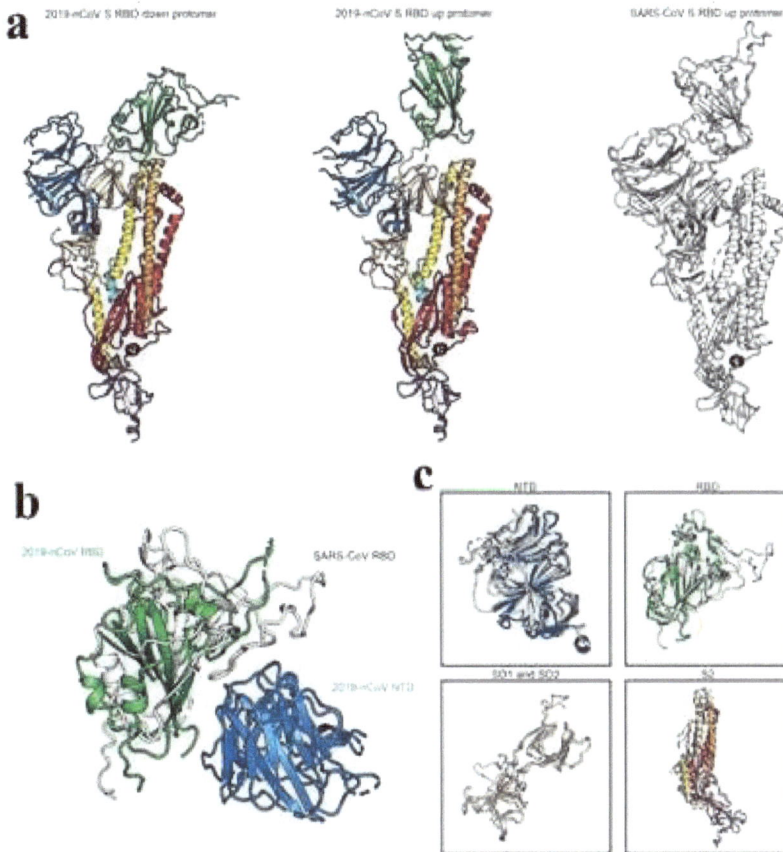

Fig. (11). Structural comparison between SARS-CoV-2 S and SARS-CoV S.

Although both SARS-CoV-2 and SARS-CoV S allocate high amino acid sequence identities among their RBDs, the NTDs display around 53% of analogy. NTDs of the various CoVs S-glycoproteins have been demonstrated to bind differing sugar. While NTD of MERS-CoV favors α2,3-linked sialic acid over α2,6-linked sialic acid, NTDs of human CoVs OC43 and HKU1 connect to 9---acetylated sialic acids 48,49. No reports claim a sugar-binding for NTD of SARS-CoV and SARS-CoV-2 [36]. Cryo-EM studies demonstrated that the RBD of the S1 subunits of the SARS-CoV, SARS-CoV-2, and MERS S-glycoproteins could exist in at least two conformations by undergoing a hinge-like movement. These structural conformations are essential for receptor attachment of all three viruses and are essential to commence the fusogenic changes [43]. The most notable topological variation between SARS-CoV, SARS-CoV-2 is the location of the RBDs in their down conformations (Fig. **11a**). The down conformation in SARS-CoV RBD holds firmly opposed to the NTD of the adjacent protomer. In the meantime, the down conformation of SARS-CoV-2 RBD is angularly located in proximity to the core void of the trimer (Fig. **11b**). The individual structural domains of SARS-CoV-2 S align with their homologous from SARS-CoV S, even with spotted conformational variance. They illustrate the large extent of structural harmony among both proteins, with the NTDs, RBDs, subdomains 1 and 2 (SD1 and SD2), and S2 subunits are yielding individual RMSD values of 2.6 Å, 3.0 Å, 2.7 Å, and 2.0 Å, respectively (Fig. **11c**) [30].

Another important topological variance among SARS-CoV and SARS-CoV-2 S-glycoproteins is the addition of an S1/S2 protease cleavage site that generates an "amino acids 682-685, RRAR" furin recognition site in SARS-CoV-2 as a substitute for the lone arginine residue in SARS-CoV [36]. The furin preactivation endows SARS-CoV-2 with the feature of less dependency on target cell proteases. It can then sustain a high ability of infection while maintaining the RBD less accessible by enhancing the admission into host cells, particularly cells that have rather small expressions of TMPRSS2 and/or lysosomal cathepsins [44].

Despite the general superimposition similarity in complexation with ACE2 between SARS-CoV and SARS-CoV-2 RBDs (Fig. **12a**). Many residues alterations may reinforce the connections between SARS-CoV-2 RBD and ACE2 and others that can change the affinity compared with SARS-CoV-RBD and ACE2. From the available crystallized structures, it was possible to highlight the differences between SARS-CoV and SARS-CoV-2 RBD residues involved in the binding of the hACE2. For instance, At the N-terminus of α1, the mutations R426→N439 (salt bridge with E329 and a hydrogen bond with Q325 on ACE2) abolished the strong polar interactions, Y484→Q498, and T487→N501 at similar locations are noticed between SARS-CoV RBD and SARS-CoV-2 RBD (Fig. **12b**). Additional alterations are detected in the central bridge. The most notable variation on β6 is replacing V404 in the SARS-CoV RBD with K417 in the SARS-CoV-2 RBD, which may induce a more firm connection due to the salt bridge development between K417 and D30 of ACE2 recovering the binding ability. Furthermore, from SARS-CoV RBD to SARS-CoV-2 RBD, the replacement of boundary residues Y442→L455, L443→F456, F460→Y473, and N479→Q493 could also alter the affinity for ACE2 (Fig. **12c**). At the C-terminus of α1, L472 in the SARS-CoV RBD is substituted by F486 in the SARS-CoV-2 RBD (Fig. **12d**). The alteration from L472 to F486 may also induce a tighter Van der Waals to attach with M82 (Fig. **12d**). Nevertheless, altering R426 with N439 seems to impair the interface by removing one vital salt bridge with D329 on ACE2 (Fig. **12b**) [38].

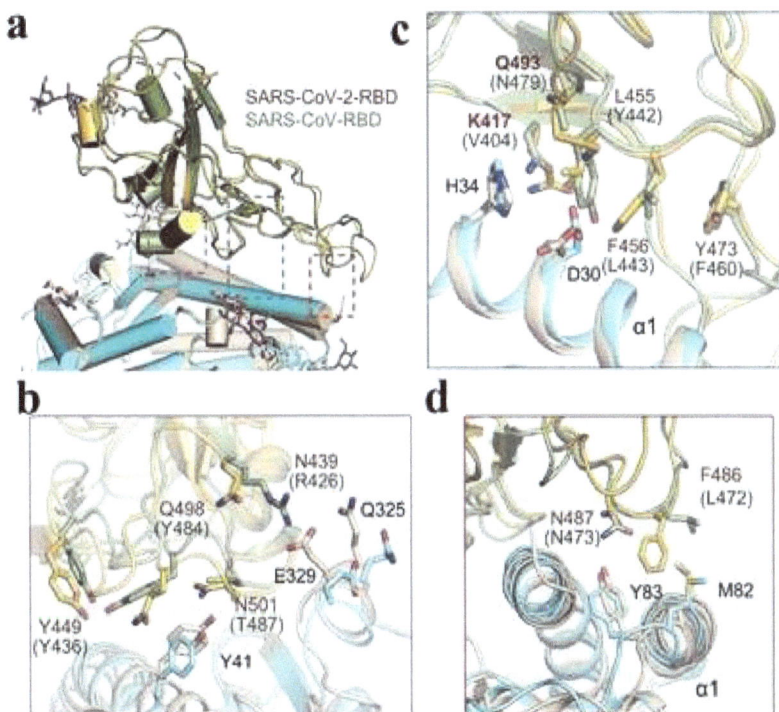

Fig. (12). Interface comparison between SARS-CoV-2-RBD and SARS-CoV-RBD with ACE2.

Regarding S2 subunit X-ray crystallographic analysis, the complex 6-HB fusion core structure of SARS-CoV-2 is similar to those of SARS-CoV and MERS-CoV. Comparing the sequence alignment of the S2 subunits in both SARS-CoV-2 and SARS-CoV shows that they are noticeably preserved, the amino acid sequence of the HR2 domain is entirely matched. At the same time, several residue alterations arise in the HR1 domain of SARS-CoV-2 with 92.6% overall homology. There are a total of 8 different residues within the central fusion region of HR1 domains (Fig. **13**), which can participate in the improved contacts amongst HR1 and HR2 and keep the 6-HB conformation of SARS-CoV-2 stable when compared with those of SARS-CoV. The K991→S929 alteration in HR1 brought a new firm hydrogen bond to be established in SARS-CoV-2 instead of the salt bridge in SARS-CoV. A new interaction in SARS-CoV-2 HR2 occurred between K933 and the carbonyl oxygen of N1192 *via* a salt bridge. It does not exist in SARS-CoV HR2. Between E918-R1166 and K929-E1163 in the HR1-HR2 domains of SARS-CoV were enhanced in SARS-CoV-2 through a weak salt bridge, where E918 mutated to D936. It bonded to R1185 in the HR2 domain through a strong salt bridge. Also, when T925 mutated to S943, it could bind to E1182 in the HR2 domain with a hydrogen bond. K947 could also attach to E1182 through a salt bridge. The various substitutions in the HR1 domain of emergent SARS-CoV-2 virus imply that this new HCoV has evolved with the enhanced binding affinity between HR1 and HR2 domains to stabilize further the 6-HB structure, which possibly will speed up the viral membrane fusion progression and boost viral contagion or transmittance ability [33].

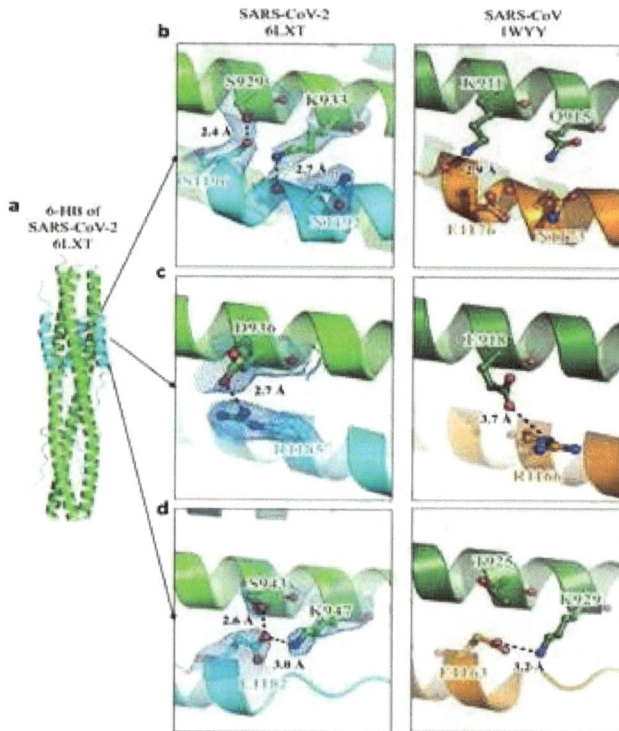

Fig. (13). Interaction between HR1 and HR2 of SARS-CoV-2 and SARS-CoV.

In terms of glycosylation, it is well-established that coronavirus S-glycoproteins are highly furnished by heterogeneous N-linked glycans emerging from the trimer surface. These oligosaccharides contribute to S folding, influence initiation by host proteases, and may modify antibody identification. SARS-CoV-2 S encompasses 22 N-linked glycosylation sequons per protomer and oligosaccharides are determined in the cryo-EM map for 16 of these sites (Fig. **14**). Whereas SARS-CoV S holds 23 N-linked glycosylation sequons per protomer, 19 of them are glycosylated. In total, 20 out of 22 SARS-CoV-2 S N-linked glycosylation sequons are preserved in SARS-CoV S. In particular, 9 out of 13 glycans in the S1 subunit and all 9 glycans in the S2 subunit are preserved amongst SARS-CoV-2 S and SARS-CoV S. Additionally, S2 N-linked glycosylation sequons are generally preserved crosswise SARSr-CoV S-glycoprotein, signifying that convenience of the fusion machinery to Abs will be analogous between these viruses [31].

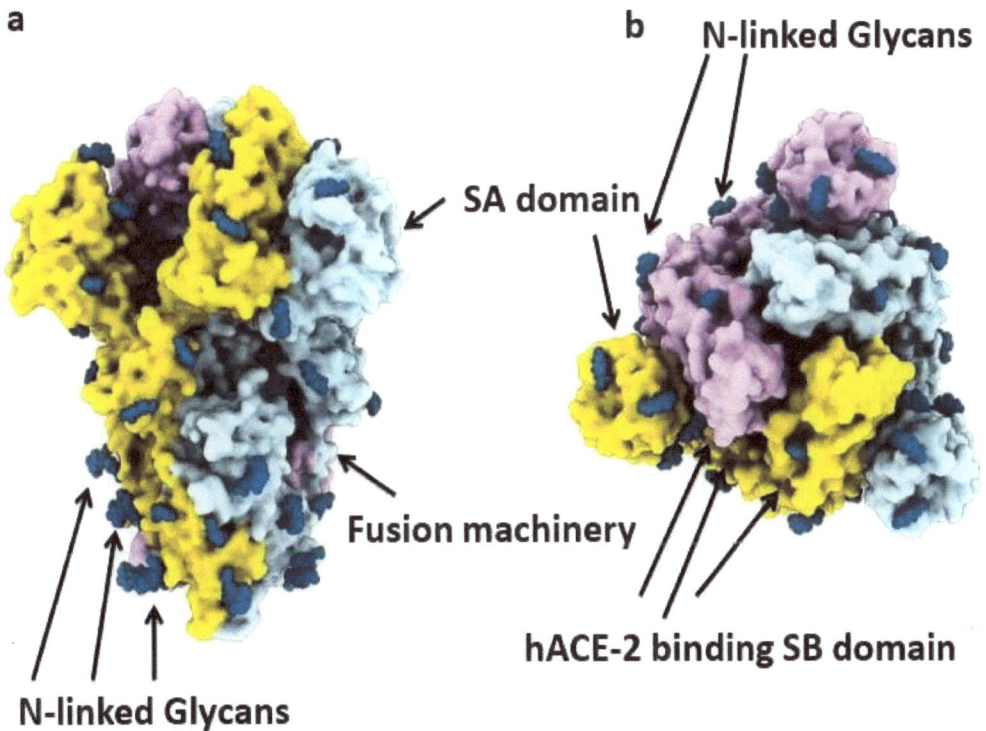

Fig. (14). Organization of the SARS-CoV-2 S N-Linked Glycans.

Conclusively, the total structural resemblance in hACE2 binding by SARS-CoV-2 and SARS-CoV confirms a tight evolutionary association among the two viruses [38].

SARS-CoV-2 S-Glycoprotein Potential Therapeutic Implications

Despite the high pathogenicity of zoonotic MERS-CoV, SARS-CoV, and SARS-CoV-2, up to the present time, no therapeutically active agents or vaccines have gain approval for treatment of any coronavirus of the human-infecting type. Biotechnology laboratories are working around the clock to develop therapeutic antibodies and antiviral drugs for curing people with COVID-19. Among the prophylactic and therapeutic interventions suggested to counter the SARS-CoV-2 effect, we can mention:

1. RNA-dependent RNA polymerase (RdRp) inhibitors: RdRp is an essential viral enzyme in the replication process of RNA viruses; thus, it became among the key targets of nucleoside analog antiviral drugs used for Ebola, Dengue, hepatitis C, Zika, and coronaviruses complications. The active RdRp site is well preserved, containing a couple of surface affordable consecutive aspartate residues in a β-turn assembly. Examples of this category include Ribavirin, Remdesivir, Sofosbuvir, Galidesivir, and Tenofovir, which have exhibited exciting results. As well, IDX-184, Setrobuvir, and YAK compounds displayed admirable outcomes for binding SARS-CoV-2 RdRp [45].
2. Anti-inflammatory antibodies/drugs in combination with anticoagulant molecules: might be utilized to prevent coagulopathy [46 - 48] and cytokine signaling outstandingly prompted by SARS-CoV-2 infection [49 - 51].
3. ACE2-mediated SARS-CoV-2 binding/fusion/entry inhibitors.

Generally, four possible approaches may be employed to tackle ACE2-interfaced SARS-CoV-2 (Fig. **15**) [9].

A. Spike Glycoprotein-based Vaccine

The viral S-glycoprotein that interacts with ACE2 receptors triggering fusion actions and facilitating the virus penetration into the human host cells is an important target for pharmacological interference. Specifically, RBD is the predominant immunogenic section of the entire spike. Yet, the veiling feature of RBD poses a difficulty in developing vaccination and antibodies due to the inadequate access area. One approach to overcome this issue is developing antibodies to bind the RBD very firmly during limited exposure. The opportunity of using the recombinant ACE2 for triggering an immune response and blocking SARS-CoV-2 RBD by targeting antibodies with a much higher RBD binding affinity than ACE2 is an optimistic approach to prevent and treat COVID-19 [44, 52]. Vaccines can also be adapted to inhibit the viral fusing capability of the S2 subunit. Still, such an approach might be of minor concern as the S2 subunit is lower in immunogenicity than the RBD [53].

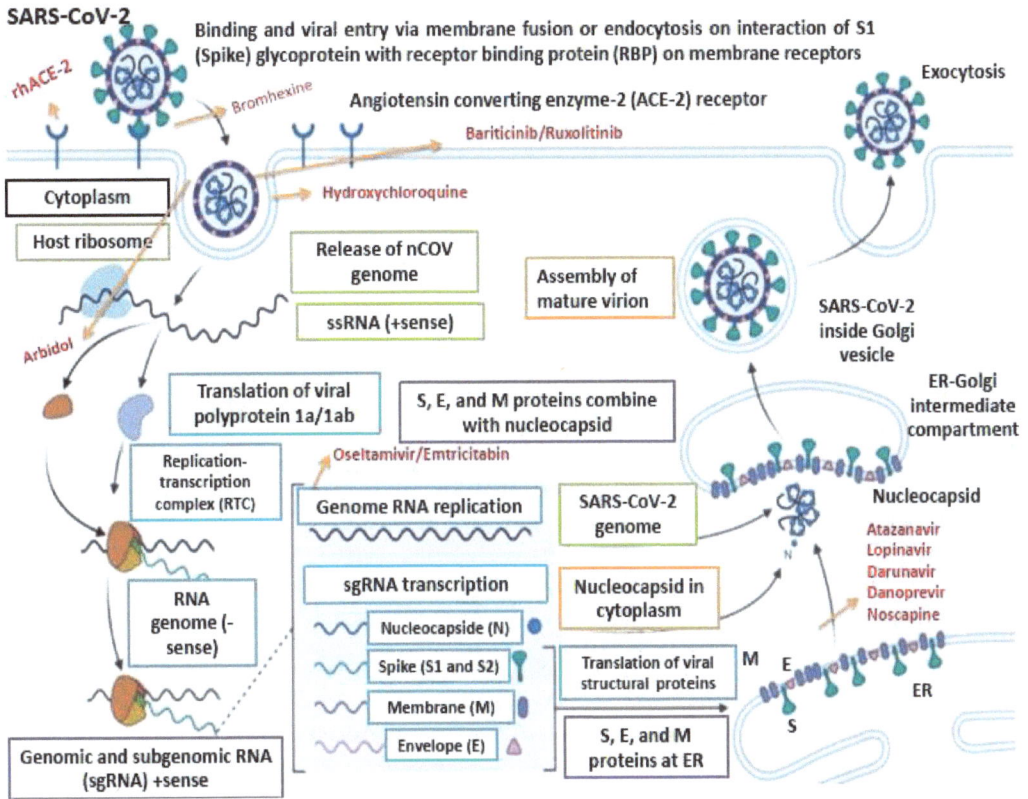

Fig. (15). Potential approaches to address ACE2-mediated COVID-19 following SARS-CoV-2 infection.

B. Inhibition of proteases activity

It has been established that initial spike protein cleavage by proteases, following ACE2 binding, is vital for viral fusion with host cell membranes and then spreading viral proteins inside. Some serine and cysteine protease inhibitors such as camostat mesylate are promising candidates [54, 55]. Camostat was developed to treat other diseases and has proved to inhibit TMPRSS2 function [56]. It has previously significantly reduced mortality in BALB/c mice following SARS-CoV infection and was recently confirmed to effectively block SARS-CoV-2 entry into lung cells [57, 58]. Nafamostat mesylate is the other TMPRSS2 inhibitor with therapeutic potential against SARS-CoV-2 invasion. FDA initially approved as a short-acting anticoagulant and then was identified as a potent inhibitor of S-mediated membrane fusion of MERS-CoV and blocked MERS-CoV infection in vitro [59]. A recent study stated that nafamostat inhibited SARS-CoV-2 entry into host cells with 5-fold higher efficiency than camostat. It blocked SARS-CoV-2 infection of human lung cells with noticeably higher efficacy camostat mesylate [60].

The host cell proteases, coronavirus Mpro and PLpro are attractive therapeutic targets because the viral replication and maturation inside the host cells significantly depend on them. Using lopinavir–ritonavir, protease inhibitors clinically available for HIV-1 infection, as an initial treatment of SARS-CoV in 2003 was associated with a reduction in the overall death rate and intubation rate. Thus, lopinavir–ritonavir was among the initial drug candidates to treat COVID-19 patients. However, in an open-label randomized study in Wuhan, China, 14 days of lopinavir-ritonavir therapy did not differ from standard care regarding clinical improvement or decreased viral RNA load. Lopinavir–ritonavir have not shown to be effective enough for SARS-CoV-2 infected patients, even though it has revealed *in vitro* effectivity for SARS-CoV [61]. This set of results suggested that lopinavir–ritonavir may have only a limited role in treating severely ill COVID-19 patients and may be used to treat mild or moderate COVID-19 patients, for example, as part of the initial treatment. Besides lopinavir–ritonavir, many other protease inhibitor drugs were examined, including favipiravir and oseltamivir, which are used for influenza. Besides, darunavir, danoprevir used for HIV, and hepatitis C infection are also effective against COVID-19, respectively [62]. Proteases are promising drug targets for the antiviral treatment of COVID-19, but the drug development and therapeutics toward them could be a highly complex process. It should be taken into account the efficacy and toxicity profile of protease modulators at the enzymatic, cellular, organ, as well as system levels.

C. Blocking the ACE2 receptor

Now that the interface between ACE2 and SARS-CoV-2 has been well-identified at the atomic level, antibodies or small peptides might be developed to target this interaction site.

D. Providing plenty of soluble forms of ACE2

SARS-CoV-2 suppresses ACE2 dimer, with no effect on ACE, by engaging its S-glycoprotein, leading eventually to severe lung damage. Thus, introducing a large quantity of ACE2 soluble forms might antagonistically bind with SARS-CoV-2 to inhibit the virus from infecting hACE2 and maintain ACE2 to function in adversely regulating the renin-angiotensin system and keep the lung intact from damage [9].

Neutralizing Antibodies (nABs) for targeting SARS-CoV-2 S-glycoprotein

CoV nAbs prompted by vaccines, or infected viruses have pivotal roles in restraining virus-mediated diseases. nABs under development mainly comprise monoclonal antibodies (mAbs), their functional antigen-binding fragment (Fab), the single-chain variable region fragment (scFv), or single-domain antibodies [nanobodies (Nbs)]. nABs is developed against the trimeric S-glycoprotein S1 subunit (S1-RBD and S1-NTD attachments) and S2 (membrane fusion subunit), inhibiting the virus from binding to hACE2 and disable virus-receptor interactions that usually ends with membrane fusion and entrance to the affected cell (Fig. **16**), *i.e.* viral infection [63, 64].

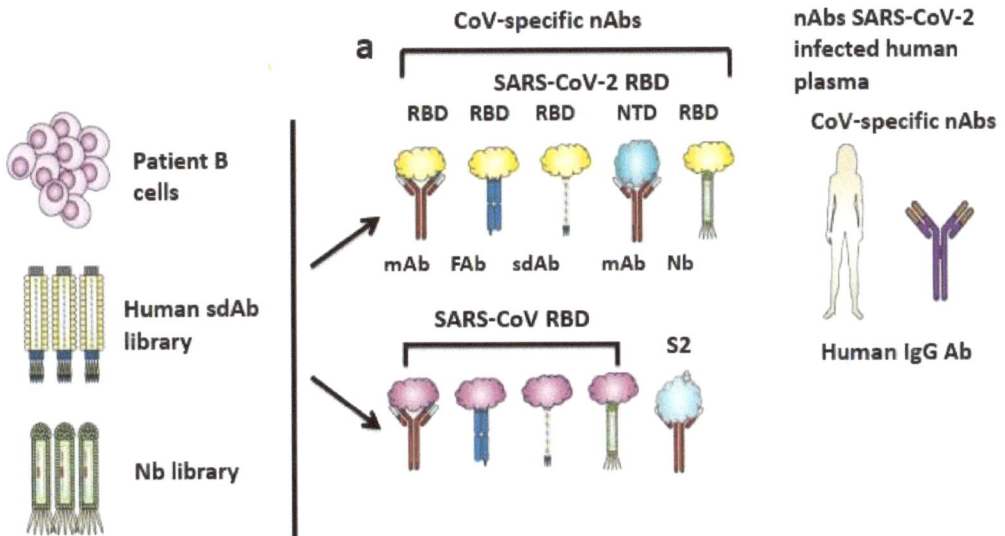

Fig. (16). Specific Neutralizing Antibodies (nAbs) against Coronaviruses.

Comprehended atomic-level structure of SARS-CoV-2 S-glycoprotein and identifying the functionally important epitopes in its RBM suggest this region as the prime candidate for structure-based design of highly effective vaccines that can trigger strong immune responses [38]. Some polyclonal antibodies from recovered COVID-19 patients have been isolated and applied to other patients with SARS-CoV-2 infection. Hitherto, no SARS-CoV-2 specific nAbs is available. Luckily, the S-glycoproteins of SARS-CoV-2 and SARS-CoV share around 77.5% amino acid sequence and are structurally very similar. So, SARS-CoV and MERS-CoV specific nAbs from the perspective of their possible cross-interactivity and/or cross-neutralizing activity against SARS-CoV-2 infection might be introduced. Very hard and extensive work is devoted to developing such mAbs and/or their functional fragments. It will be active prophylactically or therapeutically agents to prohibit or treat COVID-19. However, such agents might take years to be available for human use as they need first *in vitro* assays for neutralizing and/or cross-neutralizing activity. *In vivo* modeling is the next step, then preclinical studies are required, and finally, clinical trials are required for testing safety and efficiency.

An example of mAbs developed earlier against SARS-CoV RBD is CR3022. It could engage SARS-CoV-2 RBD with high affinity and identify an epitope on the RBD that does not superimpose with the ACE2-binding site. The crystal framework of the CR3022/SARS-CoV-2 RBD interface has been recently determined. CR3022 binds with the RBD utilizing both heavy and light chains (Fig. **17a**) along with all six-complementarity determining region (CDR) loops (Fig. **17b**). Hydrophobic interactions were shown to dominate SARS-CoV-2 recognition by CR3022 (Fig. **17d**). Among all residues in the epitope, 86% were preserved amongst SARSCoV-2 and SARS-CoV clarifying the cross-reactivity of CR3022.

Nevertheless, the non-conserved RBD epitopes caused CR3022 Fab to bind with a much higher affinity to SARS-CoV than it does to SARS-CoV-2 RBD. *In vitro* analysis showed that CR3022 could deactivate SARS-CoV but was inactive against SARS-CoV-2 even when a high concentration was applied (400 mg/ml). Such findings are in line with the low binding affinity of CR3022 to SARS-CoV-2 [65].

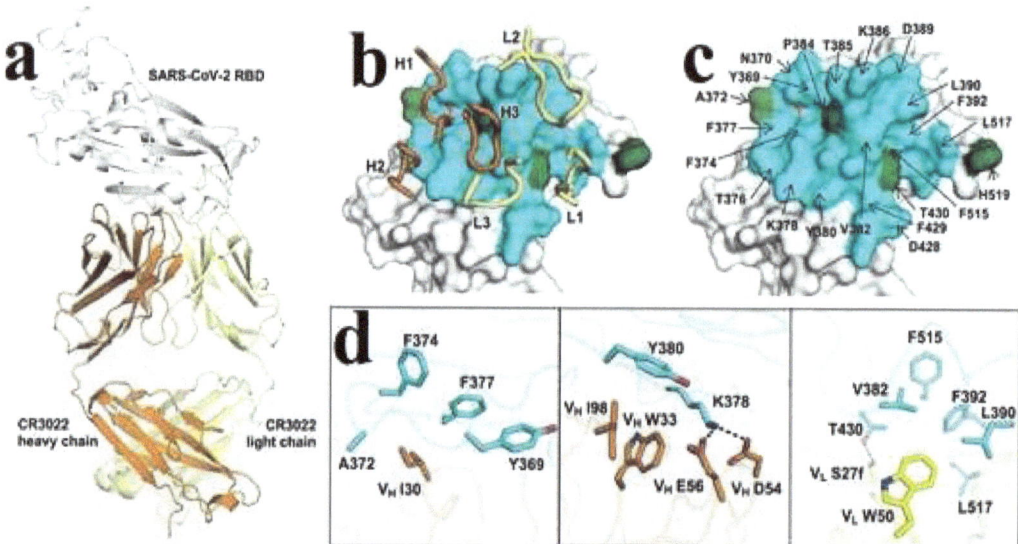

Fig. (17). Crystal structure of CR3022 in complex with SARS-CoV-2 RBD.

Still, CR3022 is among the most potential candidates, which solely or combined with other nABs to be used prophylactically or therapeutically against COVID-19 infection [66]. Likewise, the SARS-CoV nAb 47D11 cross-bind the viral S1 on a

SARS-CoV-1/SARS-CoV-2 conserved epitope away from the virus-receptor binding interface. It has consequently no influence on RBD-ACE2 interaction, avoiding the competition issues and making it feasible for Abs combinations to target non-overlapping epitopes and lowering the dose to mitigate the risk of immune escape [67]. Noteworthy, many of the most effective SARS-CoV-specific nAb (*e.g.*, m396, CR3014) acting on the SARS-CoV/ACE2 interface could not bind SARS-CoV-2 S-glycoprotein [66]. Consistently, polyclonal rabbit anti-SARS S1 antibodies T62 prevent entrance of SARS-CoV S but not SARS-CoV-2 S pseudovirions. The analysis revealed that the chief immune-epitopes for T62 antibodies are possibly locating in the area of SARS-CoV NTD. Amongst the crucial residues of SARS-CoV RBD for receptor binding and virus entering process, seven residues have changed among SARS-CoV and SARS-CoV-2 RBDs [36]. By combining a cholesterol fragment to the EK1 peptide developed earlier and directed toward the HR1 domain of the S2 subunit to inhibit infection by SARS-CoV and MERS-CoV. The compound EK1C4 was generated and found as the most potent fusion inhibitor against SARS-CoV-2 S protein-mediated membrane fusion. It is approximately 241-fold higher potency than the original EK1 peptide. It also indicate that EK1C4 might be helpful in the prevention and treat infection by presently socializing SARS-CoV-2 and other emergent SARS-CoVs [33].

The above findings imply that the modification in structures among SARS-CoV and SARS-CoV-2 has a decisive influence over the cross-interactivity of nAbs, and it is of great importance to prepare new monoclonal antibodies that can bind principally to SARS-CoV-2.

CONCLUSIONS

The trimeric S-glycoprotein of SARS-CoV-2 is responsible for binding the virus to its host cell receptor, ACE2, *via* its RBD. The high-resolution crystal structure of the RBD complexed with the PD of hACE2 exhibits that the RBD displays a softly concave surface, which frameworks the N-terminal lobe of the peptidase primarily through polar interactions. Afterward, the interface is proteolytically activated by human proteases, and the 6-HB fusion core fetches viral and hosts cell membranes into nearby juxtaposition to facilitate cell entry. Determining the detailed atomic interface between RBD/PD explained many new aspects of the novel virus in comparison with SARS-CoV and MERS-CoV: SARS-CoV-2 RBD binds as a minimum of 10-20 times more firmly than the matching RBD of SARS-CoV. Nevertheless, the whole SARS-CoV-2 S-glycoprotein has a comparable or lower affinity than the entire SARS-CoV spike due to less exposed surface for binding.

Most importantly, hidden RBD SARS-CoV-2 S-glycoprotein endows the virus with effectual cell entry while avoiding immune response. On the other hand, the cell entering the process of SARS-CoV-2 is triggered by furin-like cleavage, decreasing the need for cell proteases for entry. These aspects may promote effective cross-species infection and among human beings spreading. Finally, the detailed structure proposes methods to benefit RBD as a vital target for probable treatments and diagnosis studies. A universal vaccine is the most urgent goal at the moment. Luckily, the availability of conserved epitopes allowed many antibodies developed originally to inhibit SARS-CoV to show promising results against the novel virus.

CONSENT FOR PUBLICATION

Not Applicable.

CONFLICT OF INTEREST

The author confirms that this chapter contents have no conflict of interest.

ACKNOWLEDGEMENT

Declared none.

REFERENCES

[1]   World Health Organization. Prioritizing diseases for research and development in emergency contexts https://www.who.int/activities/prioritizing-diseases-for-research-anddevelopment-in-eme-gency-contexts

[2]   Zhu N, Zhang D, Wang W, *et al.* China novel coronavirus investigating and research team. A Novel Coronavirus from Patients with Pneumonia in China, 2019. N Engl J Med 2020; 382(8): 727-33. [http://dx.doi.org/10.1056/NEJMoa2001017] [PMID: 31978945]

[3]   Gorbalenya AE, Baker SC, Baric RS, *et al.* Coronaviridae Study Group of the International Committee on Taxonomy of Viruses. The species Severe acute respiratory syndrome-related coronavirus: classifying 2019-nCoV and naming it SARS-CoV-2. Nat Microbiol 2020; 5(4): 536-44. [http://dx.doi.org/10.1038/s41564-020-0695-z] [PMID: 32123347]

[4]   Jiang S, Du L, Shi Z. An emerging coronavirus causing pneumonia outbreak in Wuhan, China: calling for developing therapeutic and prophylactic strategies. Emerg Microbes Infect 2020; 9(1): 275-7. [http://dx.doi.org/10.1080/22221751.2020.1723441] [PMID: 32005086]

[5]   Xiong JS, Branigan D, Li M. Deciphering the MSG controversy. Int J Clin Exp Med 2009; 2(4): 329-36. [PMID: 20057976]

[6]   Jaimes JA, André NM, Chappie JS, Millet JK, Whittaker GR. Phylogenetic analysis and structural modeling of SARS-CoV-2 spike protein reveals an evolutionary distinct and proteolytically sensitive activation loop. J Mol Biol 2020; 432(10): 3309-25. [http://dx.doi.org/10.1016/j.jmb.2020.04.009] [PMID: 32320687]

[7]   Zhu S, Gouaux E. Structure and symmetry inform gating principles of ionotropic glutamate receptors. Neuropharmacology 2017; 112(Pt A): 11-5.

[http://dx.doi.org/10.1016/j.neuropharm.2016.08.034] [PMID: 27663701]

[8]	Huang C, Wang Y, Li X, *et al.* Clinical features of patients infected with 2019 novel coronavirus in Wuhan, China. Lancet 2020; 395(10223): 497-506.
[http://dx.doi.org/10.1016/S0140-6736(20)30183-5] [PMID: 31986264]

[9]	Zhang H, Penninger JM, Li Y, Zhong N, Slutsky AS. Angiotensin-converting enzyme 2 (ACE2) as a SARS-CoV-2 receptor: molecular mechanisms and potential therapeutic target. Intensive Care Med 2020; 46(4): 586-90.
[http://dx.doi.org/10.1007/s00134-020-05985-9] [PMID: 32125455]

[10]	Guo Y-R, Cao Q-D, Hong Z-S, *et al.* The origin, transmission and clinical therapies on coronavirus disease 2019 (COVID-19) outbreak - an update on the status. Mil Med Res 2020; 7(1): 11.
[http://dx.doi.org/10.1186/s40779-020-00240-0] [PMID: 32169119]

[11]	Shereen MA, Khan S, Kazmi A, Bashir N, Siddique R. COVID-19 infection: Origin, transmission, and characteristics of human coronaviruses. J Adv Res 2020; 24: 91-8.
[http://dx.doi.org/10.1016/j.jare.2020.03.005] [PMID: 32257431]

[12]	Li G, De Clercq E. Nature Publishing Group. 2020.

[13]	Kang S, Yang M, Hong Z, *et al.* Crystal structure of SARS-CoV-2 nucleocapsid protein RNA binding domain reveals potential unique drug targeting sites. Acta Pharm Sin B 2020; 10(7): 1228-38.
[http://dx.doi.org/10.1016/j.apsb.2020.04.009] [PMID: 32363136]

[14]	Belouzard S, Millet JK, Licitra BN, Whittaker GR. Mechanisms of coronavirus cell entry mediated by the viral spike protein. Viruses 2012; 4(6): 1011-33.
[http://dx.doi.org/10.3390/v4061011] [PMID: 22816037]

[15]	Chen SH, Young MT, Gounley J, Stanley C, Bhowmik D. Distinct structural flexibility within SARS-CoV-2 spike protein reveals potential therapeutic targets bioRxiv 2020.2020.2004.2017.047548
[http://dx.doi.org/10.1101/2020.04.17.047548]

[16]	Liu Z, Xiao X, Wei X, *et al.* Composition and divergence of coronavirus spike proteins and host ACE2 receptors predict potential intermediate hosts of SARS-CoV-2. J Med Virol 2020; 92(6): 595-601.
[http://dx.doi.org/10.1002/jmv.25726] [PMID: 32100877]

[17]	Wang Q, Zhang Y, Wu L, *et al.* Structural and functional basis of SARS-CoV-2 entry by using human ACE2. Cell 2020; 181(4): 894-904.e9.
[http://dx.doi.org/10.1016/j.cell.2020.03.045] [PMID: 32275855]

[18]	Lan J, Ge J, Yu J, *et al.* Structure of the SARS-CoV-2 spike receptor-binding domain bound to the ACE2 receptor. Nature 2020; 581(7807): 215-20.
[http://dx.doi.org/10.1038/s41586-020-2180-5] [PMID: 32225176]

[19]	Melin AD, Janiak MC, Marrone F, Arora PS, Higham JP. Comparative ACE2 variation and primate COVID-19 risk. bioRxiv 2020.2020.2004.2009.034967

[20]	Lu G, Wang Q, Gao GF. Bat-to-human: spike features determining 'host jump' of coronaviruses SARS-CoV, MERS-CoV, and beyond. Trends Microbiol 2015; 23(8): 468-78.
[http://dx.doi.org/10.1016/j.tim.2015.06.003] [PMID: 26206723]

[21]	Li Z, Tomlinson AC, Wong AH, *et al.* The human coronavirus HCoV-229E S-protein structure and receptor binding. eLife 2019; 8e51230
[http://dx.doi.org/10.7554/eLife.51230] [PMID: 31650956]

[22]	Lu G, Hu Y, Wang Q, *et al.* Molecular basis of binding between novel human coronavirus MERS-CoV and its receptor CD26. Nature 2013; 500(7461): 227-31.
[http://dx.doi.org/10.1038/nature12328] [PMID: 23831647]

[23]	Zhou P, Yang X-L, Wang X-G, *et al.* A pneumonia outbreak associated with a new coronavirus of probable bat origin. Nature 2020; 579(7798): 270-3.

[http://dx.doi.org/10.1038/s41586-020-2012-7] [PMID: 32015507]

[24]   Babak N, Avrin G, Kasra G, Negin N. The Effect of ACE2 Inhibitor MLN-4760 on the Interaction of SARS-CoV-2 Spike Protein with Human ACE2: A Molecular Dynamics Study 2020.

[25]   Donoghue M, Hsieh F, Baronas E, *et al.* A novel angiotensin-converting enzyme-related carboxypeptidase (ACE2) converts angiotensin I to angiotensin 1-9. Circ Res 2000; 87(5): E1-9.
[http://dx.doi.org/10.1161/01.RES.87.5.e1] [PMID: 10969042]

[26]   Hamming I, Cooper ME, Haagmans BL, *et al.* The emerging role of ACE2 in physiology and disease. J Pathol 2007; 212(1): 1-11.
[http://dx.doi.org/10.1002/path.2162] [PMID: 17464936]

[27]   Li F. Receptor recognition and cross-species infections of SARS coronavirus. Antiviral Res 2013; 100(1): 246-54.
[http://dx.doi.org/10.1016/j.antiviral.2013.08.014] [PMID: 23994189]

[28]   Towler P, Staker B, Prasad SG, *et al.* ACE2 X-ray structures reveal a large hinge-bending motion important for inhibitor binding and catalysis. J Biol Chem 2004; 279(17): 17996-8007.
[http://dx.doi.org/10.1074/jbc.M311191200] [PMID: 14754895]

[29]   Li F. Structure, Function, and Evolution of Coronavirus Spike Proteins. Annu Rev Virol 2016; 3(1): 237-61.
[http://dx.doi.org/10.1146/annurev-virology-110615-042301] [PMID: 27578435]

[30]   Wrapp D, Wang N, Corbett KS, *et al.* Cryo-EM structure of the 2019-nCoV spike in the prefusion conformation. Science 2020; 367(6483): 1260-3.
[http://dx.doi.org/10.1126/science.abb2507] [PMID: 32075877]

[31]   Walls AC, Park Y-J, Tortorici MA, Wall A, McGuire AT, Veesler D. Structure, function, and antigenicity of the SARS-CoV-2 spike glycoprotein. Cell 2020; 181(2): 281-292.e6.
[http://dx.doi.org/10.1016/j.cell.2020.02.058] [PMID: 32155444]

[32]   Bertram S, Glowacka I, Müller MA, *et al.* Cleavage and activation of the severe acute respiratory syndrome coronavirus spike protein by human airway trypsin-like protease. J Virol 2011; 85(24): 13363-72.
[http://dx.doi.org/10.1128/JVI.05300-11] [PMID: 21994442]

[33]   Xia S, Liu M, Wang C, *et al.* Inhibition of SARS-CoV-2 (previously 2019-nCoV) infection by a highly potent pan-coronavirus fusion inhibitor targeting its spike protein that harbors a high capacity to mediate membrane fusion. Cell Res 2020; 30(4): 343-55.
[http://dx.doi.org/10.1038/s41422-020-0305-x] [PMID: 32231345]

[34]   Gui M, Song W, Zhou H, *et al.* Cryo-electron microscopy structures of the SARS-CoV spike glycoprotein reveal a prerequisite conformational state for receptor binding. Cell Res 2017; 27(1): 119-29.
[http://dx.doi.org/10.1038/cr.2016.152] [PMID: 28008928]

[35]   Pallesen J, Wang N, Corbett KS, *et al.* Immunogenicity and structures of a rationally designed prefusion MERS-CoV spike antigen. Proc Natl Acad Sci USA 2017; 114(35): E7348-57.
[http://dx.doi.org/10.1073/pnas.1707304114] [PMID: 28807998]

[36]   Ou X, Liu Y, Lei X, *et al.* Characterization of spike glycoprotein of SARS-CoV-2 on virus entry and its immune cross-reactivity with SARS-CoV. Nat Commun 2020; 11(1): 1620.
[http://dx.doi.org/10.1038/s41467-020-15562-9] [PMID: 32221306]

[37]   Lan J, Ge J, Yu J, *et al.* Crystal structure of the 2019-nCoV spike receptor-binding domain bound with the ACE2 receptor. bioRxiv 2020.
[http://dx.doi.org/10.1101/2020.02.19.956235]

[38]   Yan R, Zhang Y, Li Y, Xia L, Guo Y, Zhou Q. Structural basis for the recognition of SARS-CoV-2 by full-length human ACE2. Science 2020; 367(6485): 1444-8.
[http://dx.doi.org/10.1126/science.abb2762] [PMID: 32132184]

[39]   Chan JF-W, Yuan S, Kok K-H, *et al.* A familial cluster of pneumonia associated with the 2019 novel coronavirus indicating person-to-person transmission: a study of a family cluster. Lancet 2020; 395(10223): 514-23.
[http://dx.doi.org/10.1016/S0140-6736(20)30154-9] [PMID: 31986261]

[40]   Petrosillo N, Viceconte G, Ergonul O, Ippolito G, Petersen E. COVID-19, SARS and MERS: are they closely related? Clin Microbiol Infect 2020; 26(6): 729-34.
[http://dx.doi.org/10.1016/j.cmi.2020.03.026] [PMID: 32234451]

[41]   Wu A, Peng Y, Huang B, *et al.* Genome composition and divergence of the novel coronavirus (2019-nCoV) originating in china. Cell Host Microbe 2020; 27(3): 325-8.
[http://dx.doi.org/10.1016/j.chom.2020.02.001] [PMID: 32035028]

[42]   Sun C, Chen L, Yang J, *et al.* SARS-CoV-2 and SARS-CoV Spike-RBD Structure and Receptor Binding Comparison and Potential Implications on Neutralizing Antibody and Vaccine Development. bioRxiv 2020.
[http://dx.doi.org/10.1101/2020.02.16.951723]

[43]   Yuan Y, Cao D, Zhang Y, *et al.* Cryo-EM structures of MERS-CoV and SARS-CoV spike glycoproteins reveal the dynamic receptor binding domains. Nat Commun 2017; 8(1): 15092.
[http://dx.doi.org/10.1038/ncomms15092] [PMID: 28393837]

[44]   Shang J, Wan Y, Luo C, *et al.* Cell entry mechanisms of SARS-CoV-2. Proc Natl Acad Sci USA 2020; 117(21): 11727-34.
[http://dx.doi.org/10.1073/pnas.2003138117] [PMID: 32376634]

[45]   Elfiky AA. Ribavirin, Remdesivir, Sofosbuvir, Galidesivir, and Tenofovir against SARS-CoV-2 RNA dependent RNA polymerase (RdRp): A molecular docking study. Life Sci 2020; 253117592
[http://dx.doi.org/10.1016/j.lfs.2020.117592] [PMID: 32222463]

[46]   Tang N, Bai H, Chen X, Gong J, Li D, Sun Z. Anticoagulant treatment is associated with decreased mortality in severe coronavirus disease 2019 patients with coagulopathy. J Thromb Haemost 2020; 18(5): 1094-9.
[http://dx.doi.org/10.1111/jth.14817] [PMID: 32220112]

[47]   Han H, Yang L, Liu R, *et al.* Prominent changes in blood coagulation of patients with SARS-CoV-2 infection. Clin Chem Lab Med 2020; 58(7): 1116-20. [CCLM].
[http://dx.doi.org/10.1515/cclm-2020-0188] [PMID: 32172226]

[48]   Tang N, Li D, Wang X, Sun Z. Abnormal coagulation parameters are associated with poor prognosis in patients with novel coronavirus pneumonia. J Thromb Haemost 2020; 18(4): 844-7.
[http://dx.doi.org/10.1111/jth.14768] [PMID: 32073213]

[49]   Mehta P, McAuley DF, Brown M, Sanchez E, Tattersall RS, Manson JJ. HLH Across Speciality Collaboration, UK. COVID-19: consider cytokine storm syndromes and immunosuppression. Lancet 2020; 395(10229): 1033-4.
[http://dx.doi.org/10.1016/S0140-6736(20)30628-0] [PMID: 32192578]

[50]   Clerkin KJ, Fried JA, Raikhelkar J, *et al.* COVID-19 and Cardiovascular Disease. Circulation 2020; 141(20): 1648-55.
[http://dx.doi.org/10.1161/CIRCULATIONAHA.120.046941] [PMID: 32200663]

[51]   Sodhi M, Etminan M. Safety of Ibuprofen in Patients With COVID-19: Causal or Confounded? Chest 2020; 158(1): 55-6.
[http://dx.doi.org/10.1016/j.chest.2020.03.040] [PMID: 32243944]

[52]   Mercurio I, Tragni V, Busco F, De Grassi A, Pierri CL. Protein structure analysis of the interactions between SARS-CoV-2 spike protein and the human ACE2 receptor: from conformational changes to novel neutralizing antibodies. bioRxiv 2020.
[http://dx.doi.org/10.1101/2020.04.17.046185]

[53]   Du L, He Y, Zhou Y, Liu S, Zheng BJ, Jiang S. The spike protein of SARS-CoV--a target for vaccine

and therapeutic development. Nat Rev Microbiol 2009; 7(3): 226-36.
[http://dx.doi.org/10.1038/nrmicro2090] [PMID: 19198616]

[54]   Kawase M, Shirato K, van der Hoek L, Taguchi F, Matsuyama S. Simultaneous treatment of human bronchial epithelial cells with serine and cysteine protease inhibitors prevents severe acute respiratory syndrome coronavirus entry. J Virol 2012; 86(12): 6537-45.
[http://dx.doi.org/10.1128/JVI.00094-12] [PMID: 22496216]

[55]   Zhou Y, Vedantham P, Lu K, *et al.* Protease inhibitors targeting coronavirus and filovirus entry. Antiviral Res 2015; 116: 76-84.
[http://dx.doi.org/10.1016/j.antiviral.2015.01.011] [PMID: 25666761]

[56]   Ragia G, Manolopoulos VG. Inhibition of SARS-CoV-2 entry through the ACE2/TMPRSS2 pathway: a promising approach for uncovering early COVID-19 drug therapies. Eur J Clin Pharmacol 2020; 76(12): 1623-30.
[http://dx.doi.org/10.1007/s00228-020-02963-4] [PMID: 32696234]

[57]   Zhou Y, Vedantham P, Lu K, *et al.* Protease inhibitors targeting coronavirus and filovirus entry. Antiviral Res 2015; 116: 76-84.
[http://dx.doi.org/10.1016/j.antiviral.2015.01.011] [PMID: 25666761]

[58]   Hoffmann M, Kleine-Weber H, Schroeder S, *et al.* SARS-CoV-2 Cell Entry Depends on ACE2 and TMPRSS2 and Is Blocked by a Clinically Proven Protease Inhibitor. Cell 2020; 181(2): 271-280.e8.
[http://dx.doi.org/10.1016/j.cell.2020.02.052] [PMID: 32142651]

[59]   Yamamoto M, Matsuyama S, Li X, *et al.* Identification of Nafamostat as a Potent Inhibitor of Middle East Respiratory Syndrome Coronavirus S Protein-Mediated Membrane Fusion Using the Split-Protein-Based Cell-Cell Fusion Assay. Antimicrob Agents Chemother 2016; 60(11): 6532-9.
[http://dx.doi.org/10.1128/AAC.01043-16] [PMID: 27550352]

[60]   Hoffmann M, Schroeder S, Kleine-Weber H, Müller MA, Drosten C, Pöhlmann S. Nafamostat mesylate blocks activation of SARS-CoV-2: New treatment option for COVID-19. Antimicrob Agents Chemother 2020; 64(6)e00754-20
[http://dx.doi.org/10.1128/AAC.00754-20] [PMID: 32312781]

[61]   Baden LR, Rubin EJ. Covid-19 - The Search for Effective Therapy. N Engl J Med 2020; 382(19): 1851-2.
[http://dx.doi.org/10.1056/NEJMe2005477] [PMID: 32187463]

[62]   Luan B, Huynh T, Cheng X, Lan G, Wang H-R. Targeting Proteases for Treating COVID-19. J Proteome Res 2020; 19(11): 4316-26.
[http://dx.doi.org/10.1021/acs.jproteome.0c00430] [PMID: 33090793]

[63]   Jiang S, Hillyer C, Du L. Neutralizing Antibodies against SARS-CoV-2 and Other Human Coronaviruses. Trends Immunol 2020; 41(5): 355-9.
[http://dx.doi.org/10.1016/j.it.2020.03.007] [PMID: 32249063]

[64]   Wang C, Li W, Drabek D, *et al.* A human monoclonal antibody blocking SARS-CoV-2 infection. Nat Commun 2020; 11(1): 2251.
[http://dx.doi.org/10.1038/s41467-020-16256-y] [PMID: 32366817]

[65]   Yuan M, Wu NC, Zhu X, *et al.* A highly conserved cryptic epitope in the receptor binding domains of SARS-CoV-2 and SARS-CoV. Science 2020; 368(6491): 630-3.
[http://dx.doi.org/10.1126/science.abb7269] [PMID: 32245784]

[66]   Tian X, Li C, Huang A, *et al.* Potent binding of 2019 novel coronavirus spike protein by a SARS coronavirus-specific human monoclonal antibody. Emerg Microbes Infect 2020; 9(1): 382-5.
[http://dx.doi.org/10.1080/22221751.2020.1729069] [PMID: 32065055]

[67]   Wang C, Li W, Drabek D, *et al.* A human monoclonal antibody blocking SARS-CoV-2 infection. Nat Commun 2020; 11(1): 2251.
[http://dx.doi.org/10.1038/s41467-020-16256-y] [PMID: 32366817]

CHAPTER 8

Structural Elucidation of SARS-CoV-2 Accessory Proteins

Tahir Shah[1,*] and **Kamal Niaz**[2]

¹ Department of Animal Science, Faculty of Agriculture, Ege University, İzmir, Turkey

² Department of Pharmacology & Toxicology, Faculty of Bio-Sciences, Cholistan University of Veterinary and Animal Sciences, Bahawalpur-63100, Pakistan

Abstract: The coronaviruses (CoVs) are a huge family of positive-sense RNA viruses with a single-strand. These CoVs consist of 38% G+C content and around 29,900 nucleotides, which encodes about 9,860 amino acids. It includes open reading frames yielding two polyproteins which are cleaved into 16 nonstructural proteins (nsps) proteolytically. These nsps play pivotal roles inside the lifestyles cycle of CoVs. To deal with the present-day outbreak, using wide-spectrum inhibiting drugs against CoVs is an appealing tactic. Still, for this reason, the knowledge of specific target places of nsps within the CoVs genus is necessary. The position of each nsp is well defined. The main protease (Mpro) forms replicase polyprotein complex. The papain-like protein (PLpro) also suppresses type 1 interferon signaling, thus risking the host's immunity. The NSP-3 takes part in the processing of polyprotein as a protease. Also, the NSP-8 and NSP-9 attach to the *cis*-acting parts of RNA of the virus. NSP-10 is a vital cofactor forming compounds with NSP-14 and 16. The NSP-12 encodes RNA-dependent RNA polymerase (RdRp). At the same time, the catalyzing and unwinding of duplex oligonucleotides into single strands is done by NSP-13 helicase. The NSP-14 of CoVs is important for viral replication and transcription, and NSP-16 is activated when the bond with NSP-10 preventing host recognition and decreasing the immune response. The purpose of this chapter is to elucidate the accessory proteins of SARS-CoV-2 structurally. Also explains the inflammatory cytokines produced due to SARS-CoV-2, residues involved in the interaction between viral spike and ACE2, the structure of receptor-binding domain (RBD) of ACE2 in SARS-CoV-2, and possible potential compounds that have been studied and found effective against SARS-CoV-2.

Keywords: Coronaviruses, Mpro, Nonstructural proteins, PLpro, RNA-dependent RNA polymerase.

** **Corresponding author Tahir Shah:** Department of Animal Science, Faculty of Agriculture, Ege University, İzmir, Turkey, E-mail:t.shah@aup.edu.pk*

Kamal Niaz & Muhammad Farrukh Nisar (Eds.)

INTRODUCTION

Coronaviruses (CoVs) are a huge family of positive-sense RNA viruses that are single-stranded and having 5′-cap and 3′poly-A tail belonging to the family of coronaviridae in the order Nidovirales [1, 2]. CoVs consist of 38% G+C content and around 29,900 nucleotides, which encodes about 9,860 amino acids with a 26-31 kb lengthy RNA genome. The replicase gene of CoVs includes open reading frames (ORFs) 1a and 1b. Two polyproteins are yield from these two ORFs, *i.e.*, pp1a and pp1ab. It is sliced into 16 nsps (NSP 1-16) that bring together to shape the replication-transcription complex (RTC) or has a vital role inside the lifestyles cycle of CoVs [2]. The constituents of the RTC encompass enzymes that modify mRNA and genomic RNA synthesis, proofreading, and mRNA maturation. Two of those enzymes are crucial for capping viral mRNAs, a tactic employed with the aid of more than one RNA viruses to avoid immune detection through toll-like receptors 7 (TLR7) and 8 (TLR8) [3, 4].

Spike (S), membrane (M), envelope (E), and nucleocapsid (N) proteins are 4 vital structural proteins encoded by the ORFs near the 3′-end of the genome. In CoVs replication, the nonstructural proteins are well known to play an important role. However, for establishing the virion assemblies to cause CoV infection, the structural proteins play an important role. In addition, the CoV genome encodes the accessory proteins such as HE protein [2]. Comparing SARS-CoV-2 and already existing SARS concludes that nucleotide identification was ~80% identical [5].

An appealing strategy to deal with the current outbreak of SARS-CoV-2 is important to develop wide-spectrum inhibiting drugs against CoVs associated pandemic. Still, for this reason, the knowing and identification of specific target places of nsps within CoVs genus are necessary [6, 7]. The target regions among structural proteins (S, E, M, HE, and N proteins) of CoVs have been reported with variable versions [8 - 10] therefore, adding extra complexity towards the identity of SARS-CoV-2 inhibitors. The nonstructural proteins constitute enormously conserved regions amongst CoVs that can be targeted [11]. This chapter describes the structural detail of nsps and its binding sites, inflammatory cytokines produced due to SARS-CoV-2, residues involved in the interaction between viral spike and ACE2, the structure of receptor-binding domain (RBD) of ACE2 in SARS-CoV-2, and possible potential compounds that have been studied and found effective against SARS-CoV-2.

Structural Interpretation of Vital Proteins

It is necessary to know its structural composition and what happens to the shape of the virus ewhile it enters the host cell to understand the pathogenesis of SARS-

CoV-2. The viral nucleocapsid of the virus is released to the cytoplasm once it manages to enter the host cell. Viruses exploit the host's replication machinery due to the nature of their genome. mRNA of the viruses is identical to the single-stranded RNA. There is an exact amount of nucleotide collection in a positive sense strand as in mRNA, responsible for encoding a functional protein. The genomic RNA carries out the services of being a template, and the encoding of polyproteins pp1a and pp1ab are performed at the start. These polyproteins are further cleaved utilizing virally produced chymotrypsin-like protease (3CLpro) or Mpro and one or papain-like protease to shape 16 nsps. These 16 nsps participate in RNA synthesis, genome replication, and subgenomic RNA [12]. The viral RNA synthesis occurs by a number of these nsps, the N protein, the host proteins, and the endoplasmic reticulum (ER) [13]. The positions of the nsps are known, *e.g.,* NSP-12 encodes the RdRp [14], the polyprotein processing as a protease is done with the help of NSP-3, the viral RNA binding to cis-acting elements is due to NSP-8 and NSP-9 [15, 16].

Although the viral replicas are used to catalyze the replication and transcription process of the genome, while some times the host machinery is involved in doing it. A complementary negative-sense RNA molecule is used as an intermediate to replicate the full-length gRNA. At the same time, structural and accessory proteins are produced by the smaller RNA molecules (subgenomic RNA). Mature virions are secreted while the new virions are formed in the endoplasmic reticulum [12]. It is obvious that in genome replication and virus formation nsps play a very important role. Viable alterations in the genome structure of SARS-CoV-2 were lately observed by the analysis of ORF1ab because of particular strain on the virus. Specifically, alterations were found in the role of NSP-2 protein at position 321 and NSP-3 protein at positions 192 and 543 in the recent analysis. The differences between SARS-CoV-2 and SARS-CoV resulted in the said alterations [17, 18].

To clearly understand the viral activity in the human body, we need to know that in the eukaryotic cells, RNA triphosphatase (TPase) initiates the mRNA capping. It results in the removal of γ-phosphate from the 5'-end of the nascent mRNA transcript, which generates a diphosphate 5'-ppN end. Hydrolysis of pyrophosphate (PPi) is catalyzed by RNA guanylyltransferase (GTase), creating a GMP from a guanidine triphosphate (GTP) molecule. Before forming the cap core structure, referred to as GpppN, the diphosphate 5'-ppN transcript end receives the α-phosphate of guanidine monophosphate (GMP). After the N7-methylation by guanine-N7-methyltransferase (N7-MTase) of the guanylate cap to form the Cap-0, the GpppN is formed. Further, Cap-1 and Cap-2 (sometimes) are generated when the methylation at the ribose 2'-O position. It occurs when first nucleotide of the RNA is catalyzed with the help of ribose 2'-O-methyltransferases (2'--

-MTase) [19]. S-adenosyl-L-methionine (SAM) is used as a methyl group donor by both the N7-MTase and 2'-O-MTase [19, 20].

The generation of the Cap-0 is an indication of CoV mRNA maturation, the viral nonstructural protein 14 (NSP-14) N7-MTase activity, and guanylation of the 5'-end of the nascent mRNA takes place in the TPases and GTase of the host cell [19]. In addition to the N7-MTase domain of NSP-14, an exonuclease domain makes NSP-14 a bifunctional enzyme [21]. The small viral protein modulates the activity of CoVs by binding to NSP-10. There is no effect on the N7-MTase activity of the virus, but stimulation of its exonuclease activity occurs [20]. The viral NSP-16 modifies the CoV mRNAs to have a Cap-1. NSP-16 is an m7GpppA-specific, SAM-dependent, 2'-O-MTase [22, 23], and its activation is done by NSP-10 binding to NSP-16 [24]. NSP-10 can self-dimerize as it is a stable protein [25] forming dodecamers with NSP-11 [26], but it has the function to modulate NSP-14 and NSP-16 activity [27]. The fold of NSP-10 is unique, and no specific enzymatic activity has been observed yet. NSP-10 also recognized as a zinc-binding protein, binds nonspecifically to RNA and can stabilize the SAM binding pocket in NSP-16, creating a stable complex [24]. Prevention of host recognition and decreasing immune response takes place by NSP-10- NSP-1--mediated 2'-O-methylation of CoV RNA, but the viral RNA is translated [20, 22, 28].

Main protease (Mpro)

On January 7, 2020, Chinese scientists extracted SARS-CoV-2 and sequenced the genome of SARS-CoV- 2 [29]. Liu *et al.* [30], a Chinese scientist, demonstrated the crystallized form of COVID-19 Mpro. Liu *et al.* [30] suggested that Mpro is a potential drug target protein for the inhibition of SARS-CoV-2 replication. The Mpro of SARS-CoV-2 is a 67.6 kDa homodimeric cysteine10 protease. It has about 97% sequence identity with the corresponding Mpro protease of the SARS–CoV virus responsible for the severe acute respiratory syndrome CoV (SARS) pandemic. Not surprisingly, the recent 1.75 Å X-ray crystal structure of SARS–CoV-2 Mpro protease [31, 32] demonstrates its structure is very similar to this SARS – CoV Mpro protease [33, 34]. Both of these Mpro proteases contain three similar domains. Domains I and II adopt a double β - barrel fold, with the substrate-binding site located in a shallow cleft between two anti-parallel β-barrels of Domain I and II. These Mpro proteases also have an additional C terminal helical - bundle domain, Domain III, which stabilizes their active homodimer forms. The Mpro is an essential protein required for the proteolytic maturation of the virus [35]. It is also named chymotrypsin-like protease (3CLpro). Mpro cleaves most of the sites in the polyproteins, and the products are nsps which assemble into the RTC. Thus, targeting Mpro can provide effective treatment against SARS-CoV-2 by inhibiting the viral polypeptide cleavage [35].

Proteins that are considered essential Mpro along with PLpro where these proteins also form a part of the replicase polyprotein complex in replication of SARS-CoV-2. To hamper the replication of SARS-CoV-2, the action of Mpro should be blocked because it operates at least 11 active sites of the polyprotein 1ab [36].

Papain-like protease (PLpro)

The N-terminus of the replicase polyprotein of SARS-CoV-2 is cleaved by PLpro. It works with Mpro to cleave the polyproteins into nsps and thus produce NSP- 1-2-3. Due to this action, it is considered to be an important aspect of viral replication. Type 1 interferon signaling is also considered to be suppressed by this protein which plays a significant role in reducing the host immunity [37]. The targeting of this protein is necessary for all the above-discussed reasons to inhibit viral replication [36].

Nonstructural protein 3 (NSP-3)

NSP-3 is one of the nsps containingwell-preserved macro domains, and the polypeptide 1a of SARS-CoV-2 makes this NSP-3 [38]. The ADP ribose phosphatase macro domains of NSP-3 are understood to take part in different pathways. Such as modification of post-translational protein and metabolism of ADP-ribose. The phosphatase activity of the SARS NSP-3 domain is confirmed by readily removing the 1" phosphate group from Appr-1"-p *in vitro* assays [36, 39].

Nonstructural protein 9 (NSP-9)

It is evident from above that NSP-9 is an essential component of the RNA-polymerase complex [40]. NSP-9 interacts with NSP-8 and is also known to take place in the binding of RNA strands and RNA-Polymerase. The viral replication can be stopped by inhibiting the action of NSP-9, which will prevent the binding of RNA-polymerase to the RNA strand.

Nonstructural protein 10 (NSP-10)

NSP-10 is a vital cofactor of SARS-CoVs and forms a compound with NSP-14 and 16. The structure of SARS-CoV-2 NSP-10 contains residues 19-133 (residues 4272-4392 of pp1a). It includes a positively charged and hydrophobic surface that collaborates with a hydrophobic pocket and a negatively charged surface from NSP-16, which adds to the equilibrium of the SAM binding site. The structure of NSP-10 of SARS-CoV-2 is comprised of a central anti-parallel couple of β-strands enclosed on one side by a crossover big loop. The other side is a helical domain with loops that form two zinc slices. These structures are engaged in the non-specific binding of RNA in former CoVs [19, 41]. The Zn-binding site 1 is organized by the residues C74, C77, H83, and C90. The Zn-binding site 2 is organized by C117, C120, C128, and C130.

Nonstructural protein 12 (NSP-12)

In the replication and transcription of the viral genome, NSP-1 plays an important role. NSP-12 bounds to NSP-7 and NSP-8, which are its essential cofactors. The structure of RdRp has two small-molecule docking sites based on RdRp of the SARS CoV virus. One structure is RNA from its homolog protein (3H5Y), while the other has no RNA [42].

Nonstructural protein 13 (NSP-13) helicase

NSP-13 helicase catalyzes the unwinding of duplex oligonucleotides into single strands in an NTP-dependent manner. In all CoV species, NSP-13 has a conserved sequence 'that's why it is an ideal target for developing antiviral drugs. The structure of helicase in SARS-CoVs has two sites for small molecule docking. The ADP binding site and the nucleic acid binding site [42].

Nonstructural protein 14 (NSP-14)

For viral replication and transcription of CoVs, NSP-14 is a critical component. The prevention of lethal mutagenesis is carried out by the N-terminal exoribonuclease (ExoN) domain. For mRNA capping, the C-terminal domain functions as a guanine-N7 methyltransferase (N7-MTase). The structure of NSP-14 in SARS-CoV had two sites for small molecule docking known as an active site of ExoN and N7-MTase.

Nonstructural protein 16 (NSP-16)

NSP-16 is an S-adenosylmethionine (SAM) dependent nucleoside-2'-O methyltransferase. It is only active with the binding of NSP-10. Prevention of host recognition and decreasing immune response occurs by NSP-10- NSP-1--mediated 2'-O-methylation of CoV RNA, but the viral RNA is translated [20, 22]. The NSP-16 structure is composed of 298 residues (orf1ab residues 6799-7096). The Serine-Asparagine-Alanine residues are present at the N-terminus of NSP-16 extracted from the tobacco etch virus (TEV) protease cleavage site. The NSP-16 structure constitutes the 2'-O-MTase catalytic core, which has eleven α-helices, seven β-strands, and loops in the Rossmann-like β-sheet fold. The β-sheet of the SARS-CoV-2 NSP-16 fold is arranged as a canonical 3-2-1-4-5-7-6 way, β7 being the long anti-parallel strand. The loops and α-helices sandwich this β-sheet. In the Rossmann-like fold, the β1 and β2 strands bind to the catalytic core to one molecule of SAM. By the loops 71-79, 100-108, and 130-148, the SAM binding pocket is formed, which is negatively charged. Residues Lys-46, Asp-130, Lys-170, and Glu-203, including the canonical SAM MTase motif, are near to the SAM methyl group that is catalytically transported to the 2-O sugar [19, 20, 23, 43]

Heptad repeat 1 (HR1) and Heptad repeat 2 (HR2)

The entrance of SARS-CoV-2 into the host cell is still completely unknown. Similar to SARS-CoV, on the viral membrane, the spike protein (S protein) of SARS-CoV-2 comprises of S1 and S2 subunits. The S1 subunit contains the RBD to bind to the cellular receptor of the host. The presence of a cell surface protein known as Furin has the function to slice S protein into S1 and S2 and also helps to increase the capacity of viral combination to the host cell membrane [44]. On the other hand, fusion peptide (FP), HR1, HR2, transmembrane domain (TM), and cytoplasmic domain fusion (CP) are contained in the S2 subunit, which is responsible for intervening viral merging and entrance. The resemblance of the S2 subunit of SARS-CoV-2 to the two bats SARS-Like CoV (SL-CoV ZXC21 and ZC45) and the human SARS-Like CoV is 99% and is highly conserved.

With the infection of CoV, the target cell membrane is injected by FP of the S2 subunit. After injection of FP to form a 6-helix bundle, the exposure of HR1 and HR2 domain takes place, taking the cellular and viral lipid bilayers into proximity and the membrane fusion procedure begins. There are three different conditions of the S protein when the membrane fusion procedure takes place: a pre-fusion native state, a pre-hairpin intermediate state, and a stable post-fusion hairpin state. The S protein diminishes the pre-fusion native state before binding with the receptor. The S2 unit is exposed by breaking down the S1 subunit, which occurs when the S protein binds with the receptor. At first, the S protein is in the pre-hairpin intermediate state. Then a six-helix bundle structure is made by three pairs of HR1 and HR2, and the fusion core takes the form [45]. Afterward, it is in the stable post-fusion hairpin state. In the end, it changes into the post-fusion hairpin state by blocking peptide bind to HR1, which inhibits the viral and host cell membrane fusion; thus, viral entry into cells is inhibited [46].

Inflammatory Cytokines in SARS-CoV-2

Cytokines have a significant part in invulnerability and immunopathology for quite some time. However, dysregulated and overflowing immune reactions have been appeared to cause lung harm and lessened endurance possibly. There is a rise in IL-1b, IFN-c, IP-10, MCP-1, IL-4, and IL-10 of SARS-CoV-2–contaminated people [47]. Higher IL-6, IL-10, and TNF-α and fewer CD4$^+$ and CD8$^+$ T cells were found in patients demanding ICU admission [48]. Further, there is an inverse correlation found in the degree of IL-6, IL-10, and TNF-α, with CD4+ and CD8+ T cell count [48], the cytokine storm reduces the versatile resistance against SARS-CoV disease is affirmed by earlier animals surveys [49]. The immunological qualities among extreme and moderate COVID-19 were represented by Chen and partners [50] in the issue of the JCI. CD4+ and CD8+ T cell tallies were altogether reduced (P = 0.018 and 0.035, respectively) in extreme COVID-19 patients despite an expansion in white platelet count. SARS-CoV-2 infection is linked with lymphopenia because of the levels of serum cytokines and examination of lymphocyte configuration after infection. Cytokines were overproduced (IL-6, soluble IL-2 receptor [IL-2R], IL-10, and TNF-α), and expression of IFN-γ was reduced in CD4+ T cells in severe COVID-19. These observations are clear identification of the disease severity of COVID-19 (Fig. **1**).

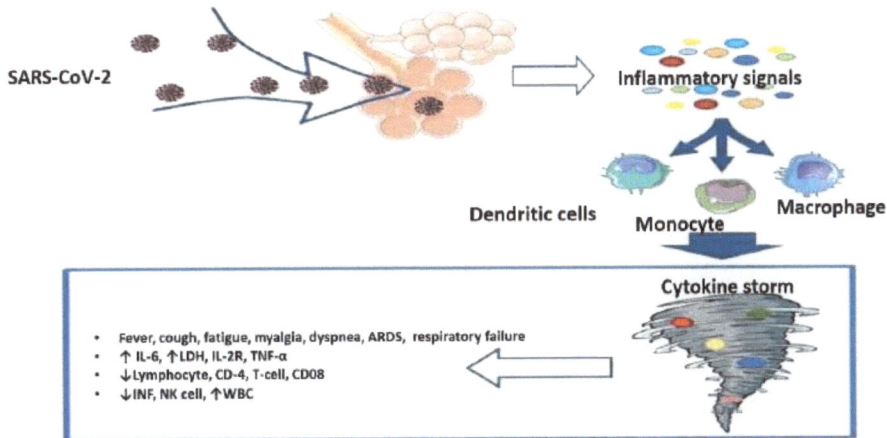

Fig. (1). The severity of COVID-19 disease is linked with Cytokine storms and T cell lymphopenia. Uninfected patient (left plate), escalation in IL-6 and shrinkage in entire T lymphocytes count, mainly CD4+ T cells and CD8+ T cells in modest COVID-19 cases (middle plate). Amplified IL-6, IL-2R, IL-10, and TNFα, while total T lymphocytes, mainly CD4+ T cells and CD8+ T cells and reduction in IFNγ-expressing CD4+ T cells show the severe COVID-19 cases (right plate).

In moderate cases, the quantities of IL-6, IL-2R, IL-10, and TNF-α were somewhat raised or inside the usual range, but in the majority of the extreme cases, the values had a significant rise. Inflammatory macrophages produce these cytokines because they are affected by the cytokine storm [51]. In moderate cases, the total lymphocyte counts, and precisely CD4+ T cells and CD8+ T cells, were somewhat lesser, considerably reduced in severe cases [50]. In patients with severe *versus* moderate COVID-19 cases, the IFN-γ expression in CD4+ T cells was lower (Although not significant, P = 0.063). COVID-19 disease severity is associated with cytokine storm [48], as demonstrated by the recent study of Diago

2020 by an increase in pulmonary pathology, depletion of T cell, and dysfunction of CD4$^+$ T cell.

Residues Involved in the Interaction between Viral Spike and ACE2

The acknowledgment of the host receptor is crucial for viral passage. For the binding to their cellular receptors, the CoVs use their homotrimeric spike glycoprotein (Comprising an S1 subunit and S2 subunit in each spike monomer) present on the envelope of the membrane. The angiotensin-converting enzyme 2 (ACE2) is recognized by the S1 protein of the SARS-CoV. Numerous investigations incorporate basic examinations that anticipate that SARS-CoV-2 likewise distinguishes ACE2 as a host receptor [52 - 54]. RBD with a center structure and a receptor-binding motif (RBM) binding to ACE2 has been uncovered by the structure examination of SARS-CoV glycoprotein. The RBM of SARS-CoV and SARS-CoV-2 was analyzed, and neither cancellations were found nor inclusions. The only main change anticipated was adding one residue further from the coupling space. Different CoVs that don't utilize ACE2 have these residues [53, 55, 56]. ACE2 is considered to be a utilitarian receptor in *in vitro* analysis. It indicated that neither aminopeptidase N (APN) nor dipeptidyl peptidase 4 (DPP4) is utilized to enter the cell during the novel infection. This has been observed in the cases of MERS-CoV [57 - 59]. Therefore, entering the SARS-CoV into the target cell, binding the virus to the ACE2 receptor is critical. The host cell most certainly has specific receptors for S protein on ACE2. CD209L, for SARS-CoV, was recently considered a putative cell receptor, human alveolar, and endothelial cells can be cured with this CD209L [60]. The same can be considered for SARS-CoV-2. An ongoing report detailed that S protein can tie to the CD147 receptor on the host cell. In light of *in vitro* analyses, CD147 refined immune response fundamentally repressed the entrance of SARS-CoV-2 into the cells [61]. The distinguishing proof of the considerable number of receptors and the specific system SARS-CoV-2 uses for cell passage will help the quest for antiviral targets [18]. ACE2 role in helping SARS-CoV-2 entrance into the host cell is of huge importance, proved by recent studies [58, 62, 63]. It was stated that host cells are vulnerable to SARS-CoV-2 infection having ACE2 while those not having ACE2 are not [58]. SARS-CoV-2 RBD binds to ACE2 was recently demonstrated by *in vitro* binding measurement, showing affinity in the low nano-molar range, demonstrating RBD is an important functional constituent within the S1 subunit that is accountable for binding of SARS-CoV-2 by ACE2 [62, 64].

Structure of RBD/ACE2 in SARS-CoV-2

The structure of the SARS-CoV-2 RBD–ACE2 complex was resolved to utilize X-beam crystallography in a recent study by Lan [65] to explain their correlation.

This basic data extraordinarily improve our comprehension of the link between SARS-CoV-2 and susceptible cells, gives an exact site to kill antibodies, and helps the structure-based immunization plan immediately required in the progressing battle against SARS-CoV-2. In the investigation of Lan [65], the SARS-CoV-2 RBD (Residues Arg319–Phe541) (Figs. **2a** and **2b**) and the N-terminal peptidase area of ACE2 (residues Ser19–Asp615) were addressed correctly (Fig.**2c**). The complex structure was controlled by atomic substitution utilizing the SARS-CoV RBD and ACE2 structures as search models [66] and refined to a goal of 2.45 Å with the last Rework and Rfree components of 19.6% and 23.7%, individually. The last model contains residues Thr333–Gly526 of the SARS-CoV-2 RBD, deposits Ser19–Asp615 of the ACE2 N-terminal peptidase area, one zinc particle, and four N-acetyl-β-glucosaminide (NAG) glycans connected to ACE2 Asn90, Asn322, and Asn546 and RBD Asn343, just as 80 water atoms.

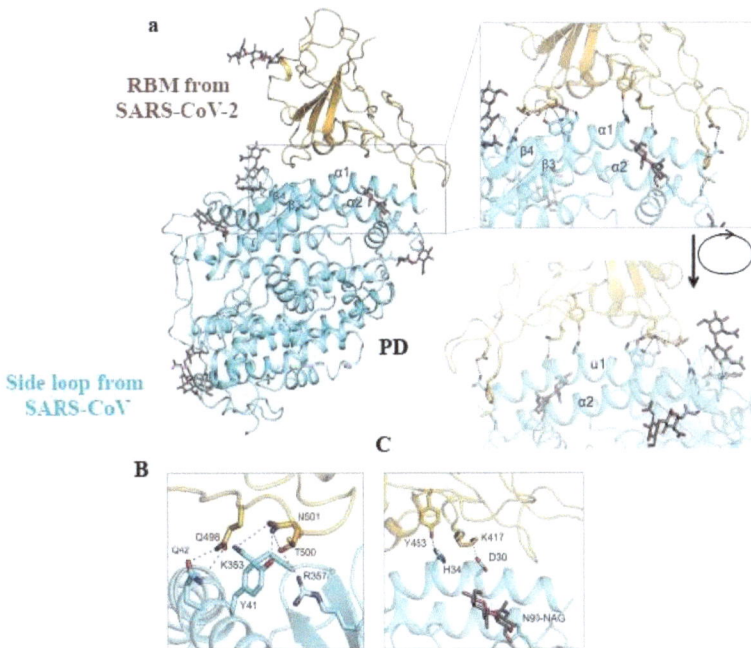

Fig. (2). Binding of SARS-CoV-2 RBD to ACE2 structure. **a**. SARS-CoV-2 spike monomer. FP; HR1; HR2; IC; NTD; SD1; SD2; TM topology. **b**. SARS-CoV-2 RBD sequence and secondary structures. **c**, binding of SARS-CoV-2 RBD to ACE2 structure.

The center of SARS-CoV-2 RBD is structured with short associating helices and circles by a bent five-stranded anti-parallel β sheet (β1, β2, β3, β4, and β7) (Figs. **2b** and **2c**). The short β5 and β6 strands lie between the β4 and β7 strands in the center, α4 and α5 helices and circles (Figs. **2b** and **2c**). The RBM is the inclusion point because it contains the vast majority of the reaching residues attached to ACE2 in SARS-CoV-2. The RBD has an aggregate of 9 cysteine residues. Among these 8 structures, 4 sets of disulfide bonds. Three of these four sets are found in the center like Cys336–Cys361, Cys379–Cys432, and Cys391–Cys525 simultaneously, helping the β sheet structure to be balanced (Fig. **2c**); the rest of the pair (Cys480–Cys488) interfaces the circles in the distal finish of the RBM (Fig. **2c**). Two flaps are present in the N-terminal peptidase area of ACE2, shaping the peptide substrate restricting site. The base side of the little flap of ACE2 is contacted with RBM in the SARS-CoV-2 RBD, which assists the N-terminal helix of the ACE2, which is a hollow external surface in the RBM (Fig. **2c**). RBD general structures of SARS-CoV-2 and SARS-CoV resemble quite a lot (Fig. **3a**); having 1.2 Å root mean square deviation (r.m.s.d.) for 174 adjusted Cα particles. Indeed, with the vast succession variety in the RBM, there is exceptional comparability (r.m.s.d. of 1.3 Å) in general structure to the SARS-CoV RBD, with just a single evident conformational change the distal end (Fig. **3a**). The general restricting method of the SARS-CoV-2 RBD to ACE2 is likewise almost indistinguishable from that saw in the recently decided structure of the SARS-CoV RBD–ACE2 complex4 (Fig. **3b**).

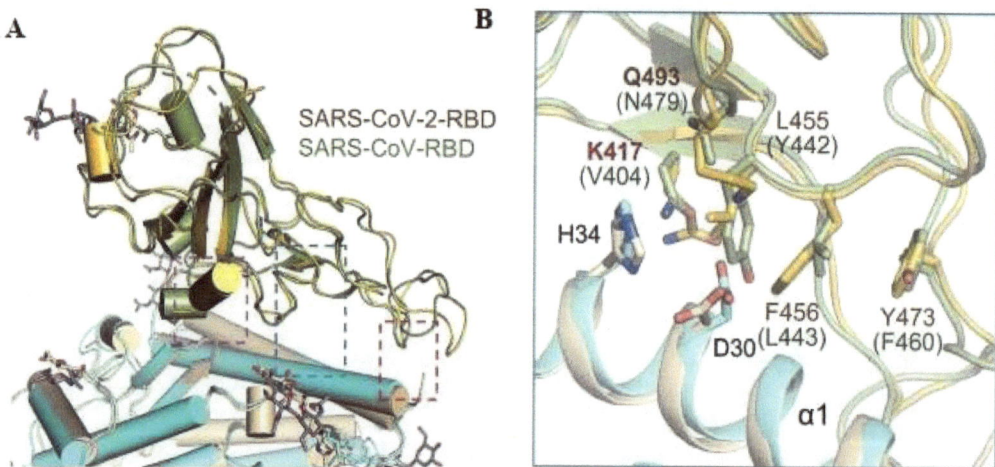

Fig. (3). Interfaces interactions comparison of SARS-CoV-2 RBD–ACE2 and SARS-CoV RBD–ACE2. **a.** SARS-CoV-2, and SARS-CoV positions interactions in the RBM around the changed residues. Cyan represents SARS-CoV-2 and SARS-CoV RBDs. Green represents ACE2. **b.** SARS-CoV-2 and SARS-CoV RBDs interactions around the K417 and V404 positions, respectively. The black arrow represents the position of K417 in the SARS-CoV-2 RBD. The green ribbon represents the N-terminal helix of ACE2.

Identification of Potential Compounds against SARS-CoV-2 Proteins

Drug identification against any specific viral disease activity can be found in two ways: 1) Direct immune response of the human immune system and 2) finding substrates that bind to specific protein sites or have an inhibitory effect on the viral activity. Due to the immune pathway's complex interplay, the first method is risky and difficult to imply, taking time to be tested and experimented before administration to human beings. However, the 2nd method is possible early in the epidemiological disease course by computational modeling and wet lab tests. Clinical testing like a randomized controlled trial can give true efficacy and side effects profile.

Presently, for SARS-CoV-2, no licensed drug or vaccine is available; therefore, current treatment focuses on relieving the patients from the symptoms such as dry cough, fever, and pneumonia. In the succeeding SARS outbreak, a series of helicase and protease inhibitors were reported to prevent viral replication [67 - 71]. For treating CoV-related pneumonia, the Chinese Center for Disease Control and Prevention (CCDC) is currently testing existing pneumonia treatments for SARS-CoV-2. Existing antivirals, including protease inhibitors (Indinavir, saquinavir, and lopinavir/ritonavir) as well as RNA polymerase inhibitors including remdesivir [72, 73], are being tested against SARS-CoV-2. Recently, the antiviral efficiency of several FAD-approved drugs, including remdesivir (EC50 = 0.77 μM) and chloroquine (EC50 = 1.13 μM) against a clinical isolate of SARS-CoV-2 *in vitro* showed potential inhibition at a low-micromolar concentration [74]. The efficacy of remdesivir is evident from a recent recovery of US patients infected with SARS-CoV-2 after intravenous treatment [75], while chloroquine is being evaluated in an open-label trial (ChiCTR2000029609). Following this, two phases of III trials (NCT04252664 and NCT04257656) were also initiated to evaluate intravenous remdesivir in patients infected with SARS-CoV-2. Others include Nafamostat (EC50 = 22.50 μM), nitazoxanide (EC50 = 2.12 μM) and favipiravir (EC50 = 61.88 μM) [74]. Randomized trials to evaluate the efficacy of favipiravir plus baloxavir marboxil (ChiCTR2000029544) and favipiravir plus interferon-α (ChiCTR2000029600) are also initiated for patients with SARS-CoV-2. Moreover, the efficacy of interferon beta and previously identified monoclonal antibodies (mAbs) is also under investigation [1] for treating SARS-CoV-2.

It was found by Saadat *et al.* [36] that the least scoring ligands on ICM and mean force scores (mfscores) contrary to PLpro protein were theasinensin A, which is a polyphenol flavonoid found in black tea (Camellia sinensis). It was found that the score of the 'ligand's oxygen-8 was around 2.9 Å and 9 amino acid residues surrounded the pocket, with G266 being the closest with a distance between them.

There were quite a few hydrophobic interactions (D164, L162, P248, Y264, N267, G163, and K157) and the ligand formed a minimum of 1 hydrogen bond with E161.

Saadat *et al.* [36], tested epigallocatechin gallate, also known as epigallocatechin-3-gallate, which is found in catechin of tea against the AMP binding site of NSP-3 protein, and the results revealed that it had the highest ICM score with extremely promising results to bind to this receptor active site. Colon cancer cells also responded positively to this drug and were proved very effective in its treatment [76]. Epigallocatechin gallate is also famous for its antioxidant properties. 6 hydrogen bonds were formed by the ligand, *i.e.*, G46, A50, G47, S128, W360, and A129, the nearest one being G46 having a distance of 2.6 Å. The following hydrophobic interactions were also present, *i.e.*, I131, A38, G130, F132, and G48 extracted from *Cimicifuga racemosa* is a notable mention for NSP-3 protein binding. In pathological or inflammation conditions, cimicifugic acid's role is well known to prevent collagen degradation by collagenases or collagenolytic enzymes activity [77]. The role of this acid is well known for its antiviral activity against enterovirus A71 infection [78].

According to Saadat *et al.* [36], theaflavin, 5,7,3′,4′-tetrahydroxy-2′-(3,3-dimethylallyl and silymarin as Mpro protein inhibitors are amongst the ligands. It has the lowest scores on ICM, and mfscore scales. A strong hydrogen bond between its hydrogen (H8) and oxygen of His41 residue was found and served as important information because it also serves a critical role in creating the active catalytic site. The active catalytic site Cys145, which was found to be in close proximity, was blocked by the ligand because of its involvement in hydrophobic interactions. Besides these, four other strong hydrogen bonds were created by theaflavin, namely T26, T24, Q189, and S46, with the closest being 2.7Å in the distance [Fig 9]. The other hydrophobic interactions found were namely M49, T25, and T45. Another study documented inferior docking scores against RNA-dependent RNA polymerase of SARS-CoV-2 [79].

Saadat *et al.* [36] reported that spike protein that binds with human ACE-2 receptor, lower value of ICM score was -19.29 with docking to C20H19F2N3O5 (Dolutegravir). In contrast, a very low mfscore of -133.7 was observed with Chebulagic. Theasinensin had good scores for its ligands on both measures included with a -19.22 score of ICM, and a -98 mfscore. Colistin has an ICM score of -16.69 mfscore of -126. Theasinensin A ligand had almost 3 hydrophobic interactions of Y505, Y495, and G496, while with 6 residues, it formed close hydrogen bonds, namely: T500, Q498, Y449, G502, N501, and R403. The closest one was 14, with a 2.47Å distance from T500. Theasinensin A is included among herbal products that already showed antiviral activity against the virus [80].

Docking results of Saadat *et al.* [36], for RNA Replicase NSP-9 displayed the lowest -26 ICM score of Epigallocatechin while Chebulagic, a benzopyran tannin, had the lowest mfscore of -117. Epigallocatechin (found in black tea) is a useful antioxidant according to several studies [81], while according to another study, the Chebulagic acid inhibits enterovirus replication [82]. Other compounds having lower ICM and mfscores were cimicifugic acid, scutellarin, and rosemarinic acid. The epigallocatechin activity resembled zinc ionophore activity seen in one of the studies [81] because of its herbal origin. Higher concentrations can be used to get improved inhibition compared to chloroquine. In both of the metrics, epigallocatechin was observed to have the lowest overall score. 2 hydrophobic interactions, namely T77 and V76. 4 hydrogen bonds, *i.e.*, R111, D78, A107, and V110, were formed by it, R111 having the shortest distance of 2.8Å with it.

According to Saadat *et al.* [36], suitable target pockets for ligand docking were found in the A-chain of NSP-16 molecules. These molecules had a volume of 348A3. They had the highest hydrophobicity and DLID scores (Drug-Likeness) [83]. Virtual screening was carried out after choosing the specific pocket, which confirmed the antiviral nature of Favipiravir (Avigan). This Favipiravir is a novel RNA polymerase inhibitor with the highest affinity having an ICM score of 36 and mfscore of 42. Favipiravir is useful against influenza virus, even those that are resistant to neuraminidase and M2 inhibitors. Also, it is a novel broad-spectrum antiviral drug [84]. Viral infection was seen to be reduced by favipiravir in a recently published work [74]. According to Saadat *et al.* [36], analysis, Favipiravir makes 5 hydrophobic interactions that are D6897, D6898, D6912, M6929, and F6947 while 4 hydrogen bonds, *i.e.*, G6869, G6911, C6913, and S6896, 2.8Å with G6869 being the closest one of them. Amentoflavone is a biflavonoid constituent of several plants including the Chinese plant *Selaginella tamariscina* and Ginkgo biloba, which can be possible ligands for NSP-16 inhibition, having a -33 ICM score showing high affinity. Some studies have proved its antiviral and anti-cancer effects [85]. Another potential inhibitor was Theaflavin for this site. The most potent compounds with their relative binding force scores, immune effects, and sources are presented in Table **1**.

RdRp, 3CLpro, PLpro, and helicase were suggested by studies [105] to be extremely vital targets because they can form small-molecule inhibitors as their biological functions are well-known and have a vital active site enzyme. The screening outputs presented a sequence for drugs for PLpro that might have a great binding affinity. The drugs were thymidine, ribavirin, and valganciclovir, which have antiviral activity. Tigecycline, cefamandole, and chloramphenicol are anti-bacterial. Carbamate and chlorphenesin are muscle relaxants, while levodropropizine is anti-tussive. Also, some natural products showed increased affinity to PLpro protein that can be potential drugs used against the SARS-Co-

-2. These natural products are platycodin D, baicalin, sugetriol-3,9-diacetate, phaitanthrin D, and 2,2-di (3-indolyl)-3-indolone, from *Platycodon grandifloras, Scutellaria baicalensis, Cyperus rotundus,* and *Isatis indigotica,* respectively [105].

Table 1. The most potent compounds with their relative binding force scores, immune effects, and sources.

Protein	Drugs	ICM Score	mf Score	Immune Effects	Viral Effects	References
PLpro	Theasinensin A	-32.25	-119.14	Proinflammatory mediators level were less	Antiviral	[86, 87]
	Curcumin	-24.23	-24.41	Proinflammatory mediators level were less	Antiviral	[88, 89]
	Quercetin	-21.06	-58.94	Macrophage inflammation was lessened	Antiviral	[89, 90]
	Mitoxantrone	-22.83	-91.00	Proinflammatory cytokines Not effected	Antiviral	[91, 92]
	Amentoflavone	-23.21	-91.43	Proinflammatory mediators level were less	Antiviral	[93, 94]
	Colistin	-11.42	-168.50	Proinflammatory cytokines	Not Known	[95]
ADP Ribose	Epigallocatechin	-43.68	-18.75	Proinflammatory mediators level were less	Antiviral	[96, 97]
	Cimicifugic acid	-36.47	-96.23	Proinflammatory mediators level were less	Antiviral	[78, 98]
	Quercetin	-36.43	-52.34	Macrophage inflammation reduced	Antiviral	[89, 90]
Mpro	Theaflavin	-25.07	-78.31	Proinflammatory mediators level were less	Antiviral	[99, 100]
	Silymarin	-23.86	-110.89	Proinflammatory mediators level were less	Antiviral	[30, 101]
Spike protein	Theasinensin A	-19.21	-98.12	Proinflammatory mediators level were less	Antiviral	[86 87]
	Chebulagic	-12.95	-133.70	Proinflammatory mediators level were less	Antiviral	[37, 80]
	Dolutegravir	-19.28	-37.62	Unknown	Anti-retroviral	[102]
	Colistin	-16.69	-126.28	Proinflammatory cytokines increased	Unknown	[95]
NSP-9	Epigallocatechin	-26.68	-11.13	Proinflammatory mediators level were less	Antiviral	[96, 97]
	Chebulagic	-16.45	-29.97	Proinflammatory mediators level were less	Antiviral	[80, 103]

(Table 1) cont.....

Protein	Drugs	ICM Score	mf Score	Immune Effects	Viral Effects	References
NSP-16	Favipiravir	-36.04	-42.26	Proinflammatory mediators level were less	Antiviral	[84, 104]
	Amentoflavone	-33.1	-117.56	Proinflammatory mediators level were less	Antiviral	[93, 94]
	Cimicifugic acid	-29.28	-109.08	Proinflammatory mediators level were less	Antiviral	[78, 98]

3CLpro has an increased binding affinity to all the natural compounds and derivatives that exhibit antiviral or anti-inflammatory effects, a. A series of derivatives from andrographolide that can be used are chrysin-7-O-b-glucuronide, betulonal, isodecortinol, and cerevisterol, hesperidin, and neohesperidin, kouitchenside I and deacetylcentapicrin from *S. baicalensis, Cassine xylocarpa, Viola diffusa, Citrus aurantium,* and the plants of Swertia genus, respectively. 3CLpro has an active site just in-between the I and II domains having a catalytic dyad of CysHis *i.e.* Cys145 and His41 [34]. The maximum binding affinity to 3CLpro is shown by lymecycline, demeclocycline, doxycycline, oxytetracycline (anti-bacterial), nicardipine, and telmisartan (anti-hypertensive), and conivaptan treating hyponatremia. The results above suggest that 3CLpro inhibitors (discussed above the small-molecule compounds) can be possible treating agents for treating SARS-CoV-2 [105].

Drugs having a mfscores lesser than 110 through the virtual screening of RdRp might be potential inhibitors against SARS-CoV-2, such as itraconazole (antifungal), novobiocin (anti-bacterial), cortisone (anti-allergic), idarubicin (anti-tumor), silybin (hepatoprotective), pancuronium bromide (muscle relaxant), and dabigatran etexilate (chronic enteritis, anticoagulant) drugs. RdRp has an increased binding affinity to the natural compounds and derivatives that exhibit anti-viral or anti-inflammatory and anti-tumor effects, such as betulonal, gnidicin and gniditrin, 2b, 30b-dihydroxy-3, 4-seco-friedelolactone-27-lactone, 14-deox--11,12-didehydroandrographolide, 1,7-dihydroxy-3-methoxyxanthone, theaflavin 3,30-di-O-gallate from, and (R)-((1R,5aS,6R,9aS)-1,5a-dimethyl-7-methy-ene-3-oxo-6-((E)-2-(2-oxo-2,5-dihydrofuran-3-yl)ethenyl)-ecahydro-1H-enzo[c]azepin-1-yl)methyl2-amino-3-phenylpropionate from C. xylocarpa, *Gnidia lamprantha, V. diffusa, Andrographis paniculata, Swerti apseudochinensis, Camellia sinensis* and andrographolide respectively [105].

Through virtual ligand screening helicase protein, lymecycline, cefsulodine, and rolitetracycline (anti-bacterial) itraconazole (anti-fungal), saquinavir (anti-HIV-1), dabigatran (anti-coagulant), and canrenoic acid (diuretic) drugs were considered to have a helicase inhibitor with high mfscores. The natural products, such as many flavonoids from different sources (a-glucosyl hesperidin, hesperidin, rutin, quercetagetin 6-O-b-D-glucopyranoside, and homovitexin), xanthones such as 3, 5-dimethoxy -1-[(6-O-b-Dxylopyranosyl- b-D-glucopyranosyl)oxy]- 9H-xanthe- -9 -one, kouitchenside H, kouitchenside A, 8, 2-dihydroxy-3, 4, 5-trimethoxy-1- [(6-O-b-D-xylopyranosyl-b-D-glucopyranosyl)oxy]-   9H-xanthen-9-one, kouitchenside D,1-hydroxy-2, 6-dimethoxy-8-[(6-O-b-Dxylopyranosyl-b -D-glucopyranosyl) oxy] -9H-xanthen-9-one and triptexanthoside D from Swertia genus, phyllaemblicin B and phyllaemblinol from *Phyllanthus emblica* showed great binding affinity to this target.

CONCLUSION

It is concluded that the nsps of SARS-CoV-2 play a vital role in the life cycle of CoVs. Therefore, 'it's necessary to structurally identify the nsps of SARS-CoV-2 and find the essential binding sites, thus knowing the mechanisms of infection and replication of SARS-CoV-2 to find effective targets for drug and vaccine development. The most important targets can be 3-chymotrypsin-like protease (3CLpro), Spike, RdRp, and PLpro. Besides these targets, NSP-3, NSP-7_ NSP-8 complex, NSP-9, NSP-10, NSP-14, and NSP-16, also play an important role in the virus RNA synthesis and replication, suggesting these proteins may be useful targets for the antiviral drug discovery.

CONSENT FOR PUBLICATION

Not Applicable.

CONFLICT OF INTEREST

The author confirms that this chapter contents have no conflict of interest.

ACKNOWLEDGEMENT

Declared none.

REFERENCES

[1]   Cui J, Li F, Shi ZL. Origin and evolution of pathogenic coronaviruses. Nat Rev Microbiol 2019; 17(3): 181-92.
[http://dx.doi.org/10.1038/s41579-018-0118-9] [PMID: 30531947]

[2]   Chen Y, Liu Q, Guo D. Emerging coronaviruses: Genome structure, replication, and pathogenesis. J Med Virol 2020; 92(4): 418-23.
[http://dx.doi.org/10.1002/jmv.25681] [PMID: 31967327]

[3]   Hyde JL, Diamond MS. Innate immune restriction and antagonism of viral RNA lacking 2'-O methylation. Virology 2015; 479-480: 66-74.
[http://dx.doi.org/10.1016/j.virol.2015.01.019] [PMID: 25682435]

[4]   Lemus MR, Minasov G, Shuvalova L, Inniss NL, Kiryukhina O, Wiersum G, *et al.* The crystal structure of nsp10-nsp16 heterodimer from SARS CoV-2 in complex with S-adenosylmethionine bioRxiv 2020.

[5]   Gralinski LE, Menachery VD. Return of the coronavirus: 2019-nCoV. Viruses 2020; 12(2): 1-8.
[http://dx.doi.org/10.3390/v12020135] [PMID: 31991541]

[6]   Yang H, Xie W, Xue X, *et al.* Design of wide-spectrum inhibitors targeting coronavirus main proteases. PLoS Biol 2005; 3(10)e324
[http://dx.doi.org/10.1371/journal.pbio.0030324] [PMID: 16128623]

[7]   De Clercq E. Potential antivirals and antiviral strategies against SARS coronavirus infections. Expert Rev Anti Infect Ther 2006; 4(2): 291-302.
[http://dx.doi.org/10.1586/14787210.4.2.291] [PMID: 16597209]

[8]   Marra MA, Jones SJM, Astell CR, Holt RA, Brooks-Wilson A, Butterfield YSN, *et al.* The genome sequence of the SARS-associated coronavirus. Science 2003; 300: 404-1399.

[9]   Rota PA, Oberste MS, Monroe SS, Nix WA, Campagnoli R, Icenogle JP, *et al.* Characterization of a novel coronavirus associated with severe acute respiratory syndrome 2003.
[http://dx.doi.org/10.1126/science.1085952]

[10]   Woo PCY, Lau SKP, Chu CM, *et al.* Characterization and complete genome sequence of a novel coronavirus, coronavirus HKU1, from patients with pneumonia. J Virol 2005; 79(2): 884-95.
[http://dx.doi.org/10.1128/JVI.79.2.884-895.2005] [PMID: 15613317]

[11]   Mirza MU, Froeyen M. Structural elucidation of SARS-CoV-2 vital proteins: Computational methods reveal potential drug candidates against main protease, Nsp12 polymerase and Nsp13 helicase. J Pharm Anal 2020; 10(4): 320-8.
[http://dx.doi.org/10.1016/j.jpha.2020.04.008] [PMID: 32346490]

[12]   Luk HKH, Li X, Fung J, Lau SKP, Woo PCY. Molecular epidemiology, evolution and phylogeny of SARS coronavirus. Infect Genet Evol 2019; 71: 21-30.
[http://dx.doi.org/10.1016/j.meegid.2019.03.001] [PMID: 30844511]

[13]   Ziebuhr J, Snijder EJ, Gorbalenya AE. Virus-encoded proteinases and proteolytic processing in the Nidovirales. J Gen Virol 2000; 81(Pt 4): 853-79.
[http://dx.doi.org/10.1099/0022-1317-81-4-853] [PMID: 10725411]

[14]   Angeletti S, Benvenuto D, Bianchi M, Giovanetti M, Pascarella S, Ciccozzi M. COVID-2019: The role of the nsp2 and nsp3 in its pathogenesis. J Med Virol 2020; 92(6): 584-8.
[http://dx.doi.org/10.1002/jmv.25719] [PMID: 32083328]

[15]   van Hemert MJ, van den Worm SHE, Knoops K, Mommaas AM, Gorbalenya AE, Snijder EJ. SARS-coronavirus replication/transcription complexes are membrane-protected and need a host factor for activity *in vitro*. PLoS Pathog 2008; 4(5)e1000054
[http://dx.doi.org/10.1371/journal.ppat.1000054] [PMID: 18451981]

[16]   Yang D, Leibowitz JL. The structure and functions of coronavirus genomic 3′ and 5′ ends. Virus Res 2015; 206: 120-33.
[http://dx.doi.org/10.1016/j.virusres.2015.02.025] [PMID: 25736566]

[17]   Watanabe R, Matsuyama S, Shirato K, *et al.* Entry from the cell surface of severe acute respiratory syndrome coronavirus with cleaved S protein as revealed by pseudotype virus bearing cleaved S protein. J Virol 2008; 82(23): 11985-91.
[http://dx.doi.org/10.1128/JVI.01412-08] [PMID: 18786990]

[18]   Anastasopoulou S, Mouzaki A. The biology of SARS-CoV-2 and the ensuing COVID-19. Achaiki Iatriki 2020; 39: 29-35.

[19]   Chen Y, Su C, Ke M, *et al.* Biochemical and structural insights into the mechanisms of SARS coronavirus RNA ribose 2′-O-methylation by nsp16/nsp10 protein complex. PLoS Pathog 2011;

7(10)e1002294
[http://dx.doi.org/10.1371/journal.ppat.1002294] [PMID: 22022266]

[20] Bouvet M, Ferron F, Imbert I, *et al.* Stratégies de formation de la structure coiffe chez les virus à ARN. Med Sci (Paris) 2012; 28(4): 423-9.
[http://dx.doi.org/10.1051/medsci/2012284021] [PMID: 22549871]

[21] Minskaia E, Hertzig T, Gorbalenya AE, *et al.* Discovery of an RNA virus 3'->5' exoribonuclease that is critically involved in coronavirus RNA synthesis. Proc Natl Acad Sci USA 2006; 103(13): 5108-13.
[http://dx.doi.org/10.1073/pnas.0508200103] [PMID: 16549795]

[22] von Grotthuss M, Wyrwicz LS, Rychlewski L. mRNA cap-1 methyltransferase in the SARS genome. Cell 2003; 113(6): 701-2.
[http://dx.doi.org/10.1016/S0092-8674(03)00424-0] [PMID: 12809601]

[23] Decroly E, Debarnot C, Ferron F, *et al.* Crystal structure and functional analysis of the SARS-coronavirus RNA cap 2'-O-methyltransferase nsp10/nsp16 complex. PLoS Pathog 2011; 7(5)e1002059
[http://dx.doi.org/10.1371/journal.ppat.1002059] [PMID: 21637813]

[24] Chen Y, Guo D. Molecular mechanisms of coronavirus RNA capping and methylation. Virol Sin 2016; 31(1): 3-11.
[http://dx.doi.org/10.1007/s12250-016-3726-4] [PMID: 26847650]

[25] Algahtani H, Subahi A, Shirah B. Neurological complications of middle east respiratory syndrome coronavirus: A report of two cases and review of the literature. Case Rep Neurol Med 2016; 20163502683
[http://dx.doi.org/10.1155/2016/3502683] [PMID: 27239356]

[26] Chau TN, Lee KC, Yao H, *et al.* SARS-associated viral hepatitis caused by a novel coronavirus: report of three cases. Hepatology 2004; 39(2): 302-10.
[http://dx.doi.org/10.1002/hep.20111] [PMID: 14767982]

[27] Pan J, Peng X, Gao Y, *et al.* Genome-wide analysis of protein-protein interactions and involvement of viral proteins in SARS-CoV replication. PLoS One 2008; 3(10)e3299
[http://dx.doi.org/10.1371/journal.pone.0003299] [PMID: 18827877]

[28] Bollati M, Milani M, Mastrangelo E, *et al.* Recognition of RNA cap in the Wesselsbron virus NS5 methyltransferase domain: implications for RNA-capping mechanisms in Flavivirus. J Mol Biol 2009; 385(1): 140-52.
[http://dx.doi.org/10.1016/j.jmb.2008.10.028] [PMID: 18976670]

[29] Lu R, Zhao X, Li J, *et al.* Genomic characterisation and epidemiology of 2019 novel coronavirus: implications for virus origins and receptor binding. Lancet 2020; 395(10224): 565-74.
[http://dx.doi.org/10.1016/S0140-6736(20)30251-8] [PMID: 32007145]

[30] Liu CH, Jassey A, Hsu HY, Lin LT. Antiviral activities of silymarin and derivatives. Molecules 2019; 24(8): 1-15.
[http://dx.doi.org/10.3390/molecules24081552] [PMID: 31010179]

[31] Zhang L, Zhou R. Binding mechanism of remdesivir to SARS-CoV-2 RNA dependent RNA polymerase Preprints 2020.

[32] Jin Z, Du X, Xu Y, Deng Y, Liu M, Zhao Y, *et al.* Structure of Mpro from COVID-19 virus and discovery of its inhibitors. Nature 2020.
[http://dx.doi.org/10.1038/s41586-020-2223-y]

[33] Anand K, Ziebuhr J, Wadhwani P, Mesters JR, Hilgenfeld R. (3CL pro) Structure : Basis for Design of Anti-SARS Drugs. Science 2003; 300(80): 7-1763.

[34] Yang H, Yang M, Ding Y, *et al.* The crystal structures of severe acute respiratory syndrome virus main protease and its complex with an inhibitor. Proc Natl Acad Sci USA 2003; 100(23): 13190-5.
[http://dx.doi.org/10.1073/pnas.1835675100] [PMID: 14585926]

[35] Adem S, Eyupoglu V, Sarfraz I, Rasul A, Ali M. Identification of Potent COVID-19 Main Protease (Mpro) Inhibitors from Natural Polyphenols: An in Silico Strategy Unveils a Hope against CORONA 2020.

[36] Saadat S, Mansoor S, Naqvi N, Fahim A, Rehman Z, Khan SY, *et al.* Structure based drug discovery by virtual screening of 3699 compounds against the crystal structures of six key SARS-CoV-2 proteins 2020.
[http://dx.doi.org/10.21203/rs.3.rs-28113/v1]

[37] Yuan L, Chen Z, Song S, *et al.* p53 degradation by a coronavirus papain-like protease suppresses type I interferon signaling. J Biol Chem 2015; 290(5): 3172-82.
[http://dx.doi.org/10.1074/jbc.M114.619890] [PMID: 25505178]

[38] Egloff M-P, Malet H, Putics A, *et al.* Structural and functional basis for ADP-ribose and poly(ADP-ribose) binding by viral macro domains. J Virol 2006; 80(17): 8493-502.
[http://dx.doi.org/10.1128/JVI.00713-06] [PMID: 16912299]

[39] Saikatendu KS, Joseph JS, Subramanian V, *et al.* Structural basis of severe acute respiratory syndrome coronavirus ADP-ribose-1″-phosphate dephosphorylation by a conserved domain of nsP3. Structure 2005; 13(11): 1665-75.
[http://dx.doi.org/10.1016/j.str.2005.07.022] [PMID: 16271890]

[40] Graham RL, Sparks JS, Eckerle LD, Sims AC, Denison MR. SARS coronavirus replicase proteins in pathogenesis. Virus Res 2008; 133(1): 88-100.
[http://dx.doi.org/10.1016/j.virusres.2007.02.017] [PMID: 17397959]

[41] Matthes N, Mesters JR, Coutard B, *et al.* The non-structural protein Nsp10 of mouse hepatitis virus binds zinc ions and nucleic acids. FEBS Lett 2006; 580(17): 4143-9.
[http://dx.doi.org/10.1016/j.febslet.2006.06.061] [PMID: 16828088]

[42] Kong R, Yang G, Xue R, Liu M, Wang F, Hu J, *et al.* COVID-19 Docking Server: An interactive server for docking small molecules, peptides and antibodies against potential targets of COVID-19 2020; (): 1-16.

[43] Schubert HL, Blumenthal RM, Cheng X. Many paths to methyltransfer: a chronicle of convergence. Trends Biochem Sci 2003; 28(6): 329-35.
[http://dx.doi.org/10.1016/S0968-0004(03)00090-2] [PMID: 12826405]

[44] Coutard B, Valle C, de Lamballerie X, Canard B, Seidah NG, Decroly E. The spike glycoprotein of the new coronavirus 2019-nCoV contains a furin-like cleavage site absent in CoV of the same clade. Antiviral Res 2020; 176104742
[http://dx.doi.org/10.1016/j.antiviral.2020.104742] [PMID: 32057769]

[45] Li F. Structure, function, and evolution of coronavirus spike proteins. Annu Rev Virol 2016; 3(1): 237-61.
[http://dx.doi.org/10.1146/annurev-virology-110615-042301] [PMID: 27578435]

[46] Ling R, Dai Y, Huang B, *et al.* In silico design of antiviral peptides targeting the spike protein of SARS-CoV-2. Peptides 2020; 130170328
[http://dx.doi.org/10.1016/j.peptides.2020.170328] [PMID: 32380200]

[47] Huang C, Wang Y, Li X, *et al.* Clinical features of patients infected with 2019 novel coronavirus in Wuhan, China. Lancet 2020; 395(10223): 497-506.
[http://dx.doi.org/10.1016/S0140-6736(20)30183-5] [PMID: 31986264]

[48] Diao B, Wang C, Tan Y, *et al.* Reduction and functional exhaustion of T cells in patients with coronavirus disease 2019 (COVID-19). Front Immunol 2020; 11: 827.
[http://dx.doi.org/10.3389/fimmu.2020.00827] [PMID: 32425950]

[49] Channappanavar R, Fehr AR, Vijay R, *et al.* Dysregulated type I interferon and inflammatory monocyte-macrophage responses cause lethal pneumonia in SARS-CoV-infected mice. Cell Host Microbe 2016; 19(2): 181-93.

[http://dx.doi.org/10.1016/j.chom.2016.01.007] [PMID: 26867177]

[50]   Chen G, Wu D, Guo W, *et al.* Clinical and immunological features of severe and moderate coronavirus disease 2019. J Clin Invest 2020; 130(5): 2620-9.
[http://dx.doi.org/10.1172/JCI137244] [PMID: 32217835]

[51]   Liao M, Liu Y, Yuan J, Wen Y, Xu G, Zhao J, *et al.* The landscape of lung bronchoalveolar immune cells in COVID-19 revealed by single-cell RNA sequencing. medRxiv 2020.
[http://dx.doi.org/10.1101/2020.02.23.20026690]

[52]   Chan JFW, Kok KH, Zhu Z, *et al.* Genomic characterization of the 2019 novel human-pathogenic coronavirus isolated from a patient with atypical pneumonia after visiting Wuhan. Emerg Microbes Infect 2020; 9(1): 221-36.
[http://dx.doi.org/10.1080/22221751.2020.1719902] [PMID: 31987001]

[53]   Wan Y, Shang J, Graham R, Baric RS, Li F. Receptor recognition by the novel coronavirus from wuhan: an analysis based on decade-long structural studies of SARS coronavirus. J Virol 2020; 94(7): 1-9.
[http://dx.doi.org/10.1128/JVI.00127-20] [PMID: 31996437]

[54]   Wu CH, Yeh SH, Tsay YG, *et al.* Glycogen synthase kinase-3 regulates the phosphorylation of severe acute respiratory syndrome coronavirus nucleocapsid protein and viral replication. J Biol Chem 2009; 284(8): 5229-39.
[http://dx.doi.org/10.1074/jbc.M805747200] [PMID: 19106108]

[55]   Millet JK, Whittaker GR. Host cell proteases: Critical determinants of coronavirus tropism and pathogenesis. Virus Res 2015; 202: 120-34.
[http://dx.doi.org/10.1016/j.virusres.2014.11.021] [PMID: 25445340]

[56]   Wang C, Liu Z, Chen Z, *et al.* The establishment of reference sequence for SARS-CoV-2 and variation analysis. J Med Virol 2020; 92(6): 667-74.
[http://dx.doi.org/10.1002/jmv.25762] [PMID: 32167180]

[57]   Corman VM, Landt O, Kaiser M, *et al.* Detection of 2019 novel coronavirus (2019-nCoV) by real-time RT-PCR. Euro Surveill 2020; 25(3): 1-8.
[http://dx.doi.org/10.2807/1560-7917.ES.2020.25.3.2000045] [PMID: 31992387]

[58]   Zhou P, Yang XL, Wang XG, *et al.* A pneumonia outbreak associated with a new coronavirus of probable bat origin. Nature 2020; 579(7798): 270-3.
[http://dx.doi.org/10.1038/s41586-020-2012-7] [PMID: 32015507]

[59]   Neuman BW, Kiss G, Kunding AH, *et al.* A structural analysis of M protein in coronavirus assembly and morphology. J Struct Biol 2011; 174(1): 11-22.
[http://dx.doi.org/10.1016/j.jsb.2010.11.021] [PMID: 21130884]

[60]   Jeffers SA, Tusell SM, Gillim-Ross L, *et al.* CD209L (L-SIGN) is a receptor for severe acute respiratory syndrome coronavirus. Proc Natl Acad Sci USA 2004; 101(44): 15748-53.
[http://dx.doi.org/10.1073/pnas.0403812101] [PMID: 15496474]

[61]   Ross J, Weill PR. Summary for Policymakers. In: Intergovernmental Panel on Climate ChangeClimate Change 2013 - The Physical Science Basis. 1-30.

[62]   Walls AC, Park YJ, Tortorici MA, Wall A, McGuire AT, Veesler D. Structure, function, and antigenicity of the SARS-CoV-2 spike glycoprotein. Cell 2020; 181(2): 281-292.e6.
[http://dx.doi.org/10.1016/j.cell.2020.02.058] [PMID: 32155444]

[63]   Letko M, Marzi A, Munster V. Functional assessment of cell entry and receptor usage for SARS-Co-2 and other lineage B betacoronaviruses. Nat Microbiol 2020; 5(4): 562-9.
[http://dx.doi.org/10.1038/s41564-020-0688-y] [PMID: 32094589]

[64]   Tian X, Li C, Huang A, *et al.* Potent binding of 2019 novel coronavirus spike protein by a SARS coronavirus-specific human monoclonal antibody. Emerg Microbes Infect 2020; 9(1): 382-5.
[http://dx.doi.org/10.1080/22221751.2020.1729069] [PMID: 32065055]

[65]   Lan J, Ge J, Yu J, *et al.* Structure of the SARS-CoV-2 spike receptor-binding domain bound to the ACE2 receptor. Nature 2020; 581(7807): 215-20.
[http://dx.doi.org/10.1038/s41586-020-2180-5] [PMID: 32225176]

[66]   Zhu N, Zhang D, Wang W, *et al.* A novel coronavirus from patients with pneumonia in China, 2019. N Engl J Med 2020; 382(8): 727-33.
[http://dx.doi.org/10.1056/NEJMoa2001017] [PMID: 31978945]

[67]   Rehman HM, Mirza MU, Saleem M, Froeyen M, Ahmad S, Gul R, *et al.* A putative prophylactic solution for COVID-19: Development of novel multiepitope vaccine candidate against SARS-COV-2 by comprehensive immunoinformatic and molecular modelling approach 2020.

[68]   Bhardwaj VK, Singh R, Sharma J, Rajendran V, Purohit R, Kumar S. Identification of bioactive molecules from tea plant as SARS-CoV-2 main protease inhibitors. J Biomol Struct Dyn 2020; 0: 1-10.
[PMID: 32397940]

[69]   Jain RP, Pettersson HI, Zhang J, *et al.* Synthesis and evaluation of keto-glutamine analogues as potent inhibitors of severe acute respiratory syndrome 3CLpro. J Med Chem 2004; 47(25): 6113-6.
[http://dx.doi.org/10.1021/jm0494873] [PMID: 15566280]

[70]   Kao RY, Tsui WHW, Lee TSW, *et al.* Identification of novel small-molecule inhibitors of severe acute respiratory syndrome-associated coronavirus by chemical genetics. Chem Biol 2004; 11(9): 1293-9.
[http://dx.doi.org/10.1016/j.chembiol.2004.07.013] [PMID: 15380189]

[71]   Tanner JA, Zheng BJ, Zhou J, *et al.* The adamantane-derived bananins are potent inhibitors of the helicase activities and replication of SARS coronavirus. Chem Biol 2005; 12(3): 303-11.
[http://dx.doi.org/10.1016/j.chembiol.2005.01.006] [PMID: 15797214]

[72]   Li G, De Clercq E. Therapeutic options for the 2019 novel coronavirus (2019-nCoV). Nat Rev Drug Discov 2020; 19(3): 149-50.
[http://dx.doi.org/10.1038/d41573-020-00016-0] [PMID: 32127666]

[73]   Morse JS, Lalonde T, Xu S, Liu WR. Learning from the Past: Possible Urgent Prevention and Treatment Options for Severe Acute Respiratory Infections Caused by 2019-nCoV. ChemBioChem 2020; 21(5): 730-8.
[http://dx.doi.org/10.1002/cbic.202000047] [PMID: 32022370]

[74]   Wang M, Cao R, Zhang L, *et al.* Remdesivir and chloroquine effectively inhibit the recently emerged novel coronavirus (2019-nCoV) *in vitro*. Cell Res 2020; 30(3): 269-71.
[http://dx.doi.org/10.1038/s41422-020-0282-0] [PMID: 32020029]

[75]   Holshue ML, DeBolt C, Lindquist S, *et al.* First case of 2019 novel coronavirus in the United States. N Engl J Med 2020; 382(10): 929-36.
[http://dx.doi.org/10.1056/NEJMoa2001191] [PMID: 32004427]

[76]   Du GJ, Zhang Z, Wen XD, *et al.* Epigallocatechin Gallate (EGCG) is the most effective cancer chemopreventive polyphenol in green tea. Nutrients 2012; 4(11): 1679-91.
[http://dx.doi.org/10.3390/nu4111679] [PMID: 23201840]

[77]   Kusano A, Seyama Y, Nagai M, Shibano M, Kusano G. Effects of fukinolic acid and cimicifugic acids from Cimicifuga species on collagenolytic activity. Biol Pharm Bull 2001; 24(10): 1198-201.
[http://dx.doi.org/10.1248/bpb.24.1198] [PMID: 11642333]

[78]   Ma Y, Cong W, Huang H, *et al.* Identification of fukinolic acid from Cimicifuga heracleifolia and its derivatives as novel antiviral compounds against enterovirus A71 infection. Int J Antimicrob Agents 2019; 53(2): 128-36.
[http://dx.doi.org/10.1016/j.ijantimicag.2018.07.014] [PMID: 30063999]

[79]   Lung J, Lin YS, Yang YH, *et al.* The potential chemical structure of anti-SARS-CoV-2 RNA-dependent RNA polymerase. J Med Virol 2020; 92(6): 693-7.
[http://dx.doi.org/10.1002/jmv.25761] [PMID: 32167173]

[80]   Lin LT, Hsu WC, Lin CC. Antiviral natural products and herbal medicines. J Tradit Complement Med 2014; 4(1): 24-35.
[http://dx.doi.org/10.4103/2225-4110.124335] [PMID: 24872930]

[81]   Dabbagh-Bazarbachi H, Clergeaud G, Quesada IM, Ortiz M, O'Sullivan CK, Fernández-Larrea JB. Zinc ionophore activity of quercetin and epigallocatechin-gallate: from Hepa 1-6 cells to a liposome model. J Agric Food Chem 2014; 62(32): 8085-93.
[http://dx.doi.org/10.1021/jf5014633] [PMID: 25050823]

[82]   Yang Y, Xiu J, Liu J, *et al.* Chebulagic acid, a hydrolyzable tannin, exhibited antiviral activity *in vitro* and *in vivo* against human enterovirus 71. Int J Mol Sci 2013; 14(5): 9618-27.
[http://dx.doi.org/10.3390/ijms14059618] [PMID: 23644889]

[83]   Sheridan RP, Maiorov VN, Holloway MK, Cornell WD, Gao YD. Drug-like density: a method of quantifying the "bindability" of a protein target based on a very large set of pockets and drug-like ligands from the Protein Data Bank. J Chem Inf Model 2010; 50(11): 2029-40.
[http://dx.doi.org/10.1021/ci100312t] [PMID: 20977231]

[84]   Furuta Y, Komeno T, Nakamura T. Favipiravir (T-705), a broad spectrum inhibitor of viral RNA polymerase. Proc Jpn Acad, Ser B, Phys Biol Sci 2017; 93(7): 449-63.
[http://dx.doi.org/10.2183/pjab.93.027] [PMID: 28769016]

[85]   Ma SC, But PPH, Ooi VEC, *et al.* Antiviral amentoflavone from it Selaginella sinensis. Biol Pharm Bull 2001; 24(3): 311-2.
[http://dx.doi.org/10.1248/bpb.24.311] [PMID: 11256492]

[86]   Hisanaga A, Ishida H, Sakao K, *et al.* Anti-inflammatory activity and molecular mechanism of Oolong tea theasinensin. Food Funct 2014; 5(8): 1891-7.
[http://dx.doi.org/10.1039/C4FO00152D] [PMID: 24947273]

[87]   Isaacs CE, Xu W, Merz G, Hillier S, Rohan L, Wen GY. Digallate dimers of (-)-epigallocatechin gallate inactivate herpes simplex virus. Antimicrob Agents Chemother 2011; 55(12): 5646-53.
[http://dx.doi.org/10.1128/AAC.05531-11] [PMID: 21947401]

[88]   Yadav R, Jee B, Awasthi SK. Curcumin Suppresses the Production of Pro-inflammatory Cytokine Interleukin-18 in Lipopolysaccharide Stimulated Murine Macrophage-Like Cells. Indian J Clin Biochem 2015; 30(1): 109-12.
[http://dx.doi.org/10.1007/s12291-014-0452-2] [PMID: 25646051]

[89]   Zorofchian Moghadamtousi S, Abdul Kadir H, Hassandarvish P, Tajik H, Abubakar S, Zandi K. A review on antibacterial, antiviral, and antifungal activity of curcumin 2014.
[http://dx.doi.org/10.1155/2014/186864]

[90]   Tang J, Diao P, Shu X, Li L, Xiong L. Quercetin and quercitrin attenuates the inflammatory response and oxidative stress in LPS-induced RAW264.7 cells: *In vitro* assessment and a theoretical model. Biomed Res Int. 2019; 2019.

[91]   Angelucci F, Batocchi AP, Caggiula M, *et al. In vivo* effects of mitoxantrone on the production of pro- and anti-inflammatory cytokines by peripheral blood mononuclear cells of secondary progressive multiple sclerosis patients. Neuroimmunomodulation 2006; 13(2): 76-81.
[http://dx.doi.org/10.1159/000095762] [PMID: 16974110]

[92]   Deng L, Dai P, Ciro A, Smee DF, Djaballah H, Shuman S. Identification of novel antipoxviral agents: mitoxantrone inhibits vaccinia virus replication by blocking virion assembly. J Virol 2007; 81(24): 13392-402.
[http://dx.doi.org/10.1128/JVI.00770-07] [PMID: 17928345]

[93]   Lee E, Shin S, Kim JK, Woo ER, Kim Y. Anti-inflammatory effects of amentoflavone on modulation of signal pathways in LPS-stimulated RAW264.7 cells. Bull Korean Chem Soc 2012; 33: 2878-82.
[http://dx.doi.org/10.5012/bkcs.2012.33.9.2878]

[94]   Li F, Song X, Su G, *et al.* Amentoflavone inhibits HSV-1 and ACV-resistant strain infection by

suppressing viral early infection. Viruses 2019; 11(5): 1-16.
[http://dx.doi.org/10.3390/v11050466] [PMID: 31121928]

[95]   Wang J, Shao W, Niu H, Yang T, Wang Y, Cai Y. Immunomodulatory effects of colistin on macrophages in rats by activating the p38/MAPK pathway. Front Pharmacol 2019; 10: 729.
[http://dx.doi.org/10.3389/fphar.2019.00729] [PMID: 31297059]

[96]   Mukherjee S, Siddiqui MA, Dayal S, Ayoub YZ, Malathi K. Epigallocatechin-3-gallate suppresses proinflammatory cytokines and chemokines induced by Toll-like receptor 9 agonists in prostate cancer cells. J Inflamm Res 2014; 7: 89-101.
[PMID: 24971028]

[97]   Kaihatsu K, Yamabe M, Ebara Y. Antiviral mechanism of action of epigallocatechin-3-O-gallate and its fatty acid esters. Molecules 2018; 23(10): 15-9.
[http://dx.doi.org/10.3390/molecules23102475] [PMID: 30262731]

[98]   Schmid D, Woehs F, Svoboda M, Thalhammer T, Chiba P, Moeslinger T. Aqueous extracts of *Cimicifuga racemosa* and phenolcarboxylic constituents inhibit production of proinflammatory cytokines in LPS-stimulated human whole blood. Can J Physiol Pharmacol 2009; 87(11): 963-72.
[http://dx.doi.org/10.1139/Y09-091] [PMID: 19935904]

[99]   Huang MT, Liu Y, Ramji D, *et al.* Inhibitory effects of black tea theaflavin derivatives on 12--tetradecanoylphorbol-13-acetate-induced inflammation and arachidonic acid metabolism in mouse ears. Mol Nutr Food Res 2006; 50(2): 115-22.
[http://dx.doi.org/10.1002/mnfr.200500101] [PMID: 16404705]

[100] Zu M, Yang F, Zhou W, Liu A, Du G, Zheng L. *In vitro* anti-influenza virus and anti-inflammatory activities of theaflavin derivatives. Antiviral Res 2012; 94(3): 217-24.
[http://dx.doi.org/10.1016/j.antiviral.2012.04.001] [PMID: 22521753]

[101] Morishima C, Shuhart MC, Wang CC, *et al.* Silymarin inhibits *in vitro* T-cell proliferation and cytokine production in hepatitis C virus infection. Gastroenterology 2010; 138(2): 671-681, 681.e1-681.e2.
[http://dx.doi.org/10.1053/j.gastro.2009.09.021] [PMID: 19782083]

[102] Cruciani M, Parisi SG. Dolutegravir based antiretroviral therapy compared to other combined antiretroviral regimens for the treatment of HIV-infected naive patients: A systematic review and meta-analysis. PLoS One 2019; 14(9)e0222229
[http://dx.doi.org/10.1371/journal.pone.0222229] [PMID: 31504060]

[103] Liu Y, Bao L, Xuan L, Song B, Lin L, Han H. Chebulagic acid inhibits the LPS-induced expression of TNF-α and IL-1β in endothelial cells by suppressing MAPK activation. Exp Ther Med 2015; 10(1): 263-8.
[http://dx.doi.org/10.3892/etm.2015.2447] [PMID: 26170946]

[104] Safronetz D, Falzarano D, Scott DP, Furuta Y, Feldmann H, Gowen BB. Antiviral efficacy of favipiravir against two prominent etiological agents of hantavirus pulmonary syndrome. Antimicrob Agents Chemother 2013; 57(10): 4673-80.
[http://dx.doi.org/10.1128/AAC.00886-13] [PMID: 23856782]

[105] Wu C, Liu Y, Yang Y, *et al.* Analysis of therapeutic targets for SARS-CoV-2 and discovery of potential drugs by computational methods. Acta Pharm Sin B 2020; 10(5): 766-88.
[http://dx.doi.org/10.1016/j.apsb.2020.02.008] [PMID: 32292689]

Part III: Quantitation Analysis of SARS-CoV-2

Antigen Capture Enzyme-Linked Immunosorbent Assay (ELISA) for the Detection of the Novel SARS-CoV-2 in Humans

Muhammad Farooq[1,*] and **Zia Ullah**[2]

[1] *Faculty of Veterinary Medicine, University of Teramo, Italy*

[2] *Institute of Microbiology, University of Agriculture Faisalabad, Pakistan*

Abstract: Severe acute respiratory syndrome-coronavirus-2 (SARS-CoV-2) is the reason behind the transmission of the recently prevailing disease worldwide and is known as coronavirus disease 19 (COVID-19). Coronavirus was first diagnosed in Wuhan, China 2019, which followed a worldwide spread. Whereas assays associated with the examination of virus molecules only detect the hereditary viral substance in the patient's body. On the other hand, the novel coronavirus requires the diagnosis of high serological parameters to examine specific antibodies of SARS-CoV-2. In this case, the only solution is the -linked immunosorbent assay (ELISA) test based on hunting the antigens. In this technique, the combination of antibodies is derived from the S proteins present in the cells of infected coronavirus patients. By applying these test assays for the COVID-19 patients, it is obvious that the nature of the testing is specific and sensitive. This test allows the detection of serum through seroconverts since the visible emergence of symptoms of SARS-CoV-2 in patients. The major benefit of this method is that it takes less time during the examination. Instead, it deals with the identifications of different antigens found in the human body. These tests play a pivotal role in characterizing introduction and recognize profoundly receptive human donors. Herein, we developed an ELISA assay for the easy detection of SARS-CoV-2 and nucleocapsid protein expression levels as an early tool for this disease.

Keywords: ELISA, Molecular detection, Nucleocapsid protein, RT-PCR, SARS-CoV-2.

INTRODUCTION

The recent coronavirus disease-2019 (COVID-19) produced by severe acute respiratory syndrome-coronavirus-2 (SARS-CoV-2) is a serious threat to public health. Pneumonia like symptoms being caused by the novel coronavirus is an extremely infectious disease which later named SARS-CoV-2, and the world

---

* **Corresponding author Muhammad Farooq:** Faculty of Veterinary Medicine, University of Teramo-Italy;
E-mail: drfarooqnabi@gmail.com

Kamal Niaz & Muhammad Farrukh Nisar (Eds.)

health organization (WHO) declared this outbreak as a global health emergency [1]. Patients suffered from acute respiratory disease have been identified with novel coronavirus of zoonotic origin. Extensive human-to-human transmission is observed in health care workers [2]. The *betacoronavirus* has confirmed the lineage based on the polygenic and genome sequencing studies of SARS-CoV-2. It shows higher sequence similarities with that of bat SARS-like coronavirus and human SARS-CoV [3]. Certain proteins (M and E proteins) are necessary for the complete development of virus assembly. Still, S protein is crucial for the attachment with the host cells, where the facilitation receptor-binding domain (RBD) of S protein interacts with angiotensin-converting enzyme 2 (ACE2).

The S protein is highly immunogenic, residing on the surface of virus particles [4, 5]. The expression and replication of virus genome ribonucleic acids (RNA), the major structural N protein, is involved in packaging the encapsulated genome into virions and heavily interferes in the host cell cycle. Furthermore, in other coronaviruses, particularly SARS-CoV, high immunogenic activity is due to N protein. It is frequently articulated during infection [6]. For serodiagnosis of COVD-19 samples, both S and N proteins play an important role in detecting the antigen. Currently, numerous diagnosis tools are being used for the confirmation of COVID-19 recommended by WHO. RNA test using next-generation sequencing and real-time polymerase chain reaction (RT-PCR) is used to confirm COVID-19. The current virus shows that the lower respiratory tract is the main infection site of SARS-CoV-2. The virus RNA has been detected in nasal cavities, bronchoalveolar lavage, and pharyngeal regions [7, 8]. The collection of respiratory specimens and viral colonization of the lower respiratory tract gives false-negative results of RT-PCR to diagnose the disease's occurrence. For the time being, it's difficult to achieve a meaningful valuation of the infected patients for which rapid and accurate method is needed. This is well known during the coronavirus epidemic, serological diagnosing techniques allow to detect viral-specific IgG and immunoglobulin [9]. The active design is dependent upon an acute viral infection. As soon as the concentration of IgG is raised, and IgM level starts declining. During the acute phase of infection, the production of host antibodies to the exact virus is constant in most patients. Still, this condition is not found in those people who are immunodeficient. As the early onset of infection occurs, the IgM antibody can be detected quickly [10]. The condition for specimen quality is low standard than for RNA-based assays. As viruses are present in the respiratory tract specimens, the specific antibody can consistently be detected by avoiding false results in sample handling for diagnosis [11].

RT-PCR test is highly productive in diagnosing SARS-CoV-2, but initially, it only gives demonstrative reports during infection. In this context, RT-PCR test has been proved significant for the early identification of patients suffering from coronavirus who were infected outside of Wuhan city. This involves the aggressive behavior of this virus, affecting the minor population in Wuhan during early 2020. Consequently, it urged the scientific community, particularly the microbiologists in China, to recognize the seriousness of this disease. However, the specialists had to face severe technical and sampling problems while conducting the tests. It is further reported that some patients who were previously suffering from ground-glass opacities. It was additionally examined to detect coronavirus and quarantine at the earliest, at the beginning of February 2020. For this purpose, special ELISA kits were manufactured, which help in identifying IgG and IgM antibodies [7]. This led to great progress in fighting this COVID-19 infection and it has also been observed that the seroconversion of IgG-type antibodies happens quite late compared with IgM. The particular reagents that facilitate the expression of specific neutralizing antibodies for SARS-CoV-2 are still in the process of being identified. It may also require a series of assays to detect the precise sequence of the viral RNA.

Some other desirable techniques are to find the precise recognition of antigens that may oppose SARS-CoV after infection [12, 13]. In the majority (93%) of the patients, the response from antibodies requires 10-28 days after the onset of the symptoms. In this context, this process seems unsuitable for the initial identification of the coronavirus. On the contrary, the curing effect (65.4%) has been observed through serological tests. There is the utilization of sera taken after 5-10 days since the symptoms started to appear in the patients. It is crucial to identify N proteins of SARS-CoV-2 to analyze the infection and formulate symptomatic methodology during the early phase of infection. Moreover, recognizing the N protein in the blood serum may avoid the chances of malady during the collection of nasopharyngeal aspirates. It has also been observed that the N protein is detectable in the plasma in the patients initially caught with the virus [14].

Massive use of routine ELISA assays is being carried out, which provides more specificity about COVID-19. Furthermore, this strategy is cheaper than that of RT-PCR and requires less time to elucidate the findings. In addition to that, there is no danger of contamination ELISA assay. COVID-19 human IgG/IgA/IgM antibody ELISA unit utilizes an indirect ELISA strategy in which standard 96-well plates (twelve strips with eight wells/strip) lined with the SARS-CoV-2 N protein can combine with the sample antibodies. When a secondary anti-human antibody-horse radish peroxidase (HRP) is included, a complex antibody HRP-human IgG/IgA/IgM antibody-virus N antigen appeared on the microplate. A 3,3',5,5'-tetramethylbenzidine (TMB) substrate is also included in this mixture that gives blue coloration. The intensity of the blue color is linked with the additional sum of immune protein display of IgM, IgG, or IgA. The color of the stop solution alters this color from blue to yellow. The readings are taken at its strength is determined at 450nm [15].

In many cases, a decline in the virulence of SARS-CoV-2 may occur due to the adjustment of people. Also, this alteration may lead to significant recognition of the molecular activities of the virus RNA. The fundamental reason for virulence soreness is the efflux of cytokines in all subtypes of coronaviruses. SARS-CoV is powerful inside the overcoming antiviral insusceptibility as well as the actuation of pro-soreness effects. SARS-CoV is distinctive from that of the novel coronavirus based on soreness activation and interferon-antagonizing capabilities [16].

In this context, it can be realized that open reading frame 3a (ORF3a) and ORF8b of the SARS-CoV genome do not share similar properties with that of ORF8 and ORF3 in the present case of *betacoronavirus*. Hence, the activating proteins present in both the type of coronaviruses are responsible for modulation of pro-inflammatory responses. These activators may modulate the expression of NLRP3 soreness activity. There is a general concept that the latest strain of coronavirus, *i.e.,* SARS-CoV-2, is less productive inside the crackdown of responsive antiviral reaction and the activation of NLRP3 soreness. Still, there is a need to try for the time being [17, 18].

During the peak of disease spread, a new danger has been idealized. Coronavirus may never be getting away from this world and ultimately transform into an endemic and took long to eradicate from different communities. This danger has been felt in the range of infections. They are making trouble before and after the symptoms of this disease appear, and the disease is spreading from patient to patient just in a while. Most of the patients suffering from coronavirus feel slightly critical infectious conditions [36, 38], primarily due to the higher immunity level of the bodies. In this regard, it is also advisable to build immunization advancement to avoid the extreme conditions of this disease. For the treatment of SARS-CoV-2, the ultimate solution is the development of the vaccines at an expert level and in a massive quantity [37]. Moreover, some other risks have emerged regarding the dependence on antibodies for the down regulation of proliferation of this virus.

Along with it, safety measures should also be incorporated. Furthermore, running the DNA/RNA samples on agarose gel electrophoresis, ethidium bromide, gel red, or SYBR green dyes are used in all these processes and are not safe like ELISA. ELISA solutions and chemicals are commonly used in research and clinical laboratories that are safer to compare these diagnosis procedures [6]. It is important to note that ELISA can provide accurate and higher sensitivity for

SARS-CoV-2 diagnosis even at the initial stage of infection. The current manuscript explains the antigen capture ELISA and its complete procedure for diagnosing the COVID-19 virus.

Protocols of ELISA for Detecting SARS-CoV-2

ELISA is utilized for distinguishing an antigen and its accessibility from a sample. The antigen is disabled inside the wells of the 96-well plate by adsorption or apprehended with a bound and antigen-specific counteracting agent. A detection antibody is joined with the protein *via* a covalent bond. Protein substrate at that point included the wells creating an obvious signal related to the amount of antigen and measured by a spectrophotometer. In certain situations, an identifying antibody may act as a detector to find specific antibodies titer in the form of dimers. This technique is known as bridging ELISA, *i.e.,* the linkage between the two antibodies acts as a bridge. The most suitable example of this method is IgG and its identification [7, 15].

Basic Protocol 1: Tranferentation of Human Cell and Purgation of Protein

The protocol is utilized for RBD and S protein of the virus. Here, one vector communicates with RBD while the other with viral S protein in the form of trimers. The expression of genes is less in S proteins (4.5 mg/l) than RBD (18 mg/l). This leads to the accompanying of RBD in the initial phases of the ELISA test while the s protein is used in proving it. The expression vector development was depicted already. The genomic sequencing of the spike proteins is responsible for this kind of activity. There is the optimization of the sequencing of the cell's culture sourced from humans. The spike protein is gathered to compensate for the emptiness of the cleavage portion of the neutralizing base [15, 16].

Basic Protocol 2: Stages of ELISA and Detection of Plasma in Patients of SARS-CoV-2

In this protocol, a strategy is asserted for detecting the responsive behavior of antigen towards a combination of proteins known as RBD and the spike protein present in the plasma of coronavirus patients. This also aids in ensuring reproducibility and consistency in the results. A two-stage ELISA in which the essential arrangement joins for the major part and the detection is done by diluting plasma with RBD. This will be taken after a second stage in which positive tests from the primary stage encounter a corroborative ELISA against the full-length spike protein, which is hardly expressed and difficult to access [39]. For the second stage, a dilution pattern is performed. Usually, it remained accessible in this case, and screening ELISAs can be run within the morning (760 samples/10 plates per run), and following up ELISAs can be run within the afternoon (140 samples/10 plates per run). Herein, we delineate the tests since it is most easy to set up such an assay [18]. A plate reader and plate washer are needed without any hurdles. Conventionally it can be balanced to use with a mechanized liquid handler. In extension, one of the challenges in setting up the ELISA test is the accessibility of appropriate negative and positive controls. Negative controls are less demanding to come by and can be taken from the serum pools. Within these hard times of the disease spread, no human sera or mAbs are available. Still, mouse mAbs, mouse sera against SARS-CoV-2, other creature sera against SARS-CoV-2, or anti-His tag antibodies (the proteins are His-tagged) can be utilized [36]. However, in this case, a secondary antibody for the species from which the primary antibody is obtained. It is required to use as a positive control.

Moreover, it is endorsed by making large clumps of positive controls, which can be utilized for various runs. The positive control ought to be chosen to result in an intense hail (propose OD490 of around 2.0) and be discernable from the negative controls. ELISA can easily be run with either serum or plasma [2].

Equipment's Required to Perform ELISA Assay

- Combination of proteins of RBD
- Combination of S proteins
- 1× PBS
- Milk powder
- PBS-T
- Sample plasma
- Immunoglobulins G (IgG)
- OPD
- Distilled RNAs free water for injection (WFI) for cell culture
- 3 M hydrochloric acid
- ELISA plates: flat-bottom Immune non-sterile 96-well plates 4 HBX
- Multichannel pipettor (s) capable of pipetting 50 to 250 µl
- Sterile reservoirs
- Temperature control water bath
- Aquamax 2000 plate washer
- Timer
- Precautionary cabinet
- 1.5 mL microcentrifuge tubes
- Flat-bottom cell culture plates
- Kimberly-Clark Kim wipes
- Bioteksynergy H1 microplate reader or equivalent
- Purifying tubes
    i. 10 mL

   ii. 45 mL
- Sterile, serological pipettes
    - i. 6 mL
    - ii. 12 mL
    - iii. 26 mL
    - iv. 52 mL
- Micropipette tips
    - i. 20 µL barrier tips
    - ii. Microtips of 200 µL
    - iii. 1000 µL barrier tips
- Pipette Aid
- Micro pipettors
- Refrigerator
- Ultra freezer (-80°C)

Buffers

The buffers used for extraction (5 l)

- 32.2 g of $NaH_2PO_4:H_2O$
- 70.5 g NaCl
- 63.0 g imidazole
- 4.1 volume of water in purified form
- Conserve for 120 days at an average temperature

Use distilled water filtered using a 0.24 µm sterile vacuum filtration system.

The buffer of phosphate and saline

- 39.2 L volume of water in purified form
- 5.2 L 10× PBS
- 53 ml Tween 20
- Conserve for 120 days at room temperature

Wash buffer (5000 mL)

- 32.21 g $NaH_2PO_4 \cdot H_2O$
- 71.35 g NaCl
- 5.23 g imidazole
- 5 L volume of water in purified form
- Conserve for 120 days at a room temperature

There is two-step ELISA testing. At the first step, the rate of production of antigens is deduced attached to the S proteins present in the serum obtained for sample testing. While at the second step, the reactivity of antibodies towards the combination of proteins present in RBD and the combination of full length S proteins present within the samples of SARS-CoV-2 patients. Moreover, this method also helps ensure the consistency and uniformity of the results obtained [19]. The ELISA testing method has been bifurcated into two phases. Also, a bend of the diluted solution takes place in the other step. The first phase of this assay is the examining ELISA, while the second phase is known as the probatory ELISA [39]. Since only one step can be performed at a time, the examining ELISA step is done first starting from morning, and almost 800 samples are run using 12 plates. In the evening, the second phase starts known as probatory ELISA, in which the testing is done on 150 samples per 12 plates. In this regard, the only mechanic framework employed is to handle the fluid in a more sensitive way.

Another problem that is faced in this method is its approach towards positive as well as negative impacts. Although the possibility of negative impacts is relatively low if it happens, there will be a massive serum. On the contrary, some positive results can also emerge that include the availability of testing strength within the patient of COVID-19 and the availability of antibodies that are in the form of single clonal like CR30229,10 [40]. In the worst case, if the availability of plasma from humans is not that enough, the serum can be obtained from rats and tested against the antibodies of SARS-CoV-2 patients. But in this case, the utilization of a different antigen is required that is compatible with the primary antibody to ensure positive results. In fact, in this case, if there is only one antigen, both S proteins present in full length, and RBD can be accompanied to gain positive controls. Furthermore, this assay comprised of step A (not prescribed) or step B may be performed even the available samples are in small quantities [20].

Methods

The basis of the ELISA method begins with capturing an antibody. It is attached to a micro surface for the creation of a substantial stage. Washing the plate clears any unbound antibody, and then it is blocked using a reagent. It is taking after a clean, tests, benchmarks, and powers at that point given rise a stable stage antibody, which engulfs the analyte. An introduction of a conjugated detection counteracting agent (*e.g.,* biotin-conjugated) after washing away the unbound analyte occurs. This location antibody ties to an atom having a different determinant and is calculated afterward. In this way, this method appeared as the shape of a sandwich. After cleaning it, to get rid of any specs of antigen, it uses an area reagent. After washing the plate, hydrogen peroxide (H_2O_2) is used, followed by the coloring of the plate. After the coloration appears, its intensity can be measured using standard equations [19, 39].

Assay designing

Multiple assay designs are being used for ELISAs, such as either direct, indirect, or sandwich capture/detection methods. Still, the necessary step involved in all types is the immobilization of the antigen. The antibody present is recognized either directly (the essential antibody) or indirectly (the secondary antibody). But mostly, the sandwich ELISA test is in use whereby implication immobilizes and by implication recognizes the linkage or association of the target antigen. This sort of capture measure constitutes a "Sandwich" test, in which each recognizes a particular epitope of the antigen. The sandwich ELISA test is extensively used due to its affectability and specificity.

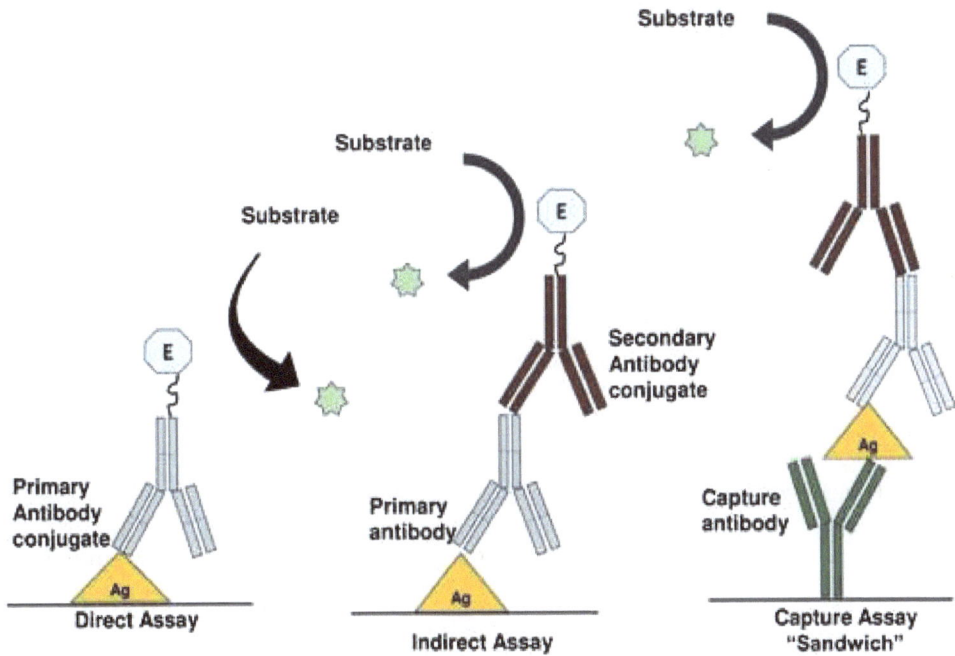

Fig. (1). Schematic diagram of various types of ELISA (direct, indirect, and sandwich assays). In the assay, the antigen of interest is immobilized by direct adsorption to the assay plate or attaching a capture antibody to the plate surface.

Among the standard measures inspected and laid out over, recognizing the techniques that are accompanied for the identification phase is crucial. The identification phase is a step that does not depend on how the antibody is conserved on the plate. This step chooses the affectability of an ELISA to an extraordinary level [38]. The identification procedure employed an antigen named with a reporter enzyme or a tag that sparks an encounter with an antibody. A special type of antigen is accompanied on the plate and kept immobile to perform a direct identification. Another type of antigen or a biotin-streptavidin complex for upgradations is employed and is the first predominant organization for ELISA using indirect detection. The secondary antibody has specificity for the primary antibody used in it. In a sandwich ELISA, the secondary antibody must be specific for disclosing the vital counteracting agent. The principal portion is typically accomplished by utilizing different types of capturing antibodies obtained from diverse species such as IgG of rabbits and mice. In sandwich ELISA tests, the utilization of secondary types of antigens can be productive for this detection. Moreover, such antibody also aids in highlighting infectious antigens that can hinder the neutralization process [21, 39].

Solution preparation

The typical specimens utilized for serological testing of COVID-19 include serum, plasma, or whole blood samples. Serum and plasma are both fluid and cell-free portions of whole blood. The serum is collected taking after coagulation of whole blood and does not contain and clotting factors. Plasma is collected by centrifugation of whole blood treated with anticoagulants and contains all the clotting factors of the blood, which is thought to make it less stable for longer storage. Antibodies are proteins that can be found in all three types of blood components. IgM antibody responses arise after a week of post-infection, which act as the first line of defense. IgM is often used as an indicator of newly acquired infection. IgM antibody responses are typically short-lived and diminish as the infection is no longer active [39, 40]. IgG antibodies appear towards the end of the active infection and persist for months or even years following infection. IgA is linked with mucosal immunity and is considered to be an important player in respiratory infections. Scientists are still learning about the natural history of COVID-19. However, preliminary serological reports suggest that the SARS-CoV-2 antibody response follows this typical pattern, with most patients seroconverting within 2-week following the appearance of symptoms and all patients seroconverting one month after symptom onset [22].

Following are the samples collection methods using ELISA

Immunizer

- Accumulate all the blood that is taken for the samples in a raw decanter such as aDE coagulant unprocessed tube. Mostly BD vacutainer tubes are used.
- Then the test tube is covered untreated for 25 mins under average temperature.
- Extraction is done by centrifugation at 31000 rpm for 15 mins to extract at 4°C.
- Measure the ingredients quickly that are present in the immunizer and place

them under -80°C. Afterward, shorten the freeze cycles.

Plasma

- Accumulate all the blood that is taken for the samples in a raw decanter such as a DE coagulant unprocessed tube. Mostly BD Immunizer Coagulation test tubes are used for this purpose. Instead of this, you can also dissolve 0.03 M of sodium citrate in 1/100 of the volume obtained at the end.
- Measure the ingredients quickly that are present in the immunizer and place them under -80°C. Extraction is done by centrifugation at 31000 rpm for 15 mins to extract at 4°C. Afterward, shorten the freeze cycles.

Serum tests were warmed at 60°C for one hour before utilizing to decrease hazard if any specs of the virus are still left in the plasma sample. A diluted solution is prepared for the test. The solution includes the plasma sample and the antigen mixed with 1% of skimmed milk powder using Tween Phosphate Buffer Saline (TPBS). The solution is then spread on the plates at a normal temperature for 2 h. About 100 mL of diluted solution is used [43]. After that, the cleaning process of the plates began, and they are washed thrice using TBPS. Another dilution (1:3000) of goat anti-human IgG-horseradish peroxidase (HRP) conjugated secondary antibody (ThermoFi3sher Logical) was prepared in 0.98% TPBS, and 1010 μL of this secondary antibody was added to each well for 1 h. Again, the process of cleaning plates takes place thrice using TPBS as soon as it dries off, 101 μL of SigmaFast OPD (Phenylenediaminedihydrochloride; Sigma-Aldrich) arrangement has been done for every well.

Moreover, the clearing of substrates also happens in this step for twelve minutes on the surface of plates. Here, the process came to an end by the dilution of 50 μL 4M HCL. After that, the measurement of the range of optical density (OD) is taken at 400 nm. The strength of OD can be measured as 500 nm of 0.13. Along with that, the value of AUC can also measure through this process. If the values of AUC drop below one, then for measuring purposes, the average range is set at 0.50. These details are examining considering the Graph pad. In few cases, the endpoint of the calculation of titers happens. The final diluted solution is considered to be the stopping point. After which, the reactivity is minimized underneath and OD 490 nm underneath 0.11 [12, 15, 40].

Sodium Dodisyl Sulphate-Polyacrylamiode Gel Electrophoresis (SDS-PAGE)

Recombinant proteins utilize another strategy known as SDS-PAGE. A gel in the SDS-PAGE that is used to examine such types of proteins and the specificity in proteins is examined. For the conduction of this method, protein is dissolved in the buffer solution with BME at a ratio of 1:1. After that, the solution is being heated at 110°C for approximately 10 mins. After that, the decolorization of gels takes place for 1-2 h, and after that, de-stained in distilled water overnight [7, 15].

Antibody Coating

The human antibody, to be specific 47D11, adheres to S proteins in both types of coronaviruses. Filtered antigens are then preserved until utilized at 4°C. The monoclonal counter-acting agent acts as a neutralizer having no restraints attached to the receptors.

Sample Processing

The ELISA convention was balanced from already set up protocols. For this step, 100 plates are coated at a mild temperature of 4.5°C. The treatments were executed at warm temperature. They were not done at high temperatures were also analyzed for comparison. Another testing technique was employed similar to the plasma technique, *i.e.,* normal human immunoglobins (NHIGs). In the initial phase of this testing method, a diluted solution of 100 µg/ml was prepared. Three non-SARS-CoV-2 receptive human mAbs and CR302220-22, a human mAb responsive to the RBD of SARS-CoV-1 and SARS-CoV-2, were utilized as controls. Again, a different ELISA test was conducted to evaluate the dissemination of the distinctive counteracting agent base utilized for the testing and led to very responsive results through the standard ELISA testing method [20]. The other ELISA test was conducted on secondary antigens 29. These antibodies include anti-human IgA (α-chain-specific) HRP antibody (Sigma A0295)(1:3,000), anti-human IgM (µ-chain-specific) HRP antibody (Sigma A6907) (1:3,000), anti-human IgG1 Fc-HRP (Southern Biotech 9054-05) (1:3,000), anti-human IgG2 Fc-HRP (Southern Biotech #9060-05) (1:3,000), anti-human IgG3hinge-HRP (Southern Biotech 9210-05) (1:3,000), and anti-humanIgG4 Fc-HRP (Southern Biotech 9200-05) [42, 43].

Dilution of Sample

Dilute sample (human serum or plasma) with measured diluents reagent (Item D) 500 times. For illustration, include 0.5 µL serum + 249.5 µL test diluent. Blend the diluted sample well and equally for taking the results.

- The user ought to calculate the sum of the test utilized for the entire test. Would you mind saving an adequate amount of samples in advance?
- Avoid utilizing tests with extreme hemolysis, precipitate, or contamination by bacteria or protein suspension.
- Use of EDTA, heparin sulfate, sodium citrate, or other anticoagulants will not

affect the results.

- In the event, buffers have some crystals that are then kept warm at room temperature and made an amalgam for dissolution.
- Turn HRP-anti positive control IgG/IgA/IgM Antibody (Item F) and include 1000 μL of test diluent (Item D) into the vial. Blow up this mixture gently before use.

Normal Human Immunoglobin (NHIG)

NHIG is a pool of IgG from thousands of healthy donors. The presentation of person givers to endemic infectious diseases, immunizations, and omnipresent microorganisms takes an interest in fighting against harmful substances inside IgG. NHIG is a potent source to cure illnesses due to soreness like leukemia and sclerosis. Moreover, it can also be used against infections and microscopic organisms such as parasites in people. Another consequence of this treatment can lead to a few unfavorable occasions related to particular immunoglobulin arrangements and individual contrasts. Still, numerous clinical and test studies appear that exchanging from NHIG to subcutaneous immunoglobulin can minimize these unfavorable conditions [25]. NHIG plays a vital part in avoiding infectious episodes in primary immunodeficient patients. The beneficial effects of these antibodies within the treatment of contagious illnesses go past straightforward neutralization of microorganisms or their poisons. Anti-inflammatory pathways are also fundamental for security against diseases. NHIG may balance the immune reaction through multiple mechanisms. It includes blocking a full cluster of proinflammatory cytokines, and Fc-gamma receptors (FcγRs). It also involves leukocyte adhesion particles that suppressing pathogenic Th1 and Th17 subsets and neutralizing pathogenic autoantibodies. NHIG can also extend administrative T-cells by accepting cyclooxygenase-2 (COX-2)-dependent prostaglandin E2 generation in dendritic cells [27, 27]. It is also showed that the advantageous impacts of NHIG were related to the suppression of inflammatory IL-6 and improvement of anti-inflammatory IL-10 within the intestines [43].

Also, NHIG treatment is driven to the expanded expression ligand-activated transcription factor that intercedes anti-inflammatory functions and resolution of aggravation, whereas TLR-4 expression, which mediates the inflammatory reaction, is decreased. In general, sera from mostly all healthy adults contain anti-coronavirus antibodies to differentiate in commercially accessible polyclonal helpful IgG products. NHIG obtained from donors with high-titer antibodies against the respiratory syncytial virus (RSV) have extraordinary potential to make strides in the result of RSV disease in immunocompromised subjects. Not only by controlling viral replication but also by lessening harm to the lung parenchyma and epithelial airway lining [27]. Presently, the meet of NHIG is restricted to the cure of the emerging coronavirus disease. Since this method for the treatment requires inflection of soreness, it can be hazardous for thepatient's body. In rare cases, some non-inflammatory types can be effective for the reduction of infection. The treatment of COVID-19 is exceptionally restricted. Moreover, NHIG also contains IgG in the dimeric form, which can cause hindrance for the naturally responsive cells used for immunity [28].

- Start of NHIG as adjuvant treatment for COVID-19 pneumonia within 48 h of affirmation to the ICU can decrease the utilization of mechanical ventilation.
- Commencement of NHIG as adjuvant treatment for COVID-19 pneumonia within 48 h of affirmation to the ICU can decrease hospital length of stay and period of stay in ICU.
- Advancement of NHIG as adjuvant treatment for COVID-19 pneumonia within 48 h of affirmation to the ICU can diminish the 28 days mortality of patients with COVID-19 severe pneumonia.

Secondary Antibody Dilution

　i. 2 h after preservation at optimal temperature.
　ii. The plates used in the ELISA test should be cleaned thrice by the automatized cleaner. This can be done with the utilization of TPBS.
　iii. Mix 1% low-fat milk with IgG antigen at special conditions through the utilization of TPBS. The ratio of diluted solution should be 3000:1.
　iv. Prepare at the slightest 5 mL per plate.
　v. Add 50 µL of the diluted solution containing antigen prepared in the above steps and spread it over the plates with the help of a pipettor.
　vi. Refrain the pipettor from making contact with the walls of the plates.
　vii. Start the stopwatch for 1 h (stay in a range of 50 to 65 min). The secondary antibody has been introduced to the first plate.
　viii. Keep plates in a 20°C (RT) incubator.

Detection *via* ELISA

A combination of nucleocapsid protein present in SARS-CoV is used to set up a method for capturing antigens known as ELISA. Antigen-capturing ELISA is a prevalent strategy for an alternative antibody test because of its quality of being effective. Another proposition of this method is that the antibodies possess the characteristic of being bivalence. The identification of the required antibody is dependent on the specificity of the antibody to the provided antigen. In this regard, the selection and decontamination of the antigen should be carried out precisely, and the test needs to be conducted exceptionally particular. Through this method, the detection of any sort of antibodies is possible [42, 43]. In this regard, the N protein attached to the antibody plays a crucial role in its detection and is also referred to as a recombinant protein to prepare the ELISA test to diagnose coronaviruses. By utilizing centrifugal force, the medium containing dissolvable S parts was deposited and washed. Afterward, the cells were cleaned thrice by using PBS at lower temperatures and preserved through applying the centrifugal force method.

Moreover, this method accompanies the ABTS substrate for the incubations of cells at a normal temperature of twelve minutes. Also, the centrifugal forces method was again accompanied to clear the substrate. With that, the calculation of OD (405 nm) was also done. After that, the cleaning of wells takes place. This was done so the substrate can be included in each well that too of 60 μL of ABTS. The calculation of OD (405 nm) takes place after twenty minutes again [20].

ELISA is the most common serological test which helps in identifying antibodies from the serum. In an ELISA, viral antigens are immobilized on a surface. Then a patient's blood or serum is added, allowing for any antibodies specific for the viral antigens to bind while all other antibodies are washed away. Then an enzyme-conjugated secondary antibody, specific for antibody isotype being targeted (*i.e.,* IgM, IgA, and IgG), is added, followed by enzyme-substrate, resulting in producing a colored product when the viral antigen-antibody complex is detected [22]. A diluted solution of the plasma of the infected person is required to perform the ELISA test. The range of the diluted solution determines AUC. Most of the plasma tests carried out for the diagnosis of SARS-CoV-2 indicated an effective response towards the S proteins and the RBD.

Moreover, the serum in the infected person was more reactive towards spike proteins than the RBD [26]. As the size of the spike protein is larger than that of the RBD, there is the possibility of the presence of more antigenic determinants in it, which consequently results in a more reactive nature. Due to this extending, epidemic tests were performed following an additional fourteen serum tests on people suffering from a minor infection of coronavirus or at an initial stage [28]. These 14 tests responded well with both S protein and RBD. Thus, the above investigation resulted in a visible difference between the plasma of participants infected with COVID-19 and has been identified positively in this regard. This comparison is made with the samples of plasma that were obtained before the virus emerged in the world [23].

Micro-Neutralization assay

Microneutralization is a profound investigation to assess those antigens that will neutralize the virus in the patients. Particularly, this analysis also leads to an accurate status that either a patient's body is capable of such antigens, which will neutralize the severity of infection or not. For neutralization assay warm unreactive plasma tests having diluted solution of concentration 10:1are serially debilitated 3-fold in 2x MEM (20%) 10× minimum basic medium(Gibco), 4YmM L-glutamine, 0.2% of sodium bicarbonate [wt/vol;Gibco],20YmM4-(--hydroxyethyl)-1-piperazine ethanesulfonic acid (HEPES, Gibco), 200YU/ml penicillin–200Yµ/ml streptomycin(Gibco), and 0.4% bovine serum egg whites (MP Biomedical)) [15]. COVID-19 virus diluted to a concentration of a hundred 50% cell culture infectious dosages (TCID$_{50}$) in 2x MEM. About 80 µL of each serum dilution and 80 µL of the infection dilution are included in a 96-well cell culture plate and permitted to incubate for one hour at room temperature. DMEM is removed from Vero. E6 cells and 120 µL of the virus-serum mixture were included in the cells, and the cells incubated at 37°C for 1 h. After 1 h incubation, the virus serum mixture removes from the cells, and 100 µL of each comparing serum dilution and 100 µL of 2x MEM containing 2% FBS added to the cells. The cells were incubated for 48 h at 37°C and after that settled with 10% paraformaldehyde (PFA) (Polysciences, Inc) for 28 h at 4°C [22]. Following fixation, the PFA was evacuated, and the cells were washed with 200 µL of PBS. The cells were permeabilized (at that point) by the expansion of 150 µL of PBS containing 0.1% Triton X-100 for 15 mins at room temperature. The plates were cleaned thrice at that point. After that, they are concealed in a solution accompanied for blocking at normal temperature for some time [16]. Afterward, they are cleaned thrice using TPBS (IgG389; Rockland Immunochemical) (diluted 1:3000) within a solution used to block the solution while placing it at normal temperature. After that, the process of washing plates occurs again, and they are cleaned thrice. This time the washing process is done with OPD substrate (SigmaFast OPD; Sigma-Aldrich) and TPBS. By collaborating four plates peruse, the OD is calculated at 490 nm. The stoppage point of OD sees a visible deviation that is thrice in every plate and can be utilized to measure the microneutralization titer [15, 29].

Formation of Recombinant Protein

Two different transformations of the S protein are generated that are present in the plasma of the person infected by COVID-19. The first transformations showed the shape of the S proteins that form trimers and are considered a more stable form [43]. On the other hand, the second transformation shows the RBD that is smaller in size than the spike proteins. The genome sequencing that was found in the earliest infection cases in January, 2020 is the basis of the order in which both these proteins are used. The genome sequencing was around 100 kbs and was also made optimized as per suiting different types of human cells. Sequencing S protein sequencing does the evacuation of the neutralizing agent's cleavage site.

Furthermore, this helps in furin detection and consists of mutations that can stable the protein. The arrangement is used to express the mammalian cell through pCAGGS, and then it is converted into a double vector [40]. In the structure of RBD, we notice that the N endpoint of the protein is linked with amino acids present in the RBD. In this way, RBD utilizes similar kinds of vectors to that of the spike proteins. The culture provided by RBD is different in human cells (20-45 mg/liter) compared to the culture produced in the cells of tiny organisms like insects (2 mg/liter). The combination of proteins present in RBD is examined under the gel of SDS-PAGE, which results in the emission of bright rays. But the process works slower while examining the proteins in the cells of tiny organisms compared to the proteins present in the cells of humans. Also, a contrast between the sizes of polysaccharides is found in the cells of both species. There are greater manifestations of frameworks in the spike protein of human cells (6 mg/liter) than that of insect cells (0.6 mg/liter) [30, 31].

Calculation of Antibodies under Different Heat Conditions within the Plasma or Serum through ELISA Assay

The calculation and detection of antigens in the body of a person infected with coronavirus is a complicated task to perform. There are chances that the vial molecules of this infection are visible within the biorepository, particularly early amid intense contamination. In this regard, the preventive measure that needs to be employed is the heating of the plasma at 65°C for 90 minutes. Through this precautionary measure, the above-mentioned hazard can be avoided. This test was carried out to evaluate if the warm temperature can detect antigens attached to the S proteins and RBD in the plasma of infected patients of SARS-CoV-2. A comparison was carried out between the heated sample of the plasma and the no-heated sample. Whereas slight contrasts are detected, there is the certainty that there is no negative result of testing while heating or providing a higher temperature during sample testing [32].

Additionally, a coordinated utilization of plasma with serum was done for the tests taken from the infected people of coronavirus, which led to irrelevant contrasts proposing that these samples can be utilized while testing. Since numerous coronaviruses are delicate to heat. The warming inactivation of tests at 56°C earlier to testing is considered a possible strategy to decrease the chance of transmission [16, 43]. However, the impact of heating on the estimation of SARS-CoV-2 antibodies is still vague. By comparing the levels of SARS-CoV-2 antibodies before and after heat inactivation of serum at 56°C for 30 minutes employing a quantitative fluorescence immunochromatographic measure. It has been shown that heat inactivation altogether interferes with the levels of antibodies to SARS-CoV-2. The IgM levels of all the 34 serum tests (100%) from

COVID-19 patients diminished by an average level of 53.56%. The IgG levels were reduced in 22 of 34 trials (64.71%) by a reasonable level of 49.54% [28]. Comparable changes can also be observed within the non-COVID-19 infections gather (n=9). Of note, 44.12% of the identified IgM levels were dropped underneath the cut-off value after warming; recommending warm inactivation can lead to false-negative comes about of these tests. Our results demonstrate that warm inactivation of serum at 56°C for 30 minutes meddling with the immune analysis of antibodies to SARS-CoV-2. Heat inactivation before immune analysis is prohibited, and the possibility of false-negative results should be considered if the test was pre-inactivated by heating [15, 32].

Antibody Isotyping, Subtyping and Neutralizing Activity

The process of classification and sub-classification of antibodies having a single clone of cells is referred to as isotyping. For example, IgM and IgG are considered the classes, while IgM1 and IgM2 are the subclasses. The process of isotyping is of fundamental importance in the reproduction of antigens. Also, it is credited vital for developing strategies for the purgation and alteration of antigens. There is the availability of several kits for isotyping on the commercial level. For carrying out immunoassays, classification through isotyping is of crucial importance since it aids in selecting the right plan through which antibodies can be cleaned and utilized [16]. To illustrate this fact, let us take the example of IgM, which the utilization will not purify G sub-protein.

Such antigens are required that are anti-immunity boosters to carry out the process of isotyping. This is necessary because only such antigens can be utilized to identify classification and sub-classification of antibodies in a single clonal form, which will further aid in reproduction. Along with that, fragmentation of IgM will be necessary to utilize it for immunity-building purposes. The process of isotyping is carried out on the commercial level to achieve this purpose. Although isotyping on a commercial level is done. It is still not easy to carry out the mass generation of antibodies and successfully get all the required antigens [14].

There are two structural designs in which the kits of isotyping are accessible. They are in the form of strip units or kits of ELISA. Ordinarily, there is the utilization of pre-coated plates, which helps capture the right antigen obtained from the sample for the test. In ELISA tests, the capturing of antigen occurs, and then it is surfaced on the plates. The plates used in the process are already coated with antibodies that are used for the process of isotyping.

Along with that, it also identifies the wells used for the capturing of such antibodies. The antibody response used for isotyping with the antibody derived as a sample for testing is placed on a cassette like a plate that produces bright colored rays on it. The use of film units can ensure the completion of the test quickly at the same time [33]. On the other hand, the use of packs of ELISA can help in carrying out the multiple numbers of the testing process at one time. Different types of antibodies belonging to various classification and sub-classification are carried out of a test based on quantities. There are chances that the results obtained from such test will be somewhat the same for all the antigens provided, and it would be difficult to differentiate among these antibodies based on specificity.

Moreover, there are cases where the isotyping of antibodies is carried out based on the ELISA testing method, but it is rare [34]. The first step is to conceal the antibody on a plate with is of micro-size to carry out this process. After that, the samples obtained for the testing are spread on wells to bind the antigens together. Secondly, the washing process takes place, discarding all the material and leaving only the antigen that is specific for the sample antibody. Lastly, the identification of antibodies takes place. In this context, make sure that only such an antibody should be utilized, specific for the isotyping of the antibody present in the sample. An isotyping and subtyping ELISA results are the utilization of S proteins present in the cells of mammals. All these tests are highly reactive, especially in the case of IgM.

Along with that, the range of reactivity is strong in IgA and IgG too. The signal of IgG1 carries out a more substantial part of the tests. It was identified that the range of reactivity is relatively slower in the case of Ig2 as well as IgG4. The type, as mentioned earlier of isotyping done through ELISA, is indicative of the results that the IgG3 subclass is the one that controls the reactivity of IgG [35, 42, 43].

CONCLUSION

COVID-19 is concluded as a promptly restrictive illness in almost 80% of patients. Severe pneumonia happened in around 15% of patients, as the data reported. The number of casualties was approximately 3.5%, and the rate of causalities remained more than 4.5% in Wuhan in the end of February 2021. Hubei province has recorded more than 4.0% of patients, while the number of patients outside Hubei province remained about 0.92%. Moreover, there is a collapse of clinics that could clarify the exceedingly high casualties in Wuhan. In addition to that, Wuhan has gone short of the kits used for sampling, resulting in fewer undiagnosed patients. As the virus is novel, so other problems in the treatments were also emerging.

Hitherto, no vaccine or certain medicine has been discovered to cure this infectious virus, which is the most problematic factor. Although medical specialists are busy inventing a vaccine, this development is not certain yet. In this regard, some other agents have also been accompanied. They may act as an antivirus and may result in a commendable examination of this virus at clinical level. ELISA encompasses a high affectability, particularly for discovering serum tests from patients. It can be a vital strategy for COVID-19 diagnosis. Notably, steroids have been tentatively utilized while curing this novel coronavirus. In addition, the doctors from China are biased towards the use of steroids for the treatment of SARS-CoV-2.

On the contrary, the chances of wellness of patients given steroids are expected relatively low. In the worst situation, this may also lead to the massive transmission of the infection and even more hazardous patients' hazardous situations. This hazard can also be illustrated through the emerging report about the patients in Wuhan who faced severe infection in the lungs due to fungal contamination. It is depicted that such a condition may have been the result of steroids for the treatment but led to negative results. The use of modern medical techniques may provide an antiviral effect against SARS-CoV-2 could be acquired to achieve better results. In this regard, specialists share the same perspective to depict the treatment of coronavirus around the world.

CONSENT FOR PUBLICATION

Not Applicable.

CONFLICT OF INTEREST

The author confirms that this chapter contents have no conflict of interest.

ACKNOWLEDGEMENT

Declared none.

REFERENCES

[1]   Coronavirus disease. 2019. [Internet]. [cited 2020 May 11]. Available from: https://www.who.int/emergencies/diseases/novel-coronavirus-2019

[2]   Chan JFW, Yuan S, Kok KH, *et al.* A familial cluster of pneumonia associated with the 2019 novel coronavirus indicating person-to-person transmission: a study of a family cluster. Lancet 2020; 395(10223): 514-23.
[http://dx.doi.org/10.1016/S0140-6736(20)30154-9] [PMID: 31986261]

[3]   Huang C, Wang Y, Li X, *et al.* Clinical features of patients infected with 2019 novel coronavirus in Wuhan, China. Lancet 2020; 395(10223): 497-506.
[http://dx.doi.org/10.1016/S0140-6736(20)30183-5] [PMID: 31986264]

[4]   National Health Commission of the PRC [Internet]. [cited 2020 May 11]. Available from: http://en.nhc.gov.cn/

[5]   Zhou P, Yang XL, Wang XG, *et al.* A pneumonia outbreak associated with a new coronavirus of probable bat origin. Nature 2020; 579(7798): 270-3.
[http://dx.doi.org/10.1038/s41586-020-2012-7] [PMID: 32015507]

[6]   Lu R, Zhao X, Li J, *et al.* Genomic characterisation and epidemiology of 2019 novel coronavirus: implications for virus origins and receptor binding. Lancet 2020; 395(10224): 565-74.
[http://dx.doi.org/10.1016/S0140-6736(20)30251-8] [PMID: 32007145]

[7]   Neuman BW, Kiss G, Kunding AH, *et al.* A structural analysis of M protein in coronavirus assembly and morphology. J Struct Biol 2011; 174(1): 11-22.
[http://dx.doi.org/10.1016/j.jsb.2010.11.021] [PMID: 21130884]

[8]   Nieto-Torres JL, DeDiego ML, Verdiá-Báguena C, Jimenez-Guardeño JM, Regla-Nava JA, Fernandez-Delgado R, *et al.* Severe Acute Respiratory Syndrome Coronavirus Envelope Protein Ion Channel Activity Promotes Virus Fitness and Pathogenesis 2014.
[http://dx.doi.org/10.1371/journal.ppat.1004077]

[9]   Woo PCY, Lau SKP, Wong BHL, *et al.* Differential sensitivities of severe acute respiratory syndrome (SARS) coronavirus spike polypeptide enzyme-linked immunosorbent assay (ELISA) and SARS coronavirus nucleocapsid protein ELISA for serodiagnosis of SARS coronavirus pneumonia. J Clin Microbiol 2005; 43(7): 3054-8.http://www.ncbi.nlm.nih.gov/pubmed/16000415 [Internet].
[http://dx.doi.org/10.1128/JCM.43.7.3054-3058.2005] [PMID: 16000415]

[10]   Hurst KR, Koetzner CA, Masters PS. Identification of *in vivo* -interacting domains of the murine coronavirus nucleocapsid protein. J Virol 2009; 83(14): 7221-34.
[http://dx.doi.org/10.1128/JVI.00440-09] [PMID: 19420077]

[11]   Cui L, Wang H, Ji Y, *et al.* The nucleocapsid protein of coronaviruses acts as a viral suppressor of RNA silencing in mammalian cells. J Virol 2015; 89(17): 9029-43. http://www.ncbi.nlm.nih.gov/pubmed/26085159 [Internet].
[http://dx.doi.org/10.1128/JVI.01331-15] [PMID: 26085159]

[12]   Perera RA, Wang P, Gomaa MR, *et al.* Seroepidemiology for MERS coronavirus using microneutralisation and pseudoparticle virus neutralisation assays reveal a high prevalence of antibody in dromedary camels in Egypt, June 2013. Euro Surveill 2013; 18(36): 20574. http://www.eurosurveillance.org/ViewArticle.aspx?ArticleId=20574 [Internet].
[http://dx.doi.org/10.2807/1560-7917.ES2013.18.36.20574] [PMID: 24079378]

[13]   Zhu N, Zhang D, Wang W, *et al.* A novel coronavirus from patients with pneumonia in China, 2019. N Engl J Med 2020; 382(8): 727-33.http://www.nejm.org/doi/10.1056/NEJMoa2001017 [Internet].
[http://dx.doi.org/10.1056/NEJMoa2001017] [PMID: 31978945]

[14]   Berry JD, Hay K, Rini JM, *et al.* Neutralizing epitopes of the SARS-CoV S-protein cluster independent of repertoire, antigen structure or mAb technology. MAbs 2010; 2(1): 53-66.http://www.ncbi.nlm.nih.gov/pubmed/20168090 [Internet].
[http://dx.doi.org/10.4161/mabs.2.1.10788] [PMID: 20168090]

[15]   Stadlbauer D, Amanat F, Chromikova V, *et al.* SARS-CoV-2 seroconversion in humans: A detailed protocol for a serological assay, antigen production, and test setup. Curr Protoc Microbiol 2020; 57(1): e100.
[http://dx.doi.org/10.1002/cpmc.100] [PMID: 32302069]

[16]   Letko M, Marzi A, Munster V. Functional assessment of cell entry and receptor usage for SARS-Co-2 and other lineage B betacoronaviruses. Nat Microbiol 2020; 5(4): 562-9.
[http://dx.doi.org/10.1038/s41564-020-0688-y] [PMID: 32094589]

[17]   Pallesen J, Wang N, Corbett KS, *et al.* Immunogenicity and structures of a rationally designed prefusion MERS-CoV spike antigen. Proc Natl Acad Sci USA 2017; 114(35): E7348-57.
[http://dx.doi.org/10.1073/pnas.1707304114] [PMID: 28807998]

[18]   Lee CYP, Lin RTP, Renia L, Ng LFP. Serological approaches for COVID-19: Epidemiologic

perspective on surveillance and control. Frontiers in Immunology. Frontiers Media S.A. 2020; Vol. 11.

[19]   Chang CK, Sue SC, Yu TH, *et al.* Modular organization of SARS coronavirus nucleocapsid protein. J Biomed Sci 2006; 13(1): 59-72.
[http://dx.doi.org/10.1007/s11373-005-9035-9] [PMID: 16228284]

[20]   Haveri A, Smura T, Kuivanen S, *et al.* Serological and molecular findings during SARS-CoV-2 infection: the first case study in Finland, January to February 2020. Euro Surveill 2020; 25(11): 2000266.https://www.eurosurveillance.org/content/10.2807/1560-7917.ES.2020.25.11.2000266 [Internet].
[http://dx.doi.org/10.2807/1560-7917.ES.2020.25.11.2000266] [PMID: 32209163]

[21]   Chu DKW, Pan Y, Cheng SMS, *et al.* Molecular diagnosis of a novel coronavirus (2019-nCoV) causing an outbreak of pneumonia. Clin Chem 2020; 66(4): 549-55.
[http://dx.doi.org/10.1093/clinchem/hvaa029] [PMID: 32031583]

[22]   Sun B, Feng Y, Mo X, *et al.* Kinetics of SARS-CoV-2 specific IgM and IgG responses in COVID-19 patients. Emerg Microbes Infect 2020; 9(1): 940-8.
[http://dx.doi.org/10.1080/22221751.2020.1762515] [PMID: 32357808]

[23]   Ching L, Chang SP, Nerurkar VR. . COVID-19 special column: principles behind the technology for detecting SARS-CoV-2, the cause of COVID-19. Hawai'i J Heal Soc Welf [Internet] 2020; 79(5): 42-136. 2020 May 1 [cited 2020 May 29]. Available from: http://www.ncbi.nlm.nih.gov/pubmed/32432217

[24]   Shen C, Wang Z, Zhao F, *et al.* Treatment of 5 critically Ill patients with COVID-19 With convalescent plasma. JAMA 2020; 323(16): 1582-9.
[http://dx.doi.org/10.1001/jama.2020.4783] [PMID: 32219428]

[25]   COVID-19. the use of intravenous immunoglobulins is also being tested - Rare Diseases Observatory [Internet]. [cited 2020 May 30]. Available from: https://www.osservatoriomalattierare.it/news/sperimentazioni/16006-covid-19-in-sperimentazione-anche-l-impiego-di-immunoglobul-ne-per-via-endovenosa

[26]   Xie Y, Cao S, Dong H, Li Q, Chen E, Zhang W, *et al.* Effect of regular intravenous immunoglobulin therapy on prognosis of severe pneumonia in patients with COVID-19 Journal of Infection. W.B. Saunders Ltd 2020.

[27]   Díez J-M, Romero C, Gajardo R. Currently available intravenous immunoglobulin contains antibodies reacting against severe acute respiratory syndrome coronavirus 2 antigens. Immunotherapy 2020; 12(8): 571-6.
[http://dx.doi.org/10.2217/imt-2020-0095] [PMID: 32397847]

[28]   Li T, Cao W, Liu X, Bai T, Fan H, Hong K, *et al.* High-Dose Intravenous Immunoglobulin as a Therapeutic Option for Deteriorating Patients With Coronavirus Disease 2019. [cited 2020 May 30]; Available from: https://academic.oup.com/ofid/article-abstract/7/3/ofaa102/5810740

[29]   Nie J, Li Q, Wu J, *et al.* Establishment and validation of a pseudovirus neutralization assay for SARS-CoV-2. Emerg Microbes Infect 2020; 9(1): 680-6.
[http://dx.doi.org/10.1080/22221751.2020.1743767] [PMID: 32207377]

[30]   Li Q, Guan X, Wu P, Wang X, Zhou L, Tong Y, *et al.* Early transmission dynamics in Wuhan, China, of novel coronavirus-infected pneumonia. New England Journal of Medicine Massachussetts Medical Society 2020; 382: 207-1199.

[31]   Khan S, Nakajima R, Jain A, de Assis RR, Jasinskas A, Obiero JM, *et al.* Analysis of Serologic Cross-Reactivity Between Common Human Coronaviruses and SARS-CoV-2 Using Coronavirus Antigen Microarray. bioRxiv 2020.https://www.biorxiv.org/content/10.1101/2020.03.24.006544v1
[http://dx.doi.org/10.1101/2020.03.24.006544]

[32]   Hu X, An T, Situ B, Hu Y, Ou Z, Li Q, *et al.* Heat inactivation of serum interferes with the immunoanalysis of antibodies to SARS-CoV-2 medRxiv 2020.

[http://dx.doi.org/10.1101/2020.03.12.20034231]

[33]   Jacofsky D, Jacofsky EM, Jacofsky M. Understanding antibody testing for COVID-19. J Arthroplasty 2020; 35(7S): S74-81.
[http://dx.doi.org/10.1016/j.arth.2020.04.055] [PMID: 32389405]

[34]   Zhao J, Yuan Q, Wang H, Liu W, Liao X, Su Y, *et al.* Antibody responses to SARS-CoV-2 in patients of novel coronavirus disease. 2019.
[http://dx.doi.org/10.1101/2020.03.02.20030189]

[35]   Wu F, Wang A, Liu M, Wang Q, Chen J, Xia S, *et al.* Neutralizing antibody responses to SARS-Co-2 in a COVID-19 recovered 1 patient cohort and their implications 2 3 medRxiv 2020.

[36]   Bermingham A, Chand MA, Brown CS, *et al.* Severe respiratory illness caused by a novel coronavirus, in a patient transferred to the United Kingdom from the Middle East, September 2012. Euro Surveill 2012; 17(40): 20290. http://www.eurosurveillance.org/ViewArticle.aspx?ArticleId=20290
[http://dx.doi.org/10.2807/ese.17.40.20290-en] [PMID: 23078800]

[37]   Assiri A, McGeer A, Perl TM, *et al.* Hospital outbreak of Middle East respiratory syndrome coronavirus. N Engl J Med 2013; 369(5): 407-16.
[http://dx.doi.org/10.1056/NEJMoa1306742] [PMID: 23782161]

[38]   Annan A, Baldwin HJ, Corman VM, *et al.* Human betacoronavirus 2c EMC/2012-related viruses in bats, Ghana and Europe. Emerg Infect Dis 2013; 19(3): 456-9.
[http://dx.doi.org/10.3201/eid1903.121503] [PMID: 23622767]

[39]   Margine I, Palese P, Krammer F. Expression of functional recombinant hemagglutinin and neuraminidase proteins from the novel H7N9 influenza virus using the baculovirus expression system. J Vis Exp 2013; (81): : e51112.
[http://dx.doi.org/10.3791/51112] [PMID: 24300384]

[40]   Hu X, *et al.* Heat inactivation of serum interferes with the immunoanalysis of antibodies to SARS-CoV-2 medRxiv 2020.
[http://dx.doi.org/10.1101/2020.03.12.20034231]

[41]   Li F, Li W, Farzan M, Harrison SC. Structure of SARS coronavirus spike receptor-binding domain complexed with receptor. Science 2005; 309(5742): 1864-8.
[http://dx.doi.org/10.1126/science.1116480] [PMID: 16166518]

[42]   Li G, De Clercq E. Therapeutic options for the 2019 novel coronavirus (2019-nCoV). Nat Rev Drug Discov 2020; 19(3): 149-50. Epub ahead of print
[http://dx.doi.org/10.1038/d41573-020-00016-0] [PMID: 32127666]

[43]   Klasse PJ. Neutralization of Virus Infectivity by Antibodies: Old Problems inNew Perspectives. Adv Biol. 2014; 2014: 157895. Coughlin MM, Prabhakar BS. Neutralizing human monoclonal antibodies tosevere acute respiratory syndrome coronavirus: target, mechanism of action,and therapeutic potential. Rev Med Virol 2012; 22: 2-17.

CHAPTER 10

Quantification of the SARS-CoV-2 RNA in Tissues by Quantitative Real Time-PCR

Abhinav Anand[1,2], Neha Sharma[1], Sonali Bajaj[1], Naman Wahal[3], Devesh Tewari[1] and Navneet Khurana[1,*]

[1] *School of Pharmaceutical Sciences, Lovely Professional University, Phagwara, Punjab, India*

[2] *CT Institute of Pharmaceutical Sciences, CT Group of Institutions, Shahpur, Jalandhar, Punjab, India*

[3] *Sardar Patel Medical College, Bikaner, Rajasthan, India*

Abstract: Severe Acute Respiratory Syndrome-coronavirus-2 (SARS-CoV-2) has become infamous recently due to its capability to cause a severe disease known as coronavirus disease-19 (COVID-19). Believed to have originated from Wuhan, Hubei province, China, SARS-CoV-2 has impacted a global scale, thereby making the World Health Organization (WHO) declare COVID-19 a pandemic. The range of R_0 values is between 2.43 and 3.10, showing the severity of the disease, highlighting this concern for health and public administration authorities. The major preventive steps from the governments and public health authorities are to conduct aggressive diagnostic tests and isolate the patients until the complete recovery of COVID-19. Out of various diagnostic methods, reverse transcription-polymerase chain reaction (RT-PCR) is an appropriate technique. The amplified RNA/DNA molecules can be quantified through quantitative real-time PCR (qRT-PCR). In this chapter, the basics of PCR shall be discussed along with the quantification of RNA from SARS-CoV-2 infected tissue samples.

Keywords: Coronavirus, COVID-19, Diagnosis, PCR, qPCR, RT-PCR.

INTRODUCTION

Human coronaviruses were first identified in the early 1960s, they have been associated with a significant incidence of infections in the upper respiratory tract. Since the beginning of the 21st century, at least five novel coronaviruses have been identified to cause severe human illnesses. It includes severe acute respiratory syndrome (SARS), Middle Eastern respiratory syndrome (MERS), and severe acute respiratory syndrome-coronavirus-2 (SARS-CoV-2), which caused

[*] **Corresponding author Navneet Khurana:** School of Pharmaceutical Sciences, Lovely Professional University, Phagwara, Punjab, India; E-mail: navi.pharmacist@gmail.com

Kamal Niaz & Muhammad Farrukh Nisar (Eds.)

remarkable mortalities [1]. Coronaviruses are members of the family Coronaviridae, subfamily Coronavirinae, and the order of Nidovirales. Four genera exist for coronaviruses *i.e.,* alphacoronavirus, betacoronavirus, deltacoronavirus, and gammacoronavirus. Genetic material contains a single positive-sense ribonucleic acid (RNA) instead of deoxyribonucleic acid (DNA). Therefore, the associated rates of mutation are higher compared to DNA viruses. This makes coronaviruses efficient for adapting and surviving for a longer time. Its genome encodes mainly four structural proteins, *i.e.,* Nucleocapsid (N), Envelope (E), Membrane (M), and Spike (S) protein, along with various other proteins that mediate the viral entry into the human cells and the subsequent replication in the host cells [2, 3]. N-proteins undergo complex formation with genomic RNA and show interaction with the viral membrane proteins while the assembly process of the virion is going on [4]. S-protein is critical for the binding of the virus to the host cell receptors. E-protein interacts with M-protein to form the viral envelope. M-protein is the central organizer of the viral assembly, and it also determines the shape of the virus envelope. It has been reported that some coronaviruses do not require a complete array of structural proteins to manufacture virions. It highlights that some proteins might be dispensable or compensated by the function of some accessory proteins [5].

SARS-CoV-2 was reported to cause severe pneumonia-like symptoms in the Wuhan city of China during December 2019. The natural reservoirs for the virus are likely the bats. It is believed that the virus started infecting humans after crossing species barriers, including other intermediate hosts like food animals and wild animals. However, the intermediate host(s) has(have) not been exactly identified to date [5, 6]. SARS-CoV-2 is rapidly contagious and spread across the globe. In January 2020, the outbreak was announced by the world health organization (WHO) as a Public Health Emergency of International Concern (PHEIC) under International Health Regulations (IHR, 2005). This was done following the reports of its spread to eighteen countries, along with human-t--human transmission. Originally, the virus was named a 2019-novel coronavirus (2019-nCoV). Later, experts from the International Committee on Taxonomy of Viruses (ICTV) officially renamed it SARS-CoV-2 as it is strikingly similar to the causative pathogen of SARS [7]. In March 2020, WHO declared COVID-19 as a pandemic. In this statement, the Director-General of WHO, General Tedros Adhanom Ghebreyesus, stated, "Let me be clear: describing this as a pandemic does not mean that countries should give up". The idea that countries should shift from containment to mitigation is wrong and dangerous [8, 9]. SARS-CoV-2, a novel human infecting betacoronavirus, binds to the angiotensin-converting enzyme 2 (ACE-2) receptor in humans [10]. The median incubation period of the disease is around five days (similar to SARS). Going by some conservative assumptions, 101 of 10,000 cases, *i.e.,* the 99th percentile, will develop clinical manifestations of the disease after fourteen days of quarantine or active monitoring [11].

The features of the spread of the virus necessitate governments and public health authorities to screen the infected persons actively. For this reason, source control measures should be adequately in place for everyone in the facility, irrespective of the symptoms. Everyone who came in contact with the patient must be identified and tested for COVID-19. Post identification, the patients can be isolated from other healthy individuals to counter pathogen and limit its transmission. If anyone reports that he/she has symptoms due to travel history of COVID-19 active nation/country/sovereignty. If he/she came in close contact with someone who has a travel history or symptoms, the person should be immediately quarantined and tested [12]. Several other diagnostic tests remain a gold standard diagnostic tool like serological antigen-antibody reaction assays, biosensor test, luminescent immunoassay, neutralization assay, lateral flow immunoassay, and reverse transcriptase-polymerase chain reaction (RT-PCR) [13]. RT-PCR is generally used to denote reverse transcriptase-polymerase chain reaction, whereas real-time PCR is usually denoted as qRT-PCR or qPCR to avoid confusion [14].

RT-PCR involves the reverse transcription of the viral RNA into cDNA, which is further amplified to make several hundred copies. It requires a very small amount of the specimen and is highly accurate. To date, the majority of the molecular diagnosis is based upon the usage of RT-PCR [13, 15]. A modification of the technology, *i.e.,* qPCR, allows us to quantitatively analyze the DNA amplicons produced in the PCR process in real-time [16]. In this chapter, we shall discuss PCR, RT-PCR, and qRT-PCR.

General Diagnostic Methods in Virology

Laboratory diagnosis of critical illnesses needs to be elaborate and accurate to enable the healthcare providers to execute effective clinical management of the disease. However, errors in diagnosis may translate to the loss of money and/or loss of life [17].

Viral infections and associated diseases (hepatitis, AIDS, influenza, SARS, MERS, and COVID-19, *etc.*) have been associated with several socioeconomic impacts. Viral diseases are difficult to treat and relatively complex to diagnose compared to bacterial diseases. Several reasons make the diagnosis of viral infections difficult. Viruses cannot be cultured on simple *in vitro* culture media; rather, highly specialized and expensive methods are needed (like cell cultures). Viruses are more prone to mutations than other pathogens. Viruses can establish an infection without significant clinical manifestations, thereby bypassing the need for medical attention. Also, viruses have high diversity amongst themselves mostly for surface glycoproteins and the parent genetic material, either DNA or the RNA) [18 - 20].

Diagnosis of viral diseases is undertaken to document a previously existing infection or provide assistance to diagnose an acute illness. Ideally, the virus's replication cycle, the appearance of associated clinical manifestations, generation of immunoglobulins (IgG and IgM), elimination/neutralization phase of the virus, and the resolution of the illness occur in a progression that can be predicted [21]. The aim and scope of the diagnosis vary from virus to virus. If the disease involves a viral replication and degeneration of the host cell, the diagnostic technique should focus on detecting the virus. In this case, efforts should be made to perform the diagnosis as early as possible, *i.e.,* when the viral titer is still high. On the other hand, some viral infections are linked with an immunological response which further mediates the disease progress. Here, the diagnostic focus should be on detecting the antibodies [22].

Several techniques are employed for the diagnosis of viral infections. The most common technique is viral isolation, wherein a conventional cell culture is utilized. The assay takes from 1 to 21 days depending upon the causative virus. The assay comes with certain merits as well as creates a possibility for isolation of several viruses, allows detection of the novel or unexpected viruses, and provides more sensitivity than antigen detection. The technique is limited by the necessity of expertise to interpret the cytopathic effect and maintain cell cultures. Also, not all viruses grow in routine cultures. This technique also creates a biohazard involving zoonotic and other novel viruses. Another variant of this technique involves rapid culture with an assay time of 1-5 days. However, it detects only targeted viruses [19, 23]. Another popularly used technique is antibody detection. Several viruses induce the production of specific antibodies, which can be detected by using several methods like enzyme-linked immunosorbent assay (ELISA) [24], enzyme immunoassay (EIA) [25], chemiluminescent immunoassay (CLIA) [26], immunofluorescence (IF) [27], immunochromatography (IC) [28], immunoblot (IB) [29], and IgG avidity assay [30]. These assays are rather rapid (assay time <30 min-24 h). These form the basis of the rapid testing kits available in the market. These can be automated and do not require special skills. However, cross-reactivity between similar viruses can occur, thereby increasing the incidence of false-positive reports. Another demerit of this technique is that immunocompromised patients may not produce antibodies. Conversely, some diagnostic tests also focus on the detection of antigens [31].

Some of the various molecular diagnostic tests for SARS-CoV-2 are summarized in Table **1** [32].

Table 1. Some of the molecular diagnostic tests for SARS-CoV-2.

Name of the Test	Type of the Test	Manufacturer/ Organization	Source of Sample	Target Gene or Region	Time for Result/Additional Information	Throughput Information
ID NOW COVID-19	Isothermal nucleic acid amplification technology	Abbot Diagnostic, Scarborough	Throat, nasal and nasopharyngeal swabs	RdRP gene	Positive: less than 5 min; Negative: 13 min	1 sample/run
iAMP COVID-19 detection kit	Real-time RT isothermal amplification test	AtilaBioSystems	Nasal, nasopharyngeal, and oropharyngeal swabs	ORF1ab, N gene	Less than 1.5 h	High throughput
BioFire COVID-19 test	Multiplex real-time RT-PCR	BioFireDefense	Nasopharyngeal swabs	ORF1ab, ORF8, N gene	About 45 min	94 samples/run
CDC 2019-Novel Coronavirus Real-Time RT-PCR Diagnostic Panel	Real-time RT-PCR	CDC-US	Aspirates/ washes and swabs from nasopharyngeal or oropharyngeal tracts/ and fluid from bronchoalveolar lavage, tracheal aspirates, sputum	N gene	Human RNase P gene (as control)	264 samples/day
CRISPR dependent tests for SARS-CoV-2	CRISPR based lateral flow assay isothermal amplification	Cepheid Sherlock Biosciences	Respiratory Samples	Viral RNA	Merges Sherlock's Cas13 and Cas12 enzymes for detection of nucleic acid with Cepheid's GeneXpert test-processing equipment	Data not available

Nucleic Acid Amplification Test (NAAT)

NAAT is an important technique in molecular biology and biotechnology. It has been widely employed in medicine, research, forensics, and agriculture. It is a highly sensitive method, especially for viruses that cannot be cultivated/grown in cell cultures. NAAT is more rapid and safer than the culturing techniques as the pathogen containing the sample is processed to deactivate and disrupt the virus [33]. The viruses contain either DNA or RNA as their genetic material. This technique is based upon amplifying the genetic material to execute the qualitative and quantitative analyses [34] effectively. The specific reaction that is used for NAAT is known as PCR. Invented by Mullis, PCR continues to be the method of choice for nucleic acid amplification [35]. Kary Mullis was awarded Nobel Prize in Chemistry in 1993 for his credit for this innovation [36].

PCR

Originally, while contemplating the process of amplifying the DNA, Kary Mullis, *et al.* [35] assumed that when the denatured DNA is subjected to the primers. They extend, and the products formed after the extension would tend to unwind from their templates, get primed again, and reiterate the extension phase. However, this did not happen. The DNA had to be subjected to immense heat, approaching the boiling temperatures after each synthesis cycle to cause denaturation of the newly formed, double-stranded DNA [37]. At such a high temperature, the DNA polymerase-I that was being utilized in the synthetic process was then inactivated, especially at the Klenow fragment. Therefore, the enzyme requirement increased at the beginning of each cycle, as Kleppe had predicted [38].

A revolutionary development that paved the way for the unequivocal usage of the PCR technique was the concept of employing a heat-tolerant DNA polymerase. The thermostable Taq DNA polymerase replaced the Klenow fragment of DNA polymerase I [39, 40]. With the introduction of Taq DNA polymerase, multiple rounds of DNA amplification were conducted in a closed tube without the addition of more enzymes. Also, the amplification of larger fragments became possible. This revolutionary concept increased the replication fidelity, allowed the direct detection of the products, and decreased the non-specificity of the product formation [41 - 43].

Components of PCR Assay

There are six critical components of a PCR assay on which the success of the assay depends [44, 45].

Template DNA

The template for PCR can be derived from any source of DNA, such as complementary DNA (cDNA), genomic DNA (gDNA), or even plasmid DNA. However, the optimal input amount varies from source to source, *e.g.,* for 50 µL of PCR volume, up to 50ng of gDNA may be required, whereas up to 1ng of plasmid DNA would suffice. In some cases, the re-amplification of PCR products is also done to increase the yield. The input amount of DNA has to be optimized well as lesser amounts decrease the yield and greater amounts elevate the risk of non-specific amplification. More often than not, the standard protocols for PCR may require the DNA input as a copy number, specifically for gDNA. The following formula can obtain copy number:

$$\text{Copy number} = L \times n$$

Where L is Avogadro's constant, n is the number of moles

DNA Polymerase

The enzyme DNA polymerase plays a pivotal role in the replication of the target DNA. The revolutionary Taq DNA polymerase has now become universally accepted for the PCR process. With a half-life of about 40 minutes at 95°C, it can amplify the lengths of approximately 5kb while incorporating approximately 60 nucleotide bases per second (70°C) [46]. In a conventional 50 µL PCR mixture, 1-2 units of DNA polymerase are adequate.

Primers

These are synthetically obtained oligonucleotides having about 15-30 bases. They are designed to form a bond (mediated through the complementarity of sequences) to the sequences. The following formula can be utilized to assess the melting temperature (T_m) of short oligonucleotides *i.e.* those with less than 25 bases [47]: It flanks the area of interest in the template.

$$T_m = 2(A+T) + 4(G+C)$$

The primers should have T_m within 5°C of each other. The primers must also exhibit sequence homology to enhance the specificity of amplification. In the reaction process, DNA polymerase acts to extend the primers from their 3' ends. The binding sites of the primers should be specific to the target with minimal or no resemblance to other sequences present on the input DNA to guarantee specific amplification. In the reaction, primers are added in the range of 0.1-1 µM. If the primer has degenerate bases, then the primer at the concentrations of 0.3-1 µ Mis generally suitable.

Deoxynucleoside Triphosphates (dNTPs)

dNTPs are the necessary building blocks for molecules of nucleic acids. They are important for the PCR process as without them, amplified DNA cannot be generated. Four individual nucleotides constitute the sequence of DNA (deoxyadenosine triphosphate-dATP, deoxythymidine triphosphate-dTTP, deoxycytosine triphosphate-dCTP, and deoxyguanosine triphosphate-dGTP). They are generally added to the PCR mix in an equimolar amount [48]. Commonly, the final concentration of each dNTP in the PCR mix is 0.2 mM. Higher concentrations of dNTPs may be added specifically to shield the process from ions like Mg^{2+} as dNTPs bind to them, thereby rendering them unavailable for incorporation. It should be noted that concentrations of dNTPs above the optimal concentration may also hinder PCR.

Magnesium Ions (Mg^{2+})

Free Mg^{2+} is essential for the activity of DNA polymerase as the ions act as a cofactor. On the other hand, Mg^{2+} can undergo complexation with DNA templates, primers, and dNTPs [49]. They help to incorporate dNTPs during the polymerization stage, where Mg^{2+} aid in catalyzing the formation of phosphodiester bonds between the phosphate group of the dNTP and the 3'-OH of the primer. Also, Mg^{2+} facilitates the complexation between DNA templates and the primer as they stabilize the negative charge due to the phosphate backbones. The Mg^{2+} ions are added to the PCR mixture in the form of an $MgCl_2$ solution. If sulfate groups are needed to provide robust and reproducible performance, Mg^{2+} ions are delivered as $MgSO_4$ solution. Typically, in the conventional PCR process, the final concentration of Mg^{2+} lies in the range of 1-4 mM. 0.5 mM titration increments are generally recommended to optimize the process.

Buffer

Generally, TNK buffers are used in the PCR process tris(T), ammonium (N), and potassium (K) as they adapt the conditions of the assay according to various primer pairs [50]. Buffers are needed to impart a conducive chemical environment to facilitate the activity of DNA polymerase. The pH of the buffer generally lies between 8-9.5 and is usually stabilized by Tris-HCl. K^+ delivered by KCl is an essential component for Taq DNA polymerase as it promotes the annealing of the primer. Ammonium ions (NH^{4+}) destabilize the weak hydrogen bonds formed due to mismatching of the primer-template base pairing, thereby improving the specificity of the reaction.

It should be noted that Mg^{2+} ions and K^+ ions have an overlapping stabilizing effect. Therefore $MgCl_2$ concentration is kept lower (1.5 ± 0.25 mM) when it is to be added to a KCl containing buffer, but higher (2.0 ± 0.5 mM) in an $(NH_4)_2SO_4$ buffer.

Apart from these 6 essential components of the PCR technique, certain additives and/or co-solvents can be employed to enhance the process [51] (Table **2**).

Table 2. Common co-solvents or additives employed to enhance PCR.

Name of Additive/co-solvent	Recommended Concentration
Dimethyl sulfoxide (DMSO)	1 to 10%
Glycerol	5 to 20%
Formamide	1.25 to 10%
Bovine Serum Albumin (BSA)	10 to 100 µg/mL
Ammonium sulphate	15 to 30 mM
Polyethylene glycol (PEG)	5 to 15%
Gelatin	0.01%
Non-ionic detergents	0.05 to 1%
N,N,N-trimethylglycine	1 to 3M

The Process of PCR

A conventional cycle of PCR consists of 3 broad steps, as illustrated in Fig. (**1**):

1. **Initial denaturation**: The reaction temperature is elevated to 95 °C, the reaction mixture is incubated for 2-5 minutes (maximum up to 10 minutes depending upon the template complexity and the enzyme characteristics). It is done to ensure that all the complex, double-stranded DNA (dsDNA) molecules are segregated into individual strands, which can be further amplified.
2. **Cycling**: This involves three steps.
   a. Denaturation: Just like in the initial denaturation, the temperature is elevated to 95°C to melt (Breakdown the hydrogen bonds between complementary bases) entire dsDNA into single-stranded DNA (ssDNA) molecules.
   b. Annealing: The temperature is reduced to 5°C, below the T_m of the primers (generally 45–60 °C). It is done to enhance the binding of the primer to the template.
   c. Extension: The temperature is again elevated to 72°C, which is optimized for DNA polymerase activity, which further allows the extension of the hybridized primers.
3. **Repeat**: The above cycling steps are performed repeatedly, leading to exponential amplification of the amplicon [52] (Fig. **2**).

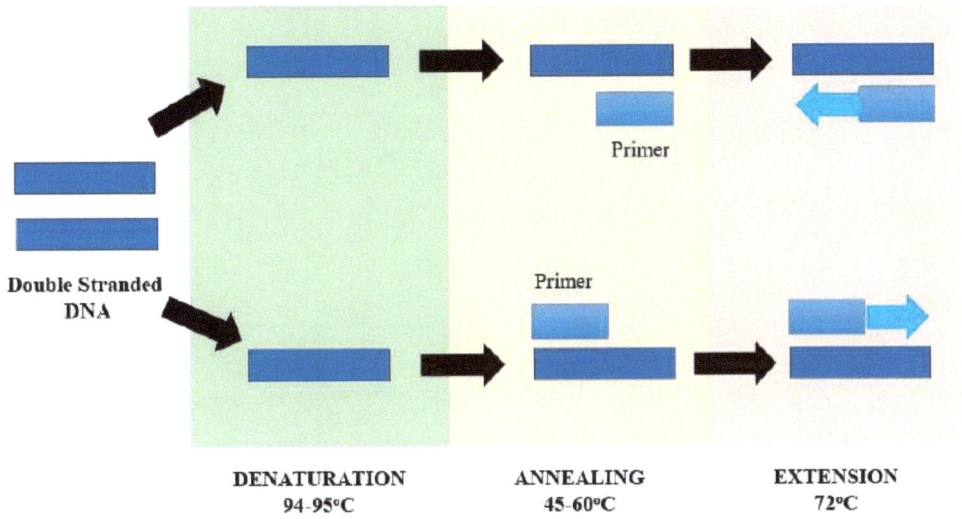

Fig. (1). The cycling of PCR.

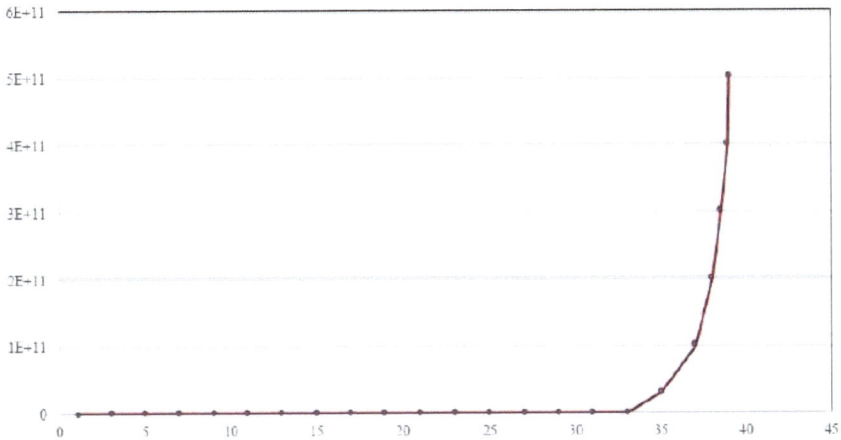

Fig. (2). Theoretical PCR amplification of a single target molecule (X-axis represents the PCR cycles. The Y-axis represents the total number of amplicon molecules).

PCR Kinetics

A traditional PCR reaction generally takes place in three stages [53]:

• the exponential phase,

• the non-exponential phase, and

• plateau or end-point phase (Fig. **3**)

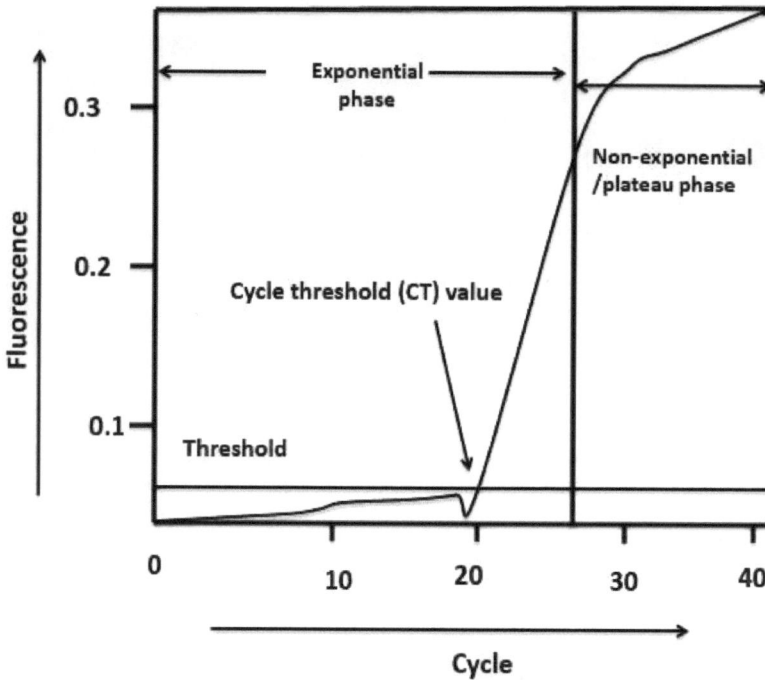

Fig. (3). Plot of amplification showing the PCR kinetics (baseline fluorescence is subtracted).

As each PCR cycle begins, all constituting elements are available in an adequately high quantity to ensure good nucleotide amplification. As the PCR proceeds and unused/unoccupied elements are available, the amplification shows an exponential trend, *i.e.,* the reaction progresses, producing double the quantity of initially present DNA with each cycle. As the cycles further proceed and the reagent elements of the reaction mixture undergo depletion, the overall reaction slows down. Here, the PCR product does not get increased by double with each cycle. The non-exponential amplification takes place where samples tend to diverge in their respective quantities. Following multiple cycles of being amplified, the PCR no longer produces a template due to the limitation of critical elements' reaction. This phase is generally referred to as the end-point or the plateau phase of the PCR. Some studies have also emphasized that the primary reason behind PCR plateau formation is depletion of the primer and not the degradation of reagents or product accumulation [54, 55].

Reverse Transcription PCR (RT-PCR)

SARS-CoV-2, previously named 2019-nCOV, is the causative pathogen behind the COVID-19 pandemic [56]. After intense research, it was reported that SARS-CoV-2 is a single-stranded, positive-sense RNA virus categorized under the genus betacoronavirus [10, 57, 58]. RT-PCR is a sensitive technique to detect and quantify the RNA from a single cell sample [59]. Some other techniques can be used to quantify mRNAs, like nuclease protection assay and Northern blot analysis. However, these techniques need larger amounts of RNA [60, 61]. During RT-PCR, the RNA sample is added along with the enzyme reverse transcriptase. These are added to the standard PCR components. The PCR mixture is subjected to a temperature of 37°C, which initiates the reverse transcription of the RNA sample to cDNA. The formed cDNA undergoes annealing to one of the primers, causing the synthesis of the first strand. Standard PCR progresses to yield dsDNA [62] (Fig. **4**). RT-PCR is a routine diagnostic tool in virology and is often used in association with qRT-PCR. Therefore, combining the two techniques allows the quantification of transcript levels of RNA in the isolated cells/tissues [63].

RT-PCR for SARS-CoV-2

For running a diagnostic test of SARS-CoV-2 respiratory material should be collected, at a minimum. In ambulatory patients, nasopharyngeal and oropharyngeal wash or swab can be collected. Also, bronchoalveolar lavage or sputum and endotracheal aspirate can be collected in patients in a more severe stage of the associated respiratory disorder. The collected samples should reach the virology laboratory as soon as possible. During transportation, correct handling of the samples is necessary. If the samples can be delivered to the testing laboratory readily, they should be stored and transported at 2-8 °C. If the laboratory is far from where the sample has to be shipped, a viral transport medium is essential. Alternatively, the samples can be subjected to freezing between -20 °C to -70 °C and shipped in a container having an ample amount of dry ice. If the shipment is expected to delay, then, repeated freezing and thawing of the samples should be avoided. A routine confirmatory test of COVID-19 is conducted to detect certain unique sequences of viral RNA by NAAT.

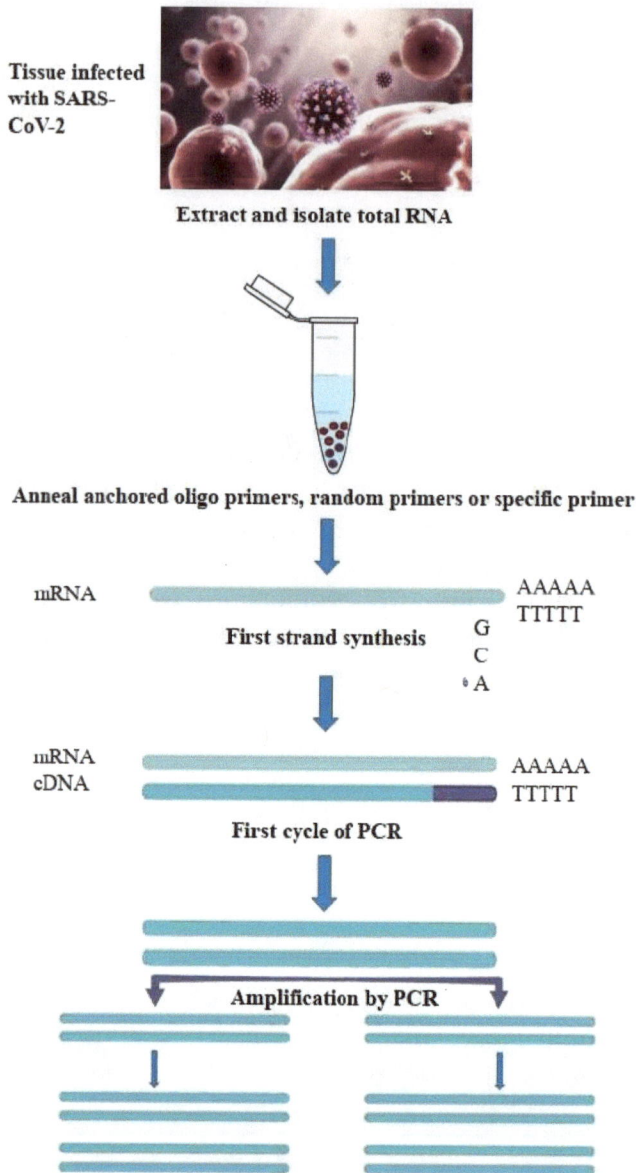

Fig. (4). The schematic representation of the steps involved in RT-PCR.

Additionally, nucleic acid sequencing can be done to solidify the diagnosis. The viral genes usually the target for diagnosis are the N, E, S, and RNA-dependent RNA polymerase (rDRP) genes. The extraction process should be carried out inside a biosafety hood present in a Biosafety Level-2 (BSL-2) facility. The sample should not be heated before the extraction of RNA [64 - 66].

The diagnosis can also produce false-negative results in certain conditions [64]:

- An objectionable quality of the collected sample containing insufficient material from the patient
- Collection of the sample too early or too late during the cycle of infection
- Mishandling of the sample during the transportation
- Technical reasons such as inhibition of PCR or viral mutation.

It is understood that the interpretation of the results as qualitative, quantitative, or semi-quantitative is essential. A minimum of two molecular targets must be analyzed during the PCR process to avoid the possibility of cross-reaction with other endemic coronaviruses along with the probable genetic drift of SARS-Co--2. The ideal approach would be the inclusion ofo include at least one specific region and one conserved region to minimize/abolish the effects of genetic drift, specifically if the virus undergoes evolution as it passes through different populations [67]. As the CT value in RT-PCR can vary due to batch effect, such alterations amidst different cycles of runs should be closely assessed [15, 68, 69].

Real-time PCR/Quantitative PCR (qPCR)

The qRT-PCR is a detection technique that allows the quantitative analysis of the PCR product in real-time. qRT-PCR does not take the support of any downstream method like densitometry or electrophoresis. It is very versatile. It enables the researchers to assess multiple targets at the same time [70]. qRT-PCR was developed as an efficient, rapid, and precise method under NAAT. It offers a few advantages over the conventional PCR, like:

- qRT-PCR merges the amplification and detection of nucleic acids into a single step
- qRT-PCR requires lesser amounts of starting material as compared to traditional PCR
- qRT-PCR offers the possibility of quantifying the product based on fluorescence detection
- In qRT-PCR, there is no need for the post-amplification process.

Detecting the template DNA (or RNA if subjected to RT before amplification) happens in real-time and is based on when the PCR product gets amplified beyond the threshold of CT number. Key applications of qPCR include - mRNA (gene expression) analysis, non-coding and micro RNA analyses, detection of genetic variations and mutations, single nucleotide polymorphism analysis, genotyping, and allelic discrimination [71, 72].

It was a great achievement in PCR usage when the concept of real-time analysis of DNA amplification by monitoring the fluorescence was introduced [73, 74]. In qRT-PCR, after each cycle, the fluorescence is noted. Its intensity indicates the number of DNA amplicons present in the specimen during that time. Initially, the fluorescent signals are too weak to be differentiated from the background. The point where the intensity of the fluorescent signals goes beyond the detectable level relates proportionally to the initial amount of DNA in the specimen. This particular point is known as the quantification cycle (C_q). C_q makes it possible to determine the absolute amount of the target DNA molecules in the specimen as per the standard calibration curve made using serial dilutions of the reference samples with known copy numbers or concentrations. qRT-PCR is also capable of delivering semi-quantitative results without using the reference but using controls as standards. Here, the results are generally given as lesser or greater multiples with standard to control [75 - 77].

Live visualization of the amplified DNA molecules/fragments can be done in two ways, *i.e.,* by using oligonucleotide probes labeled with fluorescent material or using non-specific fluorescent DNA dyes [73, 74]. A singleplex qPCR process only one gene- either the control or the target gene is amplified in each equipment well. In multiplexing, the amount of specimen needed for qPCR reaction can be decreased by recording the expression of multiple genes simultaneously. Multiplexing does not compromise the accuracy of the assay but is a fairly complex method [78, 79].

There are numerous accessory equipment available in the market for qRT-PCR, varying in terms of cycle time, cost, flexibility, and throughput. An ideal qRT-PCR instrument must provide the possibility of temperature control for DNA amplification, light excitation, and collection of fluorescent signals of apt wavelength (λ). The equipment may vary in terms of the following factors:

- Rates of heating and cooling (reaction speed)
- Uniformity and precision in controlling the temperature
- Throughput
- Range of excitation λ
- Range of detection λ
- Sensitivity
- Ease of use
- Pricing

The choice of equipment is dictated by the desired application/output of the assay [80].

Kralik and Ricchi [81] have described the mathematical principle behind qRT-PCR. Theoretically, the amount of DNA molecules doubled proceeding each cycle (In 100% efficiency) in PCR. Usually, the following equation describes the amplification reaction:

$$N_n = N_0 \, (\eta + 1)^n \tag{1}$$

Where N_n = amount of amplicons generated post n number of cycles of PCR

N_0 = starting amount of template copies in the specimen

η = Efficiency of the PCR, which can have values 0-1 (0-100%)

n = Number of cycles

Assumingly, if N_0 is taken as 1 and η is taken as 100%, the equation can be re-written as:

$$N_n = (2)^n \tag{2}$$

If a standard calibration curve is constructed, generally, 10X serial dilutions are utilized. The difference in C_q values between two 10X serial dilutions can be written as:

$$10 = (2)^n \tag{3}$$

Therefore, n equals 3.322. If η is to be determined and the equation (1) is taken as the starting point, then:

$$\eta = 10^{-(1/n)} - 1$$

Therefore, if n is 3.322, then η is =1 *i.e.* 100%

Another way to determine the relative expression (R) of genes is the Livak-Schmittgen method [82]. It compares two values in the exponent that represent normalized expression value for a target gene in specimen A compared to specimen B.

$$R = 2^{-[(Cq;TGA - Cq;REFA) - (Cq;TGB - Cq;REFB)]} = 2^{-(\Delta Cq;A - \Delta Cq;B)} = 2^{-\Delta\Delta Cq}$$

Where TG is the target gene, REF is a reference/standard gene. The exponential base of 2 applied in this equation is representative of an assumption that the process is 100% efficient for both genes. This equation has an obvious limitation of ignoring the actual efficiency of the process. Therefore, it may lead to inaccuracies in the results [83 - 85].

Addressing this issue, Pfaffl later published an expression to calculate R factoring in the efficiencies between two specimen types [86]:

$$R = \eta_{TG}^{-\Delta Cq;TG} / \eta_{REF}^{-\Delta Cq;REF}$$

There are online resources that give free pre-made Microsoft Excel templates which allow the users to enter the value obtained in the assay and deliver the results based upon Pfaffl's method [87] (Fig. **5**).

Instructions
1. Calculate the primer efficiencies for the gene of interest (GOI) and housekeeping gene (HKG). Click here for a how-to guide on this. Enter these into the red boxes below
2. Calculate the average Ct values for all GOI samples and insert them into the 'GOI average Ct' column.
3. Calculate the average Ct values for HKG for all samples and insert them into the 'HKG average Ct' column.
4. Do not change any of the other cells.
5. The 'gene expression ratio' should be calculated for you (in the green box).

Primer efficiencies:	Efficiency %	Converted efficiency E
Gene of interest (GOI)		1
Housekeeping gene (HKG)		1

$$Gene\ expression\ ratio = \frac{(E_{GOI})^{\Delta Ct\ GOI}}{(E_{HKG})^{\Delta Ct\ HKG}}$$

Sample	GOI average Ct	ΔCt GOI	HKG average Ct	ΔCt HKG	Gene expression ratio
Control 1		=DIV/0!		=DIV/0!	=DIV/0!
Control 2		=DIV/0!		=DIV/0!	=DIV/0!
Control 3		=DIV/0!		=DIV/0!	=DIV/0!
Treated 1		=DIV/0!		=DIV/0!	=DIV/0!
Treated 2		=DIV/0!		=DIV/0!	=DIV/0!
Treated 3		=DIV/0!		=DIV/0!	=DIV/0!

Group	Average	Standard deviation	Standard error
Control	=DIV/0!	=DIV/0!	=DIV/0!
Treated	=DIV/0!	=DIV/0!	=DIV/0!

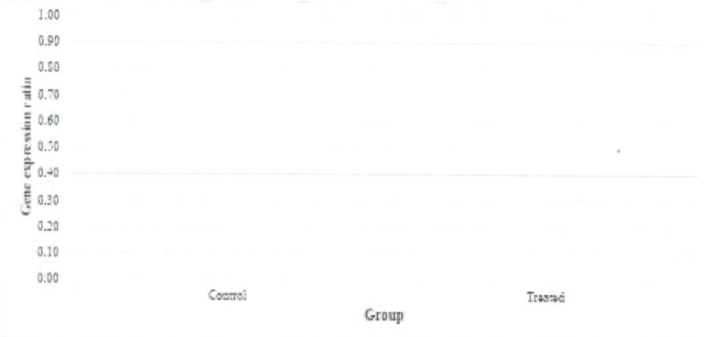

Fig. (5). Template for calculation of R based upon Pfaffl's method.

The Efficiency of the Assay: The Mathematical Model

The mathematical model of Booth *et al.* [88] makes the following assumptions:

- Symmetry exists in sense and antisense molecules. Therefore, the forward and reverse primers are present in equal amounts, and they undergo annealing to an equal amount of sense and antisense ssDNA strands.
- The efficiencies of DNA damage and polymerase damage are not different for each cycle of PCR.
- The temperature at which annealing occurs is adequately below the melting temperature of the primer, and that the annealing reactions cannot be reversed.
- No untoward reactions such as mispriming and primer-dimer formation are taken into account.

1. Efficiency of denaturing

dsDNA yields ssDNA, which is susceptible to depurination, oxidation, and hydrolytic attack. Consequently, a loss of template can happen during this step [89 - 93]. The denaturing efficiency $\eta_d \leq 1$ can be defined; so that after the denaturation, the amount of undamaged ssDNA which can undergo annealing is:

$$\overline{S_0^j} = \eta_d \, \overline{D_e^{j-1}}$$

Where S is the number of full-length top/bottom ssDNA templates, η is efficiency, D is the number of dsDNA molecules, j is the cycle number.

2. Efficiency of annealing

The competitive binding dictates the annealing efficiency- 5'-3' ssDNA (Sj$_0$). It may bind either complementary 3'-5' ssDNA strands to generate dsDNA or to the primers (Pj$_0$) to yield binary complexes. The ratio between templates to primers at the commencement of the stage of annealing in the jth cycle is defined as:

$$\gamma^j = \overline{S_0^j} \, / \, \overline{P_0^j}$$

Where γ is the ratio of template to primers, S is the number of full-length top/bottom ssDNA template molecules, P is the number of forward/reverse primer molecules, j is the cycle number.

The ratio is less in the initial cycles ($\gamma^j \ll 10^{-2}$). In contrast, the primers are utilized, and there is an increase in the number of templates. Therefore, cycle number γ^j also increases.

3. The efficiency of primer annealing

The following equation gives the expression for efficiency of annealing:

$$\eta_a^j = \frac{1}{\gamma_j} - \delta^j$$

Where η is the efficiency, γ is the ratio of template to primers, δ is the least amount of primer remaining post the annealing period, j is the cycle number.

4. The efficiency of polymerase binding

The following equation gives the efficiency of polymerase binding:

$$\eta_E^j = \frac{\text{Total ternary complexes formed at the end of elongation}}{\text{Total binary and ternary complexes formed}}$$

$$= \frac{C^j(\tau_e)}{B^j(\tau_e) + C^j(\tau_e)}$$

Where η is the efficiency, τ_e is the dimensionless time at the end of the elongation period, C is the number of ternary complexes (primer-ssDNA template-polymerase), B is the number of binary complexes (primer-ssDNA template), j is the cycle number.

5. Efficiency of elongation

The elongation efficiency can be defined as the ratio of the ternary complexes that extend fully to all ternary complexes formed.

$$\eta_e^j = \frac{C^j(\tau_c)}{C^j(\tau_e)}$$

Where η is the efficiency, τ_e is the dimensionless time at the end of the elongation period, τ_c is the dimensionless form of the cut-off time, C is the number of ternary complexes (primer-ssDNA template-polymerase), and j is the cycle number.

Accuracy of qPCR

The following points deal with the comparison of standard materials or methods with novel qPCR methods. Accuracy is a desirable factor of any diagnostic assay. Accuracy may be simply defined as the degree of agreement between measured and standard values. In binary classification assays (qualitative), the specimens processed *via* a novel assay method that needs to be verified are categorized as per their agreement with the standard method in four classes (Table **3**). This classification is based upon the statistical tool referred to as the error matrix and permits the estimation of various parameters that describe the potential of the qPCR assay [81].

Table 3. Parameters to compare qPCR results with a standard method presented as a 2X2 error matric contingency table.

		Reference Method	
		Positive	Negative
Alternative method	Positive	True positive (TP)	False-positive (FP)
	Negative	False-negative (FN)	True Negative (TN)

Diagnostic sensitivity = TP/(TP+FN)

It refers to the capability of the novel test to accurately identify specimens recognized by the standard method. Lesser diagnostic sensitivity corresponds to poor inclusivity of the tested qPCR.

Diagnostic specificity= TN/(FP+TN)

It refers to the capability of the test to accurately identify the specimens which were reported to be negative by the standard method. Lesser diagnostic specificity corresponds to a poor exclusivity of the tested qPCR.

Relative accuracy= (TN+TP)/ (FP+FN+TP+TN)

It elucidates the proportion of all accurately identified specimens amongst all specimens. If FN and FP are not detected, then the relative accuracy is 100%. In every other scenario, it is less than 100% [94].

Precision of qPCR

Precision refers to the extent of agreement between measurements under particular conditions. The statistical descriptors of precision are confidence limit or standard deviation (SD). Also, some assays use variance to describe the precision/imprecision of the assay. Variance is nothing but the square of SD. Generally, an assumption is made in laboratory conditions that the variance follows a normal distribution upon repeated analysis. It is also termed as Laplace-Gaussian distribution. Therefore, applying the principle of analysis of variance (ANOVA), the following equation holds:

$$\sigma^2_{total} = \sigma^2_{within\ run} + \sigma^2_{between\ run}$$

Where σ is the SD and σ^2 is the variance.

When something has to be measured in a matrix, the SD (σ) and the mean (μ) is unknown and therefore can only be subjected to estimation. The estimates of σ and μ are generally expressed as s and $\bar{x}$, respectively. In the case of 'n' measurements:

$$\bar{x} = \Sigma x/n$$

$$s^2 = \Sigma(x - \bar{x})^2/n\text{-}1$$

The coefficient of variation (CV) is expressed as:

$$CV = [(s/x)]\ 100\%$$

The term precision is related to the concept of variation around a central value; what is measured is imprecision [95]. The determination of qRT-PCR precision needs quantitative data. On the other hand, it is also possible to determine the precision of the process qualitatively. The results are assessed objectively, *i.e.,* negative/positive. Such an approach can be utilized to validate a specific, novel qRT-PCR method in different laboratory set-ups [81].

Validation of a novel qPCR assay

It is important to validate a novel qPCR assay to ascertain the performance and scope. The characteristics of performance that need to evaluated are given in Table **4** [80, 96]:

Table 4. Validation parameters for novel qPCR assay.

Characteristic of Performance	Performance of qPCR Assay	Experimental Process
Dynamic range	Concentrations over which the assay presents linearity	Serial dilutions from a known concentration of DNA
Repeatability	Variations in result under strictly controlled conditions	The same analyst repeating the same analysis on the same specimen using the same equipment in the same laboratory over time
Reproducibility	Variation in result under varying conditions	Different analysts repeating the same analysis on the same specimen but by using different equipment in different laboratories over time
Bias	Persistent under or overestimation of the actual result	The assigned value is compared to the mean measured value of a standard material
Specificity	The capability of the assay in terms of detection of a molecule of interest but no other compounds present in the specimen	Performance of the assay in the presence of various related targets to screen the occurrence of FP signals
Sensitivity (Limit of Detection; LOD / Limit of Quantitation; LOQ)	The least amount of the target which is reliably detectable/quantifiable	The assay is executed on increasing dilutions of the analyte to ascertain the LOD/linearity

CONCLUDING REMARKS

Aggressive diagnosis and subsequent isolation of the patients is a major task and probably the most important way to contain the spread of SARS-CoV-2. Each individual is responsible for keeping himself/herself safe from being infected by using masks, hand sanitizer, washing hands, and maintaining social distancing. However, owing to the community spread, screening of people at large is required. In spite of multiple diagnostic tools, RT-PCR is a standardized test for the detection of COVID-19. It may not be as rapid as other options available, but it delivers extreme precision in the results. Its modification into qRT-PCR has ushered in an era of powerful and impactful microbial diagnostics. In the case of viral infections, the appropriateness of this test is beyond any doubt. It provides superlative sensitivity and specificity to the target molecule amidst a mixed background. The samples processed in qRT-PCR bypass the need for post-PCR analytical tests. Also, the qRT-PCR process is carried out in the same tube throughout instead of the conventional PCR.

Consequently, it becomes nearly impossible to contaminate the product. qRT-PCR has emerged as a boon to the field of molecular diagnostics, especially for viral diagnostics. The improvements in technology have popularized qRT-PCR in the analytical community, however, several challenges are still there.

CONSENT FOR PUBLICATION

Not Applicable.

CONFLICT OF INTEREST

The author confirms that this chapter contents have no conflict of interest.

ACKNOWLEDGEMENT

Declared none.

REFERENCES

[1]   Kahn JS, McIntosh K. History and recent advances in coronavirus discovery. Pediatr Infect Dis J 2005; 24(11) (Suppl.): S223-7.
        [http://dx.doi.org/10.1097/01.inf.0000188166.17324.60] [PMID: 16378050]

[2]   Chen Y, Liu Q, Guo D. Emerging coronaviruses: Genome structure, replication, and pathogenesis. J Med Virol 2020; 92(4): 418-23.
        [http://dx.doi.org/10.1002/jmv.25681] [PMID: 31967327]

[3]   Schoeman D, Fielding BC. Coronavirus envelope protein: current knowledge. Virol J 2019; 16(1): 69.
        [http://dx.doi.org/10.1186/s12985-019-1182-0] [PMID: 31133031]

[4]   McBride R, van Zyl M, Fielding BC. The coronavirus nucleocapsid is a multifunctional protein. Viruses 2014; 6(8): 2991-3018.
        [http://dx.doi.org/10.3390/v6082991] [PMID: 25105276]

[5]   Seah I, Su X, Lingam G. Revisiting the dangers of the coronavirus in the ophthalmology practice. Eye (Lond) 2020; 34(7): 1155-7.
        [http://dx.doi.org/10.1038/s41433-020-0790-7] [PMID: 32029919]

[6]   World Health Organization (WHO). Situation Report-32 2020.

[7]   Cascella M, Rajnik M, Cuomo A, Dulebohn SC, Di Napoli R. Features, Evaluation and Treatment Coronavirus (COVID-19). StatPearls Publishing 2020.

[8]   World Health Organization (WHO). WHO announces COVID-19 outbreak a pandemic 2020. http://www.euro.who.int/en/health-topics/health-emergencies/coronavirus-covid-19/news/news/2020/3/who-announces-covid-19-outbreak-a-pandemic (accessed June 19, 2020).

[9]   Coronavirus NPR. 2020. https://www.npr.org/sections/goatsandsoda/2020/03/11/814474930/coronavirus-covid-19-is-now-officially-a-pandemic-who-says (accessed June 19, 2020).

[10]   Lu R, Zhao X, Li J, *et al.* Genomic characterisation and epidemiology of 2019 novel coronavirus: implications for virus origins and receptor binding. Lancet 2020; 395(10224): 565-74.
        [http://dx.doi.org/10.1016/S0140-6736(20)30251-8] [PMID: 32007145]

[11]   Lauer SA, Grantz KH, Bi Q, *et al.* The incubation period of coronavirus disease 2019 (CoVID-19) from publicly reported confirmed cases: Estimation and application. Ann Intern Med 2020; 172(9): 577-82.

[http://dx.doi.org/10.7326/M20-0504] [PMID: 32150748]

[12]   Centers for Disease Control and Prevention (CDC). Screening and Triage at Intake nd https://www.cdc.gov/coronavirus/2019-ncov/hcp/dialysis/screening.html(accessed June 20, 2020).

[13]   Carter LJ, Garner LV, Smoot JW, *et al.* Assay techniques and test development for COVID-19 diagnosis. ACS Cent Sci 2020; 6(5): 591-605.
[http://dx.doi.org/10.1021/acscentsci.0c00501] [PMID: 32382657]

[14]   Jalali M, Zaborowska J, Jalali M. The polymerase chain reaction: PCR, qPCR, and RT-PCR basic Sci Methods clin res. Elsevier Inc. 2017; pp. 1-18.
[http://dx.doi.org/10.1016/B978-0-12-803077-6.00001-1]

[15]   Han MS, Byun JH, Cho Y, Rim JH. RT-PCR for SARS-CoV-2: quantitative *versus* qualitative. Lancet Infect Dis 2020; 0
[http://dx.doi.org/10.1016/S1473-3099(20)30424-2] [PMID: 32445709]

[16]   Kim DW. [Real time quantitative PCR]. Exp Mol Med 2001; 33(1) (Suppl.): 101-9.
[http://dx.doi.org/10.1101/gr.6.10.986] [PMID: 11708318]

[17]   Souf S. Recent advances in diagnostic testing for viral infections. Biosci Horizons Int J Student Res 2016; 9
[http://dx.doi.org/10.1093/biohorizons/hzw010]

[18]   Duffy S. Why are RNA virus mutation rates so damn high? PLoS Biol 2018; 16(8)e3000003
[http://dx.doi.org/10.1371/journal.pbio.3000003] [PMID: 30102691]

[19]   Hematian A, Sadeghifard N, Mohebi R, *et al.* Traditional and Modern Cell Culture in Virus Diagnosis. Osong Public Health Res Perspect 2016; 7(2): 77-82.
[http://dx.doi.org/10.1016/j.phrp.2015.11.011] [PMID: 27169004]

[20]   Gentile G, Micozzi A. Speculations on the clinical significance of asymptomatic viral infections. Clin Microbiol Infect 2016; 22(7): 585-8.
[http://dx.doi.org/10.1016/j.cmi.2016.07.016] [PMID: 27450587]

[21]   Virus - The cycle of infection | Britannica n.d.   https://www.britannica.com/science/virus/The-cycl--of-infection (accessed June 16, 2020).

[22]   Storch GA. Diagnostic virology. Clin Infect Dis 2000; 31(3): 739-51.
[http://dx.doi.org/10.1086/314015] [PMID: 11017824]

[23]   Leland DS, Ginocchio CC. Role of cell culture for virus detection in the age of technology. Clin Microbiol Rev 2007; 20(1): 49-78.
[http://dx.doi.org/10.1128/CMR.00002-06] [PMID: 17223623]

[24]   Alhajj M, Farhana A. Enzyme Linked Immunosorbent Assay (ELISA). StatPearls Publishing 2020.

[25]   Lequin RM. Enzyme immunoassay (EIA)/enzyme-linked immunosorbent assay (ELISA). Clin Chem 2005; 51(12): 2415-8.
[http://dx.doi.org/10.1373/clinchem.2005.051532] [PMID: 16179424]

[26]   Cinquanta L, Fontana DE, Bizzaro N. Chemiluminescent immunoassay technology: what does it change in autoantibody detection? Auto Immun Highlights 2017; 8(1): 9.
[http://dx.doi.org/10.1007/s13317-017-0097-2] [PMID: 28647912]

[27]   Donaldson JG. Immunofluorescence Staining. Curr Protoc Cell Biol 1998; 0: 4.3.1-6.
[http://dx.doi.org/10.1002/0471143030.cb0403s00]

[28]   Enzyme Immunochromatography--A Quantitative Immunoassay Requiring No Instrumentation - PubMed. n.d.   https://pubmed.ncbi.nlm.nih.gov/3891138/(accessed June 17, 2020).

[29]   Gallagher S, Chakavarti D. Immunoblot analysis. J Vis Exp 2008; (16): 759.
[http://dx.doi.org/10.3791/759] [PMID: 19066547]

[30]   IgG Avidity Assay: A Tool for Excluding Acute Toxoplasmosis in Prolonged IgM Titer Sera From

Pregnant Women - PubMed n.d.. https://pubmed.ncbi.nlm.nih.gov/25776588/(accessed June 17, 2020).

[31]   Grandien M. Viral diagnosis by antigen detection techniques. Clin Diagn Virol 1996; 5(2-3): 81-90.
        [http://dx.doi.org/10.1016/0928-0197(96)00209-7] [PMID: 15566866]

[32]   United states food and drug administration (us-fda). Fda Combating Covid-19 With Medical Devices 2020.

[33]   Fakruddin M, Mannan KSB, Chowdhury A, *et al.* Nucleic acid amplification: Alternative methods of polymerase chain reaction. J Pharm Bioallied Sci 2013; 5(4): 245-52.
        [http://dx.doi.org/10.4103/0975-7406.120066] [PMID: 24302831]

[34]   McCulloh RJ, Koster M, Chapin K. Respiratory viral testing: new frontiers in diagnostics and implications for antimicrobial stewardship. Virulence 2013; 4(1): 1-2.
        [http://dx.doi.org/10.4161/viru.22788] [PMID: 23314568]

[35]   Mullis KB. The unusual origin of the polymerase chain reaction. Sci Am 1990; 262(4): 56-61, 64-65.
        [http://dx.doi.org/10.1038/scientificamerican0490-56] [PMID: 2315679]

[36]   Kary B. https://www.nobelprize.org/prizes/chemistry/1993/mullis/facts/

[37]   Kary B. Mullis - Nobel Lecture: The Polymerase Chain Reaction n.d. https://www.nobelprize.org/prizes/chemistry/1993/mullis/lecture/ (accessed June 17, 2020).

[38]   Kleppe K, Ohtsuka E, Kleppe R, Molineux I, Khorana HG. Studies on polynucleotides. XCVI. Repair replications of short synthetic DNA's as catalyzed by DNA polymerases. J Mol Biol 1971; 56(2): 341-61.
        [http://dx.doi.org/10.1016/0022-2836(71)90469-4] [PMID: 4927950]

[39]   Lawyer FC, Stoffel S, Saiki RK, *et al.* High-level expression, purification, and enzymatic characterization of full-length Thermus aquaticus DNA polymerase and a truncated form deficient in 5′ to 3′ exonuclease activity. PCR Methods Appl 1993; 2(4): 275-87.
        [http://dx.doi.org/10.1101/gr.2.4.275] [PMID: 8324500]

[40]   Saiki R, Gelfand D, Stoffel S, Scharf S, Higuchi R, Horn G, *et al.* Primer-directed enzymatic amplification of DNA with a thermostable DNA polymerase 1988.
        [http://dx.doi.org/10.1126/science.239.4839.487]

[41]   Saiki RK, Scharf S, Faloona F, Mullis KB, Horn GT, Erlich HA, *et al.* Enzymatic amplification of β-globin genomic sequences and restriction site analysis for diagnosis of sickle cell anemia 1985.
        [http://dx.doi.org/10.1126/science.2999980]

[42]   Mullis K, Faloona F, Scharf S, Saiki R, Horn G, Erlich H. Specific enzymatic amplification of DNA *in vitro* : the polymerase chain reaction. Cold Spring Harb Symp Quant Biol 1986; 51(Pt 1): 263-73.
        [http://dx.doi.org/10.1101/SQB.1986.051.01.032] [PMID: 3472723]

[43]   Mullis KB, Faloona FA. Specific synthesis of DNA *in vitro* via a polymerase-catalyzed chain reaction. Methods Enzymol 1987; 155: 335-50.
        [http://dx.doi.org/10.1016/0076-6879(87)55023-6] [PMID: 3431465]

[44]   PCR Setup—Six Critical Components to Consider | Thermo Fisher Scientific - IN n.d. https://www.thermofisher.com/in/en/home/life-science/cloning/cloning-learning-center/invitrogen-school-of-molecular-biology/pcr-education/pcr-reagents-enzymes/pcr-component-considerations.html (accessed June 17, 2020).

[45]   Pestana E, Belak S, Diallo A, Crowther JR, Viljoen GJ, Pestana EA, *et al.* Real-Time PCR – The Basic Principles Early, rapid sensitive Vet Mol diagnostics - real time PCR Appl. Springer Netherlands 2009; pp. 27-46.
        [http://dx.doi.org/10.1007/978-90-481-3132-7_3]

[46]   van Pelt-Verkuil E, van Belkum A, Hays JP, Eds. The Polymerase Chain Reaction BT - Principles and Technical Aspects of PCR Amplification. Springer Netherlands 2008; pp. 1-7.

[http://dx.doi.org/10.1007/978-1-4020-6241-4]

[47]   Hybridization of Synthetic Oligodeoxyribonucleotides to Phi Chi 174 DNA: The Effect of Single Base Pair Mismatch - PubMed n.d. https://pubmed.ncbi.nlm.nih.gov/158748/ (accessed June 17, 2020).

[48]   van Pelt-Verkuil E, van Belkum A, Hays JP. Deoxynucleotide Triphosphates and Buffer Components Princ Tech Asp PCR Amplif. Springer Netherlands 2008; pp. 91-101.
        [http://dx.doi.org/10.1007/978-1-4020-6241-4_6]

[49]   Ely JJ, Reeves-Daniel A, Campbell ML, Kohler S, Stone WH. Influence of magnesium ion concentration and PCR amplification conditions on cross-species PCR. Biotechniques 1998; 25(1): 38-40, 42.
        [http://dx.doi.org/10.2144/98251bm07] [PMID: 9668972]

[50]   Blanchard MM, Taillon-Miller P, Nowotny P, Nowotny V. PCR buffer optimization with uniform temperature regimen to facilitate automation. PCR Methods Appl 1993; 2(3): 234-40.
        [http://dx.doi.org/10.1101/gr.2.3.234] [PMID: 8443576]

[51]   Bartlett JMS, Stirling D. Methods in Molecular Biology PCR Protocols 2003.

[52]   Polymerase Chain Reaction PCR Process & Guide Sigma-Aldrich n.d. https://www.sigmaaldrich.com/technical-documents /articles/biology/polymerase-chain-reaction.html (accessed June 17, 2020).

[53]   Rutledge RG, Stewart D. A kinetic-based sigmoidal model for the polymerase chain reaction and its application to high-capacity absolute quantitative real-time PCR. BMC Biotechnol 2008; 8: 47.
        [http://dx.doi.org/10.1186/1472-6750-8-47] [PMID: 18466619]

[54]   Jansson L, Hedman J. Challenging the proposed causes of the PCR plateau phase. Biomol Detect Quantif 2019; 17100082
        [http://dx.doi.org/10.1016/j.bdq.2019.100082] [PMID: 30886826]

[55]   Morrison C, Gannon F. The impact of the PCR plateau phase on quantitative PCR 1994.
        [http://dx.doi.org/10.1016/0167-4781(94)90076-0]

[56]   Lai CC, Shih TP, Ko WC, Tang HJ, Hsueh PR. Severe acute respiratory syndrome coronavirus 2 (SARS-CoV-2) and coronavirus disease-2019 (COVID-19): The epidemic and the challenges. Int J Antimicrob Agents 2020; 55(3)105924
        [http://dx.doi.org/10.1016/j.ijantimicag.2020.105924] [PMID: 32081636]

[57]   Chan JF-W, Kok K-H, Zhu Z, *et al.* Genomic characterization of the 2019 novel human-pathogenic coronavirus isolated from a patient with atypical pneumonia after visiting Wuhan. Emerg Microbes Infect 2020; 9(1): 221-36.
        [http://dx.doi.org/10.1080/22221751.2020.1719902] [PMID: 31987001]

[58]   Zhu N, Zhang D, Wang W, *et al.* China Novel Coronavirus Investigating and Research Team. A novel coronavirus from patients with pneumonia in China, 2019. N Engl J Med 2020; 382(8): 727-33.
        [http://dx.doi.org/10.1056/NEJMoa2001017] [PMID: 31978945]

[59]   Álvarez-Fernández R. Explanatory chapter: PCR primer design Methods Enzymol. Academic Press Inc. 2013; 529: pp. 1-21.
        [http://dx.doi.org/10.1016/B978-0-12-418687-3.00001-X]

[60]   Reue K. mRNA quantitation techniques: considerations for experimental design and application. J Nutr 1998; 128(11): 2038-44.
        [http://dx.doi.org/10.1093/jn/128.11.2038] [PMID: 9808663]

[61]   Strategies for Detecting mRNA | Thermo Fisher Scientific - IN n.d. https://www.thermofisher.com (accessed June 18, 2020).

[62]   RT-PCR | Reverse Transcription PCR | Sigma-Aldrich n.d. https://www.sigmaaldrich.com (accessed June 18, 2020).

[63]   Walker JM, Raply R. Molecular Biology and Biotechnology. 5th ed., RSC Publishing 2003.

[64] Laboratory testing for 2019 novel coronavirus (2019-nCoV) in suspected human cases n.d 2019. https://www.who.int/publications/i/item/laboratory-testing-for-2019-novel-coronavirus-in- suspected-human-cases-20200117(accessed June 18, 2020).

[65] Corman VM, Landt O, Kaiser M, *et al.* Detection of 2019 novel coronavirus (2019-nCoV) by real-time RT-PCR. Euro Surveill 2020; 25: 3.
[http://dx.doi.org/10.2807/1560-7917.ES.2020.25.3.2000045] [PMID: 31992387]

[66] Hong KH, Lee SW, Kim TS, *et al.* Guidelines for laboratory diagnosis of coronavirus disease 2019 (COVID-19) in korea. Ann Lab Med 2020; 40(5): 351-60.
[http://dx.doi.org/10.3343/alm.2020.40.5.351] [PMID: 32237288]

[67] Tang YW, Schmitz JE, Persing DH, Stratton CW. Laboratory diagnosis of COVID-19: current issues and challenges. J Clin Microbiol 2020; 58(6)e00512-20
[http://dx.doi.org/10.1128/JCM.00512-20] [PMID: 32245835]

[68] Zou L, Ruan F, Huang M, *et al.* al. et. SARS-CoV-2 viral load in upper respiratory specimens of infected patients. N Engl J Med 2020; 382(12): 1177-9.
[http://dx.doi.org/10.1056/NEJMc2001737] [PMID: 32074444]

[69] Shen C, Wang Z, Zhao F. al. et. Treatment of 5 critically ill patients with COVID-19 with convalescent plasma. JAMA 2020.
[http://dx.doi.org/10.1001/jama.2020.4783]

[70] Maddocks S, Jenkins R. Quantitative PCR: Things to consider. Underst PCR 2017; pp. 45-52.
[http://dx.doi.org/10.1016/B978-0-12-802683-0.00004-6]

[71] Quantitative PCR (qPCR) | Biocompare n.d. https://www.biocompare.com/PCR-Real-Time-PCR/7217-Real-Time-PCR/(accessed June 19, 2020).

[72] Smith CJ, Osborn AM. Advantages and limitations of quantitative PCR (Q-PCR)-based approaches in microbial ecology. FEMS Microbiol Ecol 2009; 67(1): 6-20.
[http://dx.doi.org/10.1111/j.1574-6941.2008.00629.x] [PMID: 19120456]

[73] Holland PM, Abramson RD, Watson R, Gelfand DH. Detection of specific polymerase chain reaction product by utilizing the 5′----3′ exonuclease activity of Thermus aquaticus DNA polymerase. Proc Natl Acad Sci USA 1991; 88(16): 7276-80.
[http://dx.doi.org/10.1073/pnas.88.16.7276] [PMID: 1871133]

[74] Higuchi R, Dollinger G, Walsh PS, Griffith R. Simultaneous amplification and detection of specific DNA sequences. Biotechnology (N Y) 1992; 10(4): 413-7.
[http://dx.doi.org/10.1038/nbt0492-413] [PMID: 1368485]

[75] Yang S, Rothman RE. PCR-based diagnostics for infectious diseases: uses, limitations, and future applications in acute-care settings. Lancet Infect Dis 2004; 4(6): 337-48.
[http://dx.doi.org/10.1016/S1473-3099(04)01044-8] [PMID: 15172342]

[76] Bustin SA, Benes V, Garson JA, *et al.* The MIQE guidelines: minimum information for publication of quantitative real-time PCR experiments. Clin Chem 2009; 55(4): 611-22.
[http://dx.doi.org/10.1373/clinchem.2008.112797] [PMID: 19246619]

[77] Kubista M, Andrade JM, Bengtsson M, *et al.* The real-time polymerase chain reaction. Mol Aspects Med 2006; 27(2-3): 95-125.
[http://dx.doi.org/10.1016/j.mam.2005.12.007] [PMID: 16460794]

[78] ThermoFisher Scientific What is multiplexing? nd

[79] Henegariu O, Heerema NA, Dlouhy SR, Vance GH, Vogt PH. Multiplex PCR: critical parameters and step-by-step protocol. Biotechniques 1997; 23(3): 504-11.
[http://dx.doi.org/10.2144/97233rr01] [PMID: 9298224]

[80] Keer JT. Quantitative Real-time PCR Analysis. Essentials Nucleic Acid Anal. A Robust Approach 2008; pp. 132-66.

[81]   Kralik P, Ricchi M. A Basic guide to real time PCR in microbial diagnostics: Definitions, Parameters, and Everything. Front Microbiol 2017; 8: 108.
[http://dx.doi.org/10.3389/fmicb.2017.00108] [PMID: 28210243]

[82]   Livak KJ, Schmittgen TD. Analysis of relative gene expression data using real-time quantitative PCR and the 2(-Δ Δ C(T)) Method. Methods 2001; 25(4): 402-8.
[http://dx.doi.org/10.1006/meth.2001.1262] [PMID: 11846609]

[83]   Schefe JH, Lehmann KE, Buschmann IR, Unger T, Funke-Kaiser H. Quantitative real-time RT-PCR data analysis: current concepts and the novel "gene expression's CT difference" formula. J Mol Med (Berl) 2006; 84(11): 901-10.
[http://dx.doi.org/10.1007/s00109-006-0097-6] [PMID: 16972087]

[84]   Yuan JS, Wang D, Stewart CN Jr. Statistical methods for efficiency adjusted real-time PCR quantification. Biotechnol J 2008; 3(1): 112-23.
[http://dx.doi.org/10.1002/biot.200700169] [PMID: 18074404]

[85]   Ganger MT, Dietz GD, Ewing SJ. A common base method for analysis of qPCR data and the application of simple blocking in qPCR experiments. BMC Bioinformatics 2017; 18(1): 534.
[http://dx.doi.org/10.1186/s12859-017-1949-5] [PMID: 29191175]

[86]   Pfaffl MW. A new mathematical model for relative quantification in real-time RT-PCR. 2001; 29.

[87]   Perform HT. The Pfaffl Method For qPCR nd https://toptipbio.com/pfaffl-method-qpcr/ (accessed June 20, 2020).

[88]   Booth CS, Pienaar E, Termaat JR, Whitney SE, Louw TM, Viljoen HJ. Efficiency of the polymerase chain reaction. Chem Eng Sci 2010; 65(17): 4996-5006.
[http://dx.doi.org/10.1016/j.ces.2010.05.046] [PMID: 21799540]

[89]   Cadet J, Bellon S, Berger M, *et al.* Recent aspects of oxidative DNA damage: guanine lesions, measurement and substrate specificity of DNA repair glycosylases. Biol Chem 2002; 383(6): 933-43.
[http://dx.doi.org/10.1515/BC.2002.100] [PMID: 12222683]

[90]   Hsu GW, Ober M, Carell T, Beese LS. Error-prone replication of oxidatively damaged DNA by a high-fidelity DNA polymerase. Nature 2004; 431(7005): 217-21.
[http://dx.doi.org/10.1038/nature02908] [PMID: 15322558]

[91]   Lindahl T, Nyberg B. Rate of depurination of native deoxyribonucleic acid. Biochemistry 1972; 11(19): 3610-8.
[http://dx.doi.org/10.1021/bi00769a018] [PMID: 4626532]

[92]   Lindahl T, Nyberg B. Heat-induced deamination of cytosine residues in deoxyribonucleic acid. Biochemistry 1974; 13(16): 3405-10.
[http://dx.doi.org/10.1021/bi00713a035] [PMID: 4601435]

[93]   Pienaar E, Theron M, Nelson M, Viljoen HJ. A quantitative model of error accumulation during PCR amplification. Comput Biol Chem 2006; 30(2): 102-11.
[http://dx.doi.org/10.1016/j.compbiolchem.2005.11.002] [PMID: 16412692]

[94]   Qvist S. NordVal: A Nordic system for validation of alternative microbiological methods. Food Control 2007; 18: 113-7.
[http://dx.doi.org/10.1016/j.foodcont.2005.09.001]

[95]   Chesher D. Evaluating assay precision. Clin Biochem Rev 2008; 29 (Suppl. 1): S23-6.
[PMID: 18852851]

[96]   Broeders S, Huber I, Grohmann L, Berben G, Taverniers I, Mazzara M, *et al.* Guidelines for validation of qualitative real-time PCR methods. Trends Food Sci Technol 2014; 37: 115-26.
[http://dx.doi.org/10.1016/j.tifs.2014.03.008]

CHAPTER 11

Evaluation of SARS-CoV-2 Neutralizing Antibodies in Sera Using Live Virus Microneutralization Assay

Shaukat Hussain Munawar[1,*], Zahid Manzoor[1], Muhammad Farrukh Nisar[2], Muhammad Yasir Waqas[2] and **Imran Ahmad Khan[3]**

[1] *Department of Pharmacology and Toxicology, Faculty of Bio-Sciences, Cholistan University of Veterinary and Animal Sciences, Bahawalpur-63100, Pakistan*

[2] *Department of Physiology & Bio-Chemistry, Faculty of Bio-Sciences, Cholistan University of Veterinary and Animal Sciences, Bahawalpur-63100, Pakistan*

[3] *Faculty of Pharmacy and Alternative Medicine IUB Bahawalpur, Pakistan*

Abstract: Neutralizing antibodies (nAbs) make a defense line against viral attacks by binding to viruses to shield infections. A neutralizing antibody interferes with the virus in different ways as it may block the cell receptor or bind to viral capsid by inhibiting genome un-coating. The micro-neutralization (MN) assay is a basic technique for detecting viruses in epidemiological, immunological, virological studies, and vaccine assessment tests. The underlying mechanism of this assay is based on the detection of specific antigen-antibody reactions. It only detects the antibodies involved in the blockage of the virus replication. This technique is specifically helpful in evaluating specific micro-organism serotype neutralizing antibodies in the sera of humans and animals. It describes the neutralization or inhibition of replicating virus strains by antibodies in the sera of humans and animals. But highly constraint provisions may be required while working with live virus-based micro-neutralization techniques, particularly when handling precarious micro-organisms like severe acute respiratory syndrome-coronavirus-2 (SARS-CoV-2). Herein, all the possible data regarding isolation, amplification, and titration of SARS-CoV-2 and MN assay to measure nAbs level in the sera of mammalian species have been summarized.

Keywords: Antibodies, Microneutralization, Neutralization, SARS-CoV-2.

INTRODUCTION

Respiratory disease patients of unrevealed causes were reported in China on 31 December 2019 [1 - 3]. On 7 January 2020, Chinese scientists named severe acute

* **Corresponding author Shaukat Hussain Munawar:** Department of Pharmacology and Toxicology, Faculty of Bio-Sciences, Cholistan University of Veterinary and Animal Sciences, Bahawalpur-63100, Pakistan. E-mail: shaukathussainmunawar@cuvas.edu.pk

Kamal Niaz & Muhammad Farrukh Nisar (Eds.)

respiratory syndrome-coronavirus-2 (SARS-CoV-2) [4]. Because of causing agent of this disease, it is named "coronavirus disease-19" which is pandemic to date. Coronavirus has a single haploid set of chromosomes of 30 Kbp. There are seven coronavirus strains infecting humans to date [1, 5]. They cause infections of the respiratory system, especially the lower respiratory tract, digestive system, kidney, liver, circulatory system, mainly heart and brain. Outbreaks of SARS and MERS in human beings over the past 23 years [5, 6] have indicated the possibility that one of these micro-organisms may cause a future pandemic [7].

The SARS-CoV-2is a novel zoonotic disease. SARS-CoV-2 shows different indications such as nonspecific infections, mild or severe type symptoms of respiratory disease. Coronavirus has four types of structural proteins, *i.e.,* spike (S), membrane (M), envelop (E), and nucleocapsid (N) proteins [7 - 9]. Different studies describe humoral immunity responses by immunoglobulins G, M, and A to severe acute respiratory syndrome corona virus-2 [10, 11]. Moreover, limited studies have been found about the responses of neutralizing antibodies during natural infection [12, 13]. In humans and/or animals, the detection of anti-SAR--CoV-2 antibodies is an important tool in diagnosis [14, 15].

Furthermore, it is also used as a valuable tool in studies of epidemiology, virology, and immunology, including the determination of immunogenicity of the vaccine [16, 17]. Immunological tests use for SARS-CoV-2 detection are enzyme-linked immunosorbent assays (ELISA), pseudovirus-based neutralization assays, protein microarrays, and immunofluorescence assays [18 - 22]. There are many drawbacks and limitations in most of these assays. The required instruments and reagents are more specific and expensive. These assays have low specificity and low sensitivity, and the requirement of technically expert staff could limit the use of these assays. However, microneutralization assay dealing with the live virus is a specific and delicate method for quantifying neutralizing antibodies related to that virus [23, 24]. The assay has many advantages, such as special chemicals and equipment are not required.

Moreover, virus-specific neutralizing antibodies can be detected more precisely by this assay. Furthermore, it can control the changes because of strain-specific antigens. The main objective of the present chapter is to summarize the existing major steps involve in the isolation, amplification, titration, and neutralization of SARS-CoV-2. Also, the MN assay is suitable for the quantitative measurement of the concentration of nAbs in the sera of divergent mammalians.

MATERIALS

General Materials [24, 25]

Vero E6 cells.

Water bath (37°C).

Biosafety cabinet.

5% CO_2 humidified incubator.

Centrifuge machine (low speed).

Microscope (Inverted).

Hemocytometer or cell counter.

Laminar flow hood (biosafety cabinet).

2% DMEM, FBS (10%), l-glutamine (1%), and penicillin/streptomycin solution (1%).

70% ethyl alcohol.

Sterile pipettes of different volumes and multichannel pipettes.

Sterile DPBS.

Sterile 1× trypsin-ethylenediaminetetraacetic acid (EDTA) in DPBS.

Sterile tissue culture flasks T25, T75, and T175 with filter screw caps.

Sterile falcon tubes of 1.5 ml and 15 ml.

Sterile replaceable aerosol filter pipette tips.

Sterile syringe filters of 0.22 μm in size and exposed with gamma rays.

SARS-CoV-2 Isolation, Amplification, Titration, and Microneutralization

All handling during work with SARS-CoV-2 should be done in biosafety level 3 (BSL-3) containment laboratories. It is important to inactivate this virus *via* gamma irradiation at 2×10^6 rads/h before its use. The instructions and rules set by the institute for working in biosafety BSL-3 should be followed [25].

Convergent Vero E6 cells are grown in M-10 media using T75 culture flasks.

Sterile 96-well tissue culture plates.

Sterile plates of U-shape with 96-wells.

A sample having SARS-CoV-2 should be filtered by sterile syringes filters with a 0.22 μm size and gamma-irradiated (for separation of the virus).

Separated SARS-CoV-2 (amplified/concentrated).

For microneutralization assay, titrate the SARS-CoV-2.

Test all the samples of the serum.

METHODS

Continuous Culture of Vero E6 Cells

Sterile apparatus and solutions must be used when dealing with Vero E6 cells. All methods carefully are done in aseptic conditions. Incubate the cells at 37°C with 5% CO_2 at optimum humidity levels and normalized reagents [26].

Thaw Vero E6 cells less than one minute after removing Vero E6 cells vial from cryogenic liquid nitrogen (-195.79°C). Cryovials are free from contamination, sterilized, so the O-ring and cap of the cryovials should not be in the water.

After thawing, transfer it into a safety cabinet. Then, use 70% ethanol to disinfect the vial along with the besch and the equipment being used.

Transfer all the vial volume after removing dimethyl sulfoxide (DMSO) into a sterilized 55mm falcon tube with fresh M-10 media.

Centrifuge the tube containing cellular material at 200-500×*g* for 5 minutes at room temperature.

After centrifugation, remove the supernatant carefully with no disturbance to the pellet at the bottom.

Resuspend the cells gently in 10mm of M-10 media. Then by using a sterile 10 mm pipette, transfer it into cell culture flasks (T75).

Using a sterile 10 mm serological pipette, transfer the cell suspension to the T75 tissue culture flask.

Put the flask for incubation at 37°C adjusted at 5% CO_2.

Use an inverted microscope to examine the Vero E6 cells daily. If required, then change culture media every three to four days to recover Vero E6 cells slow after cooling and may require about 07 days for passage.

Passage the cells into new culture flasks at a ratio of 1:5 to 1:10 when the cells reach >90–95% confluency. Monitoring of Vero E6 cells is important, and usually, their passage is required 2-3 times per week.

After removing long-time storage and before their usage, maintain the cultures of Vero E6 cells and passage these cells two to three times a week.

Use a hemocytometer or cell counter for counting Vero E6 cells and prepare a cell suspension of 5×10^5 cells per mm in M-10 media.

Necessarily Vero E6 cells seeding density is changed when the cells are more or less confluent. Seed 5 mm (~2.5×10^6 cells) of cell suspension into T25 tissue culture flasks or 20 mm (~1×10^7 cells) of cell suspension into T175 culture flasks, then after 24h cells approach 90-95% confluency.

Keep the flasks in the incubator at 37°C with 5% CO_2 overnight.

CHange the media with the fresh medium, *e.g.,* add 2 mm freshly prepared M-2 media (pre-warmed) into a T25 tissue culture flask or 5 mm of freshly prepared M-2 media into T175 cellular culturing flask.

When using a positive SARS-CoV-2 sample, before inoculation onto Vero E6 cells, filter-sterilized samples using 0.22 μm filters and exposed to the gamma rays.

Add 0.5-1 mm of the virus or +ve sample after filtration to Vero E6 cells.

Evenly distribute SARS-COV-2 over Vero E6 cells then incubate for an hour at 37°C with 5% CO_2.

Prepare 5 mm media in the T25 tissue culture flask or 20 mm in the T175 flasks.

Incubate the flask at 37°C with 5% CO_2 for 2-3 days or until a marked cytopathic effect is seen (Fig.**1**).

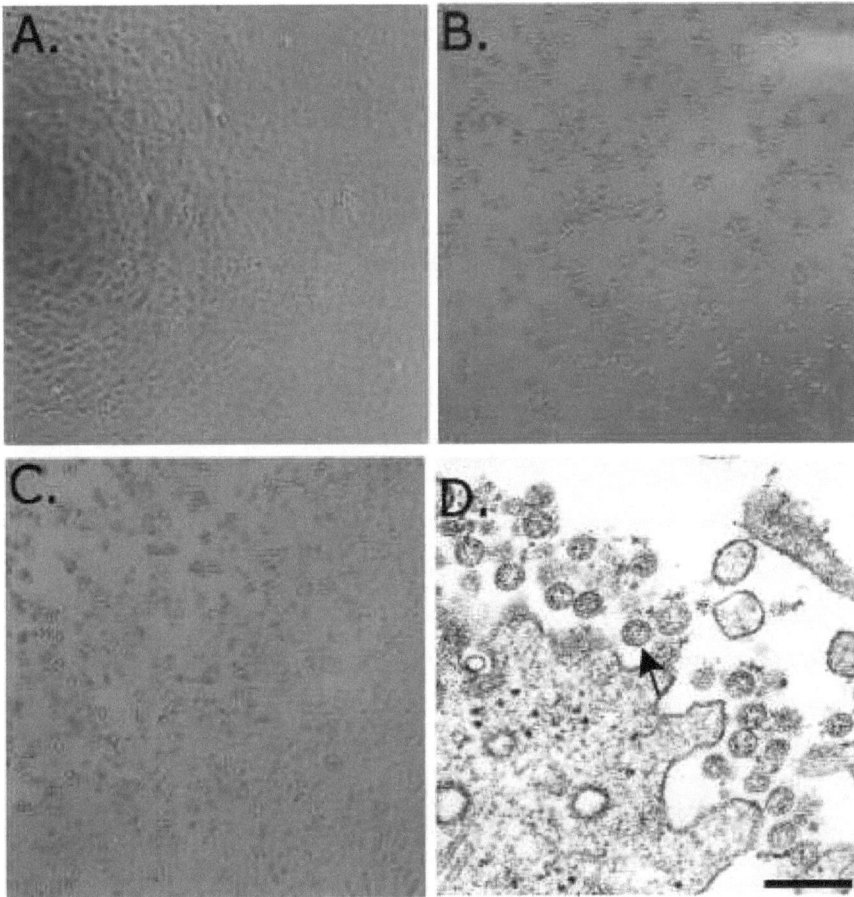

Fig. (1). (A–C) 10X phase-contrast images of Vero monolayers at 3 days post inoculation. Panels shown are (A) mock, (B) nasopharyngeal, and (C) oropharyngeal. (D) Electron microscopic image of the viral isolate showing extracellular spherical particles with cross-sections through the nucleocapsids, seen as black dots.

Examine the flask daily after SARS-CoV-2 infection as the cytopathic effect (CPE) depends on seed virus starting titer and strain.

Collect supernatant from the flask when the cytopathic effect is >50%, and for removal of cellular debris, centrifuge at 500×g for five minutes (Fig. **1**).

Aliquot the collected supernatant in hundred micro-liter or 1 mm aliquots in sterilized 1.0 and 0.5 mm tubes and place it at -80°C. Remember that each tube should be used once only as the virus titer can decrease significantly to avoid the freeze and thaw process. To amplify the virus, use 1 mm aliquot tubes.

Isolation and Amplification of SARS-CoV-2

For harvesting Vero E6 cells from T75 tissue culture flask, wash (with sterile DPBS) the sub-confluent cell monolayer twice, add two to five mm 1x trypsin-EDTA in Dulbeccos' phosphate-buffered saline (PBS) to the washed cell monolayer, and for detaching of cells, incubate it for five to ten minutes at 37°C with 5% CO_2. After detaching cells, add 5 mm 10% FBS M-10 media to inactivate trypsin. Then, collect detached cells in a 15 ml sterile falcon tube, then centrifuge these cells after and add new 1-2 mm M-10 media (pre-warmed at 37°C). Finally, use pipette re-suspend the Vero E6 cells for homogenous preparation of cell suspension.

Titration SARS-CoV-2by Tissue Culture Infective Dose 50 (TCID$_{50}$)

For harvesting Vero E6 cells from T75 flasks, first of all, wash (with sterile DPBS) the sub-confluent cell monolayer twice. Then, add 2-5 mm 1x trypsin-EDTA in prepared PBS to the washed cell monolayer, and for detaching cells, incubate it for 5-10 minutes at 37°C with 5% CO_2. After detaching cells, add 5 mm 10% FBS containing M-10 media to the flask to inactivate trypsin activity. Collect detached cells in 15 mm tubes, then centrifuge these cells following the addition of a new 1-2 mm 10% (FBS) M-10 media (pre-warmed). With the help of a pipette, re-suspend the Vero E6 cells for homogenous preparation of cell suspension.

Using a hemocytometer or cell counter, count the cells and make 1×10^5 cells/mm suspension of cells in 10% (FBS) M-10 media (pre-warmed). In each 96-well plate, 1×10^6 cells are suspended again in 10 mm.

In every well of sterile 96-well plate, seed 1×10^4 cells (100 µl) so that on the next day, the cells are over 90% confluent. Seeding density should be change accordingly when Vero E6 cells are less or more confluent.

Incubate the sterile 96-well plate at 37°C with 5% CO_2 overnight.

Add 135 µl M-2 media to all wells of the new sterile plate (U-shaped) on the next day (Fig. **2**).

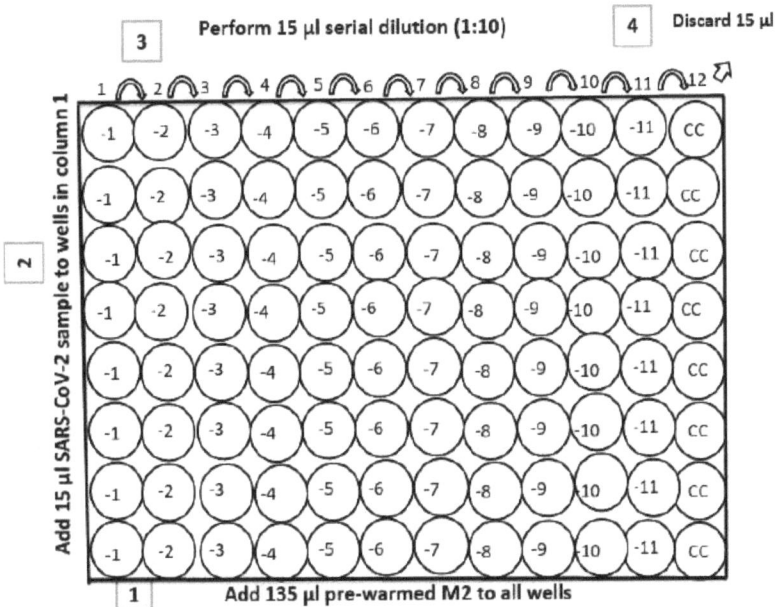

Fig. (2). Illustrative diagram of the preparation of virus dilution for SARS-CoV-2 titration by $TCID_{50}$. Numbered boxes mention the plate preparation stepwise. After completion, by using a multichannel pipette, transfer 100 µl from the 96-well U-bottom plate having diluted SARS-CoV-2 sample to Vero E6 cells in each corresponding well in the 96-well plate. CC is indicating cell control wells of the 96-well plate.

Add 15 µl of SARS-CoV-2 in each well of the first column separately to have a dilution of 1:10 (Fig. **2**).

Using a multichannel pipette, prepare tenfold serial (log_{10}) dilution by gradual column to column transfer of 15 µl (Fig. **2**). Other dilutions can be used, such as ½ log10.

Homogenize properly by pipetting few times up and down during each dilution step. Pipette tips should be changed between wells.

All wells of column twelve should not have the virus (control cells) so, discard the final 15 µl after column 11.

Aspirate the media after removal of the 96-well plate having confluent cells. Minimize the time between the aspiration of media and the addition of the inoculated virus or the mixture of serum and virus to avoid cell death.

With the help of a pipette, transfer 100 µl of diluted SARS-CoV-2 sample from 96-well plate to Vero E6 cells in each proper well of the 96-well plate.

Incubate the 96-well plate at 37°C with 5% CO_2 for 3 days.

Observe 96-well plate under an inverted microscope after the incubation period for the positive and negative SARS-CoV-2 control. Remember that alternative removes media from the Vero E6 cells and at room temperature, do cells fixation for 5 minutes with 100 µl ice-chilled 4% paraformaldehyde (PFA). Then stain cells with 100µl crystal violet (0.05% w/v) in 20% methyl alcohol after removal of fixative for 30 minutes at room temperature, and washed the cells using tap water. If cells do not stain with crystal violet, score wells as positive for SARS-CoV-2, and when staining of cells with crystal violet, score the wells as negative for SARS-CoV-2.

Calculate tissue culture infective dose 50 by using the Reed–Muench equation.

$\log_{10}$ 50% endpoint dilution $= \log_{10}$ of dilution showing mortality next above 50% - (difference of logarithms × logarithm of dilution factor).

SARS-CoV-2 Microneutralization Assay [24]

1. For harvesting Vero E6 cells from T75 tissue culture flask, first of all, wash (with sterile DPBS) the sub-confluent cell monolayer twice, add 2-5 milliliters 1× trypsin-EDTA in PBS to the washed cell monolayer and for detaching of cells, incubate it for five to ten minutes at 37°C with 5% CO_2. After detaching cells, add 5 mm 10% (FBS) M-10 media to the flask for inactivating trypsinization. Collect the detached cells in 15 mm sterile falcon tube. Then centrifuge these cells, afterward add to a new 1-2 mm 10% M-10 media (pre-warmed). With the help of a pipette, re-suspend the Vero E6 cells for homogenous preparation of cell suspension.

2. Using a hemocytometer or cell counter, count the cells and make 1×10^5 cells/mm suspend cells in M-10 media (pre-warmed). In each 96-well plate, 1×10^6 cells are suspended again in 10 mm.

3. In every well of sterile 96-well plate, seed 1×10^4 cells (100 µl) so that on the next day, the cells reached over 90% confluency. Seeding density should be change when Vero E6 cells are less or more confluent.

4. Place the flasks for incubation at 37°C with 5% CO_2 overnight.

5. Use heat-inactivate test sera for virus microneutralization by incubation for 30 minutes at 56°C on the following day.

6. Add 60 µl of 10% M-2 media (pre-warmed) to all wells of the new sterile 96-well plate (Fig. **3**).

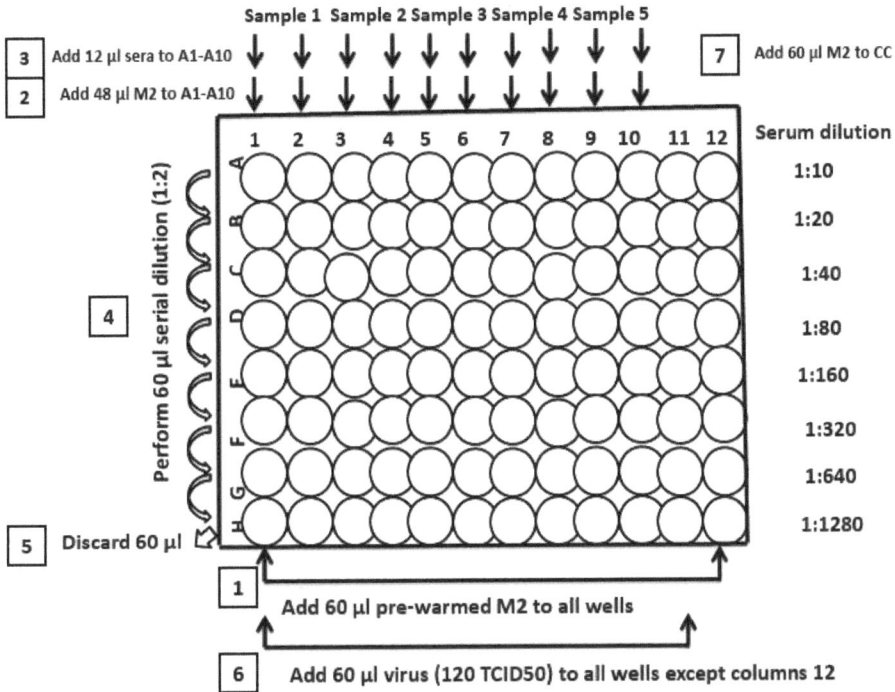

Fig. (3). Shows preparation of plate for SARS-CoV-2 microneutralization assay. Numbered boxes illustrate the preparatory steps for the SARS-CoV-2 microneutralization assay plate. Then incubation of serum-virus mixture (for one hour in 37°C temperature with 5% CO_2) after using the multichannel pipette, transfer 100 µl from the U-shaped 96-well plate having diluted SARS-CoV-2 sample to Vero E6 cells in each corresponding well in the 96-well plate. VC stands for virus control, and CC stands for cell control wells.

7. In row A, add 48 µl of 10% M-2 media (Pre-warmed) to wells A1–A10 (Fig. **3**).

8. Add 12 µl of heat-inactivated serum in each well from A1 to A10 in row A to have 1:10 dilution (Fig. **3**). The wells A11 and A12 remain without serum in row A. As for each serum sample, 12µl is the requirement for a single test, but the test for sera should be repeated twice tested, so more volume is required. When the microneutralization test is performed against various virus strains, new different plates are recommended.

9. With the help of a multichannel pipette, make two-fold serial dilutions on added serum samples by transferring 60 µl from row to row (*i.e.,* A1 to H1) successively (Fig. **3**). Using a multichannel pipette, make ten-fold serial (log10) dilutions on added serum samples by transferring 60 µl from row to row (*i.e.,* A1 to B1, *etc.* up to G1 to H1) successively (Fig. **3**).

10. Mix appropriately by using a pipette several times up and down during each dilution step. Pipette tips should be changed between wells.

11. After row H, remove the final 60 µl.

12. Make virus suspension in 10% M-2 media in a way that 60 µl (repeated four times per dilution) contains 2×10^3 $TCID_{50}$ per mm (*i.e.,* 120 $TCID_{50}$). The approximate requirement is 6 mm per plate.

13. Except for all cell control wells of column 12, add 60 µl diluted viruses to all plate wells.

14. Add 60 µl of 10% M-2 media to all cell control wells in column twelve.

15. Incubate the mixtures of serum and virus for an hour at 37°C with 5% CO_2.

16. Aspirate the media just after removing the 96-well plate having confluent cells. Cell dying should be avoided by minimizing the time between aspiring the media and the addition of virus inoculum or the mixtures of the virus with serum.

17. Using a multichannel pipette, transfer 100 µl from the U-shaped 96-well plate to Vero E6 cells in each corresponding well of the 96-well plate. Pipette tips should be changed between wells.

18. Incubate the 96-well plate for three days at 37°C with 5% CO_2. After incubation, inspect by an inverted microscope and calculate MN_{50} or MN_{100} titers of each serum sample as the highest serum dilution that completely protects the cells from cytopathic effect in 50 or 100% wells (all wells), respectively.

CONCLUSION

It is concluded that the different techniques have been discussed for the isolation, amplification, and titration of SARS-CoV-2. These all are suitable for the quantification and neutralization of antibodies titer in the sera. Therefore, it should also be implemented in the diagnosis, seroepidemiological, and immunogenicity SARS-CoV-2 vaccine along with ELISA assay. However, the use of BSL-3 and -4 laboratories will be a restrictive factor for the neutralization of such wild-type viruses. Still, due to the most consistent outcome/result, the use of this technique is appropriate.

CONSENT FOR PUBLICATION

Not Applicable.

CONFLICT OF INTEREST

The author confirms that this chapter contents have no conflict of interest.

ACKNOWLEDGEMENT

Declared none.

REFERENCES

[1]   Zhu N, Zhang D, Wang W, *et al.* China novel coronavirus investigating and research team. A novel coronavirus from patients with pneumonia in China, 2019. N Engl J Med 2020; 382(8): 727-33.
[http://dx.doi.org/10.1056/NEJMoa2001017] [PMID: 31978945]

[2]   Organization WH.

[3]   Park WB, Kwon N-J, Choi S-J, *et al.* Virus isolation from the first patient with SARS-CoV-2 in Korea. J Korean Med Sci 2020; 35(7)e84
[http://dx.doi.org/10.3346/jkms.2020.35.e84] [PMID: 32080990]

[4]   Coronaviridae Study Group of the International Committee on Taxonomy of Viruses. The species Severe acute respiratory syndrome-related coronavirus: classifying 2019-nCoV and naming it SARS-CoV-2. Nat Microbiol 2020; 5(4): 536-44.
[http://dx.doi.org/10.1038/s41564-020-0695-z] [PMID: 32123347]

[5]   Chen W, Xu Z, Mu J, *et al.* Antibody response and viraemia during the course of severe acute respiratory syndrome (SARS)-associated coronavirus infection. J Med Microbiol 2004; 53(Pt 5): 435-8.
[http://dx.doi.org/10.1099/jmm.0.45561-0] [PMID: 15096554]

[6]   Prompetchara E, Ketloy C, Palaga T. Immune responses in COVID-19 and potential vaccines: Lessons learned from SARS and MERS epidemic. Asian Pac J Allergy Immunol 2020; 38(1): 1-9.
[PMID: 32105090]

[7]   Müller MA, Meyer B, Corman VM, *et al.* Presence of Middle East respiratory syndrome coronavirus antibodies in Saudi Arabia: a nationwide, cross-sectional, serological study. Lancet Infect Dis 2015; 15(5): 559-64.
[http://dx.doi.org/10.1016/S1473-3099(15)70090-3] [PMID: 25863564]

[8]   Woo PC, Lau SK, Wong BH, *et al.* Detection of specific antibodies to severe acute respiratory syndrome (SARS) coronavirus nucleocapsid protein for serodiagnosis of SARS coronavirus pneumonia. J Clin Microbiol 2004; 42(5): 2306-9.
[http://dx.doi.org/10.1128/JCM.42.5.2306-2309.2004] [PMID: 15131220]

[9]   Woo PC, Lau SK, Wong BH, *et al.* Longitudinal profile of immunoglobulin G (IgG), IgM, and IgA antibodies against the severe acute respiratory syndrome (SARS) coronavirus nucleocapsid protein in patients with pneumonia due to the SARS coronavirus. Clin Diagn Lab Immunol 2004; 11(4): 665-8.
[PMID: 15242938]

[10]   Bauer G. The variability of the serological response to SARS corona virus-2: Potential resolution of ambiguity through determination of avidity (functional affinity). J Med Virol 2020.
[http://dx.doi.org/10.1002/jmv.26262] [PMID: 32633840]

[11]   Zhang G, Nie S, Zhang Z, Zhang Z. Longitudinal change of severe acute respiratory syndrome coronavirus 2 antibodies in patients with coronavirus disease 2019. J Infect Dis 2020; 222(2): 183-8.
[http://dx.doi.org/10.1093/infdis/jiaa229] [PMID: 32358956]

[12]   Wang D, Li F, Freed DC, *et al.* Quantitative analysis of neutralizing antibody response to human cytomegalovirus in natural infection. Vaccine 2011; 29(48): 9075-80.
[http://dx.doi.org/10.1016/j.vaccine.2011.09.056] [PMID: 21945962]

[13] Rogers TF, Zhao F, Huang D, *et al.* Isolation of potent SARS-CoV-2 neutralizing antibodies and protection from disease in a small animal model. Science 2020; 369(6506): 956-63.
[http://dx.doi.org/10.1126/science.abc7520] [PMID: 32540903]

[14] Tan CW, Chia WN, Chen MI, *et al.* A SARS-CoV-2 surrogate virus neutralization test (sVNT) based on antibody-mediated blockage of ACE2-spike (RBD) protein-protein interaction 2020.

[15] Imai M, Iwatsuki-Horimoto K, Hatta M, *et al.* Syrian hamsters as a small animal model for SARS-CoV-2 infection and countermeasure development. Proc Natl Acad Sci USA 2020; 117(28): 16587-95.
[PMID: 32571934]

[16] Ahmed SF, Quadeer AA, McKay MR. Preliminary identification of potential vaccine targets for the COVID-19 coronavirus (SARS-CoV-2) based on SARS-CoV immunological studies. Viruses 2020; 12(3): 254.
[http://dx.doi.org/10.3390/v12030254] [PMID: 32106567]

[17] Zimmermann P, Curtis N. Coronavirus infections in children including COVID-19: an overview of the epidemiology, clinical features, diagnosis, treatment and prevention options in children. Pediatr Infect Dis J 2020; 39(5): 355-68.
[http://dx.doi.org/10.1097/INF.0000000000002660] [PMID: 32310621]

[18] Hashem AM, Al-Amri SS, Al-Subhi TL, *et al.* Development and validation of different indirect ELISAs for MERS-CoV serological testing. J Immunol Methods 2019; 466: 41-6.
[http://dx.doi.org/10.1016/j.jim.2019.01.005] [PMID: 30659836]

[19] Nie J, Li Q, Wu J, *et al.* Establishment and validation of a pseudovirus neutralization assay for SARS-CoV-2. Emerg Microbes Infect 2020; 9(1): 680-6.
[http://dx.doi.org/10.1080/22221751.2020.1743767] [PMID: 32207377]

[20] Jiang HW, Li Y, Zhang HN, *et al.* SARS-CoV-2 proteome microarray for global profiling of COVID-19 specific IgG and IgM responses. Nat Commun 2020; 11(1): 3581.
[http://dx.doi.org/10.1038/s41467-020-17488-8] [PMID: 32665645]

[21] Meyer B, Torriani G, Yerly S, *et al.* Geneva Center for Emerging Viral Diseases. Validation of a commercially available SARS-CoV-2 serological immunoassay. Clin Microbiol Infect 2020; 26(10): 1386-94.
[http://dx.doi.org/10.1016/j.cmi.2020.06.024] [PMID: 32603801]

[22] Liu I-J, Chen P-J, Yeh S-H, *et al.* SARS Research Group of the National Taiwan University College of Medicine-National Taiwan University Hospital. Immunofluorescence assay for detection of the nucleocapsid antigen of the severe acute respiratory syndrome (SARS)-associated coronavirus in cells derived from throat wash samples of patients with SARS. J Clin Microbiol 2005; 43(5): 2444-8.
[http://dx.doi.org/10.1128/JCM.43.5.2444-2448.2005] [PMID: 15872279]

[23] Amanat F, White KM, Miorin L, *et al.* An in vitro microneutralization assay for SARS-CoV-2 serology and drug screening. Curr Protoc Microbiol 2020; 58(1)e108
[http://dx.doi.org/10.1002/cpmc.108] [PMID: 32585083]

[24] Manenti A, Maggetti M, Casa E, *et al.* Evaluation of SARS-CoV-2 neutralizing antibodies using a CPE-based colorimetric live virus micro-neutralization assay in human serum samples. J Med Virol 2020; 92(10): 2096-104.
[http://dx.doi.org/10.1002/jmv.25986] [PMID: 32383254]

[25] Algaissi A. Hashem, A.M.MERS Coronavirus. Springer 2020; pp. 107-16.
[http://dx.doi.org/10.1007/978-1-0716-0211-9_9]

[26] Yamate M, Yamashita M, Goto T, *et al.* Establishment of Vero E6 cell clones persistently infected with severe acute respiratory syndrome coronavirus. Microbes Infect 2005; 7(15): 1530-40.
[http://dx.doi.org/10.1016/j.micinf.2005.05.013] [PMID: 16269264]

CHAPTER 12

Pseudovirus Neutralization Assay for SARS-CoV-2

Ankush Sharma¹, Sneha Joshi², Pooja Patni¹, Navneet Khurana¹ and **Devesh Tewari**[1,*]

¹ School of Pharmaceutical Sciences, Lovely Professional University, Phagwara-144411, Punjab, India

² Department of Pharmaceutical Chemistry, PCTE Group of Institutions, Ludhiana, Punjab, India

Abstract: The World Health Organization (WHO) has indicated coronavirus disease-19 (COVID-19) as a global pandemic. A virus that is formed by the recombination process and whose genetic material as well as protein-rich envelope are resulting out of various viruses is known as pseudovirus. There are certain advantages of using pseudovirus over native viruses. Due to several novel viruses *e.g.,* Marburg virus, Ebola virus, Lassa fever virus, immunodeficiency virus, and coronavirus, there is a development of numerous packing arrangements to produce pseudotype virus having envelope in their structure. This chapter deals with various virus packaging systems with a focus on production and neutralization assay of pseudovirus.

Keywords: Assay, COVID-19, Pseudovirus, SARS.

INTRODUCTION

The World Health Organization (WHO) has indicated coronavirus disease-19 (COVID-19) as a global pandemic. The causative virus associated with COVID-19 is causing the pneumonia-associated respiratory syndrome, and the virus is attributed to severe acute respiratory syndrome coronavirus-2 (SARS-CoV-2) [1]. There are seven recognized coronavirus species which can infect human:

Common Human Coronaviruses

It usually causes cold symptoms in an infected person.

1. 229E (Alpha coronavirus)

2. NL63 (Alpha coronavirus)

3. OC43 (Beta coronavirus)

* **Corresponding author Devesh Tewari:** School of Pharmaceutical Sciences, Lovely Professional University, Phagwara- 144411, Punjab, India; E-mail: dtewari3@gmail.com

Kamal Niaz & Muhammad Farrukh Nisar (Eds.)

4. HKU1 (Beta coronavirus)

Another human coronaviruses

It usually causes respiratory syndrome in an infected person.

5. MERS-CoV [Beta coronavirus responsible for Middle East Respiratory Syndrome (MERS)]

6. SARS-CoV (beta coronavirus that causes severe acute respiratory syndrome, or SARS)

7. SARS-CoV-2 (Novel coronavirus responsible for coronavirus disease 2019 or COVID-19)

After entering the host body, the virus enters the lungs' alveoli through the angiotensin-converting enzyme 2 (ACE-2) receptor following un-coating. The genome associated with SARS-CoV-2 has a minimum of 10 open reading frames (ORFs) that can be translated [2]. The first one ORFs (ORF1a/b), which is around two-third of virus ribonucleic acid (RNA), undergoes translation to form polyproteins (pp)-1α) and pp-1β. It further undergoes processing to form 16 non-structural proteins (nsp1-nsp16) and helps in viral replicase transcriptase complex formation. The membranes from the rough endoplasmic reticulum (RER) with the help of nsps are rearranged into vesicles with two biomembranes, where the replication and transcription of the virus occur. Other ORFs present on the genome contains four structural proteins viz. spike (S), envelope (E), nucleocapsid (N), and membrane (M) proteins. After entering into host cells, the antigen binds to the antigen-presenting cells (APC). It leads to the formation of a major histocompatibility complex which is further identified through cytotoxic T lymphocytes. Afterward, there is a stimulation of humoral immunity and cellular immunity, which are mediated through specific B cells and T cells, leading to IgG and IgM antibody production. There is the production of pro-inflammatory cytokines (IFN-α, IFN-g, IL-1β, IL-6, IL-12, IL-18, IL-33, TNF-α, and TGFβ, *etc.*) and chemokines (CCL2, CCL3, CCL5, CXCL8, CXCL9, CXCL10, *etc.*). In the serum of patients, there are high amounts of IL-6, IFN-α, and CCL5, along with CXCL8 and CXCL-10 has been found1. The cytokine storm, due to cytokine, will activate a vicious attack through the immune system to the body, at last leading to acute respiratory distress syndrome, failure to multiple organs, and fatal [3, 4].

Pseudovirus: An Overview

A virus formed by the recombination process and whose genetic material and protein-rich envelope are resulting out of various viruses is known as pseudovirus [5]. Furthermore, to make them incapable of producing the surface proteins independently, the genetic material present within the pseudovirus is generally altered. To produce the pseudovirus a supplementary plasmid is also required [6]. Pseudoviruses can infect disposed cells, and they can only replicate once in the host cells that are infected [5, 7].

There are certain advantages of using pseudovirus over the native virus, such as (i) pseudoviruses are safe and are effortlessly managed in biosafety level (BSL)-2 laboratories [8]. It is manipulated experimentally in an easy manner contrary to wild-type viruses. (ii) The indigenous virus proteins and pseudo viral proteins present on the surface have a high resemblance in their conformational structure and help facilitate the entry of the virus inside the host cells. Hence, pseudovirus is extensively utilized in cell tropism [9], identification of receptor [10], suppression of virus [11], and for the production and evaluation of antibodies [12] and vaccines [13]. (iii) The results from *ex vivo* pseudovirus-dependent antiviral assays and live viruses are relatable [14, 15]. (iv) To carry the reporter genes, encoding whether an enzyme or a fluorescent protein, the genetic engineering of pseudovirus is done, which helps to carry out quantitative analysis with viruses easily [16], and the reporter gene expression is directly dependent on the number of pseudovirus-infected cells [17].

CLASSIFICATION OF THE PACKAGING SYSTEMS FOR ENVELOPE PSEUDOTYPED VIRUSES

Due to outbreak of numerous novel viruses, such as the Ebola virus, Marburg virus, Lassa fever virus, immunodeficiency virus, and coronavirus, numerous systems are developing for producing pseudotype virus having envelope in their structure [5, 18, 19]. Some of the prime packaging systems are mentioned herein.

Lentiviral Vector Packaging Systems

Lentivirus has a long incubation period and is used to deliver a huge quantity of genetic information into the deoxyribonucleic acid (DNA) of the host. Examples of lentiviruses- Human immunodeficiency virus (HIV), simian immunodeficiency virus, and feline immunodeficiency virus (https://www.genetherapynet.com/viral-vector/lentiviruses.html). Lentiviral vectors are considered the foremost option for packaging systems due to their high efficacy to produce enveloped pseudotype viruses [5].

The Human Immunodeficiency Virus Packaging System

The utmost utilized pseudovirus packaging system is HIV-1. The packaging system is made by cloning HIV genes with DNA vectors. There is no conversion back of pseudovirus to wild-type virus due to minimalize the viral gene recombination. It also utilizes 2 to 4 number plasmids as vector systems. The HIV 2-plasmid arrangement includes an envelope plasmid in addition to that one HIV-1 backbone plasmid, *i.e.,* pSG3Δenv and pNL4-3 [20]. Due to very low viral yield, this system is not perfect, and hence modifications are done by adding other sequences to get reporter gene expression which is far better, so that yield can be improved. For example, after the insertion of firefly luciferase (Fluc) as a reporter gene inside pSG3Δenv in between Env and nef. There is the production of pSG3Δenv.Fluc.Δnef [13]. This helps to produce numerous HIV pseudoviruses. It carry the envelope proteins such as MERS-CoV, rabies virus (RV), EBOV, MARV, LASV, Nipahvirus (NiV) as well as chikungunya virus [21].

The HIV 3-plasmid system includes three kinds of plasmids: the plasmid, which aids in packaging, a plasmid that aids in the transfer of genetic material comprising the marker gene, and a plasmid that expresses the E-proteins. There is a splitting of the backbone of the HIV-1 into distinct packaging and plasmids in this system. It aids in the transfer of genetic material. The plasmid, which aids in packaging, shows an expression of gag protein. It also pol proteins and the plasmid that aids in the transfer of genetic material. It has cis-regulatory components (required for HIV reverse transcription process, integration, packaging), multiple cloning sites, and marker genes. The plasmid that expresses the envelope has a vector that carries the envelope genetic factor obtained from the cytomegalovirus promoter [22 - 24].

HIV 4-plasmid arrangement depends on the three-plasmid arrangement. This packaging system includes- 1 packaging plasmid, which shows the expression of gag protein, as well as pol protein, the plasmid which aids in packaging, encodes for Rev protein, a plasmid that forms the wild type envelope, and a plasmid which aids in the transfer of genetic material [25].

There is the introduction of SIV vectors to evaluate whether these vectors can be used for the transfer of genes due to safety concerns. There is the development of a 3-plasmid system. The blood leucocytes and CD34+ cells display high transduction efficiency due to SIV-based pseudoviruses [26]. The vector pR4SA having green fluorescent protein. Also, a pseudovirus SIV 3+ packaging vector helped determine various features that will help in cellular membrane development in case of numerous viruses that are to be targeted and estimation of their yield [27]. A pseudotype virus for the SARS-CoV was developed by Moore and colleagues by using an SIV packaging system to monitor the anti-SARS-CoV compounds [5, 28, 29].

There is a significant improvement of spike protein expression by codon maximization of the SARS-CoV S-protein gene. SIV expresses the green fluorescent protein when pseudotype with the SARS-CoV S-protein, proficiently infects HEK293T cells expressing ACE-2. The enzymatic activity of ACE-2 is having no role in S-protein-mediated infection [28]. Pseudoviruses have simplified preclinical studies in antiviral screening and studies related to gene therapy [5, 28].

The Feline Immunodeficiency Virus Packaging System

The system established on the Feline immunodeficiency virus is one of the promising methods which were used to produce pseudotyped Ebola virus. The packaging plasmid and transfer vector of feline immunodeficiency virus were used. It showed a higher titer compared to the Ebola pseudovirus packaged with the HIV system. Higher pseudo viral titers have resulted by causing mutation in glycoproteins, leading to higher safety of pseudoviruses [30]. The production of several pseudotyped viruses, such as SARS-CoV, vesicular stomatitis virus (VSV), and Ross river virus could happen with the help of the FIV packaging system. These viral particles are utilized to study gene transduction and viral receptor recognition [31, 32].

The Vesicular Stomatitis Virus Packaging System

This packaging arrangement possesses no rigid selectiveness for the proteins having envelope in their structure. It is a multipurpose tool used to develop pseudotyped viruses with the advantage. These produced viruses can be maintained under BSL-2 laboratories. After introducing VSV and virus conjointly to produce co-infection in the cells, there was the production of the pseudotyped virus, which carried the VSV nucleus along with the protein comprising envelope [33]. A stable VSV was produced for the first time by Stillman and colleagues, who cloned the genetic material of VSV inside a plasmid [34]. This VSV help to produce pseudovirus, which carries heterogeneous glycoproteins [35, 36]. Numerous reporter genes were inserted into its plasmid to facilitate easy detection [37, 38]. Examples of pseudovirus packaged by the VSV system are Ebola virus glycoprotein (EBOV GP), Hantavirus G1/G2, measles virus, Arenavirus glycoprotein, avian influenza virus, and Nipah virus. There is a possibility that residual VSV virus mixed with pseudoviruses while making it with the help of the VSV packaging system. In doing so, the neutralization assay results can be complicated, and it may show false-positive results. The amount of vesicular stomatitis virus use should be minimized to avoid such complications. If the extra

VSV is supposed to be interrupted with an assay, the pseudovirus preparation can be treated with a VSV neutralizing antibody.

The Murine Leukemia Virus Packaging System

Murine leukemia virus packaging system with vesicular stomatitis virus causes infection in the cells. It leads to the production of pseudovirus that can be used in the neutralization of antibody assay [39]. Murine leukemia virus packaging arrangement, even known as a retroviral arrangement, is generally employed for the production of pseudovirus such a: Ebola virus glycoprotein (EBOV GP), La Crosse virus (G1/G2), Hantavirus (G1/G2), human immunodeficiency virus -1 envelope (HIV-1 Env), human immunodeficiency virus -2 envelope (HIV-2 Env), Visna virus Env, Ross river virus glycoprotein (RRV GP), Simian immunodeficiency virus (SIV), SARS-CoVs, MERS-CoVs, Vesicular stomatitis virus glycoprotein (VSV GP) Arenavirus glycoprotein, and Influenza virus hemaglutinin.

The genome of the murine leukemia virus is split into 2 parts to produce the highly efficient packaging system: reporter gene and an encoding gag-pol, which were further cloned into the plasmids [40]. Several cell lines were developed to enhance the stability of the MLV packaging system. Compared to the HIV packaging system, murine leukemia virus is an excellent choice in few cases, such as studying Lassa mammarenavirus (LASV) mediated entry into the host cells. Also, the MLV system is 5-fold more effective as compared to the HIV system [41].

Other Packaging Systems

The abovementioned pseudovirus-based arrangements are not necessarily effective in the production of a few pseudoviruses. During these situations, reverse genetics may be helpful. Hu and colleagues used the human immunodeficiency virus system to develop the pseudotype dengue virus (DENV) types 1-4. Its titer was unsatisfactorily high [42]. Reporter genes had been inserted to develop a plasmid-based, self-organized, and pseudotype flavivirus with the help of reverse genetics into the viral genome. Other few instances of this are the West Nile virus (WNV) and the Japanese encephalitis virus.

Mechanistic Study of Viral Infection

Recently, single-strand RNA (ssRNA) *betacoronavirus* has been recognized, which involves few other viruses, *i.e.,* SARS, MERS, and SARS-CoV-2. Current learning concludes the similarity between SARS coronavirus and novel coronavirus based on genetic material. It has been proven that novel coronavirus is 96% similar to bat coronavirus. It shows the 90% sequence similarity in essential enzymes like 3CL pro (3CL protease), PL pro (Papain-like proteinase), RNA-dependent RNA polymerase, along withspike glycoprotein [43]. Its size range between 60-140 nm, and consider its spherical shape. The mechanism regarding access of virus into the host cell can be either by endocytosis (receptor-mediated) or by plasma membrane direct fusion [44]. Coronavirus is composed of quartet proteins such as M (membrane), S (spike), E (envelope), and N (nucleocapsid). The spike polypeptide is mainly accountable for the affixing virus through which it enters inside the target cell; as a result, it causes the infection process. Therefore these proteins account for the chief intent for coronavirus drug formation and immunization [45].

Large homogenous proteins, generally known as spike proteins, are important for host cell interactions. The cell responsible for forming the viral cell membrane (epithelial) is parabronchial and pulmonary cells. Furthermore, this epithelial cell has an abundant ACE-2, which is attacked by the virus. Transfer of coronavirus into the human circulatory system generally takes place by recognition of ACE-2 by S protein. In a recent study, it is being said that the ACE-2 is the novel coronavirus receptor and is requisite for cell entry. This virus is a family of single-stranded RNA that replicates virus genes by benefiting from the host cell.

Moreover, elaborating the process, once the virus has proceeded towards the cell organelle (ribosome) of living host cells, it utilizes the organelle of the living cell for replicating polyprotein (PP). The process of imitation and formation of parent polyprotein takes place in epithelia. Once polyprotein is formed, the two enzymes, *i.e.,* 3CLpro and PLpro are responsible for rending the polyprotein into much smaller products used to replicate the new virus. The enzyme RNA-dependent RNA polymerase is a paramount biocatalyst responsible for the generation of the daughter RNA genome by catalyzing the genesis of RNA strand (complementary) with the help of the virus RNA template [43].

Another structural protein, hemaglutinin (HA), has a crucial job in the attachment of the virus to the receptor, entry of virus, and the fusion of membrane in influenza. Throughout the time of virus inflammation, HA effectuates attachment of virus following its entry into the target cells. Therefore, for persuading immunity against the influenza virus primary target is HA protein [46]. Several other viral proteins are responsible for the release of coronavirus. The twin proteins M and E had an indispensable role in the assembly of coronavirus. The inter-relationship connecting the M and S protein as well as M and N protein is responsible for the recruitment of structural components. The M protein controls homotypic interactions, which serves as a platform for viral assemblage and ontogenesis in impaired cells. Co-articulation of the two proteins, *i.e.,* envelope and nucleocapsid, accompanied by membrane protein, lead to the development and exemption of VLP's (Virus-like particles), later the transfection process of Vero E6 cells. Particles of coronavirus can also be budded inside the host cell by ER Golgi intermediate compartment (ERGIC). These particles enter the smooth wall vesicle, which is then transferred into the specific pathway liberating the virus through the process of exocytosis [43].

It has already been mentioned that S-protein is mainly in charge of mediating virus entry inside the living cell. The S-protein comprises three components, *i.e.,* a membrane (single pass), tail (short intracellular), and ectodomain. Component ectodomain may be further segregated into two subunits which include receptor binding and membrane fusion. The receptor-binding subunit 1 consists of dyad autonomous domains, NTD (N- terminal domain), and C-domain. The current virus condition will either bind with NTD or C-domain or intermittently to both and functions like RBD (receptor-binding domain). The host ACE-2 is recognized as a receptor by S1 C-domain, which is considered as RBD. The primary function of ACE-2 is to regulate the pathway (renin-angiotensin), which modulates the pressure level of blood. ACE-2 also consists of two domains which are the C-terminal collectrin domain and the N-terminal peptidase domain. The binding interactions of ACE-2 and SARS-CoV RBD mainly depend on the range of cell and living host species to which the virus infects [47].

Another mechanism related to S-protein emphasizes the involvement of other cell organelles, *i.e.,* Golgi complex and rough endoplasmic reticulum (RER). S-protein is transferred to polysomes (membrane-bound), then incorporated into RER, and finally moves to the Golgi complex. S-protein is integrated into virus particles during the transport, which is positioned between the Golgi complex and RER. Secretary vesicles carry entire virus particles from the Golgi complex to the cytoplasmic membrane. The release of these virions takes place when vesicles fuse (virions containing vesicles) with the plasma membrane. Thus protein is attached with virions gets shifted to the surface of the membrane. SARS-CoV S-protein is 1255 amino acids long which has13 amino acid signal peptides, a single ectodomain that contains 1182 amino acids, and a transmembrane region (28 residues) [48]. Considering the examples of SAR-CoV virus in 2003 and HCOV-NL 63 (human coronavirus NL63) recognized in 2004 generally attached to the ACE-2 receptor. It initiates the process of endocytosis through which the virus enters inside the host cell. The coronavirus entry in human cells occurred *via* two important mechanisms: caveolae-independent endocytosis and clathrin-mediated endocytosis. It was anticipated that novel coronavirus might use the same mechanistic approach for cell entry [44].

Recent studies emphasize glycogen synthase kinase3 (GSK3) which introduces phosphoryl group by the process of phosphorylation to N protein of coronavirus by repressing GSK 3 the viral replication in Vero E6 cells can be inhibited. Another important factor for viral synthesis is hnRNPA1 (heterogeneous nuclear ribonucleoprotein A1), associated with the splicing of pre-existing m-RNA in the center of the cell, *i.e.,* nucleus along with injunction in the host cell. It is worth noting that nucleocapsid polypeptide of coronavirus can bind with human hnRNPA1. On account of these findings, we may conclude that hnRNPA1 can bind with coronavirus protein to form the replication complex, which generally controls the synthesis of viral RNA [43].

Pseudoviral System Application to Neutralize Antibody and Antibody-Dependent Cell-Mediated Cytotoxicity Assay

The most vital protective mechanism against viral infection *in vivo* is antibody-dependent cellular cytotoxicity (ADCC). The antibodies that conciliate ADCC activity can lead to several conducive circumstances, including lowering the risk of infection, decreased load of the virus, reduced transmission rate, and slower disease progression. Comparing the case of neutralizing and non-neutralizing HIV-1 monoclonal antibodies, the former does not confirm the activity of antibody-dependent cell-mediated cytotoxicity. At the same time, the latter mediates high activity, indicating the difference between epitopes of neutralizing antibodies and ADCC. More than a dozen of neutralizing antibodies have been outlined from ADCC epitopes [49].

Neutralizing antibodies (Nabs) have an important role in protecting one from different viral diseases. The Nab responses are checked in patients infected with the virus to ensure the protection of individuals through immunity. Besides, it is also considered to be a crucial part of the development of the vaccine process. Traditionally these neutralizing assay uses replication-competent retrovirus, for many anti-sera analyzing through neutralizing assay is off-putting due to safety concerns [48].

Antibody-dependent Cellular Cytotoxicity (ADCC)

TF228 cell lines were kept in RPMI 1640 growth medium. The used blood sample was heparinized by centrifugation technique using Ficoll density gradient separation to isolate human PBMC's (peripheral blood mononuclear cells). Based on flow cytometry, ADCC assay uses TF228 cell lines as target cells and PBMC as effector cells in the T/E ratio of 1/50., Two fluorescent dyes were used to differentiate between live and dead cells. A membrane labeling dye PKH-67 is utilized to ascertain the TF228 target cells. PKH-67 dye progressively binds to the cytoplasmic membrane, and even after cell death, it remains attached to the membrane, which avoids any contamination with effector cells. TF228 target cells were tinted with PKH-67 at room temperature for 10 min, and 3 mL of FBS was added to cease the reaction. 'PBMC's were prepared by five healthy donors continued to be kept in RPMI 1640 growth medium, which contains 100 µg/mL streptomycin and 100 U/mL penicillin. TF228 cells were placed in 96-well plates round-bottomed of 50 µL capacity dispensed with a 1640 growth medium. Antibodies were placed in the well for 15 mins at 37°C in a CO_2 incubator. 'PBMC's were also put into each well and kept at 37°C for 4 hours in the CO_2 incubator. One microliter of 7 7-amino actinomycin D a DNA dye (-AAD solution) was added up and placed for 15 mins in an incubator at 4°C. The analysis of mixtures was performed by flow cytometry. Percent of ADCC was calculated [49].

Drug Screening

A wide range of approaches is applied to generate various preventive and curative measures to treat this novel coronavirus pandemic. The different processes are designed to target the S-protein which includes, subunit vaccines, viral vectored vaccines, vaccines based on RNA, neutralizing antibodies (specifically monoclonal). It is also necessary that novel coronavirus could be managed by BSL-3 [45].

As of now, there is no rectified treatment of coronavirus; hence some broad-spectrum inhibitors can be helpful to treat this pandemic. Some new compounds have been identified derived from screening assay. For example, high throughput screening by using the compound library, which exhibits antiviral activity against coronavirus. An alkaloid lycorine isolated from *Lycorisradiata* family *Amaryllidaceae* showed potency against coronaviruses. Another compound is emetine which generally hinders both RNA and DNA replication of viruses; along with that, it also displays potent anti COV activity. Mycophenolic acid (an immunosuppressant) derivative Mycophenolatemofetil reported stronger activity against coronavirus. Phenazopyridine which is used as a urinary analgesic,has found to exhibit broad-spectrum inhibitory activity. The FDA-approved drug pyrviniumpamoate is used as an anthelminthic, which also shows inhibition of viral replication and low toxicity. Though several drugs either inhibit the entry or replication of the virus, still the *in vivo* antiviral efficiency remains unknown. A combination of different antiviral drugs may result in synergistic effects of COV infections [50].

A recent study on natural products also suggests antiviral activity. Two natural compounds which are flavone and coumarin show promising results as proteinase inhibitors of SARS-CoV-2. Some more natural product extracts which have shown effective results against HIV are *Tordyliumpersicum* Boiss. and Hausskn extracts along with this *Cuscuta compestris* which effectively inhibits HIV replication. Some Chinese traditional medicines, such as *polygonum cuspidatum* may have some components that need to be checked in clinical trials [43].

Chloroquine is included by the federal guidelines useful for the cure of novel SARS-CoV-2, which is generally found based on preclinical trials. Although the drug lies in the nascent stage of the clinical trial, it is important to be conscious about the preventive and analeptic clinical protocols, which include disease stage, dosing, and patient population. According to the latest study, hydroxychloroquine is considered safe along that it also has corresponding anti-CoV-2 results *in vitro* in comparison with the former drug. Several other findings also revealed that drugs that have shown good results in preclinical trials have conflicting results in animal studies. Therefore, one should be cautious before prescribing these drugs [44].

Another set of research also focuses on the use of Ibuprofen which worsens the disease. In France, the database study revealed that the patients who were pre-hospitalized for community-acquired pneumonia were administered with non-steroidal anti-inflammatory drugs due to which they develop more severe pneumonia. An additional study was untaken on children's, unveiling the risk factors for Ibuprofen and acetaminophen [51].

Previously, several drugs were utilized to cure MERS-CoV and SARS. These drugs might have potency against SARS-CoV-2, such as ribavirin, ritonavir, lopinavir, and favipiravir. In the recent scenario of COVID-19, there is no effective drug to treat this pandemic; however, reports suggest that one patient has been successfully treated with Remdesivir in the US. Current studies indicate that the combination of a small molecule of Remdesivirand chloroquine successfully suppresses the SARS-COV-2 replication *in vitro*. The initial development of remdesivir was done to analyze drug efficacy on inhibition of EBOV (Ebola virus) replication. The latest computational studies ascertained few more drugs are capable of binding with SARS-COV-2 protease. They include lopinavir, oseltamivir, and ritonavir. β-D-N4-hydroxycytidine (NHC, EIDD-1931) is a broad-spectrum antiviral drug that shows antagonistic effects on various RNA viruses such as Ebola. Current research suggests that NHC can effectively inhibit MERS-COV and novel coronavirus. NHC has shown effective results to prevent virus replication in COV, novel coronavirus, and MERS. In addition to that NHC also inhibit the replication of Remdesivir (RDV) resistant virus. Pro-drug β-D--4-hydroxycytidine-5'-isopropyl ester was developed to enhance *in vivo* pharmacokinetic profile. The ongoing clinical trials on several nucleotide substrate analogs may have improved antiviral activity against novel coronavirus.

Few nucleotide substrate analogs are given below in Table **1** [43].

Table 1. Structure and chemical properties of nucleotide substrate analogs.

Drug	Drug Profile	Structure
Remdesivir (GS-5734, Gilead)	**Formula:** C27H35N6O8P **MW:** 602.6g/mole	
Ribavirin (an adenosine analog, nucleotide inhibitor)	**Formula:** C8H12N4O5 **MW:** 244.21g/mole	

(Table 1) cont.....

Drug	Drug Profile	Structure
Galidesivir (BCX-4430) an adenosine analog	**Formula:** C11H15N5O3 **MW:** 256.27 g/mole	
Favipiravir (T705)	**Formula:** C5H4FN3O2 **MW:** 157.1 g/mole	

Pseudo Virus-Based Neutralization Assay: Protocols and Neutralization Assaysof SARS-CoV-2

SARS-pseudo virus infects Vero E6 cells and coronavirus S-glycoprotein murine leukemia virus (MuLV). There is no requirement of low pH for infection; hence the virus can enter by direct fusion. The SARS pseudovirus which was produced can be retarded by the serum obtained recovered patient from coronavirus. This also indicates that S-glycoprotein present in SARS-CoV can be the target of neutralizing antibodies. The main purpose of producing SARS pseudovirus was to prepare an assay for determining virus-neutralizing antibodies. After 9 days of illness, the antibodies against the SARS protein appear, so on that account, high throughput serology-based diagnosis should be developed, which could complement PCR-based analysis. For enhancing the accuracy of early diagnosis, a virus-neutralizing assay can also be used. Since neutralizing antibodies is a key factor for virus clearance, this procedure can also be used to determine the prognosis of the disease [48]. SARS pseudovirus could also be used to assess the potency of vaccines based on various S-glycoprotein.

Production of SARS-COV Pseudo-virus

Transfection of the MuLV cell line, *i.e.,* TELCeB6, was done with pHCMV-S, pcDNA-S, pHCMV-G, or pLTR-gp140 any of the two methods, which include either lipofection or calcium phosphate precipitation. Two days after post-transfection, cell medium was harvested, and centrifugation was done to remove cell debris. The supernatant liquid was removed and stored by using a virus stock at -80°C. Titers were performed in the cell. For example, SARS-S and VSV-G have Vero E6 cells, and HIV-1 gp140 has HOS-CD4-CCR5. Cell infection was done by 60-80 infections units kept for 36 hours. Phosphate-buffered saline(PBS) was used for cell washing, which was incubated by mixing 1% formaldehyde and 0.05% glutaraldehyde along with PBS kept for 10 mins at room temperature. The cell washing process was again followed along with incubation by a fresh staining solution. It contains PBS, 5mM of potassium ferricyanide and potassium ferrocyanide, 1mg/ml of X-Gal, and 2mM $MgCl_2$ kept for less than two hours at 37°C.M

The analysis was performed by manually counting stained blue cells with the help of the inverted microscope. pH dependency of viral entry is determined by the culture media technique in which Vero E6 was placed in media comprising chloroquine of 0-100 μM for 1 hour at 37°C. Pseudovirus VSV-G or SARS-S absorb the cells without chloroquine under similar time and temperature conditions. After removing the virus, inoculum cells were washed. Then, the infection proceeded for 36 h again in chloroquine absence. The infections were performed in duplicates [48].

During the pseudovirus production, cell lines that were tested include Hela, A549, 293 T, and BS-C-1. The BS-C-1cells are the kidney cells of African green monkeys, which were earlier not sensitive enough, but when infections were performed with high multiplicity, the detection of infected BS-C-1 was feasible. As a result of cell division which follows the integration of MuLV pseudovirus genome encoding, the beta-galactosidase pseudovirus appears to be doublet. Yet, these duos are calculated as a solo unit. On comparing the output of severe acute respiratory syndrome pseudovirus, the vectors pHCMV-S and pcDNA-3 show different results as the former yield was about $2x10^4$; however, the latter has 5-fold greater yield.

The vesicular stomatitis virus G protein lies in the range between $3×104$ and $9×104$. Further, the yields of various other pseudovirus are as HIV-1 lies between $2×103$ and $2×104$. The cationic lipid method, *i.e.,* lipofection, is considered more efficient than the calcium phosphate method for the production of the SARS pseudovirus [48].

Plasmid encoding Env-defective was used for co-transfection of 293T cells along with pNL4-3. Luc.RE (Luciferase-expressing HIV-1). It also includes 10 µg of 6 plasmids HK97 HA, QH-HA, 1194-HA, Xj-HA, AH-HA, and H1N1-HA. By using the calcium phosphate method, they were transferred to 100mm of dishes. After 8 hours cells changed to 'Dulbecco's modified eagle medium (DMEM) and neuraminidase (NA) from *vibrio cholerae*were added after 24 and 48 hours post-transfection at 4.8µg/ml concentration control transfection was formed without NA addition. The volume of supernatant liquid that contains HA pseudovirus was harvested for 72 hours post-transfection, which was then utilized for solo cycle infection. Vectors like HIV-1, VSV-G, VSV-G-pcDNA3.1, and pc-DNA3.1 are utilized for co-transfecting with pNL4-3. Luc.RE for the generation of VSV-G pseudovirus and as control pseudovirus without Env. For titration, the 293 pseudovirus cells were infected with 100µl and bi-fold dilution in culture plates (96-well), leading to luciferase activity detection after 72 hours. RLU (relative luciferase unit) is considered for the expression of pseudovirus titer [46].

Neutralization Assay of Pseudovirus

TZM.bL and 293T/17 cell lines were procured and kept in Dulbecco's modified eagle's medium (D-MEM), containing 10% fetal bovine serum inactivated by heat with that 50 µg/mL gentamicin and HEPES which is of 25 mM. The EDTA solution did cell harvesting. Cell lines were kept at a specific temperature of 37°C in a humidifier that contains 5% CO_2. The neutralization assay of the virus was measured with the help of luciferase assay in cell TZM.bL. During this process, luciferase reduction is measured, which follows the solo cycle of virus infection. Serum sample dilution was performed in 10% DMEM growth medium (100µL/well), and 50 µL of 200 TCID50 (tissue culture infection dose) of the virus was put onto each well, also kept in incubation for 1 h at 37°C. After that cell, TZM.bL was added to the DMEM growth medium (10%) containing 11µg/mL DEAE dextran (diethyl aminoethyl). After 48 h of incubation at 37°C, addition of 100 µL luciferase reagent (bright glow) takes place, thereby removing 150 µL of assay medium. For 2 mins, cells were lysed after that cell lysate of 150 µL quantity was moved to the plates. The luminescence was measured using victor 3 luminometer. The data was analyzed by using neutralizing antibody analysis software [52]. Another pseudo-virus-neutralizing assay, which contains supernatant liquid and about 1 h at 37°C they were incubated by H5N1 HA monoclonal antibodies before the addition to 293T cell plate (96-well culture plates), where 33G4 monoclonal antibodies were used as the negative control. After 24 h, fresh medium was added to cells, and further lysing buffer and lysate were also put into 96-well plates. In addition to the luciferase substrate to the plates, relative luciferase activity was determined using ultra 384 luminometers. Calculation of HA pseudovirus neutralization was presented as neutralizing antibody titer in 50% value, *i.e.*, NT_{50} [46].

Infections unit of the pseudovirus near about 60-80 diluted by convalescent sera and incubated for 1 h at 37°C. The amalgam was prepended into Vero E6 cells which include VSV-G or HOS-CD4/CCR5. Inflammation continued for 36 h, and neutralizing activity was carried out by moderate or no serum controls. Neutralizing tests are also performed by using convalescent sera after 13-50 days of symptoms onset.

High throughput Evaluation of Infections (pseudovirus)

Pseudovirus neutralization testing is a quantitative, secured, and tactful process. Still, it owns a limitation, *i.e.,* X-Gal stained cells are counted individually by microscope. ELISPOT reader was used as an automating data collector to surpass this issue. However, this instrument utilizes to appraise T cell antigen-specific cytokine responses. This instrument efficiently calculates spots at solo cell resolution and precisely processing 96-well plates in less than 20 mins.

Protein Expression, cell Culture, and Western Blot Assay for Bhk-21 and other Cell Lines

Except for Vero E6, all cell lines were maintained in DMEM along with 10% fetal bovine serum, L-glutamine as 2 mM, and antibiotics, including streptomycin and penicillin. Same supplements were used for cells Vero E6 but kept in 'Eagle's minimum essential medium (EMEM) containing 0.1mM amino acids (non-essential). Cultured at a temperature of 37°C, incubated with 5% CO_2 and cells were transferred by calcium phosphate precipitation method with a plasmid for expression of S-protein. 0.5ml of 0.25M $CaCl_2$ solution containing 30 μg of plasmid was combined with 1.5 mM sodium hydrogen phosphate, 280 mM of NaCl, and 50 mM of 4-(2-hydroxy ethyl)-1-piperazine ethane sulfonic acid is maintained at pH 7.1 and was prepended to the cell. For overnight incubation, culture media was returned and again incubated for two more consecutive days. Infections of cells were done by vTF7-3, which includes pTM-S and pTM-eSHis. Hypotonic buffer is used for the process of cell lysis, which contains (10 mM NaCl, 1.5 mM $MgCl_2$, 10 mM of tris buffer, and 1% NP-40) after the following 2 days of infection. Insoluble debris and nuclei were removed by centrifugation. Further lysates of cells were exposed to western blot and sodium dodecyl sulfate-polyacrylamide gel electrophoresis (SDS-PAGE). Detection of S-protein was done with the help of monoclonal antibody (1:3000 dilution), convalescent sera (1:100 dilution), or IgG antibody discretely. Protein bands were visualized by using the chemiluminescence detection system [48].

HIV-1p24 and HA were determined by SDS-PAGE, which is followed by western blot. The lysed pseudoviruses were resolved by adding 10-20% tricine gel after that shifted to the membrane of nitrocellulose, by using 5% non-fat milk blocking was performed and kept all-night at 4°C. Anti-HIV-1 p24 and HA did the incubation of blots at dilution of 1:1000. After washing blots three times, HRP-conjugated anti-mouse IgG (1:5000) was used for incubation kept at room temperature for about an hour. Visualization was performed by using western blot substrate reagents [46].

BHK-21 cells are susceptive to various viruses, including human adenovirus D, reovirus, vesicular stomatitis virus, *etc.* BHK-21 cells were lysed incubating in 0.5% NP-40 buffer at 4°c for 30 mins. Separations of lysates were moved to a nitrocellulose membrane by electrophoresis (SDS-PAGE), accompanied by blocking with skim milk (5%) for 60 mins in PBS. Then, it was incubated with primary antibody overnight at 4°C. Tween 20 buffer and PBS were used to wash. Then, again the membrane was incubated by antibody (secondary) for about an hour. Scanning was done by utilizing an infrared imaging system [50].

ELISA for Detection of p24

Enzyme-linked immunosorbent assay (ELISA) measures p24 pseudovirus. This method plates (96-well) were coated previously with anti-HIV-1 P24 (5µg/ml), which was kept overnight at 4°c and inhibited or blocked by 2% non-fat milk for 2 h at 37°C. After the process of washing is complete, HIV-IgG sera (1µg/mL) was added, incubated at 37°C· and kept for 1 h. Further, subsequent incubation with biotin-labeled goat antihuman IgG (1:10,000) along with horseradish peroxidase (HRP) (1:10,000) for 1 h at 37°C temperature was done. Further, the substrate, *i.e.,* TMB 3,3´, 5,5'tetramethylbenzidine, was put onto the plates, and termination of the reaction was done by 1 N H_2SO_4. ELISA plate reader was used to measure absorbance at 450 nm [46].

Cell Viability Assays

To assess cell viability, methyl-thiazolyl-tetrazolium (MTT) assay was applied. To the final concentration (0.5 mg/mL), MTT was included, and cells were incubated in 5% CO_2 at 37°C for 3 h. The plates were centrifuged, and the supernatant liquid was removed with the help of a micropipette. Further, 100 µL of DMSO (dimethyl sulfoxide) was added, and plates were shaken gently. The absorbance was detected at 580 nm with the help of the Microelisa Auto Reader MR 580 spectrometer.

Coronavirus Entry Inhibition Assay for MERS

Previously inhibiting coronavirus entry was generally determined by using pseudoviruses. The co-transfection of 293F T cells was done by using plasmids which are PNL4-3.luc.RE and pVRC-MERS-S, the culture supernatant liquid was collected 72 h later. After attaining a density of 5000 in 96-well plates, the dipeptidyl peptidase 4 (DPP4) was infected with 200 TCID50. The culture was resuscitated by adding 2% fetal bovine serum (FBS), *i.e.,* fresh medium. After the incubation for 48 h, finally, luciferase activity was determined by using a luminometer.

Immunofluorescence Assay

In this process, BHK-21 cells were infected by HCoV-OC43-WT, along with 10 µM indicator inhibitor with chloroquine as positive and DMSO as negative controls. 72 h later, 4% formaldehyde was added, which was permeabilized in Triton X-100 (0.5%), and 5% bovine serum albumin was used for blocking. The examination was done by nucleocapsid protein antibody (anti-HCoV-OC43) kept for 1 h at normal room temperature. Washing of cells was done three times using PBS, incubated with fluorescein isothiocyanate labeled IgG (1:100) for 1 h. Cells were washed again for the nuclei detection by staining it with 4,6-diamidino-2-phenylindole. Images were obtained and analyzed with the help of a video documentation system using a fluorescence microscope [50].

CRISPR Technology

CRISPR is clustered regularly interspaced short palindromic repeats. It is a very basic and potent tool that is designed to modify mammalian cell genomes. Due to the development of low-cost-sensitive RNA detection methods, this is rapid and may help in virus detection, genotyping along with disease progression monitoring. CRISPR diagnostic assay uses Cas enzymology, which targets Orflab or spike gene, and pre-amplification of nucleic acid to establish the desired RNA sequence. One more factor for targeting spike and ORFlab gene is gRNA (guide RNA) and isothermal primers which may be designed for effective CRISPR. This is a rapid diagnostic assay and can provide results in an hour with RNA detection, having even single base pair mismatch capability. Hence, it is important to develop such a diagnostic assay that is rapid and robust in such a pandemic situation [43].

CONCLUSION

Due to several emerging viruses, such as the Ebola virus, Marburg virus, Lassa fever virus, immunodeficiency virus, and coronavirus, several packaging systems are developing to produce envelope pseudotyped viruses. Different assays are being developed as neutralization assays of pseudovirus. Still, there is an emerging need for the development of neutralization assays of pseudovirus.

CONSENT FOR PUBLICATION

Not Applicable.

CONFLICT OF INTEREST

The author confirms that this chapter contents have no conflict of interest.

ACKNOWLEDGEMENT

Declared none.

REFERENCES

[1]   Zhou P, Yang X-L, Wang X-G, *et al.* A pneumonia outbreak associated with a new coronavirus of probable bat origin. Nature 2020; 579(7798): 270-3.
[http://dx.doi.org/10.1038/s41586-020-2012-7] [PMID: 32015507]

[2]   Kim D, Lee J-Y, Yang J-S, Kim JW, Kim VN, Chang H. The architecture of SARS-CoV-2 transcriptome. Cell 2020; 181(4): 914-921.e10.
[http://dx.doi.org/10.1016/j.cell.2020.04.011] [PMID: 32330414]

[3]   Rothan HA, Byrareddy SN. The epidemiology and pathogenesis of coronavirus disease (COVID-19) outbreak. J Autoimmun 2020; 109102433
[http://dx.doi.org/10.1016/j.jaut.2020.102433] [PMID: 32113704]

[4]   Cascella M, Rajnik M, Cuomo A, *et al.* Features, evaluation and treatment coronavirus (COVID-19). Statpearls [internet]: StatPearls Publishing 2020.

[5]   Li Q, Liu Q, Huang W, Li X, Wang Y. Current status on the development of pseudoviruses for enveloped viruses. Rev Med Virol 2018; 28(1)e1963
[http://dx.doi.org/10.1002/rmv.1963] [PMID: 29218769]

[6]   Clapham PR. Vesicular Stomatitis Virus Pseudotypes of Retroviruses BT - Practical Molecular Virology: Viral Vectors for Gene Expression.95-102.

[7]   Zhang L, Li Q, Liu Q, Huang W, Nie J, Wang Y. A bioluminescent imaging mouse model for Marburg virus based on a pseudovirus system. Hum Vaccin Immunother 2017; 13(8): 1811-7.
[http://dx.doi.org/10.1080/21645515.2017.1325050] [PMID: 28481728]

[8]   Welch SR, Guerrero LW, Chakrabarti AK, *et al.* Lassa and Ebola virus inhibitors identified using minigenome and recombinant virus reporter systems. Antiviral Res 2016; 136: 9-18.
[http://dx.doi.org/10.1016/j.antiviral.2016.10.007] [PMID: 27771389]

[9]   Bartosch B, Dubuisson J, Cosset F-L. Infectious hepatitis C virus pseudo-particles containing functional E1-E2 envelope protein complexes. J Exp Med 2003; 197(5): 633-42.
[http://dx.doi.org/10.1084/jem.20021756] [PMID: 12615904]

[10]   Radoshitzky SR, Abraham J, Spiropoulou CF, *et al.* Transferrin receptor 1 is a cellular receptor for New World haemorrhagic fever arenaviruses. Nature 2007; 446(7131): 92-6.
[http://dx.doi.org/10.1038/nature05539] [PMID: 17287727]

[11]   Wang J, Cheng H, Ratia K, *et al.* A comparative high-throughput screening protocol to identify entry

inhibitors of enveloped viruses. J Biomol Screen 2014; 19(1): 100-7.
[http://dx.doi.org/10.1177/1087057113494405] [PMID: 23821643]

[12]　Robinson JE, Hastie KM, Cross RW, *et al.* Most neutralizing human monoclonal antibodies target novel epitopes requiring both Lassa virus glycoprotein subunits. Nat Commun 2016; 7: 11544.
[http://dx.doi.org/10.1038/ncomms11544] [PMID: 27161536]

[13]　Nie J, Wu X, Ma J, *et al.* Development of *in vitro* and *in vivo* rabies virus neutralization assays based on a high-titer pseudovirus system. Sci Rep 2017; 7: 42769.
[http://dx.doi.org/10.1038/srep42769] [PMID: 28218278]

[14]　Wright E, Temperton NJ, Marston DA, McElhinney LM, Fooks AR, Weiss RA. Investigating antibody neutralization of lyssaviruses using lentiviral pseudotypes: a cross-species comparison. J Gen Virol 2008; 89(Pt 9): 2204-13.
[PMID: 18753230]

[15]　Zhou S, Liu Q, Wu X, *et al.* A safe and sensitive enterovirus A71 infection model based on human SCARB2 knock-in mice. Vaccine 2016; 34(24): 2729-36.
[http://dx.doi.org/10.1016/j.vaccine.2016.04.029] [PMID: 27102822]

[16]　Liu Q, Nie J, Huang W, *et al.* Comparison of two high-throughput assays for quantification of adenovirus type 5 neutralizing antibodies in a population of donors in China. PLoS One 2012; 7(5): e37532-2.
[http://dx.doi.org/10.1371/journal.pone.0037532] [PMID: 22655054]

[17]　Chan E, Heilek-Snyder G, Cammack N, Sankuratri S, Ji C. Development of a Moloney murine leukemia virus-based pseudotype anti-HIV assay suitable for accurate and rapid evaluation of HIV entry inhibitors. J Biomol Screen 2006; 11(6): 652-63.
[http://dx.doi.org/10.1177/1087057106288881] [PMID: 16844967]

[18]　Sakuma T, De Ravin SS, Tonne JM, *et al.* Characterization of retroviral and lentiviral vectors pseudotyped with xenotropic murine leukemia virus-related virus envelope glycoprotein. Hum Gene Ther 2010; 21(12): 1665-73.
[http://dx.doi.org/10.1089/hum.2010.063] [PMID: 20507233]

[19]　Nie J, Liu Y, Huang W, Wang Y. Development of a triple-color pseudovirion-based assay to detect neutralizing antibodies against human papillomavirus. Viruses 2016; 8(4): 107.
[http://dx.doi.org/10.3390/v8040107] [PMID: 27120611]

[20]　Bosch V, Pawlita M. Mutational analysis of the human immunodeficiency virus type 1 env gene product proteolytic cleavage site. J Virol 1990; 64: 2337-44.

[21]　Liu Q, Fan C, Li Q, *et al.* Antibody-dependent-cellular-cytotoxicity-inducing antibodies significantly affect the post-exposure treatment of Ebola virus infection. Sci Rep 2017; 7: 45552.
[http://dx.doi.org/10.1038/srep45552] [PMID: 28358050]

[22]　Ao Z, Patel A, Tran K, *et al.* Characterization of a trypsin-dependent avian influenza H5N1-pseudotyped HIV vector system for high throughput screening of inhibitory molecules. Antiviral Res 2008; 79(1): 12-8.
[http://dx.doi.org/10.1016/j.antiviral.2008.02.001] [PMID: 18359097]

[23]　Guo Y, Rumschlag-Booms E, Wang J, *et al.* Analysis of hemagglutinin-mediated entry tropism of H5N1 avian influenza. Virol J 2009; 6: 39.
[http://dx.doi.org/10.1186/1743-422X-6-39] [PMID: 19341465]

[24]　Ferrara F, Molesti E, Böttcher-Friebertshäuser E, *et al.* The human Transmembrane Protease Serine 2 is necessary for the production of Group 2 influenza A virus pseudotypes. J Mol Genet Med 2012; 7: 309-14.
[PMID: 23577043]

[25]　Dull T, Zufferey R, Kelly M, *et al.* A third-generation lentivirus vector with a conditional packaging system. J Virol 1998; 72: 8463-71.

[26]　Sandrin V, Boson B, Salmon P, *et al.* Lentiviral vectors pseudotyped with a modified RD114 envelope glycoprotein show increased stability in sera and augmented transduction of primary lymphocytes and CD34+ cells derived from human and nonhuman primates. Blood 2002; 100(3): 823-32.
[http://dx.doi.org/10.1182/blood-2001-11-0042] [PMID: 12130492]

[27]　Sandrin V, Cosset F-L. Intracellular *versus* cell surface assembly of retroviral pseudotypes is determined by the cellular localization of the viral glycoprotein, its capacity to interact with Gag, and the expression of the Nef protein. J Biol Chem 2006; 281(1): 528-42.
[http://dx.doi.org/10.1074/jbc.M506070200] [PMID: 16195228]

[28]　Moore MJ, Dorfman T, Li W, *et al.* Retroviruses pseudotyped with the severe acute respiratory syndrome coronavirus spike protein efficiently infect cells expressing angiotensin-converting enzyme 2. J Virol 2004; 78: 10628-35.

[29]　Schnell T, Foley P, Wirth M, Münch J, Uberla K. Development of a self-inactivating, minimal lentivirus vector based on simian immunodeficiency virus. Hum Gene Ther 2000; 11(3): 439-47.
[http://dx.doi.org/10.1089/10430340050015905] [PMID: 10697118]

[30]　Medina MF, Kobinger GP, Rux J, *et al.* Lentiviral vectors pseudotyped with minimal filovirus envelopes increased gene transfer in murine lung. Mol Ther 2003; 8(5): 777-89.
[http://dx.doi.org/10.1016/j.ymthe.2003.07.003] [PMID: 14599811]

[31]　Jia HP, Look DC, Shi L, *et al.* ACE2 receptor expression and severe acute respiratory syndrome coronavirus infection depend on differentiation of human airway epithelia. J Virol 2005; 79: 14614-21.

[32]　AU - Mendenhall A Packaging HIV- or FIV-based Lentivector expression constructs & transduction of VSV-G pseudotyped viral particles. JoVE 2012; e3171.. 2012.

[33]　Huang AS, Palma EL, Hewlett N, Roizman B. Pseudotype formation between enveloped RNA and DNA viruses. Nature 1974; 252(5485): 743-5.
[http://dx.doi.org/10.1038/252743a0] [PMID: 4373658]

[34]　Stillman EA, Rose JK, Whitt MA. Replication and amplification of novel vesicular stomatitis virus minigenomes encoding viral structural proteins. J Virol 1995; 69: 2946-53.

[35]　Schnell MJ, Buonocore L, Kretzschmar E, *et al.* Foreign glycoproteins expressed from recombinant vesicular stomatitis viruses are incorporated efficiently into virus particles 1996.
[http://dx.doi.org/10.1073/pnas.93.21.11359]

[36]　Whitt MA. Generation of VSV pseudotypes using recombinant ΔG-VSV for studies on virus entry, identification of entry inhibitors, and immune responses to vaccines. J Virol Methods 2010; 169(2): 365-74.
[http://dx.doi.org/10.1016/j.jviromet.2010.08.006] [PMID: 20709108]

[37]　Moeschler S, Locher S, Conzelmann K-K, Krämer B, Zimmer G. Quantification of lyssavirus-neutralizing antibodies using vesicular stomatitis virus pseudotype particles. Viruses 2016; 8(9): 254.
[http://dx.doi.org/10.3390/v8090254] [PMID: 27649230]

[38]　Kaku Y, Noguchi A, Marsh GA, *et al.* Second generation of pseudotype-based serum neutralization assay for Nipah virus antibodies: sensitive and high-throughput analysis utilizing secreted alkaline phosphatase. J Virol Methods 2012; 179(1): 226-32.
[http://dx.doi.org/10.1016/j.jviromet.2011.11.003] [PMID: 22115786]

[39]　Witte ON, Baltimore D. Mechanism of formation of pseudotypes between vesicular stomatitis virus and murine leukemia virus. Cell 1977; 11(3): 505-11.
[http://dx.doi.org/10.1016/0092-8674(77)90068-X] [PMID: 195740]

[40]　Soneoka Y, Cannon PM, Ramsdale EE, *et al.* A transient three-plasmid expression system for the production of high titer retroviral vectors. Nucleic Acids Res 1995; 23(4): 628-33.
[http://dx.doi.org/10.1093/nar/23.4.628] [PMID: 7899083]

[41] Cosset F-L, Marianneau P, Verney G, *et al.* Characterization of lassa virus cell entry and neutralization with lassa virus pseudoparticles. J Virol 2009; 83: 3228-37.

[42] Hu H-P, Hsieh S-C, King C-C, Wang WK. Characterization of retrovirus-based reporter viruses pseudotyped with the precursor membrane and envelope glycoproteins of four serotypes of dengue viruses. Virology 2007; 368(2): 376-87.
[http://dx.doi.org/10.1016/j.virol.2007.06.026] [PMID: 17662331]

[43] Huang J, Song W, Huang H, Sun Q. Pharmacological therapeutics targeting RNA-dependent RNA polymerase, proteinase and spike protein: From mechanistic studies to clinical trials for COVID-19. J Clin Med 2020; 9(4): 1131.
[http://dx.doi.org/10.3390/jcm9041131] [PMID: 32326602]

[44] Hu TY, Frieman M, Wolfram J. Insights from nanomedicine into chloroquine efficacy against COVID-19. Nat Nanotechnol 2020; 15(4): 247-9.
[http://dx.doi.org/10.1038/s41565-020-0674-9] [PMID: 32203437]

[45] Nie J, Li Q, Wu J, *et al.* Establishment and validation of a pseudovirus neutralization assay for SARS-CoV-2. Emerg Microbes Infect 2020; 9(1): 680-6.
[http://dx.doi.org/10.1080/22221751.2020.1743767] [PMID: 32207377]

[46] Du L, Zhao G, Zhang X, *et al.* Development of a safe and convenient neutralization assay for rapid screening of influenza HA-specific neutralizing monoclonal antibodies. Biochem Biophys Res Commun 2010; 397(3): 580-5.
[http://dx.doi.org/10.1016/j.bbrc.2010.05.161] [PMID: 20617558]

[47] Li F. Receptor recognition and cross-species infections of SARS coronavirus. Antiviral Res 2013; 100(1): 246-54.
[http://dx.doi.org/10.1016/j.antiviral.2013.08.014] [PMID: 23994189]

[48] Han DP, Kim HG, Kim YB, Poon LL, Cho MW. Development of a safe neutralization assay for SARS-CoV and characterization of S-glycoprotein. Virology 2004; 326(1): 140-9.
[http://dx.doi.org/10.1016/j.virol.2004.05.017] [PMID: 15262502]

[49] Yang Z, Liu X, Sun Z, *et al.* Identification of a HIV Gp41-Specific human monoclonal antibody with potent antibody-dependent cellular cytotoxicity. Front Immunol 2018; 9: 2613.
[http://dx.doi.org/10.3389/fimmu.2018.02613] [PMID: 30519238]

[50] Shen L, Niu J, Wang C, *et al.* High-throughput screening and identification of potent broad-spectrum inhibitors of coronaviruses. J Virol 2019; 93(12): e00023-19.
[http://dx.doi.org/10.1128/JVI.00023-19] [PMID: 30918074]

[51] Sodhi M, Etminan M. Safety of ibuprofen in patients with COVID-19 Causal or Confounded? Chest 2020; S0012-3692(20): 9-30572.

[52] Seaman MS, Janes H, Hawkins N, *et al.* Tiered categorization of a diverse panel of HIV-1 Env pseudoviruses for assessment of neutralizing antibodies. J Virol 2010; 84(3): 1439-52.
[http://dx.doi.org/10.1128/JVI.02108-09] [PMID: 19939925]

CHAPTER 13

Quantitative and Qualitative Determination of COVID-19 (SARS-CoV-2) Specific Antibodies Using ELISA

Mohammad Ejaz[1], Shahzad Ali[2] and Muhammad Ali Syed[1],*

[1] *Department of Microbiology, The University of Haripur, Haripur, Pakistan*

[2] *Department of Wildlife and Ecology, University of Veterinary & Animal Sciences, Lahore, Pakistan*

Abstract: After the emergence of coronavirus disease-19 (COVID-19) in late 2019 spread to different countries, becoming a global health concern. It belongs to the betacoronavirus family notorious for causing two outbreaks of severe acute respiratory syndrome (SARS-CoV) and the Middle East respiratory syndrome (MERS-CoV) in the last decade, causing huge morbidities and mortalities in a large number of population. For the current pandemic of COVID-19, accurate and precise diagnosis and surveillance of the infected individuals must be tackled by providing healthcare facilities and preventive measures in hotspot regions. COVID-19 patients were observed with non-specific symptoms like dry cough, sore throat, and fever in the early phase of infection that can worsen to serve acute respiratory syndrome and shock in the later phase of infection. Besides clinical symptoms, the radiographical finding of lungs and other definitive tests like real-time-polymerase chain reaction (RT-PCR) confirms the presence of a causative agent of COVID-19. After the infection of COVID-19, the human immune system activates and tries to neutralize the infection by forming virus-specific neutralizing antibodies. These antibodies can be detected in the patient's serum and can serve as the diagnostic biomarker. Several different types of serological assays, including enzyme-linked immunosorbent assay (ELISA), immunofluorescence assay, chemiluminescence enzyme immunoassays, immunofluorescence assay, and lateral flow immune assay, used to detect the presence of antibodies in the serum of infected individuals. This chapter will focus on the quantitative and qualitative determination of SARS-CoV-2 specific antibodies by different serological assays like ELISA in COVID-19 patients.

Keywords: Antibodies, COVID-19, ELISA, Severe Acute Respiratory Syndrome-2, Serological Tests.

---

* **Corresponding author Muhammad Ali Syed:** Infectious Diseases Research Group, Department of Microbiology University of Haripur, Pakistan; Tel: +92-332 5256722; E-mails: syedali@uoh.edu.pk and mirwah2000@yahoo.de

Kamal Niaz & Muhammad Farrukh Nisar (Eds.)

INTRODUCTION

By March 11, 2020, the World Health Organization (WHO) has declared a public health emergency worldwide due to the pandemic of COVID-19 (coronavirus disease-2019) caused by SARS- CoV-2 [1]. Since the first reported case of the novel coronavirus on December 31, 2019, the virus has rapidly spread worldwide in Wuhan, China. To date, the pandemic has spread to the whole world with 12,552,765 confirmed cases and 561,617 deaths. The most affected countries include the USA with confirmed cases of 3,163,581 and 133,486 deaths, France having 161,275 confirmed cases and 29,907 deaths, Italy with confirmed cases 242,827 and 34,905 death, the United Kingdom with 288,958 confirmed cases and 44,798 reported deaths, China with 85,522 cases and 4,648 reported deaths [2]. However, these number of cases and deaths are increasing continuously with a fatality rate of approximately 4.4% [2] compared to 34.4% of Middle Eastern respiratory syndrome (MERS) [3] and 9.6% of severe acute respiratory syndrome (SARS) [4]. The SARS-CoV-2 has shown the mean incubation periods of 5.2 days and 14 days of median duration from post symptoms onset to death and the mortality rate is alarming in the patients with age more than 70 years as they have a median duration of 11.5 days from the initial onset of the symptoms to the death [5].

The early studies reported the zoonotic transfer of virus in the live market of animals in Wuhan, China [6]. The virus spread in a local transmission from person to person *via* infectious aerosol inhalation. The international committee on taxonomy of virus (ICTV) officially classified the novel COVID-19 as SARS-CoV-2 [7]. The studies showed a higher reproductive number of 2.2 and shorter expected serial interval distribution of 7.5 days of SARS-CoV-2 than MERS-CoV that has a 0.9 reproductive number and 12.6 days of serial interval distributions [8]. The causative agent of COVID-19 related phylogenetically to SARS-CoV, sharing 79.6% sequence homology and angiotensin-converting enzyme 2 (ACE-2) receptor. Despite sharing sequence homology, the clinical outcomes of COVID-19 not only include viral pneumonia but also involve milder illness or even asymptomatic infections [5, 9, 10]. The disease ranges from mild to severe illness that subsequently leads to death in critical cases. The virus mainly infects the lower respiratory tract leading to atypical pneumonia. The radiographical finding shows the formation of ground-glass opacities, bilateral and peripheral distribution in the lungs. It also includes consolidation in the lungs [11]. Non-specific symptoms associated with infection include myalgia, dry cough, hypoxemia, difficulty breathing, and dyspnea [5]. In most cases, laboratory findings showed an elevated C-reactive protein, lymphopenia, elevated creatine phosphokinase, lactate dehydrogenates D-dimers, alanine transaminase, and creatine kinase, prolong thrombin time. The erythrocytes sedimentation rate can subsequently lead to multiple organ failure, acute distress respiratory syndrome (ADRS), kidney injury, and other comorbidities. The critical patients' plasma was observed with a higher MIP1A, IP10, IL2, and IL7 [12].

Moreover, the laboratory diagnosis includes detection of viral RNA by nucleocapsid-based RT-PCR in the sputum assay, throat swab, and bronchoalveolar lavage (BAL) collected from infected patients. The results of studies reported the peaked viral load of 10^4 to 10^7 copies/ml after 5-6 days of symptoms onset [13]. The sample from bronchoalveolar lavage aspirate is considered an ideal specimen for detecting the virus in the infected individual. It yields a higher positive rate in the nucleic acid test. However, collecting the sample by bronchoscopy requires the experienced staff and has a high potential of health risk of health care workers during sampling [14]. The nucleic acid detection by quantitative RT-PCR is considered the gold standard, but there are certain limitations as RT-PCR may give false-positive and false-negative results. Therefore, other assays need validation to diagnose COVID-19 disease with high accuracy and sensitivity. Several alternative assays have been developed for SARS-CoV-2 detection, including CRISPER-based detection and antigen-based immunoassays like lateral flow immunoassay (LFIA). It also includes immunofluorescence assay (IFA), chemiluminescence enzyme immunoassay (CLIA), and enzyme-linked immunosorbent assay (ELISA). Different assays have different specificity, sensitivity, significance, and drawbacks, and people choose assay following their demands. Serological assays play a major role in diagnosing SARS-CoV-2 in infected individuals. It is easier to detect the antibodies in a patient's blood and serum with a low risk for healthcare personnel more stable than viral RNA. Antibodies can be detected even after the clearance of the virus from the body and help in serosurveys to determine the accurate number of infected individuals. Antibodies are produced in response to viral infection by the human immune system. After entry of the virus into cells, the body's immune system activates to produce cell or humoral-mediated immunity to clear the virus. Humoral-mediated immunity involves producing antibodies specific to SARS-CoV-2 to neutralize its infection in COVID-19 patients [15].

After the emergence of COVID-19 caused by SARS-CoV-2, it has spread worldwide. It becomes a global public health concern, scientists throughout the world sparing all their efforts to diagnose and determine SARS-CoV-2 in COVID-19 patients. For more rapid SARS-CoV-2 antibody detection (IgM, IgA, and IgG), serological assays can be a high throughput alternative [16]. This chapter aims to give a detailed account of the SARS-CoV-2 specific antibodies detection in COVID-19 patients with a particular focus on quantitative and qualitative diagnosis of antibodies to SARS-COV-2 using ELISA techniques.

Diagnostic Approaches for Detection of Coronavirus

After its spread in late December 2019, scientists have adopted various diagnostic methods to find out the cause of atypical pneumonia. The accurate and rapid diagnosis of COVID-19 cases contributes to disease and outbreak management by enabling prompt public health surveillance, prevention, and control measures. Diagnosis of SARS-CoV-2 is typically based on clinical findings and physical examination followed by the radiological finding. It shows ground-glass opacities (GGO), focal consolidation, and paving patterns due to superimposed interlobular reticulations in the lungs [11]. Several diagnostic approaches have been adopted for the definitive detection of SARS-CoV-2, as depicted in Table **1**.

Table 1. Diagnostic approaches for the detection of SARS-CoV-2 in COVID-19 infected patients.

Agents	Assay	Detection Performance	Limitations
Virus	Viral culture	Low sensitivity	BSL III required with Experienced researchers and technologists
Nucleic acid (RNA)	RT-PCR	High sensitivity Several targets, including polymerase, nucleocapsid, and spike genes with SARS-CoV-2 specific primers	False-negative results when viral load is below the detection level
Antibodies	ELISA	Detection of SARS-CoV-2 specific IgM, IgA, and IgG	Cannot detect antibodies in the first week of illness Cross-reactivity with other coronaviruses
	Western Blot	Detection of IgM, IgA, and IgG	Expensive and Labor intensive
	Immunofluorescence assay (IFA)	Detection of IgM and IgG, rapid detection	Requires fluorescent microscope and expensive method
	Neutralization	Determines the neutralizing titer of antibodies	Requires BSL III, expensive, Labor intensive, and reference test only
	Lateral flow immunoassay (LFIA)	Detection of IgM and IgG	Low specificity and sensitivity
CRISPER	Crisper-Cas12	Rapid detection of viral RNA, high sensitivity	Experienced technologists required off-targets can exist

For definitive identification of SARS-CoV-2, viral isolation in cell culture is required. Still, due to lack of permissible cell lines, BSL-3, expertise requirements, time-consuming, labor-intensive method, and viral culture are not adopted commercially [17, 18]. SARS-CoV, MERS-CoV, and SARS-CoV-2 grow in cell lines such as Huh7, Vero, U251, LLCMK2, and non-human primate cell lines [18, 19]. Despite that, cell culture is critical to get isolates for the development of therapeutic agents and vaccines. The standard gold method for detecting SARS-CoV-2 in COVID-19 patients is RT-PCR based on spike and nucleocapsid genes. RT-PCR detects the viral RNA with probes or primers such as N gene, S gene, E gene, ORF1ab, and RdRP, specifically targeting the SARS-CoV-2 genome [20, 21]. However, RT-PCR-based diagnosis has certain limitations, such as a short detection window of oropharyngeal and nasopharyngeal swabs, cross-contamination of samples, false sampling, false positive and false negative results [22, 23].

Serological assays such as ELISA, IFA, and CLIA were used to detect SARS-CoV-2 specific antibodies. ELISA-based detection has many advantages over RT-PCR-based detection. It is less stringent to collect blood samples than oropharyngeal, nasopharyngeal, or bronchoalveolar lavage, and antibodies remain for a long time even after the clearance of viral infection. Serological assays detect the presence of IgM and IgG antibodies specific to COVID-19 based on recombinant antigens like spike protein and nucleocapsid protein [24, 25].

Physical Examination and Clinical Manifestation

The patients suffering from SARS-CoV-2 develop mild symptoms like fever, sore throat, myalgia, nasal congestion, vomiting, diarrhea, and dry cough. However, some infected patients develop fatal complications like severe pneumonia, pulmonary edema, acute respiratory distress syndrome (ARDS), septic shock, and organ failure [26]. Some studies also report the infection in kidneys and testis due to COVID-19 [27]. Intensive care is needed for older patients that are prone to infection because of multiple other comorbidities like cerebrovascular, cardiovascular, digestive, and/or respiratory diseases. The fatality rate in patients with different conditions such as cardiovascular diseases, respiratory diseases, hypertension, oncological complications, and diabetes is 10.5%, 6.5%, 6%, 5.6%, and 7.3%, respectively. In contrast, the case fatality rate is lower in the patients without such comorbidities (0.9%) [28]. The patients that need intensive care are more likely to be observed with dyspnea, dizziness, anorexia, and abdominal pain [29]. The critical patients have been reported with higher levels of different cytokines/mediators such as tumor necrosis factor-α (TNF-α), interferon gamma-induced protein 10 (IP10), macrophage inflammatory protein alpha (MIPIA), interleukin (IL)-2, IL-7, and IL-10, granulocyte colony-stimulating factor (GCSF) and monocyte chemotactic protein 1 (MCP1) [30]. WHO and the Center for Disease Control and Prevention (CDC) have issued guidance on the epidemiological risks and clinical findings of COVID-19 infected individuals [31, 32]. The infected person may have lymphopenia, elevated creatine phosphokinases, elevated C-reactive protein, elevated lactate dehydrogenates, prolonged thrombin time, and elevated hepatic transaminases [12, 33].

Importance of Serological Assays

Serological assays are blood-based tests used to identify the exposure of people to certain infections. Serological tests use whole blood serum that contains antibodies produced when exposed to certain antigens. The first antibody that appeared in response to the infection is IgM in the acute phase. In comparison, IgG antibody appears later after the onset of infection and could be detected in the patient's serum in the convalescent phase (10-14 days). If the antibody titer is four-fold higher in the convalescent phase than the acute phase, the patient is considered infected with the pathogen [34]. The serological assays are important to determine the seroprevalence and fatality rate of COVID-19 in an affected area. They allow us to know precisely the immune response against a pathogen. Serological assays can determine whether an individual is immune or not. It can identify the individual who mounted an intense antibodies immune response and serves as a donor in convalescent plasma therapy. The most commonly used serological assay for detecting infections includes neutralization, western blotting, and ELISA, *etc.*

The neutralization test is the reaction of a virus with a specific homologous antibody. It helps to lose infectivity. Therefore, homologous antibodies are the neutralizing antibodies in an antigen-antibody reaction that neutralize the biological and pathophysiological effects of the virus. The most common neutralization test for the virus is a viral haemagglutination inhibition test. It is used for the detection of Influenza virus [35], measles virus and mumps virus [36, 37], and coronavirus infection [38].

ELISA is a commonly used analytical assay in biochemistry, invented by Perlmann and Engvall [39]. ELISA is an immunological procedure in which an enzyme measurement detects antigen-antibody reaction. ELISA is a laboratory technique that quantifies antibodies, peptides, hormones, or proteins of the biological system. ELISA has a wide range of applications in medicine, forensic science, food science, toxicology, and immunology. It is the diagnostic tool used for determining the presence of antibodies of HIV [40], hepatitis B, and hepatitis C in the patient's serum [41]. It is also used for the detection of *Rotavirus* and enterotoxin produced by *E.coli* in the feces [42, 43], serological testing of celiac diseases [44, 45], detection of blistering autoimmune disease [46], and diagnosis of disseminated candidiasis [47].

Western blotting (immunoblotting) is an important serological assay used to identify specific proteins in a mixture to diagnose infection. When the protein to be identified is an antibody, it helps a lot in diagnosis [48]. Towbin *et al.* [49] and Burnette [50] first described the technique that relies on the interaction of specific antibodies with targeted antigens in the sample. It is a significant technique to determine the presence of protein, its relative mass, abundance, protein-protein interaction, and post-translational modification [51]. The western blotting technique is used as the diagnostic test of HIV, detection of Lyme disease [52], and the definitive test of bovine spongiform encephalopathy [53]. The world anti-doping agency also uses the western blotting technique to detect the use of illegal substances in the blood of athletes [54].

Qualitative Detection of SARS-CoV-2-Specific Antibodies

A better understanding of viral protein to which immune response occurs is essential to develop any serological assay. SARS-CoV-2 has four structural proteins, including Nucleocapsid (N), Membrane (M), Envelope (E), and Spike (S) proteins, 15 non-structural proteins, and 8 accessory proteins [55]. Once identified, the protein of interest is produced in large quantities to provide the coating or anchor of ELISA or other assays. Secondary antibodies could be created to react to human antibodies bounded to the anchor of an assay. It will create fluorometric or colorimetric detection. The ideal viral protein against which antibodies can develop is the S-protein since spike protein plays a major role in viral entry into the host cell *via* the receptor-binding domain (RBD) [56]. Besides S protein, nucleocapsid protein could also use in diagnosing antibody response against SARS-CoV-2, as it is present at a high level in virus-infected cells. E and M proteins are involved in viral assembly before releasing from an infected cell and can be used in the diagnosis of antibody response [57]. Most of the studies reported that Spike (S) antigen-based tests are more sensitive than N antigen-based tests in detecting SARS-CoV-2 [58]. Similar studies compared the seropositivity of the RBD of spike protein and nucleocapsid protein using enzyme immunoassay (EIA). The comparison results revealed that the onset of seropositivity is earlier for anti-RBD than anti-NP for IgM (26% and 17%, respectively) and IgG (43% and 4%, respectively). The seropositivity after 14 days or even more was 94% for anti-RBD IgM and 100% for anti-RBD IgG while 88% for anti-NP IgM and 94% for anti-NP IgG [59].

Serological assays can detect antibodies (qualitative detection) or the amount/titer of antibodies in the serum (quantitative detection). The qualitative detection of antibodies involves the assays like EIA or qualitative ELISA, CLIA, LFIA, IFA, and neutralization test. Among them, the most reliable and widely used detection method is ELISA that diagnoses/detects IgM, IgG, and IgA in the serum. A meta-analysis of different studies shows higher specificity with ELISA and LFIA, reaching about 99% specificity. The sensitivity of ELISA and CLIA based detection method is about 90-94%, followed by LIFA and IFA method with a sensitivity of 80-86% [58]. ELISA-based antibody detection using recombinant protein is well known for its higher reproducibility, less labor-intensive, and easier to standardize than IFA and ELISA detection with culture extract.

ELISA-based detection of antibodies (IgM and IgG) performed by a research group using recombinant spike (rS) and recombinant nucleocapsid (rN) proteins. The cutoff value was calculated by taking the average of A_{450} of negative control and summing 0.130. When OD of A_{450} equal to or more than the cutoff value sample considered positive, but when below the cutoff considered negative. The results report the overall positivity rate of 82.2% and 80.4% for spike protein and nucleocapsid protein, respectively. The study included 214 patients with PCR confirmed samples. They were diagnosed with rS-based IgM and IgG 77.1% and 74.3%, respectively, and with rN-based IgM and IgG antibodies are 68.2% and 70.1%, respectively. The sensitivity of rS based IgM ELISA was higher compared to rN based IgM ELISA. In contrast, no significant difference was observed for IgG ELISA of both recombinant antigens [60].

Xiang *et al.* [61] used both ELISA and lateral flow colloidal gold immunochromatographic assay (GICA) to detect specific antibodies in SARS-CoV-2 infected individuals. The method adopted for the preparation of IgM capture ELISA involves adding a diluted sample to the microtiter plate coated with mouse anti-human IgM monoclonal antibodies. After incubation of 60 min at 37°C, the microtiter plate was washed to remove unbounded antibodies. The enzyme-linked antibody is then added to detect the presence of IgM. Similarly, IgG indirect ELISA was performed by adding a sample to the microplate coated with a recombinant antigen of SARS-CoV-2, incubated for 60 minutes, and washed. Then enzyme-labeled monoclonal mouse anti-human IgG was added to detect the presence of IgG after adding the respective substrate. For the colloidal gold assay, added a diluted sample to the pad of the testing strip. The sample moves through a gold-labeled pad, testing area to quality control area, and finally to the adsorption area. The results were monitored after 10 minutes by the color of tests and control lines. ELISA results show specificity, sensitivity, and accuracy of 100%, 87.3%, and 91.8%, respectively, for total antibodies (IgM+ IgG), while GICA shows specificity, sensitivity, and accuracy of 100% 82.45, and 87.3% respectively for total antibodies.

Guo and co-workers [62] studied the host's humoral response against COVID-19 by using an ELISA-based assay on the recombinant nucleocapsid protein of SARS-CoV-2. The study reports the positivity rate of 92.7%, 85.2%, and 77.9% for IgA, IgM, and IgG, respectively, and observed the median duration for detecting IgA and IgM antibodies was five days while for IgG was 14 days post symptoms onset. Another ELISA assay was developed to detect IgM and IgG specific to SARS-CoV-2 based on the RBD of the spike protein. The assay combines with confirmatory plaque reduction neutralization test 90% ($PRNT_{90}$) and microneutralization (MN) using live viruses were evaluated in BSL-3. The corresponding cutoff values for IgM and IgG were OD >0.67 and OD> 0.40, respectively. All serum samples collected were positive for IgG and IgM in RBD-based ELISA, $PRNT_{90}$, and MN after 29 days. The $PRNT_{90}$ titers and the microneutralization antibody titer ranging from 1:10 to 1:1280 were seropositive, and 1:10 to 1:320 for seropositive samples, respectively. The $PRNT_{90}$ titers were more sensitive in antibody detection than microneutralization assay. They were 4-fold higher in serum than those of microneutralization assay carried out with conventional $TCID_{100}$ [63].

Immunochromatographic assay testing is ideal for prompt detection of SARS-CoV-2. For this purpose, Pan *et al.* [64] reported the use of colloidal gold ICG that detects SARS-CoV-2 specific IgM and IgG antibodies. The sensitivity of ICG in early 1-7 days of infection was low with 11.1% sensitivity, that increase to 92.9% in 8-14 days of symptoms onset, reaching 96.8% after 15 days of illness. Li and co-workers [65] developed a point of care lateral flow immunoassay for the rapid detection of SARS-CoV-2 specific IgM and IgG antibodies within 15 minutes. The recombinant antigen (MK201027) belongs to the receptor-binding domain of the SARS-CoV-2 spike protein used for the qualitative detection of antibodies to SARS-CoV-2. The developed kit had specificity and sensitivity of 90.63% and 88.66%, respectively. In a mimicking study, García with colleagues [66] develops a rapid diagnostic kit to detect IgM and IgG in SARS-CoV-2 patients based on the principle of the immunochromatographic test. The study reports an overall specificity of 100% and sensitivity of 47%, 74%, and 89% after 11, 14, and 17 days, respectively, of symptoms onset.

A study conducted to detect antibodies against spike protein of SARS-CoV-2 by using CLIA reports the seroconversion of IgA was 2 days post symptoms onset. Seroconversion of IgM and IgG was after 5 days of initial symptoms. The study reported a positivity rate of 93.4%, 98.9%, and 95.1% for IgM, IgA, and IgG, respectively. After 32 days, the seroconversion rate is 100% for all the antibodies [67]. In a similar study, serum IgM and IgG antibodies were detected using GICA that reported the sensitivity of 23.0% for IgM, 53.8% for IgG. However, during the early course of the disease, it increased up to 55.2% and 91.3% for IgM and IgG, respectively, after 15 days of illness [68].

End-Point Titration of SARS-CoV-2-Specific Antibodies

Conventional serological assays have a high-throughput significance for detecting IgM and IgG antibodies compared to the RT-PCR method. It gives false-negative results when viral load is low. Quantitative ELISA-based detection of antibodies determines the titer of IgM, IgA, and IgG antibodies in the patients' serum/plasma. The end-point titration is considered the reciprocal of the highest serial dilution that determines the minimum activity of the antibody. The concentration of antibodies in the serum sample monitored by a standard curve when tested by quantitative ELISA. For prompt diagnosis of COVID-19, many research groups developed different quantitative diagnostic methods, including ELISA, CLIA, and IFA, to observe the antibody titers in different phases of coronavirus infection.

In another attempt, Zhong and co-workers [69] develop ELISA and CLIA based techniques to detect SARS-CoV-2 specific antibodies in serum for recombinant S and N proteins. The study shows that area under the ROC curve (AUC) of rN protein-based IgG reached 0.999 while the AUC of recombinant spike protein (rS) based IgG reached 0.949. The optimal cutoff value of rN based IgG is 0.443 with specificity and sensitivity of 99.7% and 97.9%, respectively. The cutoff value of rS-based IgG was 0.176 with specificity and sensitivity of 85.7% 95.7%, respectively. For rN-based IgM, the cutoff value was 0.994 with specificity and sensitivity of 99.7% and 97.9%, respectively, and for rS-based IgM-based IgM, the specificity and sensitivity are 97.0% and 89.1%, with a cutoff value of 0.167. The study also determines the results of the chemiluminescence assay by analyzing the receiver operating characteristic (ROC) curve. The ROC ' 'curve's analysis for IgM showed the optimal cutoff value of 0.230 with specificity and sensitivity of 95.2% and 97.7%, respectively. For IgG, the cutoff value was 0.199 with specificity and sensitivity of 96.6% and 95.6%.

An ELISA-based end-point titer of antibodies response and their kinetics were determined using nucleocapsid protein of SARS-CoV-2. The OD value at 450-630 was measured and titer calculated to determine the dynamics of antibodies in the infected individuals. The optimal dilution was 1:100 for IgM and 1:20 for IgG. The study categorizes the patients into three categories: strong responders with peak titer of more than 2-fold of cutoff value, a responder with peak titer 1-2 fold of cutoff values, and non-responder with peak titer below cutoff value. For IgM and IgG antibodies, the study report 31.1% and 22.2% positivity for the strong responder, 17.2%, and 61.1% for the responder. It also showed 51.7% and 16.7% for the non-responder. IgM antibodies appear on day 7, peaked at day 28, while IgG antibodies appear after day 10, and peaked on day 49 after the onset of symptoms. IgM and IgG antibodies in serve patients respond early, and titer is reported to be significantly higher than less serve cases of COVID-19 [70].

Another study that shows more sensitivity than RT-PCR in the diagnosis of the SARS-CoV-2 patients is ELISA-based detection of antibodies. The concentration unit of antibodies present in the sample (AU/ml>10) was positive. IgM concentration in patients was 40.76 AU/ml in severe cases, 29.19 AU/ml in moderate cases, and 23.25 AU/ml in critical cases. In the meantime, the concentration of IgG was 148.63 AU/ml in severe cases, 147.73 AU/ml in moderate cases, and 140.40 AU/ml in critical cases, respectively. The total positive cases by RT-PCR were 68.42%, while 78.95% are positive for the presence of antibodies specific to SARS-CoV-2 depict higher sensitivity [71].

Chemiluminescence immunoassay is also used for the detection of antibodies titer in patients infected with SARS-CoV-2. Magnetic particle coated antigen having SARS-CoV-2 Nucleocapsid protein and Envelope protein used to identify the presence of IgM and IgG antibodies specific to SARS-CoV-2. A positive correlation between the amount of SARS-CoV-2 specific antibodies in the sample and relative luminescence intensity (RLU) was observed. The concentration of antibodies (AU/ml) was calculated according to RLU and built-in calibration curve considering 10.0 AU/ml as a positive value. The study found the optimum cutoff value of 10.14 and 15.99 for IgM and IgG, respectively, and AUC was 0.988 and 1.000 [72]. In a similar study, a chemiluminescence assay using recombinant nucleocapsid protein (YP_009724397.2) was used for the detection of IgM and IgG antibodies specific to SARS-CoV-2. The average RLU (relative length unit) values of IgM were observed to be 6 to 8 fold higher in SARS-CoV-2 infected individuals than healthy individuals.

In contrast, IgG average RLU values were observed 60 to 70 times higher in an infected individual. The study reports the cutoff setting of (RLU 162296) for IgM and (RLU 336697) for IgG and shows the specificity of 81.25% and 97.5% for IgM and IgG, respectively. The sensitivity of IgM and IgG was 82.28% and 82.28%, respectively [73]. Moreover, the IgM and IgG antibody titer was determined in a retrospective study against nucleoprotein and spike proteins of SARS-CoV-2 using chemiluminescence assay. The immunoassay analyzer based on RLU (relative light unit) automatically calculated the IgM/IgG titer (AU/ml). The cutoff value of 10AU/ml is considered positive for IgM and IgG. The specificity of IgM and IgG was 100% and 90.9%, and sensitivity was 48.1% and 88.9%, respectively. The median titers of IgM and IgG in infected individuals were 12.1AU/ml and 132.2 AU/ml, respectively [74].

Padoan*et al* [75], evaluated the kinetics of SARS-CoV-2 specific IgA, IgM, and IgG antibodies using CLIA and ELISA. The repeatability values (CVs %) of chemiluminescent assay for IgM are 4.05%, 1.84% and 3.06% at 4.39 kAU/L, 1.84 kAU/L and 0.61 kAU/L concentration levels respectively for IgG, repeatability values are 3.18%, 3.86% and 5.69% at 10.59 kAU/L, 2.99 KAU/L and 0.48 kAU/L concentration levels, respectively. The cutoff values of IgM and IgG were 1.0 kAU/L and 1.1 kAU/L. The CVs % for IgA in ELISA-based detection was 2.4% at the ratio of 1.03 and 13.7% at the ratio of 0.20, respectively. For IgG, the CVs % were between 3.9% to 16% at the ratio of 2.36 and 0.07, respectively. The cutoff value is ≥ 1.1 for both IgA and IgG. The result reported by the study showed the average increase in the level of IgM and IgA antibodies after 6-8 days of symptoms onset. Anti-SARS-CoV-2 IgM antibody level peaked at 10-12 days and decline after 18 days post-onset of symptoms, while the IgA antibody level peaked at 20-22 days. The antibody detection assays using different SARS-CoV-2 specific antigens with their detection significance are also summarized Table **2**.

Table 2. Characteristics of detection assay with sensitivity and specificity using different antigens of SARS-CoV-2.

Assay	COVID-19/Healthy	Ascertainment	Antigen	Antibody	Positive (%)			Specificity	Sensitivity	References
					IgM	IgA	IgG			
ELISA	214/100	Clinical features/NAT	N	IgM and IgG	68.2%	NR	72.1%	NR	NR	[60]
ELISA	214/100	Clinical features/NAT	S	IgM and IgG	77.1%	NR	74.3%	NR	NR	[60]
LFIA	398/127	NAT	S	IgM and IgG	64.48%	NR	64.48%	90.63%	88.6%	[65]
ELISA	173/0	Clinical features/NAT	RBD of S	IgM and IgG	94.3%	NR	79.8%	99.1%	89.6%	[76]
CLIA	27/33	Clinical features/NAT	N and S	IgM and IgG	48.1%	NR	88.9%	IgG=100% IgM=90.5%	NR	[74]
ELISA	23/0	Clinical features/NAT	N	IgM and IgG	88%	NR	94%	NR	NR	[77]
ELISA	23/0	Clinical features/NAT	RBD	IgM and IgG	94%	NR	100%	NR	NR	[77]
ELISA	99/519	Clinical features/NAT	S	IgM and IgG	NR	NR	NR	>99%	96%	[78]
ELISA	208/0	Clinical features/NAT	N	IgM, IgA and IgG	85.4%	92.7%	77.9%	NR	NR	[62]
ELISA	47/300	Clinical features/NAT	S	IgM and IgG	NR	NR	NR	IgM=99.7% IgG=85.7%	IgM=97.9% IgG=95.7%	[69]
ELISA	47/300	Clinical features/NAT	N		NR	NR	NR	IgM=97.0% IgG=99.7%	IgM=89.1% IgG=97.9%	[69]
CLIA	47/300	Clinical features/NAT	S and N	IgM and IgG	NR	NR	NR	IgM=95.2% IgG=99.6%	IgM=97.7% IgG=95.6%	[69]
LFIA	85/371	NAT	S and N	IgM and IgG	NR	NR	NR	99.5%	82.8%	[79]
LIFA	45/118	Clinical features/NAT	N and S	IgM and IgG	39.7%	NR	88.9%	100%	73.9%	[66]
CLIA	133/0	NAT	N and S	IgM and IgG	78.95%	NR	96.8%	NR	NR	[71]

(Table 2) cont.....

Assay	COVID-19/Healthy	Ascertainment	Antigen	Antibody	Positive (%)			Specificity	Sensitivity	References
ELISA/ CLIA	79/80	Clinical features/NAT	N	IgM and IgG	NR	NR	NR	97.5%	82.28%	[73]
LFIA	38/0	NAT	N and S	IgM and IgG	50.0%	NR	92.1%	NR	IgM=52.2% IgG=91.3%	[68]
ELISA	67/0	NAT	N	IgM and IgG	57.1%	NR	86.7%	NR	NR	[70]
ELISA/ LFIA/ CLIA	80/300	Clinical features/NAT	S and N	IgM and IgG	96.7%	NR	93.3%	IgM=100% IgG=99.1%	IgM=93.8% IgG=93.8%	[80]
CLIA	348/0	Clinical features/NAT	N and S	IgM and IgG	94.1%	NR	100%	NR	NR	[81]
CLIA	222/0	Clinical features/NAT	N and S	IgM and IgG	82.0%	NR	98.6%	NR	NR	[82]
IFA	34/9	NAT	S and N	IgM and IgG	NR	NR	NR	NR	NR	[83]
CLIA	228/223	Clinical features/NAT	E and N	IgM and IgG	NR	NR	NR	97%	100%	[72]
ELISA	173/0	Clinical features/NAT	RBD of S	IgM and IgG	82.7%	NR	64.7%	IgM=98.6% IgG=99.0%	IgM=73.3% IgG=79.8%	[76]
ELISA	63/35	Clinical features/NAT	N and S	IgM and IgG	44.4%	NR	82.5%	100%	87.3%	[61]
LFIA	91/35	Clinical features/NAT	S and N	IgM and IgG	57.1%	NR	81.3%	100%	82.4%	[61]
ELISA	238/130	Clinical features/NAT	N	IgM and IgG	81.5%	NR	81.5%	NR	81.5%	[84]
ELISA	69/412	NAT	S	IgM and IgG	NR	NR	NR	97.5%	97.5%	[85]
LFIA	397/128	NAT	RBD of S	IgM and IgG	6.04%	NR	18.1%	90.6%	88.6%	[65]
LFIA	105/0	Clinical features/NAT	N and S	IgM and IgG	57.1%	NR	71.4%	NR	68.6%	[64]
LFIA	29/124	NAT	N and S	IgM and IgG	69%	NR	93.1%	IgM=100% IgG=99.2%	IgM=69.0% IgG=93.1%	[86]
ELISA	9/45	Clinical features/NAT	S	IgM and IgA	NR	NR	NR	NR	NR	[87]
ELISA	85/14	Clinical features/NAT	N	IgM and IgG	77.3%	NR	83.3%	IgM=100% IgG=95%	IgM=77.3% IgG=83.3%	[24]
LFIA	70/0	NAT	S and N	IgM and IgG	81.4%	NR	100%	NR	NR	[88]
CLIA	87/283	Clinical features/NAT	N and RBD	IgM, IgA and IgG	NR	NR	NR	IgA=98.1%, IgM=92.3% IgG=99.8%	IgA=98.6%, IgM=96.8% IgG= 96.8%	[89]
CLIA	37/0	NAT	S	IgM, IgA and IgG	93.4%	98.9%	95.1%	NR	NR	[67]

• NR=Not reported RDB= Receptor binding domain, S= Spike protein, N= Nucleocapsid protein, E= Envelope protein

Immunity to SARS-CoV-2

SARS-CoV-2 is an enveloped positive single-stranded RNA virus with a genome size of about 30,000 nucleotides, belongs to β-*cornaviridae* family. Besides SARS-CoV-2, 6 known human pathogenic coronaviruses belong to β-*cornaviridae* family, *i.e.,* SARS-CoV, MERS-CoV, HCoV-OC43, HCoV-229E, HCoV-NL63, and HCoV-HKU1 [90, 91].

The genome codes for 27 proteins. It includes four structural proteins and RNA-dependent RNA polymerase [55, 92]. The receptor-binding S-protein binds to the cellular ACE-2 receptor of coronaviruses resulting in the entry of virus particles into the cell [93, 94]. The two functional subunits of the S-protein, the S1 subunit, are responsible for binding the virus to the host cell receptor and the fusion of cellular and viral membranes. In contrast, the S2 subunit determines the viral transmission and host tropism [94]. SARS-CoV-2 enters into the host cell *via* membrane fusion, independent endocytosis, or catherin-dependent endocytosis. At the same time, MERS-CoV evolves, the two-step furin-mediated activation of S-protein results in the viral and cellular membrane fusion causing entry of the virus in the host cell [95, 96]. After its entry, viruses were recognized as foreign antigens and presented to antigen-presenting cells (APCs). The presentation of antigen brought out by major histocompatibility complex (MHC) or human leukocyte antigen (HLA) to the T-lymphocytes. The antigen is presented by MHC I in SARS-CoV-2 but can also be presented by MHC II. MHC II, such as HLA-DQB1*02:0 and HLA-DRB1*11:01 reported presenting the antigen in MERS patients [97, 98].

Cellular and Humoral Immunity Against SARS-CoV-2

Antigen presentation leads to the development of the body's immune response as cellular and humoral mediated immunity, resulting in the activation of specific T and B cells, respectively. T-lymphocytes are generally divided into cytotoxic T-lymphocytes (CD 8+) and helper T lymphocytes (CD 4+). CD 8+ or cytotoxic T cells can proliferate rapidly and differentiate into effector cells that result in the production of cytokines and killing of the targeted cells, hence involved in cellular immunity. CD 4+ or helper T lymphocytes can produce T cell-dependent virus-specific antibodies and increase the number of memory cells, which respond to the same virus's reinfection and provide immunity [99]. CD8+ cells account for approximately 80% of total infiltrated inflammatory cells in the interstitial fluid of lungs in SARS-CoV-2 infected patients and play a significant role in clearing the coronaviruses from an infected cell [100]. Recent studies show the decrease in the level of CD8+, CD4+ T cells, and INF-γ- expressing CD4+ cells in SARS-CoV-2 infected patients [101]. The lymphopenia and cytokine storm can subsequently lead to respiratory disorders like pulmonary disorders and ARDS. A study reported that SARS-CoV-2 could infect type 1pneumocytes and alveolar macrophages in the lungs [102]. CD 4+ T cells are involved in producing virus-specific antibodies by activating the T cell-dependent B-cell [103].

The formation of antibodies accomplishes the humoral mediated immunity in SARS-CoV-2 by B-cell that can be detected in the patient's serum from 7 to 11 days post symptoms onsets. The first antibody that appeared in the acute stage of infection is IgM seroconverted to IgG after few days to clear the infection. Several studies reported the development of IgM, IgA, and IgG with different titers in different phases of infection. The highest titer of IgM is observed in the acute phase of illness, while the IgG titer is at the peak level in the convalescent phase of infection [104].

Cytokines Production in SARS-CoV-2 Patients

Cytokines are soluble proteins with a low molecular weight that regulate adaptive and innate immunity against the antigen. Mononuclear phagocytes (dendritic cells and macrophages) primarily produce cytokines that regulate the innate or non-specific immunity; however, NK cells, endothelial cells, mucosal epithelial cells, and T-lymphocytes can also produce them [105, 106]. The laboratory findings by Wang *et al.* [102] found an elevated cytokine level of IL2, IL7, IL10, GSCF, IP10, MCP1, MIP1A, and TNFα in the patient's plasma suffering from SARS-CoV-2. A similar study also observed elevated chemokines and cytokines, including CXCL1, CXCL5, CXLC10, MCP1, and IL-6 in SARS-CoV-2 patients. Previous studies also found elevated cytokines such as IL-6, INF-α, and chemokines such as CXCL-8, CXCL-10, and CCL5 in MERS infected patients [107]. Chemokines and cytokines have long been considered important in regulating the immune system, but dysregulation and excessive release can lead to lung damage. The elevated cytokines in SARS-CoV-2 patients can trigger an intense immune response causing multiple organ failure and ADRS. They can lead to death as similar to SARS-CoV and MERS-CoV infections [108, 109].

Evasion of coronavirus from the immune system

Coronavirus has adopted multiple strategies to avoid the immune response, including the formation of double-membrane vesicles that lack pattern recognition receptors (PPRs), replicating in the vesicle as they cannot be recognized as pathogen-associated molecular patterns, thereby preventing the host from their detection [108]. Both innate and adaptive immune response is vital in the viral clearance. Coronavirus has developed some strategies to overcome innate immunity. Interferon (INF) is crucial in initial response; coronavirus has developed active and passive tools to counter interferon signaling and induction. INF cannot be induced in the fibroblast infected with SARS-CoV [110, 111].

Moreover, viral proteins (nsp1, nsp3, SARS-CoV accessory proteins ORF3b, ORF6, and N protein) also avert ' 'interferon's induction [112, 113]. An accessory protein 4a of MERS-CoV works as an INF antagonist by direct interaction with dsRNA [114]. Additionally, membrane proteins, ORF4a, ORFb4, and ORF 5 of MERS-CoV inhibit the activation of the INF-β promoter and nuclear transport of INF regulatory factor 3 [115]. The studies on the evasion of SARS-CoV-2 may show a similar pattern as of the other coronavirus. To date, there is hardly any study to report the molecular pattern and evasion of SARS-CoV-2 published. The protective immunity against the virus does not exist in humans. The virus can evade the innate immune response and thus cause infection in host cells, which can proliferate and result in cell death.

Consequently, cell death causes the release of the virus particles and intracellular components to extracellular spaces that result in the recruitment of immune cells. The recruitment of immune cells subsequently causes inflammatory responses by producing cytokines and chemokines, resulting in ARDS comorbidities. Immune modulating and antiviral treatments are currently under trial.

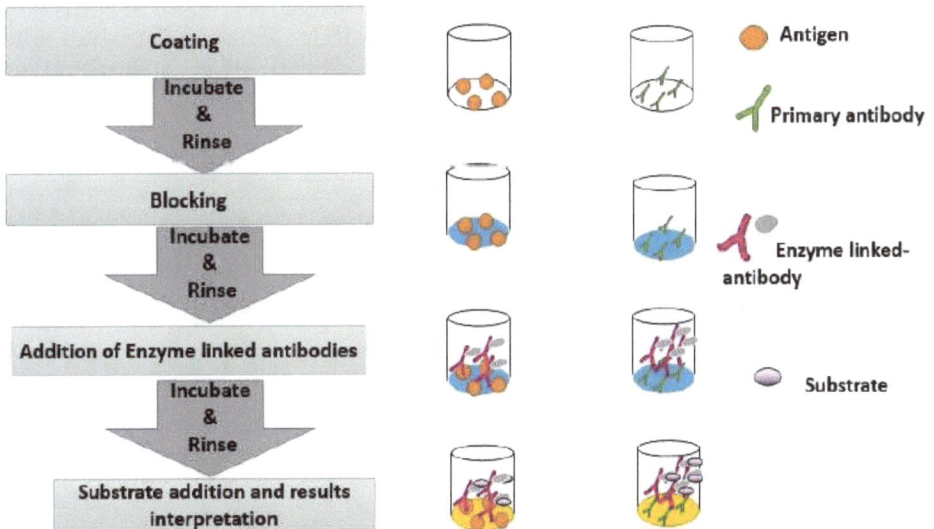

Fig. (1). General procedure of ELISA-based detection of antigen or antibodies. The first step involves the coating of antigen or antibody on microtiter well following by blocking and adding enzyme-linked antibodies. The last steps involve the addition of a substrate that results in the formation of a detectable product.

ELISA-Based Detection of SARS-CoV-2 Antibodies

The use of ELISA as a serological assay has virtually burst out from the last two decades after its discovery by Engvall [39]. ELISA is an assay technique designed to detect and quantify antibodies, hormones, proteins, and peptides. An antigen is immobilized on a solid surface in this technique and then binds with an antibody linked with an enzyme. The detection accomplished by incubating the antigen-enzyme link antibody complex with a particular substrate produces a measurable product. ELISA is typically performed in 96-well polystyrene microtiter plates that passively bind proteins and antibodies. The serum containing antigen or antibodies is incubated in the well coated with corresponding antibodies or antigen. After incubation, the microtiter plate was rinsed to remove unbounded antigens or antibodies. A secondary antibody attached to enzymes (Alkaline phosphatase or Horse reddish peroxidase) was added to detect the bound antibodies or antigen. After incubation for some time, the microtiter plates were washed to remove unbounded secondary antibodies. Then substrate was added that reacts with an enzyme to produce the measurable product, and a generalized overview of all these steps in ELISA is given in Fig. (**1**).

Based on the binding structure between antigen and antibody, ELISA is classified into four different types: direct ELISA, indirect ELISA, sandwich ELISA, and competitive ELISA (Fig. **2**). The extensively used types in the detection of SARS-CoV-2 are indirect ELISA and sandwich ELISA. Most of the studies use these techniques to determine the presence and quantification of antibodies against SARS-CoV-2 in the patient's serum.

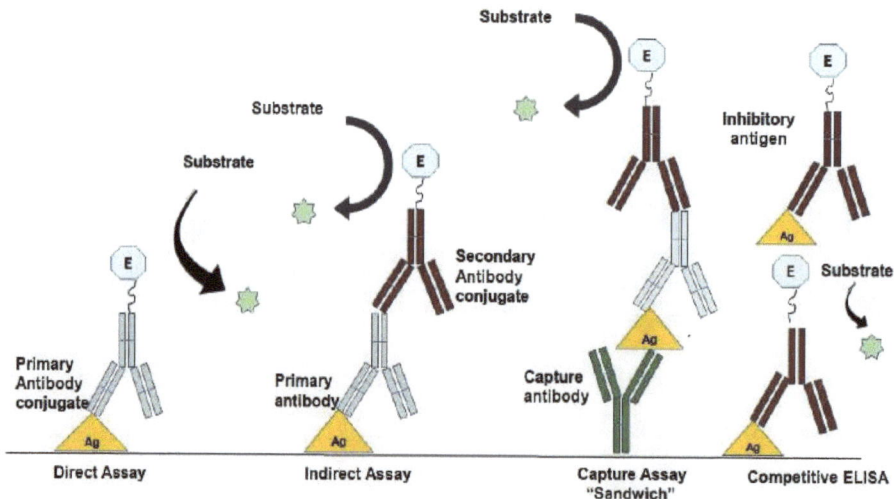

Fig. (2). Types of ELISA for the detection of antigens or antibodies in serum.

The gold standard for identification (nucleic acid testing) using RT-PCR is not ideal for determining the asymptomatic infection of SARS-COV-2 after week 3 of illness. Serological diagnosis of SARS-CoV-2 specific antibodies can fill these gaps in detection. The protocol of qualitative and quantitative techniques for the detection of antibodies was developed *via* a two-stage ELISA. The first stage includes screening samples in only one serum dilution against the receptor-binding domain, followed by the second stage, confirming a positive sample from the first stage using S-based ELISA. For the second stage, confirmatory ELISA, the dilution curve was performed to quantify the antibodies [116].

S-protein-based ELISA was used to determine the prevalence of SARS-CoV-2 specific antibodies in the serum of the patient. Receiver operator characteristic (ROC) analysis was conducted for spike protein-based ELISA using anti-human pan Ig, anti-human IgM, and anti-human IgG. Using anti-human pan Ig with serum dilution of 1:100 and 1:400 at a cutoff value of 0.4, specificity and sensitivity were 99.3% and 99.88%, respectively. The sensitivity was 94.74% and 76.19% using anti-human IgG and anti-IgM at the same cutoff and dilution, respectively [78].

In another study, antibodies were detected in the human serum. SARS-CoV-2 Rp3 nucleocapsid protein had approximately 90% sequence similarity to other coronaviruses [117]. The Sandwich ELISA technique was used to determine recombinant protein coated on the surface of the 96-well microtiter plate. After incubation and washing off excess protein, the diluted human serum was added and incubated for 1 hour that was washed again to remove unbound proteins. Then anti-human IgG antibodies labeled with an enzyme horse reddish peroxidase (HRP) were added and incubated to bind with the target. The plate was washed again, followed by the addition of substrate (3, '3', 5, 5'-tetramethylbenzidine). The enzyme reacts with the substrate to cause a color change that is detected by using an ELISA plate reader. As the patient has anti-SARS-CoV-2 IgG antibodies, it will sandwich between coated nucleoprotein and anti-human IgG probes, indicating the positivity of the sample. Similarly, IgM antibodies were detected using recombinant Nucleoprotein and anti-human IgM. The study reports the increase in IgM and IgG antibodies for the first 5 days of symptoms onset. After 5 days, the level of IgM and IgG antibodies increases to 81% and 100%, respectively.

Obka *et al.* [87] developed an ELISA assay for the detection of antibodies against spike protein including receptor-binding domain, N-terminal subunit of spike protein (S1 subunit), C- terminal subunit of spike protein (S2 subunit), domain A of spike S1 subunit (S1A subunit) and nucleocapsid protein. The study used confirmed serum samples of SARS-CoV-2 by RT-PCR and confirmed samples of other seasonal coronaviruses (HCoV-229E, OC43, NL63, SARS, and MERS), reporting the immune response against the tested proteins of SARS-CoV-2. The tested samples were seroconverted and showed IgA and IgG antibodies with varying degrees of sensitivity, IgA being more sensitive. However, the cross-reactivity of S1 and S proteins of SARS-CoV and, to some extent, MERS-CoV was observed in the study.

Used of recombinant nucleocapsid protein in sandwich ELISA assay to detect IgM and IgG antibodies of SARS-CoV-2 reported the seropositivity of 81.5% in the patients [84]. In a similar study, the seropositivity of IgM and IgG was reported to be 77.1% and 74.3%, respectively. In comparison, recombinant spike protein of SARS-CoV-2 shows the seropositivity of 80.4% and 82.2% for IgM and IgG, respectively. The positive rS-based IgM and IgG rate was less than 60% than rN-based IgM and IgG during the early stage of infection (0-10 days post-onset) after that antibodies level increase after 10 days post-onset [60].

An indirect ELISA technique was developed to detect SARS-CoV-2 specific IgM and IgG antibodies using recombinant S1 protein of SARS-CoV-2. The developed ELISA kit has parameters like 1.5µg/ml S1-His of SARS-CoV-2 for coating the microtiter plate, incubation in microplate shaker with constant rotation, and human sera dilution 1:20 using 20% CS-PBS as a specimen. The developed ELISA specificity was determined 97.5%, examining the 412 normal human sera, and sensitivity was 97.5% by testing 69 human sera having confirmed COVID-19 infection. The overall accuracy rate of the ELISA kit was determined to be 97.3% [85]. A similar study conducted by Liu *et al.* [84] reported the positivity rate of 81.5% for IgM and IgG against SARS-CoV-2 when tested using ELISA assay, which is significantly higher than the positivity rate viral RNA (64.3%). The study analyzing the specificity and sensitivity of ELISA-based detection of different companies reports the highest sensitivity and specificity for Wantai SARS-CoV-2 total Ab ELISA. The Wantai SARS-CoV-2 detection ELISA is based on the sandwich ELISA principle against RBD of S-protein [118].

Antibody Isotyping and Subtyping

Antibody isotyping is the determination of the classes and subclasses of monoclonal antibodies. The antibodies are classified into five isotypes (IgM, IgG, IgA, IgE, and IgD) that differ in their ability to deal with different antigens, half-life, biological properties, and physiological effects locations. The antibody isotype of B-cell changes during the development and activation of the cell. The naïve B cell expresses only IgM antibody isotype but can express both IgM and IgD isotypes when reaching a mature stage. B-cell activation leads to the differentiation of cells into antibody-producing plasma cells. When encountering specific signaling molecules *via* their cytokines and CD40 receptors, the activated B cell undergoes the class switching from IgM to IgG, IgE, or IgA antibodies. Class switching does not change the specificity of the antibody for an antigen. However, it rather permits to exert different biological effects. This permits different daughter cells from the same initiated B cell to give antibodies of various isotypes or subtypes (*e.g.,* IgG1, and IgG2, *etc.*) In class switching, the antibody's constant region of the antibody constant region's heavy chain is changed, but the variable region of the heavy chain remains the same [119].

The antibody isotypes present in the patients' serum can provide important information about the initial exposure to the antigen. Seroconversion of antibodies is used to understand the progression and prognosis of the disease. Of particular interest is the transition of IgM antibodies to the IgG antibodies that are progressively effector antibodies. IgM appears in primary immune response and has a pentameric structure, thus have 10 antigen-binding sites allowing the strong binding to the foreign antigen with multiple repetitive epitopes. However, IgM is unable to clear the foreign material alone. Thus, class switching occurs and converts IgM into IgG or IgA, providing better effector contrivance for clearance of antigen [120].

The serological assays like ELISA, IFA, Western blotting, and immunoblot, *etc.*, are used to determine the dynamics of antibody class switching qualitatively and quantitatively. The seroconversion rate or serosurveys are important to determine the precise infection rate.It is an essential variable to determine the morbidity and mortality rate of infection in an affected area. Previous researches conducted on SARS-CoV infection reported the appearance of IgM antibodies by 3 to 6 days, while IgG can be recognized after 8 days of onset of symptoms [121, 122]. The seroconversion profiles were also used to detect IgM, IgG, and IgA antibodies against the nucleocapsid protein of SARS-CoV [123]. The median time of seroconversion for IgM, IgG, and IgA detected by ELISA was 20.5 days, 17 days, and 17 days, respectively. The median time was the median time with the indirect immune-fluorescence assay 16.5 days, 17 days, and 17.5 days. A similar study conducted on SARS-CoV, using the nucleoprotein-fusion protein of SARS-CoV as antigen, reported that antibodies to SARS-CoV could not be detected in the patient in the first week of illness. In the second week of symptom onset, 83.3% and 66.7% were seropositivities for IgM and IgG, respectively, reaching almost 100% by the third week for both antibodies. IgG titer reached a peak value by one month after onset of symptoms and remained high for the next two months, while seropositivity of IgM decreased to 61.5% in the second month and further decreased to 38.5% in the second month week three of the post-onset [124].

Similarly, the antibodies against MERS-CoV infection were at peak titer after 6 days of symptoms onset when tested against RBD of Spike protein, while against nucleoprotein antibodies were detected after 7-12 days [125].

The first report on the profile of SARS-CoV-2 specific antibodies showed that the immune system of patients has responded to the infection, and antibodies (IgM and IgG) shown positive after 2 weeks from the onset of symptoms. The study reported the mean value of 322.80 AU/ml and 112.40 AU/ml (Reference: 10 AU/ml) of IgM and IgG in the third week after symptoms onset. The fourth week of observation found the decline in IgM and the rise in IgG level, while in the fifth week after symptoms onset, 16.7% of the patients got negative results for IgM, all the patients are positive for IgG. Over time, the IgM titer was observed with a decline rate while the IgG titer increased [126]. A study was conducted on serological isotyping and subtyping of antibodies. It uses ELISA to detect viral genetic material utilizing recombinant antigens obtained from the spike protein of SARS-CoV-2. Strong reactivity was observed in all samples for IgA IgM, IgG1, IgG3, and IgG4. An IgG1 signal was detected for most samples, while low reactivity for IgG2 and IgG4 was identified. Unlike influenza virus infection, in which IgG1 response is dominant, IgG3 response is dominant in SARS-CoV-2. The study also reported a negligible cross-reactivity with other coronaviruses [127].

Moreover, a study conducted on the response of antibodies to spike glycoprotein of SARS-CoV-2 reported the average level of antibodies (IgM and IgA) increased at 6-8 days with peak values of IgM antibody at 10-12 days with a significant decline after 18 days and 20-22 days peak value of IgA antibodies [75]. A comparable study conducted by Zhou *et al.* [76] reported the seroconversion rate of 93.1%, 82.7%, and 64.7% for Total anti-SARS-CoV-2 Ab, IgM anti-SAR--CoV-2 antibodies, and IgG anti-SARS-CoV-2 antibodies, respectively. The median for seroconversion of total antibodies, IgM, and IgG was 11, 12, and 14 days respectively. Another study reported the seroconversion rate for total Ab, IgM, and IgG in SARS-CoV-2 patients was 98.8%, 93.8%, and 93.8%, respectively. The first detectable marker is total Ab followed by IgM and IgG antibodies, with median seroconversion of 9, 10, and 12 days post symptoms onset [80]. The majority of studies reported the seroconversion of antibodies within 7 to 11 days [128].

Application of COVID-19 Antibodies Detection by ELISA

Serological testing for SARS-CoV-2 is mainly used to quantify the number of COVID-19 cases. It includes those that have recovered or may be asymptomatic. This is of great importance because diagnostic techniques like RT-PCR; viral culture currently being used can only detect viral material inactive cases. However, ELISA-based diagnosis not only detects the antibodies (IgM, IgA, and IgG) in the acute phase of illness but can also detect later in the convalescent phase. The occurrence and frequency of infection in a characterized population can be estimated by serological tests, as these assays are widely used in seroprevalence surveys. ELISA-based serological testing was found more sensitive than RT-PCR to detect SARS-CoV-2 in COVID-19 patients after the first week of illness. In Japan, cross-sectional serological testing for SARS-CoV-2 was conducted, suggesting that the number of seropositive individuals was much greater than the cases confirmed by PCR [129]. A retrospective study conducted on the comparative analysis of detection abilities of viral RNA and antibodies *via* PCR and the serological assay was reported, respectively. The higher sensitivity of serological diagnosis was seen compared to RT-PCR-based detection of SARS-CoV-2. The study reported the positivity of 71.15% samples by RT-PCR, and 82.69% were positive for the presence of antibodies [71].

ELISA-based antibody detection can also determine the seroconversion of antibodies during the acute and convalescent phases of the illness. A study in the US indicated that antibodies begin to produce within 6-10 days after infection with SARS-CoV-2 [130]. IgM seems to be at a peak level after 12 days of symptoms onset and persists in adequate amounts for up to 35 days, after which the amount declines rapidly. IgG level can be seen at peak level around 17 days after SARS-CoV-2 infection and persists for up to 49 days [70]. The clinical trial to find the prevalence of individuals with no symptoms having antibodies to SARS-CoV-2 is under process by the National Institute of Allergy and Infectious Diseases (NIAID) [131].

Quantitative ELISA could detect patients that have developed an intense immune response, and these patients can donate their plasma. One of the possible treatments can be from using the conventional method of plasma therapy as used in the previous pandemics of Influenza virus [132], SARs-CoV [133], West-Nile virus [134, 135], and Ebola virus [136]. Patients recovered from SARS-CoV-2 infection with significantly high neutralizing antibody titer can be the donor source of convalescent plasma. Neutralizing antibodies play a significant role in viral clearance and are considered key products of the immune system to protect against viral infections. Virus-specific neutralizing antibodies are induced by either viral infection or through vaccination and help in neutralizing and blocking the viral infections. Passive immunization is a method to accomplish short-term vaccination against infectious agents by regulating pathogen-specific antibodies. Artificially acquired passive immunity achieved mainly by using convalescent plasma taken from an individual who has established a strong antibody response against the causative agent and recovered from the infection. Convalescent plasma therapy is the best to diagnose and recover the patient after the onset of symptoms if it is managed right on time prophylactically [137, 138]. The antibodies present in convalescent plasma mediate their therapeutic effect by a different mechanism. Antibodies bind to the target pathogen, neutralizing infectivity of the pathogen directly. Some of the other mechanisms involve humoral mediated immunity, complement activation, and cellular cytotoxicity by helper T lymphocytes contribute to therapeutics. Non-neutralizing antibodies may also contribute to enhancing recovery and prophylaxis.

In the 21st century, convalescent plasma has been utilized for two coronavirus epidemics: SARS-CoV in 2003 and MERS-CoV in 2012. It was indicated from those outbreaks that neutralizing antibodies are present in convalescent plasma [139]. Eighty patients with SARS-CoV were treated in Hong Kong by using convalescent plasma [140]. Another data also suggested that three patients with SARS-CoV were recovered by passive antibody therapy [141]. Three patients with MERS were also treated with convalescent plasma in South Korea [142]. Convalescent plasma has additionally been used in the COVID-19 pandemic. Limited information indicates some breakthrough in clinical advantage, including a decrease in viral loads and some radiological benefits [143]. In a pilot investigation of 10 patients with severe COVID-19, transfusion of convalescent plasma with neutralizing antibody titer of 1:640 or more dilution came about in no serious adverse effect, and patients have recovered within 1-3 days of transfusion [144]. A case study reports the recovery of 5 patients *via* the transfusion of convalescent plasma (SARS-CoV-2 IgG titers >1000) as evidenced by improved oxygenation and decreased viral load in China [145].

Validation and Limitation of ELISA-Based Detection

Validation of an assay is the determination of the suitability of a test for a particular use. It is a series of experiments establishing the assay's performance characteristics such as specificity, sensitivity, accuracy, precision, variation, robustness, and detection limitation. A validated assay usually provides test results that identify whether the patient is positive or negative for a process or analyte. Intra and inter-assay precision are important in assay validation, as intra-assay validation determines the reproducibility between the well within the microtiter plate. In contrast, inter-assay precision determines the reproducibility between assays that have been done on different days. Similarly, the assay's sensitivity is the lowest level of analyte that differentiate from their background, and the specificity of an assay determines the cross-reactivity with other related molecules. The specificity of the ELISA for SARS-CoV-2 is the proportion of accurately identified participant test negative for COVID-19 while the sensitivity of an ELISA is the proportion of 'patients' accurately detected positive for COVID-19, as initially diagnosed by nucleic acid using RT-PCR.

Biomarkers play a central and significant role in diagnosing and treating patients in clinical medicine, clinical research, and the development of drugs. The wide range of such biomarkers is low-abundance proteins like antibodies, cytokines, and chemokines. For the antibody-based assay, the most widely used technique to get analytical sensitivity is ELISA. However, to get the desired and reliable results, the assay performance needs to be validated by measuring the performance characteristics [146]. ELISA has many advantages over other detection methods regarding its lower cost, less prone to sampling quality issues, and health risk for healthcare workers in collecting samples, as the serum is used that can easily be collected compared to bronchoalveolar lavage (BAL) and nasopharyngeal swabs. Besides that, it has less risk of contaminating specimens, shorter turnaround duration, and capacity of large volume processing. Serological assay like ELISA can also detect past infection as antibodies persist for a long time even after the clearance of infection [147].

Moreover, it is also validated that the analytical performance of CLIA. It was revealed that the repeatability values for IgM and IgG are <4% and <6%, respectively [75], and intermediate precision is <6% for both IgM and IgG. The sensitivity was reported 88% and 100% for IgM and IgG respectively by the 12 days of symptoms onset [148].

Besides its significance and advantages, ELISA has certain limitations such as insufficient sensitivity in detecting certain biomarkers, tedious and labor-intensive, cross-reactivity among other closely related biomolecules, and detection limitation in the acute phase of the illness. One of the major drawbacks of ELISA-based detection is that it may give false-positive or false-negative results. For instance, SARS-CoV-2 specific antibodies are undetectable in 1st week of illness and appear after 7-11 days of symptoms onset [127]. The difficulty in using such a serological assay is that some immunocompromised patients cannot mount an adequate immune response to the infection. Thus, false-negative results can occur. Similarly, false-positive results can occur due to the endemic human coronaviruses (SARS-CoV and MERS-CoV), to which the human might develop an antibody response [149].

Wan *et al.* [151] report the cross-reactivity between SARS-CoV and SARS-Co--2 due to protein structure similarity when tested by ELISA. There is a high sequence similarity of proteins between SARS-CoV-2 and other human coronaviruses. The cross-reactivity with other related sister species is highly expected and is one of the limitations in ELISA-based detection. The study reports the strong frequency of cross-reactivity against the spike protein of SARS-CoV, and SARS-CoV2 was observed in the plasma of COVID-19 patients [150]. Coronavirus antigen microarray contains important immunologic antigens such as SARS-CoV, MERS-CoV, SARS-CoV-2, and other common respiratory viruses. They have developed to determine the cross-reactivity between these viruses. The study reports the strong IgG seroreactivity in common coronaviruses. It has low IgG seroreactivity of SARS-CoV-2 with that of the nucleocapsid and S2 domain of Spike protein [152].

CONCLUSION

Detection and identification of causative agents have always been challenging tasks for centuries to diagnose diseases in newly emerged infections. Significant advances in microbiology and molecular biology have made remarkable contributions in the areas of diagnosis. Molecular diagnostic techniques offer a high-throughput and rapid diagnosis with extreme specificity and sensitivity. Among molecular diagnostic methods that have been adopted for the detection of SARS-CoV-2 includes the use of RT-PCR. Still, this approach can also give false positive, or negative results. Serological testing focused mainly on complementing molecular tests for the diagnosis of SARS-CoV-2 and providing therapeutic and prognostic information along with the diagnosis. The antibody-based diagnosis of SARS-CoV-2 by ELISA may have many other applications besides detection. It includes the diagnosis of the level of the immune response in different phases of infection, neutralizing antibodies level, the peak level of the immune response, and seroprevalence of infection. It also involves serosurveys in retrospective, cohort studies, and antibodies levels that could be used in convalescent plasma therapy. Many FDA EUA-approved serological tests for diagnosis of SARS-CoV-2 are succeeding. Certain new serological testing methods with high throughput are still in developmental stages. The development of ultra-rapid test kits and ELISA with point-of-care tests should be focused on rapid response time for therapy and eliminate the time consumption in the testing of the COVID-19 by RT-PCR. The further expansion of surveillance, investigations, testing capability, upgrading technologies, and appropriate health workforce is essential in the management of COVID-19.

CONSENT FOR PUBLICATION

Not Applicable.

CONFLICT OF INTEREST

The author confirms that this chapter contents have no conflict of interest.

ACKNOWLEDGEMENT

Declared none.

REFERENCES

[1]   WHO Director-General's opening remarks at the media briefing on COVID-19 - March 11 2020. 2020. Available from: https://www.who.int/dg/speeches/detail/who-director-general-s-opening-rema-ks-at-the-media-briefing-on-covid-19---11-march-2020

[2]   Coronavirus disease (COVID-19) Situation Report – 174. 2020. [July 17 2020]; Available from: https://www.who.int/docs/default-source/coronaviruse/situation-reports/20200712-covid-19-s-trep-174.pdf?sfvrsn=5d1c1b2c_2

[3]   Middle East respiratory syndrome coronavirus (MERS-CoV) 2020. Available from: https://www.who.int/emergencies/mers-cov/en/

[4]   Summary of probable SARS cases with onset of illness from November 1 2002 to July 31 2003. 2020. Available from: https://www.who.int/csr/sars/country/table2004_04_21/en/

[5]   Chan JF-W, Yuan S, Kok K-H, *et al.* A familial cluster of pneumonia associated with the 2019 novel coronavirus indicating person-to-person transmission: a study of a family cluster. Lancet 2020; 395(10223): 514-23.
[http://dx.doi.org/10.1016/S0140-6736(20)30154-9] [PMID: 31986261]

[6]   Phelan AL, Katz R, Gostin LO. The novel coronavirus originating in Wuhan, China: challenges for global health governance. JAMA 2020; 323(8): 709-10.
[http://dx.doi.org/10.1001/jama.2020.1097] [PMID: 31999307]

[7]   Gorbalenya AE. Severe acute respiratory syndrome-related coronavirus–the species and its viruses, a statement of the coronavirus study group. BioRxiv 2020.
[http://dx.doi.org/10.1101/2020.02.07.937862]

[8]   Song J-Y, Yun J-G, Noh J-Y, Cheong H-J, Kim W-J. Covid-19 in South Korea - Challenges of Subclinical Manifestations. N Engl J Med 2020; 382(19): 1858-9.
[http://dx.doi.org/10.1056/NEJMc2001801] [PMID: 32251568]

[9]   Zhou P, Yang X-L, Wang X-G, *et al.* A pneumonia outbreak associated with a new coronavirus of probable bat origin. Nature 2020; 579(7798): 270-3.
[http://dx.doi.org/10.1038/s41586-020-2012-7] [PMID: 32015507]

[10] Zhu N, Zhang D, Wang W, *et al.* A novel coronavirus from patients with pneumonia in China, 2019. N Engl J Med 2020; 382(8): 727-33.
[http://dx.doi.org/10.1056/NEJMoa2001017] [PMID: 31978945]

[11] Hani C, Trieu NH, Saab I, *et al.* COVID-19 pneumonia: A review of typical CT findings and differential diagnosis. Diagn Interv Imaging 2020; 101(5): 263-8.
[http://dx.doi.org/10.1016/j.diii.2020.03.014] [PMID: 32291197]

[12] Sohrabi C, Alsafi Z. World Health Organization declares global emergency: A review of the 2019 novel coronavirus (COVID-19). Int J Surg 2020.
[http://dx.doi.org/10.1016/j.ijsu.2020.02.034]

[13] Pan Y, Zhang D, Yang P, Poon LLM, Wang Q. Viral load of SARS-CoV-2 in clinical samples. Lancet Infect Dis 2020; 20(4): 411-2.
[PMID: 32105638]

[14] Gao Z. Efficient management of novel coronavirus pneumonia by efficient prevention and control in scientific manner. Chinese Journal of Tuberculosis and Respiratory Diseases 2020; 43: E001.

[15] Prompetchara E, Ketloy C, Palaga T. Immune responses in COVID-19 and potential vaccines: Lessons learned from SARS and MERS epidemic. Asian Pac J Allergy Immunol 2020; 38(1): 1-9.

[PMID: 32105090]

[16]   Tang Y-W, Schmitz JE, Persing DH, Stratton CW. Laboratory diagnosis of COVID-19: current issues and challenges. J Clin Microbiol 2020; 58(6)e00512-20
[http://dx.doi.org/10.1128/JCM.00512-20] [PMID: 32245835]

[17]   Zaki AM, van Boheemen S, Bestebroer TM, Osterhaus AD, Fouchier RA. Isolation of a novel coronavirus from a man with pneumonia in Saudi Arabia. N Engl J Med 2012; 367(19): 1814-20.
[http://dx.doi.org/10.1056/NEJMoa1211721] [PMID: 23075143]

[18]   Chu H, Chan JF-W, Yuen TT-T, *et al.* Comparative tropism, replication kinetics, and cell damage profiling of SARS-CoV-2 and SARS-CoV with implications for clinical manifestations, transmissibility, and laboratory studies of COVID-19: an observational study. Lancet Microbe 2020; 1(1): e14-23.
[http://dx.doi.org/10.1016/S2666-5247(20)30004-5] [PMID: 32835326]

[19]   Ksiazek TG, Erdman D, Goldsmith CS, *et al.* A novel coronavirus associated with severe acute respiratory syndrome. N Engl J Med 2003; 348(20): 1953-66.
[http://dx.doi.org/10.1056/NEJMoa030781] [PMID: 12690092]

[20]   Bai H, Cai X, Zhang X. Landscape Coronavirus Disease 2019 test (COVID-19 test) *in vitro*--A comparison of PCR *vs* Immunoassay *vs* Crispr-Based test. 2020.

[21]   Wang Y, Wang Y, Chen Y, Qin Q. Unique epidemiological and clinical features of the emerging 2019 novel coronavirus pneumonia (COVID-19) implicate special control measures. J Med Virol 2020; 92(6): 568-76.
[http://dx.doi.org/10.1002/jmv.25748] [PMID: 32134116]

[22]   Xiao SY, Wu Y, Liu H. Evolving status of the 2019 novel coronavirus infection: Proposal of conventional serologic assays for disease diagnosis and infection monitoring. J Med Virol 2020; 92(5): 464-7. [Commentary/Review].
[http://dx.doi.org/10.1002/jmv.25702] [PMID: 32031264]

[23]   Lan L, Xu D, Ye G, *et al.* Positive RT-PCR test results in patients recovered from COVID-19. JAMA 2020; 323(15): 1502-3.
[http://dx.doi.org/10.1001/jama.2020.2783] [PMID: 32105304]

[24]   Xiang F, Wang X, He X, Peng Z, Yang B, Zhang J, *et al.* Antibody detection and dynamic characteristics in patients with COVID-19. Clin Infect Dis 2020.

[25]   Li M, Jin R, Peng Y, Wang C, Ren W, Lv F, *et al.* Generation of antibodies against COVID-19 virus for development of diagnostic tools. medRxiv 2020.
[http://dx.doi.org/10.1101/2020.02.20.20025999]

[26]   Chen N, Zhou M, Dong X, *et al.* Epidemiological and clinical characteristics of 99 cases of 2019 novel coronavirus pneumonia in Wuhan, China: a descriptive study. Lancet 2020; 395(10223): 507-13.
[http://dx.doi.org/10.1016/S0140-6736(20)30211-7] [PMID: 32007143]

[27]   Caibin Fan KLYD. ACE2 Expression in Kidney and Testis May Cause Kidney and Testis Damage After 2019-nCoV Infection medRxiv 2020.

[28]   Hassan SA, Sheikh FN, Jamal S, Ezeh JK, Akhtar A. Coronavirus (COVID-19): a review of clinical features, diagnosis, and treatment. Cureus 2020; 12(3)e7355
[http://dx.doi.org/10.7759/cureus.7355] [PMID: 32328367]

[29]   Wang D, Hu B, Hu C, *et al.* Clinical characteristics of 138 hospitalized patients with 2019 novel coronavirus–infected pneumonia in Wuhan, China. JAMA 2020; 323(11): 1061-9.
[http://dx.doi.org/10.1001/jama.2020.1585] [PMID: 32031570]

[30]   Huang C, Wang Y, Li X, *et al.* Clinical features of patients infected with 2019 novel coronavirus in Wuhan, China. Lancet 2020; 395(10223): 497-506.
[http://dx.doi.org/10.1016/S0140-6736(20)30183-5] [PMID: 31986264]

[31]   Clinical management of severe acute respiratory infection when COVID-19 is suspected 2020. Available from: https://www.who.int/publications-detail/clinical-management-of-severe-acute-respiratory-infection-when-novel-coronavirus-(ncov)-infection-is-suspected

[32]   Coronavirus disease (COVID-19) 2020. Available from: https://www.cdc.gov/coronavirus/2019-ncov/index.html

[33]   Oberholtzer K, Sivitz L, Mack A, Lemon S, Mahmoud A, Knobler S. Learning from SARS: Preparing for the Next Disease Outbreak: Workshop Summary. National Academies Press 2004.

[34]   Levinson W, Jawetz E. Medical microbiology and immunology: examination and board review. Appleton & Lange 1996.

[35]   de Jong JC, Palache AM, Beyer WE, Rimmelzwaan GF, Boon AC, Osterhaus AD. Haemagglutination-inhibiting antibody to influenza virus. Dev Biol (Basel) 2003; 115: 63-73.
[PMID: 15088777]

[36]   Cohen BJ, Audet S, Andrews N, Beeler J. Plaque reduction neutralization test for measles antibodies: Description of a standardised laboratory method for use in immunogenicity studies of aerosol vaccination. Vaccine 2007; 26(1): 59-66.
[http://dx.doi.org/10.1016/j.vaccine.2007.10.046] [PMID: 18063236]

[37]   Mauldin J, Carbone K, Hsu H, Yolken R, Rubin S. Mumps virus-specific antibody titers from pre-vaccine era sera: comparison of the plaque reduction neutralization assay and enzyme immunoassays. J Clin Microbiol 2005; 43(9): 4847-51.
[http://dx.doi.org/10.1128/JCM.43.9.4847-4851.2005] [PMID: 16145156]

[38]   Traggiai E, Becker S, Subbarao K, *et al.* An efficient method to make human monoclonal antibodies from memory B cells: potent neutralization of SARS coronavirus. Nat Med 2004; 10(8): 871-5.
[http://dx.doi.org/10.1038/nm1080] [PMID: 15247913]

[39]   Engvall E. Enzyme immunoassay ELISA and EMIT Methods in enzymology. Elsevier 1980; pp. 419-39. [28]

[40]   Holmström P, Syrjänen S, Laine P, Valle SL, Suni J. HIV antibodies in whole saliva detected by ELISA and western blot assays. J Med Virol 1990; 30(4): 245-8.
[http://dx.doi.org/10.1002/jmv.1890300403] [PMID: 2370520]

[41]   Usuda S, Okamoto H, Iwanari H, *et al.* Serological detection of hepatitis B virus genotypes by ELISA with monoclonal antibodies to type-specific epitopes in the preS2-region product. J Virol Methods 1999; 80(1): 97-112.
[http://dx.doi.org/10.1016/S0166-0934(99)00039-7] [PMID: 10403681]

[42]   Yolken RH, Greenberg HB, Merson MH, Sack RB, Kapikian AZ. Enzyme-linked immunosorbent assay for detection of *Escherichia coli* heat-labile enterotoxin. J Clin Microbiol 1977; 6(5): 439-44.
[http://dx.doi.org/10.1128/jcm.6.5.439-444.1977] [PMID: 336638]

[43]   Sthevaan V, Swamy M, Shrivastava D, Verma Y. Prevalence of bovine rota virus infection in diarrhoeic calves. Indian J Vet Pathol 2014; 38(3): 190-2.
[http://dx.doi.org/10.5958/0973-970X.2014.01170.5]

[44]   Sblattero D, Berti I, Trevisiol C, *et al.* Human recombinant tissue transglutaminase ELISA: an innovative diagnostic assay for celiac disease. Am J Gastroenterol 2000; 95(5): 1253-7.
[http://dx.doi.org/10.1111/j.1572-0241.2000.02018.x] [PMID: 10811336]

[45]   Porcelli B, Ferretti F, Vindigni C, Terzuoli L. Assessment of a test for the screening and diagnosis of celiac disease. J Clin Lab Anal 2016; 30(1): 65-70.
[http://dx.doi.org/10.1002/jcla.21816] [PMID: 25385391]

[46]   Ishii K. Importance of serological tests in diagnosis of autoimmune blistering diseases. J Dermatol 2015; 42(1): 3-10.
[http://dx.doi.org/10.1111/1346-8138.12703] [PMID: 25558946]

[47]   Gegić M, Numanović F, Delibegović Z, Tihić N, Nurkić M, Hukić M. The importance of serological tests implementation in disseminated candidiasis diagnose. Coll Antropol 2013; 37(1): 157-63. [PMID: 23697267]

[48]   Tortora GJ, Funke BR, Case CL, Johnson TR. Microbiology: an introduction. San Francisco, CA: Benjamin Cummings 2004.

[49]   Towbin H, Staehelin T, Gordon J. Electrophoretic transfer of proteins from polyacrylamide gels to nitrocellulose sheets: procedure and some applications. Proc Natl Acad Sci USA 1979; 76(9): 4350-4. [http://dx.doi.org/10.1073/pnas.76.9.4350] [PMID: 388439]

[50]   Burnette WN. "Western blotting": electrophoretic transfer of proteins from sodium dodecyl sulfate--polyacrylamide gels to unmodified nitrocellulose and radiographic detection with antibody and radioiodinated protein A. Anal Biochem 1981; 112(2): 195-203. [http://dx.doi.org/10.1016/0003-2697(81)90281-5] [PMID: 6266278]

[51]   Pillai-Kastoori L, Schutz-Geschwender AR, Harford JA. A systematic approach to quantitative Western blot analysis. Anal Biochem 2020; 593113608 [PMID: 32007473]

[52]   Artsob H. Western Blot as a confirmatory test for Lyme disease. Can J Infect Dis 1970; 4. [PMID: 22346434]

[53]   Ingrosso L, Vetrugno V, Cardone F, Pocchiari M. Molecular diagnostics of transmissible spongiform encephalopathies. Trends Mol Med 2002; 8(6): 273-80. [http://dx.doi.org/10.1016/S1471-4914(02)02358-4] [PMID: 12067613]

[54]   Reichel C, Benetka W, Lorenc B, Thevis M. Evaluation of AMGEN clone 9G8A anti-Epo antibody for application in doping control. Drug Test Anal 2016; 8(11-12): 1131-7. [http://dx.doi.org/10.1002/dta.2057] [PMID: 27552163]

[55]   Wu A, Peng Y, Huang B, *et al.* Genome composition and divergence of the novel coronavirus (2019-nCoV) originating in China. Cell Host Microbe 2020; 27(3): 325-8. [http://dx.doi.org/10.1016/j.chom.2020.02.001] [PMID: 32035028]

[56]   Wrapp D, Wang N, Corbett KS, *et al.* Cryo-EM structure of the 2019-nCoV spike in the prefusion conformation. Science 2020; 367(6483): 1260-3. [http://dx.doi.org/10.1126/science.abb2507] [PMID: 32075877]

[57]   Chang CK, Sue S-C, Yu TH, *et al.* Modular organization of SARS coronavirus nucleocapsid protein. J Biomed Sci 2006; 13(1): 59-72. [http://dx.doi.org/10.1007/s11373-005-9035-9] [PMID: 16228284]

[58]   Kontou PI, Braliou GG, Dimou NL, Nikolopoulos G, Bagos PG. Antibody tests in detecting SARS-CoV-2 infection: a meta-analysis medRxiv 2020. [http://dx.doi.org/10.1101/2020.04.22.20074914]

[59]   To KK-WTO-Y, Tsang OT, Leung WS, *et al.* Temporal profiles of viral load in posterior oropharyngeal saliva samples and serum antibody responses during infection by SARS-CoV-2: an observational cohort study. Lancet Infect Dis 2020; 20(5): 565-74. [http://dx.doi.org/10.1016/S1473-3099(20)30196-1] [PMID: 32213337]

[60]   Liu W, Liu L, Kou G, Zheng Y, Ding Y, Ni W, *et al.* Evaluation of Nucleocapsid and Spike Protein-based ELISAs for detecting antibodies against SARS-CoV-2. J Clin Microbiol 2020. [http://dx.doi.org/10.1128/JCM.00461-20]

[61]   Xiang J, Yan M, Li H, Liu T, Lin C, Huang S, *et al.* Evaluation of Enzyme-Linked Immunoassay and Colloidal Gold-Immunochromatographic Assay Kit for Detection of Novel Coronavirus (SARS-Co-2) Causing an Outbreak of Pneumonia (COVID-19) medRxiv 2020. [http://dx.doi.org/10.1101/2020.02.27.20028787]

[62]   Guo L, Ren L, Yang S, *et al.* Profiling early humoral response to diagnose novel coronavirus disease

(COVID-19). Clin Infect Dis 2020; 71(15): 778-85.
[http://dx.doi.org/10.1093/cid/ciaa310] [PMID: 32198501]

[63] Perera RA, Mok CK, Tsang OT, *et al.* Serological assays for severe acute respiratory syndrome coronavirus 2 (SARS-CoV-2), March 2020. Euro Surveill 2020; 25(16)2000421
[http://dx.doi.org/10.2807/1560-7917.ES.2020.25.16.2000421] [PMID: 32347204]

[64] Pan Y, Li X, Yang G, *et al.* Serological immunochromatographic approach in diagnosis with SARS-CoV-2 infected COVID-19 patients. J Infect 2020; 81(1): e28-32.
[http://dx.doi.org/10.1016/j.jinf.2020.03.051] [PMID: 32283141]

[65] Li Z, Yi Y, Luo X, *et al.* Development and clinical application of a rapid IgM-IgG combined antibody test for SARS-CoV-2 infection diagnosis. J Med Virol 2020; 92(9): 1518-24.
[http://dx.doi.org/10.1002/jmv.25727] [PMID: 32104917]

[66] Garcia FP, Tanoira RP, Cabrera JPR, Serrano TA, Herruz PG, Gonzalez JC. Rapid diagnosis of SARS-CoV-2 infection by detecting IgG and IgM antibodies with an immunochromatographic device: a prospective single-center study medRxiv 2020.
[http://dx.doi.org/10.1101/2020.04.11.20062158]

[67] Yu HQ, Sun BQ, Fang ZF, *et al.* Distinct features of SARS-CoV-2-specific IgA response in COVID-19 patients. Eur Respir J 2020; 56(2)2001526
[http://dx.doi.org/10.1183/13993003.01526-2020] [PMID: 32398307]

[68] Yong G, Yi Y, Tuantuan L, *et al.* Evaluation of the auxiliary diagnostic value of antibody assays for the detection of novel coronavirus (SARS-CoV-2). J Med Virol 2020; 92(10): 1975-9.
[http://dx.doi.org/10.1002/jmv.25919] [PMID: 32320064]

[69] Zhong L, Chuan J, Gong B, *et al.* Detection of serum IgM and IgG for COVID-19 diagnosis. Sci China Life Sci 2020; 63(5): 777-80.
[http://dx.doi.org/10.1007/s11427-020-1688-9] [PMID: 32270436]

[70] Tan W, Lu Y, Zhang J, Wang J, Dan Y, Tan Z, *et al.* Viral kinetics and antibody responses in patients with COVID-19 medRxiv 2020.
[http://dx.doi.org/10.1101/2020.03.24.20042382]

[71] Liu R, Liu X, Han H, Shereen MA, Niu Z, Li D, *et al.* The comparative superiority of IgM-IgG antibody test to real-time reverse transcriptase PCR detection for SARS-CoV-2 infection diagnosis medRxiv 2020.
[http://dx.doi.org/10.1101/2020.03.28.20045765]

[72] Zhang J, Liu J, Li N, Liu Y, Ye R, Qin X, *et al.* Serological detection of 2019-nCoV respond to the epidemic: A useful complement to nucleic acid testing. medRxiv 2020.
[http://dx.doi.org/10.1101/2020.03.04.20030916]

[73] Lin D, Liu L, Zhang M, Hu Y, Yang Q, Guo J, *et al.* Evaluations of serological test in the diagnosis of 2019 novel coronavirus (SARS-CoV-2) infections during the COVID-19 outbreak medRxiv 2020.
[http://dx.doi.org/10.1101/2020.03.27.20045153]

[74] Jin Y, Wang M, Zuo Z, *et al.* Diagnostic value and dynamic variance of serum antibody in coronavirus disease 2019. Int J Infect Dis 2020; 94: 49-52.
[http://dx.doi.org/10.1016/j.ijid.2020.03.065] [PMID: 32251798]

[75] Padoan A, Sciacovelli L, Basso D, *et al.* IgA-Ab response to spike glycoprotein of SARS-CoV-2 in patients with COVID-19: A longitudinal study. Clin Chim Acta 2020; 507: 164-6.
[http://dx.doi.org/10.1016/j.cca.2020.04.026] [PMID: 32343948]

[76] Zhao J, Yuan Q, Wang H, *et al.* Antibody responses to SARS-CoV-2 in patients of novel coronavirus disease 2019. Clin Infect Dis 2020; 71(16): 2027-34.
[http://dx.doi.org/10.1093/cid/ciaa344] [PMID: 32221519]

[77] To KK-W, Tsang OT-Y, Leung W-S, *et al.* Temporal profiles of viral load in posterior oropharyngeal saliva samples and serum antibody responses during infection by SARS-CoV-2: an observational

cohort study. Lancet Infect Dis 2020; 20(5): 565-74.
[http://dx.doi.org/10.1016/S1473-3099(20)30196-1] [PMID: 32213337]

[78]   Freeman B, Lester S, Mills L, Rasheed MAU, Moye S, Abiona O, *et al.* Validation of a SARS-CoV-2 spike ELISA for use in contact investigations and serosurveillance bioRxiv 2020.

[79]   Bendavid E, Mulaney B, Sood N, Shah S, Ling E, Bromley-Dulfano R, *et al.* COVID-19 Antibody Seroprevalence in Santa Clara County, California medRxiv 2020.

[80]   Lou B, Li T, Zheng S, Su Y, Li Z, Liu W, *et al.* Serology characteristics of SARS-CoV-2 infection since the exposure and post symptoms onset medRxiv 2020.
[http://dx.doi.org/10.1101/2020.03.23.20041707]

[81]   Long Q-x, Deng H-j, Chen J, Hu J, Liu B-z, Liao P, *et al.* Antibody responses to SARS-CoV-2 in COVID-19 patients: the perspective application of serological tests in clinical practice medRxiv 2020.
[http://dx.doi.org/10.1101/2020.03.18.20038018]

[82]   Zhang B, Zhou X, Zhu C, Feng F, Qiu Y, Feng J, *et al.* Immune phenotyping based on neutrophil-t--lymphocyte ratio and IgG predicts disease severity and outcome for patients with COVID-19 medRxiv 2020.
[http://dx.doi.org/10.1101/2020.03.12.20035048]

[83]   Hu X, An T, Situ B, Hu Y, Ou Z, Li Q, *et al.* Heat inactivation of serum interferes with the immunoanalysis of antibodies to SARS-CoV-2 medRxiv 2020.
[http://dx.doi.org/10.1101/2020.03.12.20034231]

[84]   Liu L, Liu W, Wang S, Zheng S. A preliminary study on serological assay for severe acute respiratory syndrome coronavirus 2 (SARS-CoV-2) in 238 admitted hospital patients medRxiv 2020.
[http://dx.doi.org/10.1101/2020.03.06.20031856]

[85]   Zhao R, Li M, Song H, Chen J, Ren W, Feng Y, *et al.* Serological diagnostic kit of SARS-CoV-2 antibodies using CHO-expressed full-length SARS-CoV-2 S1 proteins medRxi 2020.
[http://dx.doi.org/10.1101/2020.03.26.20042184]

[86]   Hoffman T, Nissen K, Krambrich J, *et al.* Evaluation of a COVID-19 IgM and IgG rapid test; an efficient tool for assessment of past exposure to SARS-CoV-2. Infect Ecol Epidemiol 2020; 10(1)1754538
[http://dx.doi.org/10.1080/20008686.2020.1754538] [PMID: 32363011]

[87]   Okba NM, Muller MA, Li W, Wang C. GeurtsvanKessel CH, Corman VM, *et al.* SARS-CoV-2 specific antibody responses in COVID-19 patients. medRxiv 2020.

[88]   Du Z, Zhu F, Guo F, Yang B, Wang T. Detection of antibodies against SARS-CoV-2 in patients with COVID-19. J Med Virol 2020; 92(10): 1735-8.
[PMID: 32243608]

[89]   Ma H, Zeng W, He H, Zhao D, Yang Y, Jiang D, *et al.* COVID-19 diagnosis and study of serum SARS-CoV-2 specific IgA, IgM and IgG by chemiluminescence immunoanalysis medRxiv 2020.
[http://dx.doi.org/10.1101/2020.04.17.20064907]

[90]   Su S, Wong G, Shi W, *et al.* Epidemiology, genetic recombination, and pathogenesis of coronaviruses. Trends Microbiol 2016; 24(6): 490-502.
[http://dx.doi.org/10.1016/j.tim.2016.03.003] [PMID: 27012512]

[91]   Chen Y, Liu Q, Guo D. Emerging coronaviruses: Genome structure, replication, and pathogenesis. J Med Virol 2020; 92(4): 418-23.
[http://dx.doi.org/10.1002/jmv.25681] [PMID: 31967327]

[92]   Udugama B, Kadhiresan P, Kozlowski HN, *et al.* Diagnosing COVID-19: the disease and tools for detection. ACS Nano 2020; 14(4): 3822-35.
[http://dx.doi.org/10.1021/acsnano.0c02624] [PMID: 32223179]

[93]   Li W, Moore MJ, Vasilieva N, *et al.* Angiotensin-converting enzyme 2 is a functional receptor for the

SARS coronavirus. Nature 2003; 426(6965): 450-4.
[http://dx.doi.org/10.1038/nature02145] [PMID: 14647384]

[94]   Walls AC, Park Y-J, Tortorici MA, Wall A, McGuire AT, Veesler D. Structure, function, and antigenicity of the SARS-CoV-2 spike glycoprotein. Cell 2020.
[http://dx.doi.org/10.1016/j.cell.2020.11.032]

[95]   Millet JK, Whittaker GR. Host cell entry of Middle East respiratory syndrome coronavirus after two-step, furin-mediated activation of the spike protein. Proc Natl Acad Sci USA 2014; 111(42): 15214-9.
[http://dx.doi.org/10.1073/pnas.1407087111] [PMID: 25288733]

[96]   Wang H, Yang P, Liu K, *et al.* SARS coronavirus entry into host cells through a novel clathrin- and caveolae-independent endocytic pathway. Cell Res 2008; 18(2): 290-301.
[http://dx.doi.org/10.1038/cr.2008.15] [PMID: 18227861]

[97]   Liu J, Wu P, Gao F, *et al.* Novel immunodominant peptide presentation strategy: a featured HLA-A*2402-restricted cytotoxic T-lymphocyte epitope stabilized by intrachain hydrogen bonds from severe acute respiratory syndrome coronavirus nucleocapsid protein. J Virol 2010; 84(22): 11849-57.
[http://dx.doi.org/10.1128/JVI.01464-10] [PMID: 20844028]

[98]   Hajeer AH, Balkhy H, Johani S, Yousef MZ, Arabi Y. Association of human leukocyte antigen class II alleles with severe Middle East respiratory syndrome-coronavirus infection. Ann Thorac Med 2016; 11(3): 211-3.
[http://dx.doi.org/10.4103/1817-1737.185756] [PMID: 27512511]

[99]   Lu B, Tao L, Wang T, *et al.* Humoral and cellular immune responses induced by 3a DNA vaccines against severe acute respiratory syndrome (SARS) or SARS-like coronavirus in mice. Clin Vaccine Immunol 2009; 16(1): 73-7.
[http://dx.doi.org/10.1128/CVI.00261-08] [PMID: 18987164]

[100] Maloir Q, Ghysen K, von Frenckell C, Louis R, Guiot J. Acute respiratory distress revealing antisynthetase syndrome. Rev Med Liege 2018; 73(7-8): 370-5.
[PMID: 30113776]

[101] Pedersen SF, Ho Y-C. SARS-CoV-2: a storm is raging. J Clin Invest 2020; 130(5): 2202-5.
[http://dx.doi.org/10.1172/JCI137647] [PMID: 32217834]

[102] Chu H, Chan JF-W, Wang Y, *et al.* Comparative replication and immune activation profiles of SARS-CoV-2 and SARS-CoV in human lungs: an *ex vivo* study with implications for the pathogenesis of COVID-19. Clin Infect Dis 2020; 71(6): 1400-9.
[http://dx.doi.org/10.1093/cid/ciaa410] [PMID: 32270184]

[103] Camara NOS, Lepique AP, Basso AS. Lymphocyte differentiation and effector functions. Journal of Immunology Research 2012; 2012

[104] Qu J, Wu C, Li X, Zhang G, Jiang Z, Li X, *et al.* Profile of IgG and IgM antibodies against severe acute respiratory syndrome coronavirus 2 (SARS-CoV-2). Clin Infect Dis 2020.
[http://dx.doi.org/10.1093/cid/ciaa489]

[105] Iwasaki A, Medzhitov R. Regulation of adaptive immunity by the innate immune system. Science 2010; 327(5963): 291-5.
[http://dx.doi.org/10.1126/science.1183021] [PMID: 20075244]

[106] Lacy P, Stow JL. Cytokine release from innate immune cells: association with diverse membrane trafficking pathways. Blood 2011; 118(1): 9-18.
[http://dx.doi.org/10.1182/blood-2010-08-265892] [PMID: 21562044]

[107] Min C-K, Cheon S, Ha N-Y, *et al.* Comparative and kinetic analysis of viral shedding and immunological responses in MERS patients representing a broad spectrum of disease severity. Sci Rep 2016; 6(1): 25359.
[http://dx.doi.org/10.1038/srep25359] [PMID: 27146253]

[108] Li X, Geng M, Peng Y, Meng L, Lu S. Molecular immune pathogenesis and diagnosis of COVID-19. J

Pharm Anal 2020; 10(2): 102-8.
[http://dx.doi.org/10.1016/j.jpha.2020.03.001] [PMID: 32282863]

[109]   Xu Z, Shi L, Wang Y, *et al.* Pathological findings of COVID-19 associated with acute respiratory distress syndrome. Lancet Respir Med 2020; 8(4): 420-2.
[http://dx.doi.org/10.1016/S2213-2600(20)30076-X] [PMID: 32085846]

[110]   Versteeg GA, Bredenbeek PJ, van den Worm SH, Spaan WJ. Group 2 coronaviruses prevent immediate early interferon induction by protection of viral RNA from host cell recognition. Virology 2007; 361(1): 18-26.
[http://dx.doi.org/10.1016/j.virol.2007.01.020] [PMID: 17316733]

[111]   Perlman S, Netland J. Coronaviruses post-SARS: update on replication and pathogenesis. Nat Rev Microbiol 2009; 7(6): 439-50.
[http://dx.doi.org/10.1038/nrmicro2147] [PMID: 19430490]

[112]   He R, Leeson A, Andonov A, *et al.* Activation of AP-1 signal transduction pathway by SARS coronavirus nucleocapsid protein. Biochem Biophys Res Commun 2003; 311(4): 870-6.
[http://dx.doi.org/10.1016/j.bbrc.2003.10.075] [PMID: 14623261]

[113]   Kopecky-Bromberg SA, Martínez-Sobrido L, Frieman M, Baric RA, Palese P. SARS coronavirus proteins Orf 3b, Orf 6, and nucleocapsid function as interferon antagonists. J Virol 2006.

[114]   Niemeyer D, Zillinger T, Muth D, *et al.* Middle East respiratory syndrome coronavirus accessory protein 4a is a type I interferon antagonist. J Virol 2013; 87(22): 12489-95.
[http://dx.doi.org/10.1128/JVI.01845-13] [PMID: 24027320]

[115]   Yang Y, Zhang L, Geng H, *et al.* The structural and accessory proteins M, ORF 4a, ORF 4b, and ORF 5 of Middle East respiratory syndrome coronavirus (MERS-CoV) are potent interferon antagonists. Protein Cell 2013; 4(12): 951-61.
[http://dx.doi.org/10.1007/s13238-013-3096-8] [PMID: 24318862]

[116]   Stadlbauer D, Amanat F, Chromikova V, *et al.* SARS-CoV-2 Seroconversion in humans: A detailed protocol for a serological assay, antigen production, and test setup. Curr Protoc Microbiol 2020; 57(1)e100
[http://dx.doi.org/10.1002/cpmc.100] [PMID: 32302069]

[117]   Zhang W, Du R-H, Li B, *et al.* Molecular and serological investigation of 2019-nCoV infected patients: implication of multiple shedding routes. Emerg Microbes Infect 2020; 9(1): 386-9.
[http://dx.doi.org/10.1080/22221751.2020.1729071] [PMID: 32065057]

[118]   Lassaunière R, Frische A, Harboe ZB, Nielsen AC, Fomsgaard A, Krogfelt KA, *et al.* Evaluation of nine commercial SARS-CoV-2 immunoassays medRxiv 2020.

[119]   Stavnezer J, Amemiya CT, Eds. Evolution of isotype switching Seminars in immunology. Elsevier 2004.

[120]   Willey JM, Sherwood L, Woolverton CJ. Prescott, Harley, and Klein's microbiology 2008.

[121]   Lee H-K, Lee B-H, Seok S-H, *et al.* Production of specific antibodies against SARS-coronavirus nucleocapsid protein without cross reactivity with human coronaviruses 229E and OC43. J Vet Sci 2010; 11(2): 165-7.
[http://dx.doi.org/10.4142/jvs.2010.11.2.165] [PMID: 20458159]

[122]   Wan Z, Zhang X, Yan X. IFA in testing specific antibody of SARS coronavirus. S China J Prev Med 2003; 29(3): 36-7.

[123]   Woo PC, Lau SK, Wong BH, *et al.* Longitudinal profile of immunoglobulin G (IgG), IgM, and IgA antibodies against the severe acute respiratory syndrome (SARS) coronavirus nucleocapsid protein in patients with pneumonia due to the SARS coronavirus. Clin Diagn Lab Immunol 2004; 11(4): 665-8.
[PMID: 15242938]

[124]   Che X, Hao W, Qiu L, Pan Y, Liao Z, Xu H, *et al.* Antibody response of patients with severe acute

respiratory syndrome (SARS) to nucleocapsid antigen of SARS-associated coronavirus. Di 1 JuneJune yi da xue xue bao= Academic journal of the first medical college of PLA 2003; 23(7): 9-637.

[125] Wang W, Wang H, Deng Y, *et al.* Characterization of anti-MERS-CoV antibodies against various recombinant structural antigens of MERS-CoV in an imported case in China. Emerg Microbes Infect 2016; 5(11)e113
[http://dx.doi.org/10.1038/emi.2016.114] [PMID: 27826140]

[126] Xiao AT, Gao C, Zhang S. Profile of specific antibodies to SARS-CoV-2: The first report. J Infect 2020; 81(1): 147-78.
[http://dx.doi.org/10.1016/j.jinf.2020.03.012] [PMID: 32209385]

[127] Amanat F, Stadlbauer D, Strohmeier S, *et al.* A serological assay to detect SARS-CoV-2 seroconversion in humans. Nat Med 2020; 26(7): 1033-6.
[http://dx.doi.org/10.1038/s41591-020-0913-5] [PMID: 32398876]

[128] Patel R, Babady E, Theel ES, Storch GA, Pinsky BA, George KS, *et al.* Report from the American Society for Microbiology COVID-19 international summit, March 23 2020: value of diagnostic testing for SARS–CoV-2/COVID-19. Am Soc Microbiol 2020.

[129] Doi A, Iwata K, Kuroda H, Hasuike T, Nasu S, Kanda A, *et al.* Estimation of seroprevalence of novel coronavirus disease (COVID-19) using preserved serum at an outpatient setting in Kobe, Japan: A cross-sectional study medRxiv 2020.

[130] Okba NMA, Müller MA, Li W, *et al.* Severe Acute Respiratory Syndrome Coronavirus 2-Specific Antibody Responses in Coronavirus Disease Patients. Emerg Infect Dis 2020; 26(7): 1478-88.
[http://dx.doi.org/10.3201/eid2607.200841] [PMID: 32267220]

[131] Abraham EP, Chain E. An enzyme from bacteria able to destroy penicillin. 1940. Rev Infect Dis 1988; 10(4): 677-8.
[PMID: 3055168]

[132] Zhou B, Zhong N, Guan Y. Treatment with convalescent plasma for influenza A (H5N1) infection. N Engl J Med 2007; 357(14): 1450-1.
[http://dx.doi.org/10.1056/NEJMc070359] [PMID: 17914053]

[133] Mair-Jenkins J, Saavedra-Campos M, Baillie JK, *et al.* The effectiveness of convalescent plasma and hyperimmune immunoglobulin for the treatment of severe acute respiratory infections of viral etiology: a systematic review and exploratory meta-analysis. J Infect Dis 2015; 211(1): 80-90.
[http://dx.doi.org/10.1093/infdis/jiu396] [PMID: 25030060]

[134] Planitzer CB, Modrof J, Kreil TR. West Nile virus neutralization by US plasma-derived immunoglobulin products. J Infect Dis 2007; 196(3): 435-40.
[http://dx.doi.org/10.1086/519392] [PMID: 17597458]

[135] Haley M, Retter AS, Fowler D, Gea-Banacloche J, O'Grady NP. The role for intravenous immunoglobulin in the treatment of West Nile virus encephalitis. Clin Infect Dis 2003; 37(6): e88-90.
[http://dx.doi.org/10.1086/377172] [PMID: 12955669]

[136] van Griensven J, Edwards T, de Lamballerie X, *et al.* Evaluation of convalescent plasma for Ebola virus disease in Guinea. N Engl J Med 2016; 374(1): 33-42.
[http://dx.doi.org/10.1056/NEJMoa1511812] [PMID: 26735992]

[137] Casadevall A, Pirofski LA. A new synthesis for antibody-mediated immunity. Nat Immunol 2011; 13(1): 21-8.
[http://dx.doi.org/10.1038/ni.2184] [PMID: 22179281]

[138] Casadevall A, Scharff MD. Serum therapy revisited: animal models of infection and development of passive antibody therapy. Antimicrob Agents Chemother 1994; 38(8): 1695-702.
[http://dx.doi.org/10.1128/AAC.38.8.1695] [PMID: 7985997]

[139] Zhang JS, Chen JT, Liu YX, *et al.* A serological survey on neutralizing antibody titer of SARS convalescent sera. J Med Virol 2005; 77(2): 147-50.

[http://dx.doi.org/10.1002/jmv.20431] [PMID: 16121363]

[140] Cheng Y, Wong R, Soo YO, *et al.* Use of convalescent plasma therapy in SARS patients in Hong Kong. Eur J Clin Microbiol Infect Dis 2005; 24(1): 44-6.
[http://dx.doi.org/10.1007/s10096-004-1271-9] [PMID: 15616839]

[141] Yeh K-M, Chiueh T-S, Siu LK, *et al.* Experience of using convalescent plasma for severe acute respiratory syndrome among healthcare workers in a Taiwan hospital. J Antimicrob Chemother 2005; 56(5): 919-22.
[http://dx.doi.org/10.1093/jac/dki346] [PMID: 16183666]

[142] Ko J-H, Seok H, Cho SY, *et al.* Challenges of convalescent plasma infusion therapy in Middle East respiratory coronavirus infection: a single centre experience. Antivir Ther 2018; 23(7): 617-22.
[http://dx.doi.org/10.3851/IMP3243] [PMID: 29923831]

[143] Bloch EM, Shoham S, Casadevall A, *et al.* Deployment of convalescent plasma for the prevention and treatment of COVID-19. J Clin Invest 2020; 130(6): 2757-65.
[http://dx.doi.org/10.1172/JCI138745] [PMID: 32254064]

[144] Duan K, Liu B, Li C, Zhang H, Yu T, Qu J, *et al.* The feasibility of convalescent plasma therapy in severe COVID-19 patients: a pilot study medRxiv 2020.
[http://dx.doi.org/10.1101/2020.03.16.20036145]

[145] Shen C, Wang Z, Zhao F, *et al.* Treatment of 5 critically ill patients with COVID-19 with convalescent plasma. JAMA 2020; 323(16): 1582-9.
[http://dx.doi.org/10.1001/jama.2020.4783] [PMID: 32219428]

[146] Andreasson U, Perret-Liaudet A, van Waalwijk van Doorn LJ, *et al.* A practical guide to immunoassay method validation. Front Neurol 2015; 6: 179.
[http://dx.doi.org/10.3389/fneur.2015.00179] [PMID: 26347708]

[147] Bramhachari PV, Sheela GM, Prathyusha A, Madhavi M, Kumar KS, Reddy NNR, *et al.* Advanced Immunotechnological Methods for Detection and Diagnosis of Viral Infections: Current Applications and Future Challenges Dynamics of Immune Activation in Viral Diseases. Springer 2020; pp. 261-75.

[148] Padoan A, Cosma C, Sciacovelli L, Faggian D, Plebani M. Analytical performances of a chemiluminescence immunoassay for SARS-CoV-2 IgM/IgG and antibody kinetics. Clin Chem Lab Med 2020; 58(7): 1081-8. [CCLM].
[http://dx.doi.org/10.1515/cclm-2020-0443] [PMID: 32301749]

[149] Zhang JLJ, Li N, Liu Y, Ye R, Qin X, *et al.* Serological detection of 2019-nCoV respond to the epidemic: A useful complement to nucleic acid testing medRxiv 2020.
[http://dx.doi.org/10.1101/2020.03.04.20030916]

[150] Lv H, Wu NC, Tsang OT-Y, Yuan M, Perera RA, Leung WS, *et al.* Cross-reactive antibody response between SARS-CoV-2 and SARS-CoV infections. bioRxiv 2020.
[http://dx.doi.org/10.1101/2020.03.15.993097]

[151] Wan WY, Lim SH, Seng EH. Cross-reaction of sera from COVID-19 patients with SARS-CoV assays. medRxiv 2020.
[http://dx.doi.org/10.1101/2020.03.17.20034454]

[152] Saahir Khan RN, Jain A. Assis RRd, Jasinskas A, Obiero JM, Adenaiye O, *et al.* Analysis of Serologic Cross-Reactivity Between Common Human Coronaviruses and SARS-CoV-2 Using Coronavirus Antigen Microarray bioRxiv 2020.

CHAPTER 14

Chest CT Scan: An Ideal Diagnostic Tool for COVID-19

Noor Muhammad Khan[1,*], Muhammad Adil[2], Amar Nasir[3] and Arbab Sikandar[4]

[1] *University of Veterinary and Animal Sciences, Lahore Sub-campus Jhang, Pakistan*

[2] *Department of Pharmacology and Toxicology, University of Veterinary and Animal Sciences, Lahore Sub-campus Jhang, Pakistan*

[3] *Department of Clinical Sciences, University of Veterinary and Animal Sciences, Lahore Sub-campus Jhang, Pakistan*

[4] *Department of Anatomy and Histology, University of Veterinary and Animal Sciences, Lahore Sub-campus Jhang, Pakistan*

Abstract: Diagnosis of any disease requires careful assessment. Diagnostic procedures might play a pivotal role in making the treatment protocols more powerful/potent efficient, and effective by highlighting the clinical findings of the disease. Along with other diagnostic techniques, a computed tomography (CT) scan has been employed to diagnose coronavirus disease-19 (COVID-19) patients since the outbreak of this disease and therefore promises it as a crucial diagnostic tool. A CT-scan is a specialized medical imaging technique that produces cross-sectional images of specific areas of a targeted object utilizing a combination of multiple X-ray measurements taken from multiple angles. CT scan help diagnose COVID-19 individuals display severe clinical features and advanced forms of the disease. Pulmonary CT images of COVID-19 patients had common diagnostic manifestations such as ground-glass opacities (GGO), consolidation, reticular pattern, and fibrosis. It also includes nodular lesions reversed halo sign. and thickening of the pleura as the less common findings. The receiver operative characteristic (ROC) curve has been successfully applied for determining the accuracy of the CT-scan-based diagnosis of COVID-19. Artificial intelligence (AI) techniques, particularly deep learning, are extensively used for processing and evaluating imaging data, thereby improving the diagnostic performance of radiologists and clinicians. Despite its emergence as an effective method for screening COVID-19 patients, a CT scan is not recommended as a primary tool for diagnosing COVID-19 and must be used with utmost caution as it may cause the transmission of COVID-19 pathogen in the current epidemic. Overall, the current chapter focuses on CT-scan implications in diagnosing the COVID-19 infection and its comparison with the other diagnostic tools.

* **Corresponding author Noor Muhammad Khan:** University of Veterinary and Animal Sciences, Lahore Sub-campus Jhang, Pakistan; E-mail: noor.muhammad@uvas.edu.pk

Kamal Niaz & Muhammad Farrukh Nisar (Eds.)

Keywords: Computed Tomography, Consolidation, Coronavirus, COVID-19, Disease, Ground-Glass Opacity, Imaging, Receiver Operative Characteristic.

INTRODUCTION

Disease diagnosis and investigation have always remained the integral components of an effective treatment protocol for any disease. Many hallmarks of the diagnosis prevail depending upon the nature of the disease. Health experts have to choose very conscientiously/carefully among the available techniques, which can be useful in revealing the manifestations regarding the nature and severity of the anomaly. Apart from the traditional testing of samples with different origins, radiography helps in a more clear disease manifestation by providing clinical pictures of the internal organs and systems of the body. These include the traditional X-Ray photographs and ultrasound to more advanced diagnostic techniques such as magnetic resonance imaging (MRI) and computed tomography (CT) scan. Thanks to Gabriel Frank, who developed the idea of 'today's CT in the 1940s [1]. Both CT scans and MRI are the recent versions of advanced imaging techniques in the science of radiology. CT scan is usually considered the gold standard and soft tool for the morphological examination of the lungs [2].

CT scan is based on the principle of subjecting the patient to a narrow beam of X-Rays at different angles to create cross-sectional or tomographic images of the scanned object using a computer. This technique can provide an effective clinical diagnosis by scanning and obtaining images of different body organs and tissues. This technique has potentially acquired a greater consideration and scope on account of its certain advantages over traditional radiography. In the current novel coronavirus disease-19 (COVID-19) crisis, the entire focus is on containing the virus, but unfortunately, no effective treatment has been discovered so far. Accordingly, the scope and applications of CT scans have further extended to the diagnosis of COVID-19 and its comparison with other respiratory diseases.

Moreover, contemporary research has also validated the high sensitivity of chest CT scan for the diagnosis of COVID-19. The overall sensitivity of chest radiography and CT scan has been reported to be very close to RT-PCR [6]. Therefore, it is considered an effective tool for detecting COVID-19 in pandemic areas [5].

This chapter overall focuses on different aspects of CT scan with special reference to COVID-19. Moreover, the scope and applications of this technique in COVID-19, the suitability of patients, CT scan-based diagnosis, severity assessment of COVID-19, imaging manifestations, comparison of CT scan with other conventional radiological techniques, CT imaging findings of COVID-19, along with the applications of receiver operating characteristic and artificial intelligence (AI) deep learning in combating COVID-19 have also been addressed.

Types of COVID-19 Patients for which CT Scan can be Used

CT scan can be assumed as an essential tool for the diagnosis of COVID-19 patients when a series of signs and symptoms are thoroughly investigated. It is pertinent to mention that COVID-19 reflects great variations in signs and symptoms among different patients. It is a challenging task to go for diagnostic imaging for a large number of patients. Therefore, the need for diagnostic imaging arises as the disease advances. The pulmonary signs and symptoms become more evident, which is the stage when the use of chest radiography can be incorporated. Studies have suggested using the following protocols in determining the scope of chest radiography (including CT scan) in COVID-19 patients [3].

1. Imaging is not essentially indicated in suspected patients having mild clinical signs of COVID-19 and lacking the disease progression [3].
2. Chest radiography can be indicated in individuals exhibiting severe respiratory systems, *i.e.,* severe coughing and shortness of breath, which might worsen as the disease progresses [3].
3. In certain conditions, *e.g.,* lack of resources for conducting expensive tests like RT-PCR, chest radiography, or CT scan, can be employed for suspected patients showing moderate to severe COVID-19 symptoms [3].

The first scenario describes patients being presented at health care centers or telemedicine services shown in Fig. (**1**). Individuals showing mild clinical symptoms consistent with COVID-19 do not require chest imaging such as CT scan. However, careful monitoring of such patients is required. The imaging is indicated in a group of patients in which the disease progression is noticed, deduced from the worsening respiratory symptoms.

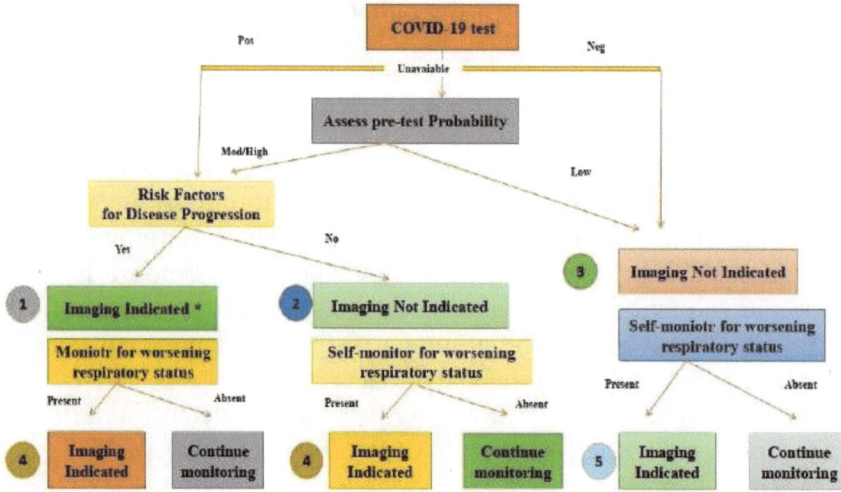

Fig. (1). Showing the different components of the first scenario in which the Chest imaging can be indicated for the diagnosis of COVID-19.

The second recommendation is about patients possessing severe respiratory symptoms consistent with COVID-19, and the symptoms aggravate with time, as shown in Fig. **(2)**.

Under such circumstances, chest imaging is highly recommended.

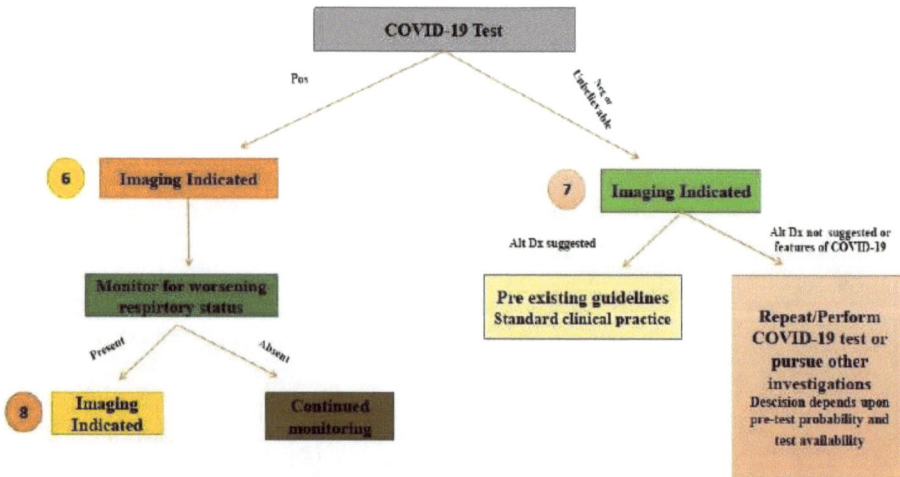

Fig. (2). Illustrating the different conditions in the second scenario in which the Chest imaging can be indicated for the diagnosis of COVID-19.

The third scenario implies whenever there are greater chances of the disease. Based upon the clinical signs and an environment that lacks sufficient resources for the effective diagnosis and management of the COVID-19 infected patients', *e.g.,* personal protective equipment (PPE), ventilators, health personals, beds, and testing facilities.

Additionally, a questionnaire was formulated and presented to a panel of radiology experts. The responses to each question were laid down on a 5-point scale, as shown in Fig. (**3**). Each member of the panel expressed different consensus concerning the conditions in which the chest imaging (Including CT scan) can be of clinical significance in the wake of the COVID-19 outbreak.

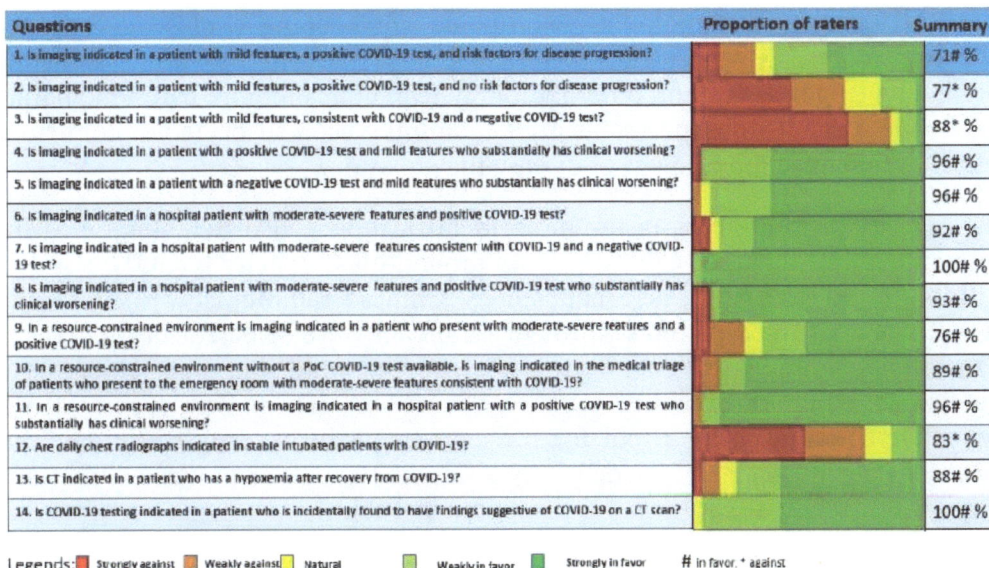

Questions	Proportion of raters	Summary
1. Is imaging indicated in a patient with mild features, a positive COVID-19 test, and risk factors for disease progression?		71# %
2. Is imaging indicated in a patient with mild features, a positive COVID-19 test, and no risk factors for disease progression?		77* %
3. Is imaging indicated in a patient with mild features, consistent with COVID-19 and a negative COVID-19 test?		88* %
4. Is imaging indicated in a patient with a positive COVID-19 test and mild features who substantially has clinical worsening?		96# %
5. Is imaging indicated in a patient with a negative COVID-19 test and mild features who substantially has clinical worsening?		96# %
6. Is imaging indicated in a hospital patient with moderate-severe features and positive COVID-19 test?		92# %
7. Is imaging indicated in a hospital patient with moderate-severe features consistent with COVID-19 and a negative COVID-19 test?		100# %
8. Is imaging indicated in a hospital patient with moderate-severe features and positive COVID-19 test who substantially has clinical worsening?		93# %
9. In a resource-constrained environment is imaging indicated in a patient who present with moderate-severe features and a positive COVID-19 test?		76# %
10. In a resource-constrained environment without a PoC COVID-19 test available, is imaging indicated in the medical triage of patients who present to the emergency room with moderate-severe features consistent with COVID-19?		89# %
11. In a resource-constrained environment is imaging indicated in a hospital patient with a positive COVID-19 test who substantially has clinical worsening?		96# %
12. Are daily chest radiographs indicated in stable intubated patients with COVID-19?		83* %
13. Is CT indicated in a patient who has a hypoxemia after recovery from COVID-19?		88# %
14. Is COVID-19 testing indicated in a patient who is incidentally found to have findings suggestive of COVID-19 on a CT scan?		100# %

Legends: ▮ Strongly against ▮ Weakly against ▮ Natural   ▮ Weakly in favor   ▮ Strongly in favor   # in favor, * against

Fig. (3). A compilation of 14 questions presented to a panel of experts in the field of Radiology. Different legends show the individual response of each expert to a specific question, while the "summary" column presents the overall response to a particular question in percentage (%).

However, the Center for Disease Control (CDC), American College of Radiology, does not currently encourage chest X-ray (CXR) or CT scan as a first option for diagnosing COVID-19. The American College of Radiology has further put forward their recommendations to using CXR and CT scan in the diagnosis of COVID-19.

1. CT scan should not be used for screening and as a first option in the diagnosis of COVID-19.
2. CT scan should be preferably used in symptomatic hospitalized patients by

adopting appropriate infection control strategies before the screening.
3. Mobile (ambulatory) radiography assembly or equipment should be used as they can be cleaned easily. The flow of patients to the radiography units can be avoided in this way.
4. Radiology personals should develop acquaintance and expertise in interpreting the CT image findings in the case of COVID-19. They must also be capable of differentiating it from similar findings in other ailments.

CT Scan Severity Score Assessment

The ongoing crisis of COVID-19 essentially requires an understanding of the nature and severity of pneumonia that constitutes a key diagnostic feature in COVID-19 patients. Radiologists worldwide are keeping a close eye on the diagnosis of this disease using CXR and CT. However, they are also facing certain challenges as CT and other radiology techniques require careful handling and frequent disinfection protocols after examining each suspected or confirmed patient to minimize the chances of disease transmission.

The severity scoring helps in the rapid identification and differentiation of the different clinical forms of COVID-19 *via* ground-glass opacity (GGO), as shown in Table **1**. A research was conducted by Chinese radiologists in which 102 COVID-19 confirmed patients (through RT-PCR) were selected for a chest CT scan. Among those, 84 patients were stable, showing mild signs and symptoms of the disease, while 18 exhibited severe cases of COVID-19. The opacity of the parenchyma was used as a tool for the assessment of severity score. For this purpose, both lungs were divided into different regions (Segments n=20) and scores were assigned as follows [4] illustrated in Table **1**.

Table 1. Severity scoring of the lungs regions in COVID -19 patients based on ground-glass opacity (GGO).

The Opacity of the Parenchyma (%)	Severity Score
0	0
<50	1
= or >50	2

CT scans were examined for pulmonary parenchymal opacity at a window width and level of 1000 to 2000 HU and -700 to -500 HU, respectively. Expert radiologists elucidated all the images. The same study has further made a comparison among the individual lung segments in the form of a table which not only mentions the individual scoring of the different segments of the lungs but also the cumulative scoring, which may range from 0-40 points [4] as shown as Table **2**.

Table 2. Comparison and severity scoring of the individual lung segments based on the presence of parenchymal opacity in CT images of 102 COVID-19 patients. The overall scoring is also mentioned.

Variable	Sample	Mild (n=84)	Severe (n=18)		P	Kappa
anterior segment (L)	-	-	-	-	-	-
0	59	53 (63.10%)	6	(33.33%)	0.002	0.648
1	41	31 (36.90%)	10 (55.56%)		-	-
2	2	0 (0.00%)	2	(11.11%)	-	-
apical segment (L)	-	-	-	-	-	-
0	56	52 (61.90%)	4	(22.22%)	<0.001	0.776
1	44	32 (38.10%)	12 (66.67%)		-	-
2	2	0 (0.00%)	2	(11.11%)	-	-
posterior segment (L)	-	-	-	-	-	-
0	34	32 (38.10%)	2	(11.11%)	<0.001	0.782
1	54	46 (54.76%)	8	(44.44%)	-	-
2	14	6 (7.14%)	8	(44.44%)	-	-
superior lingular segment (L)	-	-	-	-	-	-
0	30	29 (34.52%)	1	(5.56%)	0.002	0.829
1	65	52 (61.90%)	13 (72.22%)		-	-
2	7	3 (3.57%)	4	(22.22%)	-	-
inferior lingular segment (L)	-	-	-	-	-	-
0	39	38 (45.24%)	1	(5.56%)	<0.001	0.798
1	51	42 (50.00%)	9	(50.00%)	-	-
2	12	4 (4.76%)	8	(44.44%)	-	-
superior segment (L)	-	-	-	-	-	-
0	23	22 (26.19%)	1	(5.56%)	<0.001	0.883
1	56	51 (60.71%)	5	(27.78%)	-	-
2	23	11 (13.10%)	12 (66.67%)		-	-
anterior basal segment (L)	-	-	-	-	-	-
0	59	55 (65.48%)	4	(22.22%)	<0.001	0.687
1	37	29 (34.52%)	8	(44.44%)	-	-
2	6	0 (0.00%)	6	(33.33%)	-	-
medial basal segment (L)	-	-	-	-	-	-
0	76	69 (82.14%)	7	(38.89%)	<0.001	0.799

(Table 2) cont.....

Variable	Sample	Mild (n=84)	Severe (n=18)		P	Kappa
1	21	15 (17.86%)	6	(33.33%)	-	-
2	5	0 (0.00%)	5	(27.78%)	-	-
lateral basal segment (L)	-	-	-	-	-	-
0	23	23 (27.38%)	0	(0.00%)	<0.001	0.816
1	68	58 (69.05%)	10 (55.56%)		-	-
2	11	3 (3.57%)	8 (44.44%)		-	-
posterior basal segment (L)	-	-	-	-	-	-
0	21	21 (25.00%)	0	(0.00%)	<0.001	0.807
1	64	55 (65.48%)	9 (50.00%)		-	-
2	17	8 (9.52%)	9 (50.00%)		-	-
anterior segment (R)	-	-	-	-	-	-
0	38	36 (42.86%)	2 (11.11%)		0.006	0.757
1	61	47 (55.95%)	14 (77.78%)		-	-
2	3	1 (1.19%)	2 (11.11%)		-	-
apical segment (R)	-	-	-	-	-	-

0	60	54 (64.29%)	6 (33.33%)		0.011	0.721
1	39	29 (34.52%)	10 (55.56%)		-	-
2	3	1 (1.19%)	2 (11.11%)		-	-
posterior segment (R)	-	-	-	-	-	-
0	34	31 (36.90%)	3 (16.67%)		<0.001	0.878
1	59	51 (60.71%)	8 (44.44%)		-	-
2	9	2 (2.38%)	7 (38.89%)		-	-
medial segment (R)	-	-	-	-	-	-
0	54	50 (59.52%)	4 (22.22%)		<0.001	0.891
1	42	34 (40.48%)	8 (44.44%)		-	-
2	6	0 (0.00%)	6 (33.33%)		-	-
lateral segment (R)	-	-	-	-	-	-
0	35	33 (39.29%)	2 (11.11%)		<0.001	0.966
1	56	47 (55.95%)	9 (50.00%)		-	-
2	11	4 (4.76%)	7 (38.89%)		-	-
superior segment (R)	-	-	-	-	-	-
0	23	21 (25.00%)	2 (11.11%)		<0.001	0.858
1	63	58 (69.05%)	5 (27.78%)		-	-
2	16	5 (5.95%)	11 (61.11%)		-	-

(Table 2) cont.....

anterior basal segment (R)	-	-	-	-	-	-
0	53	49 (58.33%)	4	(22.22%)	<0.001	0.770
1	43	35 (41.67%)	8	(44.44%)	-	-
2	6	0 (0.00%)	6	(33.33%)	-	-
medial basal segment (R)	-	-	-	-	-	-
0	59	55 (65.48%)	4	(22.22%)	<0.001	0.793
1	37	28 (33.33%)	9	(50.00%)	-	-
2	6	1 (1.19%)	5	(27.78%)	-	-
lateral basal segment (R)	-	-	-	-	-	-
0	32	30 (35.71%)	2	(11.11%)	<0.001	0.664
1	58	50 (59.52%)	8	(44.44%)	-	-
2	12	4 (4.76%)	8	(44.44%)	-	-
posterior basal segment (R)	-	-	-	-	-	-
0	19	18 (21.43%)	1	(5.56%)	0.001	0.761
1	61	54 (64.29%)	7	(38.89%)	-	-
2	22	12 (14.29%)	10 (55.56%)		-	-
Score of left lung	102	6.00 (3.00, 8.00)	12.00 (9.00, 14.00)		<0.001	0.925#
Score of right lung	102	6.00 (3.45, 8.00)	12.00 (9.00, 16.05)		<0.001	0.892#
Total score	102	13.00 (6.00, 16.00)	23.50 (20.95, 30.05)		<0.001	0.990#

Where # represents the Interclass correlation coefficient
R=Right Lung
L=Left Lung

Studies have revealed that both the right and left lungs could be affected by the disease. The superior segment of the inferior lobe and the posterior segment of the superior lobe are affected. Lateral, and posterior basal segments of inferior lobes were most affected, as shown in Fig. D. Pulmonary pacifications are found more prominent in the lower lobes than the middle and upper lobes of the lungs [4]. As the disease attacks individuals irrespective of their sex, studies have suggested that the lungs of both sexes can be equally affected in an orderly fashion. Ground glass opacities and consolidations have been observed in the different pulmonary segments of female and male patients [4].

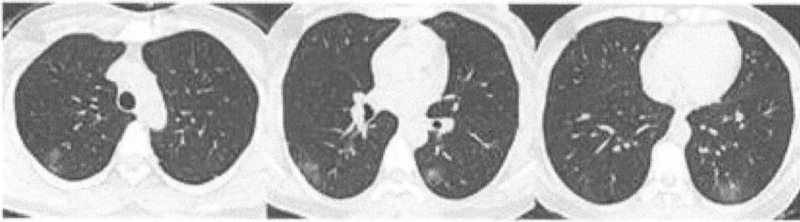

Fig. (4). CT images of the lungs showing affections (ground-glass opacities) of the posterior segment of the upper lobe (right lung), anterior segment of bilateral lungs, and posterior segments of the right-left lobe of a woman suffering from COVID-19. The Severity score is 4.

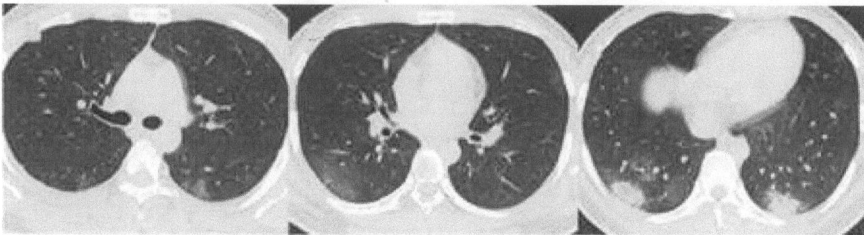

Fig. (5). CT images showing consolidation and ground-glass opacities in multiple lung segments of the 20-year man with COVID-19. The severity score is 7.

CT Imaging Manifestations

Chest imaging is of pivotal importance in diagnosing and subsequently managing the patients affected with COVID-19 infection. Plain radiography is inferior to high-resolution CT in detecting the early GGO associated with COVID-19 and non-COVID-19-pneumonia [8], as presented in Fig. **(5)**. It permits objective assessment of pulmonary lesions, thereby facilitating the better elucidation of disease pathogenesis. Sequential CT scanning can be employed for determining the occurrence, developmental pattern, and prognosis of the disease. Histopathological examination is considered of limited diagnostic value owing to the high infectivity of COVID-19 infection. Another advantage of CT scan over histopathology is that the former can evaluate entire lungs. In comparison, histopathology is characterized by inherent sampling errors with localized outcomes [9].

Imaging Manifestations in COVID-19 and their Features

Generally, the imaging features of COVID-19 strikingly resemble those of severe acute respiratory syndrome (SARS) and the Middle East respiratory syndrome (MERS) [10]. In SARS, solitary lesion involves unilateral lung with obvious sepal thickening after 14 days or so post-infection. MERS, on the other hand, inflicts a higher number of deaths [11]. Although it is hard to differentiate it from COVID-19 based on imaging, pneumothorax and pleural effusions are relatively more common in expired patients of MERS [12]. Bacterial pneumonia is commonly exhibited by nodular, patchy, or consolidation shadows, spreading along with the pulmonary segments or bronchi, and can be differentially identified [13].

The imaging manifestations in confirmed COVID-19 patients have been broadly divided into:

a. Common Imaging Manifestations
b. Uncommon Imaging Manifestations

Common Manifestations

Common manifestations are the primary and solid findings of COVID-19 and have been depicted in various studies. These include ground-glass opacities (GGO), consolidation, reticular pattern, crazy peavey pattern, air bronchogram, and fibrosis.

1. Ground Glass Opacity

Ground glass opacity was generally defined as an area with a hazy appearance and slightly increased density due to movement or displacement of air. Findings have revealed the presence of GGO in both lungs and different affecting segments, including the peripheral segments as well as subpleural segments [14]. GGO was observed in 57% of COVID-19 patients. It was regarded as one of the early findings in the CT manifestation of the disease.

2. Consolidation

When the air in alveoli is replaced by inflammatory cells, tissue, and pathological fluid, the density of parenchyma tissue in the lungs is increased. This is referred to as consolidation and among the key pathological findings in COVID-19 CT images. Depending upon nature, consolidation may be patchy, multifocal, or segmental, as presented in Fig. (**6**) [15].

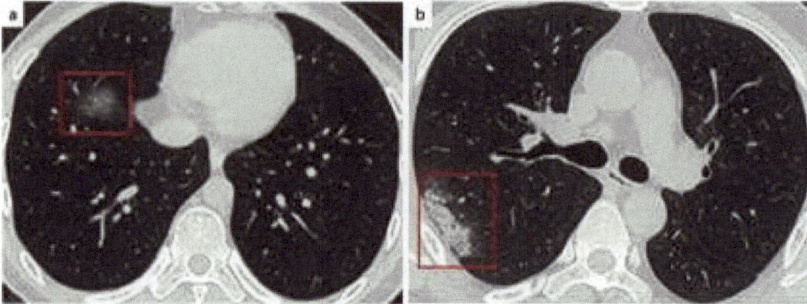

Fig. (6). (a) Ground glass opacity (GGO) in 35-Year-old male COVID-19 patient, **(b)** Consolidation in the lungs of a 47-year-old male.

3. Reticular Pattern

The thick pulmonary interstitial structures include interlobular and intraocular lines, is called the reticular pattern. It has been revealed as one of the basic findings along with GGO and consolidation in CT images of confirmed COVID-19 patients [16], as shown in Fig. (7). The greater number of interstitial lymphocyte infiltration results in interlobular septum thickening [17].

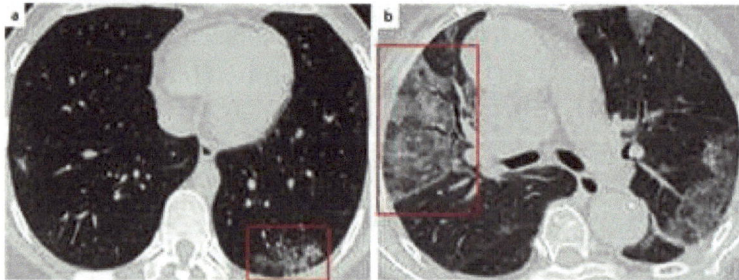

Fig. (7). (a) Slight reticular pattern shown in 34 year-old female patient, **(b)** CT image of 81 years old female showing the reticular pattern in superimposed GGO background.

4. Crazy Peavey Pattern

The thickening of the interlobular septum and intraocular lines on a superimposed GGO background resembling paving stones is called a peavey pattern, as shown in figure (Gb) [14]. This may result from alveolar edema and acute pulmonary injury.

5. Air Bronchogram

Air bronchogram is another CT finding in COVID-19. This is referred to as a visible pattern of bronchi filled with air on a background of opaque (Air-free) lung. It may be accompanied by bronchiolar dilatation (Bronchiolectasis) [18].

6. Fibrosis

Fibrosis is also a core finding in the CT images of COVID-19 patients. Fibrosis may occur due to chronic pulmonary inflammation and repair process [19, 20], as illustrated in Fig. (**8**).

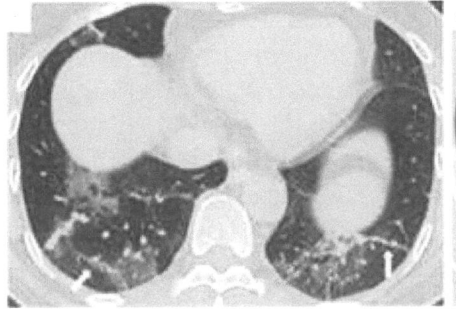

Fig. (8). CT image of 66 Year of female showing pulmonary fibrosis (white arrow).

Certain uncommon manifestation associated with COVID-19 infection includes:

1. ***Nodular Lesions***: Mostly, the nodular lesions are of mixed origin with either GGO or consolidation, while few patients manifest implenodular lessions [21].
2. ***Reversed Halo Sign***: These changes exhibit a high peripheral but low central density of lesions when examined through CT scanning. Despite being recorded in patients suffering from COVID-19, pneumonia, tuberculosis, and Cryptococcus, the exact mechanism of these non-specific imaging changes is still unknown [22].
3. ***Thickening of Adjacent Pleura***: Some patients may show thickening of the contiguous pleura, pericardial effusion, hydrothorax, and enlargement of mediastinal lymph nodes [23].
4. ***Consolidation with Cavity:*** It may be ascribed to the release of necrotic matter from bronchial lesions being a rare phenomenon [9].

CT scan as a Diagnostic Procedure and its Key Findings in COVID-19

CT scan, also known as computer-assisted tomography (CAT) scan, is a specialized medical imaging technique that produces cross-sectional (tomographic) images of specific areas of a targeted object. It utilizes a combination of multiple X-ray measurements taken from different angles. It also visualizes the inner details of the body without any surgical intervention. The technique was developed by American physicist and British electrical engineer

Allan M. Cormack and Godfrey N. Hounsfield, respectively, and awarded Nobel Prize in 1979 [24].

Radiological techniques being economical, are important diagnostic tools for various diseases and valuable for gauging therapeutics outcomes [25]. Considering the simplicity and economic aspects, the CT scan is regarded as the first-line imaging modality utilized in patients highly suspected of COVID-19 infection [26]. It is getting increasingly popular in clinical practice [23]. Studies have reported high sensitivity (98%) of chest CT scan in identifying the COVID-19 patients than RT-PCR (71% sensitive)results [27, 28]. Presently, the diagnosis of COVID-19 relies on RT-PCR of throat swab, sputum, or lower respiratory tract secretion [9]. However, these methods do not unfold the disease severity and have a long lag phase before results. CT scan is more sensitive than normal X-rays, it can detect any abnormalities in the lung tissue earlier than related techniques and has proved very sensitive in COVID-19 [18].

The quality of CT scans can be enhanced with high and sufficient radiation to manifest delicate pathological changes. Furthermore, reconstructions with thinner and thicker sections with edge-enhancing and soft algorithms are also imperative. With a low-dose technique, more chances of noise surge exist particularly during the processing of high-resolution images. Hence, the computed tomography dose index (CTDI) ranging from 5–10Gy is recommended. A contrast medium is often indicated to access detailed and specified pathological lesions. If contrast medium is not deemed feasible, spectral CT scan can decrease the requirements of contrast medium volume and provide reasonable image quality, such as in pulmonary embolisms.

A range of changes have been observed in CT scans among patients undergoing different stages of infection and are useful in assessing the intensity and prognosis of the disease. Earlier studies have evaluated chest CT scan describing features. It includes the existence of GGO, consolidation, laterality of GGOs and consolidation, the number of affected lung lobes, and the extent of involvement of individual lung lobe in the context of entire lung measured through a "total severity score" presence of nodules. It also involves pleural effusions, thoracic lymphadenopathy (when lymph node is 10 mm or greater in width), pathologies of the airways with thickened walls, bronchiectasis, and endo-luminal secretions. Axial distribution of disease and the existence of primary lung ailments like fibrosis or emphysema [14].

Certain defects, containing linear opacities, opacities with a "reverse halo" sign, opacities with rounded morphology, opacities with intra-regional cavitation, and "Crazy-paving" pattern opacities, have also been recorded among the affected patients. Hazy opacifications of lungs with augmented lung weakened with time. Its intact bronchial and vascular margins are termed ground-glass opacification. In contrast, opacification with masking of blood vessel boundaries and walls of the airway is called consolidation [14]. Human lungs are comprised of five lobes, and each lobe evaluated in earlier studies determined the degree of involvement and intensity of pathological changes. Findings are classified as No involvement (Score 0/0%), minimal involvement (Score 1/1-25%), mild involvement (Score 2/26-50%), moderate involvement (Score 3/51-75%), or severe involvement (Score 4/ 76 - 100%). An overall lung "total severity score" was obtained by adding up the scores of all the five lobes (In the range of 0-20) [29].

CT Scan Findings in COVID-19

The distinctiveness of CT scan findings in COVID-19 infection is directly associated with the duration of illness that is divided into three phases, *i.e.,* early, intermediate (from 3-5 days of apparent infection period), and a late phase. The early phase comprises of first few days without any distinct CT findings. Studies have revealed that 56% had normal CT findings among symptomatic patients during the first couple of days of infection, reducing to 9% during the next 3-5 days (2nd phase) and remaining only 4% after 6-12 days. The frequency of clinical and CT findings varies with the severity of the infection [29].

The classical CT scan findings of bilateral ground-glass opacities of pulmonary lobes with peripheral distribution mostly occur in the lower lung lobes of a COVID-19 patient (Fig. **9**) [23]. In the intermediate phase, increased consolidation of lung lobes occurs along with enhanced septation besides crazy paving indicating interstitial affection (Fig. **10**). An overall increased extension with GGOs and consolidation remained the dominant changes (Fig. **11**).

Chest imaging possesses pivotal significance in diagnosing and managing COVID-19 patients, but chances of missing the diagnosis at early stage GGOs with simple plain chest radiography are there. Thus, high-resolution CT can provide an objective and detailed evaluation of lung tissue for abnormalities and better understand the disease pathogenesis [19]. Using serial CT examinations, the incidence, pathophysiology, and disease prognosis can be perceived. Owing to the contagious nature of COVID-19, histopathological examination is strictly prohibited restricted. Contrarily, it provides limited information related to a small sample and possible sampling error, while CT can gauge the entire lungs [9].

CT Imaging findings have four distinct phases: early, progressive, severe, and dissipative phases [19]. The patients in the first (early) phase presented reasonable clinical symptoms with lesions being solitary (Fig. **9**)) or multiple (Fig. **10**), the majority of lesions lying along with the sub-pleural areas (Fig. **11**) or bronchi

[30]. Such outcomes suggested the unique features of pathological changes spreading down the airway, beginning with the penetration of bronchioles and epithelium of alveoli in the peripheral lung tissues progressively covering towards the center. The pathological changes were nodule-like or patches of GGOs, with prominent and thickened blood vessels coursing the GGO. This was also together with the thickening of intralobular and interlobular septae, along with the emergence of halo signs circling the nodules [29, 31]. The interstitial edema of the interlobular septum may be the congestion of capillaries in the alveolar septa with fluid exuded into the interstitial spaces and alveoli.

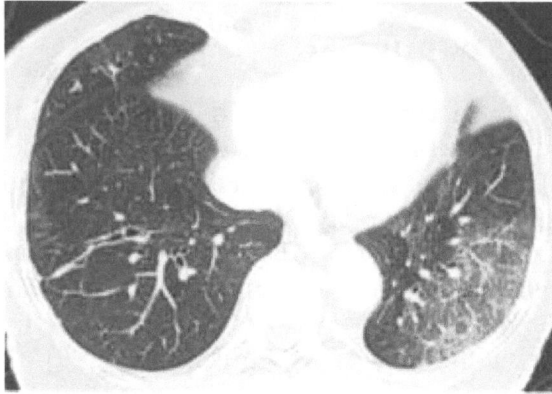

Fig. (9). Patient with COVID-19 with the reduced general condition, nausea, vomiting, syncope, and possible chills. Two days after the onset of symptoms, CT thorax shows ground-glass opacities most distinctly in the left lower lobe.

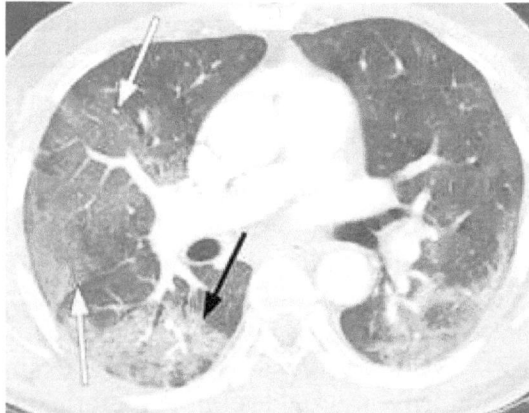

Fig. (10). Chest CT seven days after symptom onset shows extensive bilateral ground-glass opacities (white arrows), only limited consolidation (Black arrow).

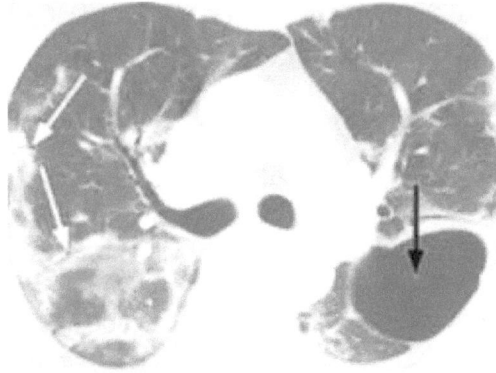

Fig. (11). Chest CT 20 days after COVID-19 symptoms onset shows bilateral opacities with the peripheral and peri-bronchovascular distribution. Bronchiectasis (white arrows)and an air-filled cavity (black arrow) in the left lung provide evidence of the organization.

The progressive phase characterized by rapidly spreading lesions corresponds to the severe type of clinical manifestations. The number and severity of lesions increased significantly during this phase [23]. The coexistence of GGOs and the consolidations showed both recently formed and primary lesions with slight dissolving. It is due to massive cellular exudate leaks out of blood vessels into nearby tissues. It causes interstitial vasodilation and exudation, resulting in alveoli fusion in the alveolar cavity. The "crazy paving appearance" is due to swollen interlobular and intralobular septae depicting interstitial lesions. Additional outcomes comprised alteration of the local lung tissues, focal atelectasis, and bronchodilation [9].

During the severe phase, pathological changes of lungs attained a peak in about 14 days of disease initiation, but a tiny number of cases developed lesions speedily. The lesions were bilateral with disseminated infiltration of the entire lung lobes manifested as "white lung". Air bronchogram revealed heavy cellular exudation in the alveolar cavity. In some cases, sub-segmental atelectasis with reduced lung volume and a little pleural fluid were seen in both the lungs [32].

After 14 days, a dissipative phase encompassing progressive resolving of the pathological changes was observed, with remnants of some high density, cord-like shadows indicating fibrosis. The imaging appearances advanced right from the early to the dissipative phase [9].

Receiver Operating Characteristic (ROC) and Curve for Computed Tomography Severity Score (CT-SS) Assessment of COVID-19

Basic principles of receiver operating characteristic analysis

Conventionally, diagnostic and imaging tests are documented in terms of dichotomous outcomes (*i.e.,* true positive, true negative, false positive, and false negative) according to a reference standard [33]. The proportions of true positive and true negative outcomes represent the core accuracy indices, referred to as sensitivity and specificity, respectively [34]. The following formulae are used for calculating the true positive, false negative, true negative, and false-positive fractions of the patient population corresponding to some standard diagnostic criteria [33, 35].

- True positive fraction (Sensitivity) = True positive / (True positive + False negative)
- False negative fraction (1-Sensitivity) = False negative / (True positive + False negative)
- True negative fraction (Specificity) = True negative / (True negative + False positive)
- False positive fraction (1-Specificity) = False positive / (True negative + False positive)

Receiver operating characteristic (ROC) is a mode of objective measurement widely used in clinical radiology to express the diagnostic accuracy of imaging examinations [36]. Lee Lusted pioneered the application of the ROC model in diagnostic radiology by re-analyzing the published data for establishing the reciprocal association between false positive and false negative cases of pulmonary tuberculosis in 1960 [37]. ROC analysis determines the correlation between sensitivity and specificity of a diagnostic test for classifying the diseased and non-diseased patients under an appropriate gold standard. The true positive fraction (TPF) and a false-positive fraction (FPF) of patients are taken into account for ROC analysis. Consequently, the ROC curve is obtained by plotting TPF (sensitivity) on the y-axis and FPF (1-specificity) on the x-axis for a range of diagnostic cutoff points [33, 38, 39]. Ranging between 0.0 and 1.0, the area under the ROC curve (AUC) indicates the average sensitivity value for all possible specificity values and vice versa. Moreover, the ROC curve area constitutes a global marker of test accuracy owing to its lack of dependency on disease prevalence and diagnostic cutoff points [40, 41].

Modified Versions and Software Packages of ROC

The assumed ROC model represents a modified form of ROC wherein the binormal distribution of test results provides a basis for making assumptions and consequently drawing the smooth or fitted ROC curve. Localization ROC (LROC) and free-response ROC (FROC) represent the modified versions for coping with the limitations of conventional ROC in terms of failure to determine the localization of abnormality and presence of more than one abnormality in an image, respectively [42]. Besides, the Jackknife AFROC (JAFROC) has been introduced to generalize the analysis concerning readers and cases [35]. Several freely accessible software programs (including CMDT, LABMRMC, and ROCKIT) and commercial packages (like AccuROC, Analyse-It, GraphROC, and MedCalc) are available for efficient ROC analysis [43, 44].

Application of ROC for CT-SS Evaluation of COVID-19

A semi-quantitative grading technique coupled with chest CT-SS utilizes the degree of lung opacification as a marker for discriminating the mild and severe types of COVID-19 patients [4]. This method is based upon the correlation of ground-glass opacity, air trapping, and interstitial opacity with clinical and laboratory findings of patients. Both lungs, each comprising 18 segments, are partitioned into 20 regions. The % parenchymal opacification of 0, <50, and ≥50 are graded as 0, 1, and 2, respectively. The overall CT-SS ranging from 0 to 40 points can be estimated for each lung. It is done *via* adding the individual scores of all 20 regions. Finally, the ROC curve analysis is conducted to estimate the diagnostic method's threshold, sensitivity, specificity, and accuracy in distinguishing the mild and severe groups of COVID-19 patients. Nevertheless, the lung opacification score has not been validated as the primary surrogate of the COVID-19 severity assessment histologically.

Another semi-quantitative scoring system of 0 to 20 points, integrated with the ROC model, can be applied to differentiate early and exacerbated stages of COVID-19 [45]. The exacerbation phase is accompanied by are remarkable elevation of clinical manifestations and laboratory findings. Likewise, the multifocal and bilateral nature of pulmonary lesions and ground-glass opacity with consolidation are detectable on CT examination. Clinical and CT attributes of proven COVID-19 patients are analyzed from the onset of the disease until exacerbation periodically. For this purpose, each lung is divided into five lobes, and main CT characteristics, including the distribution, pattern, number, and morphological aspects of pulmonary lesions as well as the number of affected lobes, are carefully recorded. CT images exhibiting typical lesions with the involvement of 0%, <25%, 25-50%, 50-75% and >75% of lung regions are assigned the scores of 0, 1, 2, 3 and 4, respectively. The prospective clinical outcome can be forecasted by estimating the cutoff point using the ROC model. This technique provides a better understanding of pulmonary lesion dynamics on account of repeated CT examinations.

CT-SS estimation involving a predefined set of atypical and representative features of COVID-19 allows the differential diagnosis of COVID-19 and non-COVID-19 (viral or community-acquired) pneumonia using ROC analysis [46]. CT scans presenting the characteristic features of COVID-19 are categorized as +1, while those illustrative of non-COVID-19 pneumonia are labeled as -1. The resultant ROC curve indicates an extrapolative cutoff value for COVID-19.

Quantitative assessment of radiologic findings has also been used for predicting mortality in COVID-19 patients [47]. CT scans reflecting normal attenuation, ground-glass attenuation, and consolidation are allocated the radiologic scores of 1, 2, and 3, respectively. After dividing both lungs into upper, middle, and lower zones. The affected parenchymal distributions of 0%, <25%, 25-50%, 50-75%, and >75% are graded as 1, 2, 3, and 4, and subsequently multiplied by the corresponding radiologic scores. The summation of the numerical points of all zones provides a cumulative score (ranging from 0 to 72) for each lung. The collected data can be utilized for estimating a predictive cutoff point of CT score through ROC analysis. The relatively small number of only inpatients used in developing this model and evidence of a strong association between mortality and co-morbidities can influence the prognostic efficacy of this model.

CT Scan and the Diagnosis of other Respiratory Diseases

The internal body comprehensive images are produced during CT. The CT deals with a sub-millimeter ranged resolution and are the preeminent model for assessing a minute intra-pulmonary and mediastinal lesions and stands superior to the chest radiography [48]. The musculoskeletal disorder like infections, tumors, blood clots, and bone fractures can be diagnosed through a CT scan. Also, this method can help in the biopsy, minor surgery, therapy through radiation; perceive cardiovascular and hepatic illness, and identify peritoneal injuries. A special CT scan is used to differentiate between high vascularized and non/less-vascularized tissues in the body, which requires a visual enhancer dye (contrast-material) [49]. This is the most suitable method to investigate pulmonary disorders like pulmonary embolism, emphysema, and fibrosis.

CT scan can be used for the diagnosis of numerous diseases affecting the respiratory system. It includes bronchitis (acute or chronic), bronchiectasis, emphysema, cystic fibrosis/bronchiectasis, pulmonary hemorrhage, pulmonary atelectasis, pulmonary emphysema, pulmonary hypertension, tuberculosis, cancer, pus, fluid, foreign bodies and fibrosis in the lungs, and COVID-19 infection.

Some common respiratory diseases which can be diagnosed through a CT scan are described below.

1. Rhinitis (common cold and is represented by a watery or seromucous secretion). By obtaining radiographs and CT images, it can help diagnose rhinitis of diverse nature.
2. Epistaxis (Bleeding from the nose). CT scans can provide an insight into the cause and severity of the nature of epistaxis.
3. Catarrhal Laryngitis (diphtheria). CT images of laryngeal regions might help depict the nature and cause of laryngitis.
4. Asthma (inflammation of intrapulmonary conducting tubes and turned to be sensitive for common allergens) can be detected through state-of-the-art CT images [50].
5. Chronic obstructive pulmonary disease (bronchitis and emphysema) can easily be diagnosed through a CT scan.

Artificial Intelligence Deep-Learning Using CT Scan for COVID-19

AI or machine intelligence refers to computer-based imitation or simulation of human cognition [51]. As a subdivision of AI, machine learning focuses on data receiving, automated learning, and algorithms (sets of well-defined procedures used for problem-solving) changing capacities of machines. Deep learning (also referred to as deep structured learning) constitutes a subset of machine learning that employs a hierarchical sequence of artificial neural networks for executing the process of machine learning. AI techniques, particularly deep learning, have been widely used for processing and evaluating imaging data, thereby improving the diagnostic performance of radiologists and clinicians. Given the current COVID-19 pandemic, several AI-aided applications have been designed to provide contactless imaging workflows, enhance diagnostic accuracy, and reduce the average diagnosis time [52].

AI-Equipped Imaging Workflows

AI-enabled imaging workflows are meant for automated imaging processes through data acquisition using visual sensors (such as Time-of-Flight pressure imaging) or thermal (Forward-looking infrared) cameras [53]. Moreover, such AI-empowered imaging workflows can estimate and determine the optimal scanning parameters, including the scan limit (implicating the starting and ending positions of CT scan) and ISO-centering (referring to aligning the target body part of the patient).

AI-Guided Image Segmentation

AI-assisted processing and evaluation of CT scans involve the critical step of segmentation for delineating the regions of interest (ROIs) regarding lesions, anomalous pulmonary regions, lobes, bronchopulmonary segments, or the entire lung [52]. Segmentation techniques used to separate the entire lung or a particular lobe from the background are termed lung-region-oriented methods. Whereas lesions, motion artifacts, or metals are located using lung-lesion-oriented methods.

Several techniques with diverse goals are available for lung segmentation. U-Net represents the most frequently applied, fully convolutional network for segmenting pulmonary regions and lesions in COVID-19 patients [54, 55]. Its U-shaped design with symmetric encoding and decoding signal pathways linked by shortcut connections facilitates better learning of visual semantics and thorough contextures. Various modified forms of U-Net have also shown acceptable segmentation of COVID-19 images. The three-dimensional version of the traditional U-Net called the 3D U-Net can use the inter-slice data [56]. Further improvements in segmentation have been ascribed to the utilization of residual blocks and typical bottleneck blocks as the main convolutional blocks of V-Net and Visual Basic (VB)-Net, respectively [57, 58]. UNet^{++} is characterized by the insertion of a nested convolutional structure between encoding and decoding pathways and can be applied for localizing pulmonary lesions associated with COVID-19 [59, 60]. Attention U-Net can be efficiently used for segmenting pulmonary nodules and lesions of COVID-19 on account of its capacity to capture delicate objects in CT scans [61].

The lack of sufficient training data for the segmentation networks has been resolved by incorporating human knowledge [52]. The Human-in-the-loop approach involving the interactive role of radiologists has been employed for training a VB-Net-assisted segmentation network [58]. Likewise, the preliminary inputs of a radiologist were integrated into the training and effective segmentation of pulmonary lesions using U-Net [54]. Diagnostic knowledge has also been applied to identify infected lung regions through the attention method [62]. Moreover, the deficiency of training data for segmentation networks can be addressed through weakly supervised, semi-supervised, and unsupervised learning procedures [55].

Image segmentation can be used for data quantification with several medical applications. Deep learning-based segmentation methods focusing on lung regions, lesions and opacities have been effectively used to forecast disease progression and hospital stay [52]. For instance, VB-Net-assisted pulmonary segmentation has been successfully applied for visualizing the distribution of lesions, providing quantification data for further studies, projecting the disease severity, and appraising the progression of COVID-19 [58]. U-Net-based segmentation of pulmonary lesions can be employed for extrapolating the hospital stay of COVID-19 patients [54].

AI-Based Diagnosis of COVID-19

Prompt diagnosis and effective treatment of COVID-19 are indispensable for presumptive patients, particularly in endemic regions. Despite being an excellent diagnostic modality, CT scans typically include many slices and require ample time for comprehensive assessment through an ordinary diagnostic approach. Furthermore, the CT scan-based conventional diagnosis is further confounded by identical imaging features of COVID-19 and other types of pneumonia. Therefore, AI-based techniques are substantially exploited for rapid, accurate, and convenient diagnosis of COVID-19.

UUNet++ assisted screening of CT scans has been successfully employed for differentiating the COVID-19 and non-COVID-19 patients based on pulmonary lesions [60]. COVID-19 detection neural network (COVNet) represents a ResNet50-based model for distinguishing COVID-19 and community-acquired pneumonia using two-dimensional slices. DeCoVNet investigates the pulmonary segmentation product of U-Net by a three-dimensional convolutional neural network (CNN)-based model for estimating the likelihood of COVID-19 [55]. Besides, ResNet50 can be used for processing U-Net++-induced segmentation and detecting COVID-19-positive slices. Deep Pneumonia is another ResNet50-based diagnostic system for diagnosing COVID-19 and bacterial pneumonia through CT scan-derived pulmonary slices [63]. Another CT-scan-dependent, VB-Net model divides the lungs into lobes and segments, followed by the estimation of infection load and ratios of anatomical subdivisions [64]. The resultant quantitative parameters are employed by an RF-based system for evaluating the severity of COVID-19.

AI-Supported Follow-up Solutions

Machine learning and visualization methods are integrated for determining the variation of density, size, and other clinically significant elements of the diseased region of the patient's body. Afterward, the recorded clinical data is compiled in terms of an automatically generated clinical report. The so-called contrastive follow-up model for COVID-19 operates by evaluating, comparing, and reflecting changes in sequential CT scans of the same patient [52].

Limitations and Future Perspectives

Although, AI has been effectively applied throughout the entire process of imaging-based diagnosis of COVID-19. Nevertheless, certain advancements are still needed to enhance deep learning expediency as the leading approach in combating COVID-19. Several existing AI-aided models are based upon transfer learning to resolve small datasets, whereas the implemented networks are pre-trained using general datasets [65]. Overfitting of data necessitates the conduction of further AI-based segmentation and diagnostic studies using larger sample sizes. Moreover, improving the interpretability of AI-assisted diagnostic models is also suggested for facilitating radiologists by providing more useful data [65].

Diagnosis of Pulmonary Diseases: What are the options we have?

A wide range of tests, including blood examination, are used to detect infection. Furthermore, chest and/or sinus X-ray imaging, electrocardiography, echocardiography, ultrasonography, scintigraphy, ventilation-perfusion scan, pulmonary angiogram, sputum cytology, lung function tests, and CT imaging are primarily used for the diagnosis of pulmonary diseases. Among these, the CT scan is generally considered a convenient tool and gold standard for the morphological examination of the lungs.

The diagnostic performance of CT technology is increasing every year, minimizing the extra usage of other risky and invasive imaging methods like angiography. Simple PPD tuberculin is being used intradermally for tuberculosis. Lung diseases can also be diagnosed through various advanced kits and molecular methods like various PCR levels and types, ELISA [66].

Diagnosing COVID-19 Using other Diagnostic Tests and Tools: Advantages and Limitations of CT Scan

As the definite vaccines or drugs for COVID-19 are not available so far, it is fundamental to identify this illness at the initial stage. For the control of COVID-19, it is crucial to diagnose the disease promptly and accurately [67]. Apart from the CT scan, various diagnostic tools are being used in the scientific community. Some of them are mentioned as under.

Nasopharyngeal and or Pharyngeal Swab

COVID-19 is diagnosed extensively through nasopharyngeal swab, or pharyngeal swab, sputum, and bronchoalveolar lavage. Let the patient sit on the chair, holding his neck gently, tilting his head towards the back, and then enter the swab stick into the nasopharynx, rotate the swab stick for around15 seconds into the mucus membrane of the nose before examination in the laboratory [68].

Point-of-Care Testing

It is performed when samples are not sent to centralized facilities, and lab infrastructure is absent. Lateral flow Antigen detection is done in it. In this test, a membrane strip is coated with double lines. Antibody conjugated with gold nanoparticles is present in one line and captures antibodies in another line. The sample is placed on a membrane, and proteins are pinched across strips [69].

COVID-19 IgM/IgG Rapid Test

It can also facilitate early diagnosis. It is initial screening by detecting anti-SARS IgM and IgG antibodies in human serum, plasma, or whole blood within 15 minutes. This method is easy to use, requires only basic equipment, and needs no extra skilled personnel. It has almost 97.1% and 97.8% sensitivity and specificity, respectively [70].

Real-time PCR or Molecular Assay for Viral Nucleic Acid

It is the most reliable and primary method for the diagnosis of COVID-19. It uses a fluorescent probe and specific primer to detect three specific regions within the SARS-CoV-2nucleocapsid protein N Gene. RT-PCR encompasses the reverse transcription of SARS-CoV-2 RNA into complementary DNA strands. Then, the amplification of detailed sections of cDNA is done. The RdRP gene (RNA-dependent RNA polymerase), E gene (envelop gene), and N gene (RP primers and probes target Human RNase P gene) are the three regions to be discovered. The two tasks are performed, including A: Primer designing and B: Assay optimization and testing (nCoVPC,2019-nCoV positive control used in the assay. The ingredients include: Primer and probe for N1 Primer and probe for N2, Primer and probe for human RNase P, buffer, dNTPs, reverse transcriptase enzyme (RT), DNA polymerase, plasmid DNA having nucleocapsid protein (target gene) with the DNA holding internal control gene fragment (RNP) and the nuclease-free water. This molecular panel helps in the detection of viral RNA from SARS-CoV-2. Kit has three primers. Primer probe set N1 and N2 specifically detect SARS-CoV-2. The kit also includes a primer-probe set, RNP, which is built-in to act as a reference to monitor the collection of samples, RNA extraction, and amplification [71].

Aridia COVID-19 Real Time PCR Test

The sample should be collected by trained personnel, and they should ensure his security by wearing all the necessary PPEs. The sample should be collected from the lower respiratory tract; it includes sputum, bronchi alveolar lavage, and tracheal aspirate. Besides, the combination of nasopharyngeal or pharyngeal swabs samples can also be used to analyze COVID-19 infection. All the samples should preserve at 4-8 degrees centigrade, and they should use within 24 hours. If we must keep the specimen for more than 24 hours, we will have to preserve it at -70ºC. It is multiplex PCR fluorescent probe technology with fast one-step RT PCR technology. This method enjoys 95.1% sensitivity, 95.9% specificity, has dual-target gene detection primer-probe, and is an open PCR system [72]. It is practical to all labs and has two types of tests: the antigen test (RT-PCR and LAMP) and the antibody test (ELISA and fluorescent antibody technique).

LAMP Test

The researchers have adopted a technique called loop-mediated isothermal amplification (LAMP) to detect coronavirus specifically. This technique amplifies the RNA virus at 65°C. The results of this test come within 40 minutes or maximum within 01 hours. The test tube containing primer, hotplate, and the thermometer pot of water is required for conducting this test. By combining primers optimized specifically for SARS-CoV-2 with the specific gene of the virus, the researchers can detect as little as 10 copies of the virus gene. The technique can combine with a pH indicator which changes the color of the reaction mix from pink (Alkaline) to yellow (Acidic) if the sample is positive for SARS-CoV-2, otherwise no color changes [73].

Antigen Test

It detects the virus present in the affected person. Samples of interest are oral and pharyngeal swabs from 3-10 days affected person. It is time-consuming technique, but WHO recommends this test as a rapid diagnostic test for coronavirus because of its good results.

Antibody Test

It detects the IgG and IgM antibodies in the serum of an already affected patient. This test can only be performed after 13 days of infection because antibodies require time to be generated against the virus.

ELISA Protocol

SARS-CoV-2 IgM ELISA kit is based on capturing ELISA to detect IgM in human plasma or serum. The monoclonal antibody is coated initially on the well. After adding the sample and incubating, the IgM antibody in the sample will bound to an anti-u monoclonal antibody. Add the enzymes labeled reagent and allow the plate for second incubation. If the sample is positive, then a complex called SARS-CoV-2 IgM antibody- SARS-CoV-2 antigen is formed. Otherwise, no complex is there. It is based on the natural interaction of antibodies with the antigen. Different kits are available in the market, but a general principle is adding the antibody to the antigen-containing wells. The antibody will bind to the antigen bound to the plate. Wash the plate to remove the unbind SARS-CoV-2 IgM. Now apply the Enzyme liked substrate to link to the bound antibodies, and the substrate will give a fluorescent or chromogenic effect. Read it *via* spectrophotometer or ELISA reader [74]. Various meta-analysis data show positive results in the laboratory, including decreased albumin, lymphopenia, high erythrocyte sedimentation rate (ESR), and high lactate dehydrogenase (LDH).

Advantages and Drawbacks of CT Scan over other Diagnostic Tests

Compared to the above-mentioned tests:

- CT imaging is a more practical, rapid, and reliable technique to identify and evaluate the COVID-19 in the epidemic region [75].
- CT scanning is a fast, painless, non-invasive, and accurate method used for lung screening.
- Effective screening of COVID-19 can be carried out using a CT scan and CXR, providing the clinical picture regarding the nature and severity of the disease.
- However, CT scan is not recommended as a first choice for screening COVID-19 patients due to the risk of transmission as its use on subsequent patients. At present, most radiological societies do not recommend going for CT testing of COVID-19 [7].

Also, one of the core shortcomings of CT is that it contains radiation. Therefore, another suitable method must be used, particularly in the case of pregnant women and children.

CONCLUSION

CT scan is considered a convenient tool and gold standard for the morphological examination of the lungs. Currently, its scope and applications have been extended to the diagnosis of COVID-19 and its differentiation from other types of pneumonic respiratory diseases. AChest CT scan has been recommended as an efficient tool for detecting COVID-19 in endemic areas based on its proven, high diagnostic sensitivity. A pulmonary CT scan is primarily indicated for patients exhibiting moderate to severe signs of COVID-19 and in circumstances when RT-PCR facilities are not available. Moreover, sequential CT scanning can be employed for determining the occurrence, developmental pattern, and prognosis of COVID-19.

Generally, the imaging features of COVID-19 strikingly resemble those of SARS and MERS. Imaging findings of confirmed COVID-19 patients are categorized into common and uncommon imaging manifestations. The primary and common manifestations are ground-glass opacities, consolidation, reticular pattern, crazy peavey pattern, air bronchogram, and fibrosis. Whereas nodular lesions, reversed halo sign, thickening of adjacent pleura, and consolidation with cavity encompass the uncommon imaging findings attributable to COVID-19. Parenchymal opacity-based severity scoring facilitates the rapid identification and discrimination of clinical forms of COVID-19 through CT scan examination.

CT Imaging findings of COVID-19 are categorized into four distinct phases. The early phase is characterized by clinical manifestations of moderate-intensity associated with solitary or multiple lesions occupying the sub-pleural or bronchial regions. This is followed by a significant rise in the extent and density of lesions during the progressive phase. Peak intensity of pulmonary lesions, attained in about 14 days, represents the hallmark of the severe phase. The dissipative phase is marked by gradual absorption and dispersion of lesions withthe likelihood of fibrosis.

ROC is a mode of objective measurement widely used in clinical radiology to express the diagnostic accuracy of imaging examinations.ROC analysis determines the correlation between sensitivity and specificity of a diagnostic test for classifying the diseased and non-diseased patients under an appropriate gold standard. Several semi-quantitative grading methods have been integrated with the ROC model and effectively applied to discriminate mild and severe types of COVID-19, differential diagnosis of COVID-19 from other pneumonic respiratory diseases, and prediction of mortality in COVID-19 patients.

AI techniques, particularly deep learning, are extensively used for processing and evaluating imaging data, thereby improving the diagnostic performance of radiologists and clinicians. Given the current COVID-19 pandemic, several AI-aided applications for contactless imaging workflows, pulmonary segmentation, diagnosis, and follow-up have been designed.

CONSENT FOR PUBLICATION

Not Applicable.

CONFLICT OF INTEREST

The author confirms that this chapter contents have no conflict of interest.

ACKNOWLEDGEMENT

Declared none.

REFERENCES

[1]   Hsieh J. Computed tomography: principles, design, artifacts, and recent advances. SPIE press 2003.

[2]   Eichinger M, Heussel CP, Kauczor HU, Tiddens H, Puderbach M. Computed tomography and magnetic resonance imaging in cystic fibrosis lung disease. J Magn Reson Imaging 2010; 32(6): 1370-8.
[http://dx.doi.org/10.1002/jmri.22374] [PMID: 21105141]

[3]   Rubin GD, Ryerson CJ, Haramati LB, *et al.* The role of chest imaging in patient management during the COVID-19 pandemic: a multinational consensus statement from the Fleischner Society. Chest 2020; 158(1): 106-16.
[http://dx.doi.org/10.1016/j.chest.2020.04.003] [PMID: 32275978]

[4]   Yang R, Li X, Liu H, *et al.* Chest CT severity score: an imaging tool for assessing severe COVID-19. Radiol Cardiothorac Imaging 2020; 2(2): e200047.
[http://dx.doi.org/10.1148/ryct.2020200047] [PMID: 33778560]

[5]   Ai T, Yang Z, Hou H, *et al.* Correlation of chest CT and RT-PCR testing in coronavirus disease 2019 (COVID-19) in China: a report of 1014 cases. Radiology 2020; 296(2): E32-40.
[http://dx.doi.org/10.1148/radiol.2020200642] [PMID: 32101510]

[6]   Wong HY, Lam HY, Fong AH, *et al.* Frequency and distribution of chest radiographic findings in COVID-19 positive patients. Radiology 2020.: 201160.
[PMID: 32216717]

[7]   Simpson S, Kay FU, Abbara S, *et al.* Radiological Society of North America Expert Consensus Document on Reporting Chest CT Findings Related to COVID-19: Endorsed by the Society of Thoracic Radiology, the American College of Radiology, and RSNA. Radiol Cardiothorac Imaging 2020; 2(2): e200152.
[http://dx.doi.org/10.1148/ryct.2020200152] [PMID: 33778571]

[8]   Pan F, Ye T, Sun P, *et al.* Zhang L andZheng C. Time course of lung changes on chest CT during recovery from 2019 novel coronavirus (COVID-19) pneumonia. Radiology 2020; 295(3): 715-21.
[http://dx.doi.org/10.1148/radiol.2020200370] [PMID: 32053470]

[9]   Li M, Lei P, Zeng B, *et al.* Coronavirus disease (covid-19): spectrum of CT findings and temporal progression of the disease. Acad Radiol 2020; 27(5): 603-8.
[http://dx.doi.org/10.1016/j.acra.2020.03.003] [PMID: 32204987]

[10]   Das KM, Lee EY, Langer RD, Larsson SG. Middle East respiratory syndrome coronavirus: what does a radiologist need to know? AJR Am J Roentgenol 2016; 206(6): 1193-201.
[http://dx.doi.org/10.2214/AJR.15.15363] [PMID: 26998804]

[11]   Ooi GC, Khong PL, Müller NL, *et al.* Severe acute respiratory syndrome: temporal lung changes at thin-section CT in 30 patients. Radiology 2004; 230(3): 836-44.
[http://dx.doi.org/10.1148/radiol.2303030853] [PMID: 14990845]

[12]   Das KM, Lee EY, Al Jawder SE, *et al.* Acute Middle East respiratory syndrome coronavirus: temporal lung changes observed on the chest radiographs of 55 patients. AJR Am J Roentgenol 2015; 205(3): W267-74.
[http://dx.doi.org/10.2214/AJR.15.14445] [PMID: 26102309]

[13]   Chen W, Xiong X, Xie B, *et al.* Pulmonary invasive fungal disease and bacterial pneumonia: a comparative study with high-resolution CT. Am J Transl Res 2019; 11(7): 4542-51.
[PMID: 31396358]

[14]   Hansell DM, Bankier AA, MacMahon H, McLoud TC, Müller NL, Remy J. Fleischner Society: glossary of terms for thoracic imaging. Radiology 2008; 246(3): 697-722.
[http://dx.doi.org/10.1148/radiol.2462070712] [PMID: 18195376]

[15]   Kanne JP. Chest CT findings in 2019 novel coronavirus (2019-nCoV) infections from Wuhan, China: key points for the radiologist. Radiology 2020; 295(1): 16-7.
[http://dx.doi.org/10.1148/radiol.2020200241] [PMID: 32017662]

[16]   Ajlan AM, Ahyad RA, Jamjoom LG, Alharthy A, Madani TA. Middle East respiratory syndrome coronavirus (MERS-CoV) infection: chest CT findings. AJR Am J Roentgenol 2014; 203(4): 782-7.
[http://dx.doi.org/10.2214/AJR.14.13021] [PMID: 24918624]

[17]   Xu Z, Shi L, Wang Y, *et al.* Pathological findings of COVID-19 associated with acute respiratory distress syndrome. Lancet Respir Med 2020; 8(4): 420-2.
[http://dx.doi.org/10.1016/S2213-2600(20)30076-X] [PMID: 32085846]

[18]   Rao TNA, Paul N, Chung T, *et al.* Value of CT in assessing probable severe acute respiratory syndrome. AJR Am J Roentgenol 2003; 181(2): 317-9.
[http://dx.doi.org/10.2214/ajr.181.2.1810317] [PMID: 12876004]

[19]   Pan Y, Guan H, Zhou S, *et al.* Initial CT findings and temporal changes in patients with the novel coronavirus pneumonia (2019-nCoV): a study of 63 patients in Wuhan, China. Eur Radiol 2020; 30(6): 3306-9.
[http://dx.doi.org/10.1007/s00330-020-06731-x] [PMID: 32055945]

[20]   Ye Z, Zhang Y, Wang Y, Huang Z, Song B. Chest CT manifestations of new coronavirus disease 2019 (COVID-19): a pictorial review. Eur Radiol 2020; 30(8): 4381-9.
[http://dx.doi.org/10.1007/s00330-020-06801-0] [PMID: 32193638]

[21]   Franquet T. Imaging of pulmonary viral pneumonia. Radiology 2011; 260(1): 18-39.
[http://dx.doi.org/10.1148/radiol.11092149] [PMID: 21697307]

[22]   Zhan X, Zhang L, Wang Z, Jin M, Liu M, Tong Z. Reversed halo sign: presents in different pulmonary diseases. PLoS One 2015; 10(6): e0128153-.
[http://dx.doi.org/10.1371/journal.pone.0128153] [PMID: 26083865]

[23]   Chung M, Bernheim A, Mei X, *et al.* CT imaging features of 2019 novel coronavirus (2019-nCoV). Radiology 2020; 295(1): 202-7.
[http://dx.doi.org/10.1148/radiol.2020200230] [PMID: 32017661]

[24]   Raju TN. The nobel chronicles. 1979: Allan macLeod cormack (b 1924); and sir godfrey newbold hounsfield (b 1919). Lancet 1999; 354(9190): 1653-6.
[http://dx.doi.org/10.1016/S0140-6736(05)77147-6] [PMID: 10560712]

[25]   Guan WJ, Ni ZY, Hu Y, *et al.* Zhu SY and Zhong NS. Clinical characteristics of coronavirus disease 2019 in China. N Engl J Med 2020; 382(18): 1708-20.
[http://dx.doi.org/10.1056/NEJMoa2002032] [PMID: 32109013]

[26]   Makhnevich A, Sinvani L, Cohen SL, *et al.* The Clinical Utility of Chest Radiography for Identifying Pneumonia: Accounting for Diagnostic Uncertainty in Radiology Reports. AJR Am J Roentgenol 2019; 213(6): 1207-12.
[http://dx.doi.org/10.2214/AJR.19.21521] [PMID: 31509449]

[27]   Fang Y, Zhang H, Xie J, *et al.* Sensitivity of chest CT for COVID-19: comparison to RT-PCR. Radiology 2020; 296(2): E115-7.
[http://dx.doi.org/10.1148/radiol.2020200432] [PMID: 32073353]

[28]   Huang P, Liu T, Huang L, *et al.* Use of chest CT in combination with negative RT-PCR assay for the 2019 novel coronavirus but high clinical suspicion. Radiology 2020; 295(1): 22-3.
[http://dx.doi.org/10.1148/radiol.2020200330] [PMID: 32049600]

[29]   Bernheim A, Mei X, Huang M, *et al.* LiK, Li S, ShanH, JacobiA and Chung M. Chest CT findings in

coronavirus disease 2019 (COVID-19): Relationship to duration of infection. Radiology 2020; 295(3): 685-91.
[PMID: 32077789]

[30]   Kim JY, Ko JH, Kim Y, *et al.* Viral load kinetics of SARS-CoV-2 infection in first two patients in Korea. J Korean Med Sci 2020; 35(7): e86.
[http://dx.doi.org/10.3346/jkms.2020.35.e86] [PMID: 32080991]

[31]   Liu K, Fang YY, Deng Y, *et al.* Clinical characteristics of novel coronavirus cases in tertiary hospitals in Hubei Province. Chin Med J (Engl) 2020; 133(9): 1025-31.
[http://dx.doi.org/10.1097/CM9.0000000000000744] [PMID: 32044814]

[32]   Chan MS, Chan IY, Fung KH, Poon E, Yam LY, Lau KY. High-resolution CT findings in patients with severe acute respiratory syndrome: a pattern-based approach 2004.
[http://dx.doi.org/10.2214/ajr.182.1.1820049]

[33]   Hajian-Tilaki K. Receiver operating characteristic (ROC) curve analysis for medical diagnostic test evaluation. Caspian J Intern Med 2013; 4(2): 627-35.
[PMID: 24009950]

[34]   Park SH, Goo JM, Jo CH. Receiver operating characteristic (ROC) curve: practical review for radiologists. Korean J Radiol 2004; 5(1): 11-8.
[http://dx.doi.org/10.3348/kjr.2004.5.1.11] [PMID: 15064554]

[35]   Krupinski EA. Receiver operating characteristic (ROC) analysis. Frontline Learn Res 2017; 5(3): 41-52.
[http://dx.doi.org/10.14786/flr.v5i2.250]

[36]   Vining DJ, Gladish GW. Receiver operating characteristic curves: a basic understanding. Radiographics 1992; 12(6): 1147-54.
[http://dx.doi.org/10.1148/radiographics.12.6.1439017] [PMID: 1439017]

[37]   Lusted LB. Logical analysis in roentgen diagnosis. Radiology 1960; 74(2): 178-93.
[http://dx.doi.org/10.1148/74.2.178] [PMID: 14419034]

[38]   Obuchowski NA, Blackmore CC, Karlik S, Reinhold C. Fundamentals of clinical research for radiologists. AJR Am J Roentgenol 2005; 184(2): 364-72.
[http://dx.doi.org/10.2214/ajr.184.2.01840364] [PMID: 15671347]

[39]   Kumar R, Indrayan A. Receiver operating characteristic (ROC) curve for medical researchers. Indian Pediatr 2011; 48(4): 277-87.
[http://dx.doi.org/10.1007/s13312-011-0055-4] [PMID: 21532099]

[40]   Hanley JA, McNeil BJ. The meaning and use of the area under a receiver operating characteristic (ROC) curve. Radiology 1982; 143(1): 29-36.
[http://dx.doi.org/10.1148/radiology.143.1.7063747] [PMID: 7063747]

[41]   Campbell G. Advances in statistical methodology for the evaluation of diagnostic and laboratory tests. Stat Med 1994; 13(5-7): 499-508.
[http://dx.doi.org/10.1002/sim.4780130513] [PMID: 8023031]

[42]   Obuchowski NA. How many observers are needed in clinical studies of medical imaging? AJR Am J Roentgenol 2004; 182(4): 867-9.
[http://dx.doi.org/10.2214/ajr.182.4.1820867] [PMID: 15039154]

[43]   Stephan C, Wesseling S, Schink T, Jung K. Comparison of eight computer programs for receiver-operating characteristic analysis. Clin Chem 2003; 49(3): 433-9.
[http://dx.doi.org/10.1373/49.3.433] [PMID: 12600955]

[44]   Lasko TA, Bhagwat JG, Zou KH, Ohno-Machado L. The use of receiver operating characteristic curves in biomedical informatics. J Biomed Inform 2005; 38(5): 404-15.
[http://dx.doi.org/10.1016/j.jbi.2005.02.008] [PMID: 16198999]

[45]   Liu J, Chen T, Yang H, *et al.* Clinical and radiological changes of hospitalized patients with COVID-19 pneumonia from disease onset to acute exacerbation: a multicenter paired cohort study. Eur Radiol 2020; 1.

[46]   Luo L, Luo Z, Jia Y, *et al.* CT differential diagnosis of COVID-19 and non-COVID-19 in symptomatic suspects: a practical scoring method. BMC Pulm Med 2020; 20(1): 129.
[http://dx.doi.org/10.1186/s12890-020-1170-6] [PMID: 32381057]

[47]   Yuan M, Yin W, Tao Z, Tan W, Hu Y. Association of radiologic findings with mortality of patients infected with 2019 novel coronavirus in Wuhan, China. PLoS One 2020; 15(3): e0230548.
[http://dx.doi.org/10.1371/journal.pone.0230548] [PMID: 32191764]

[48]   Crane CH, Koay EJ. Solutions that enable ablative radiotherapy for large liver tumors: Fractionated dose painting, simultaneous integrated protection, motion management, and computed tomography image guidance. Cancer 2016; 122(13): 1974-86.
[http://dx.doi.org/10.1002/cncr.29878] [PMID: 26950735]

[49]   Thorisdottir S, Oladottir GL, Nummela MT, Koskinen SK. Diagnostic performance of CT and the use of GI contrast material for detection of hollow viscus injury after penetrating abdominal trauma. Experience from a level 1 Nordic trauma center. Acta Radiol 2020; 61(10): 1309-15.
[http://dx.doi.org/10.1177/0284185120902389] [PMID: 32046497]

[50]   Taka S, Tzani-Tzanopoulou P, Wanstall H, Papadopoulos NG. MicroRNAs in asthma and respiratory infections: identifying common pathways. Allergy Asthma Immunol Res 2020; 12(1): 4-23.
[http://dx.doi.org/10.4168/aair.2020.12.1.4] [PMID: 31743961]

[51]   Muhammad LJ, Garba EJ, Oye ND, Wajiga GM. Modeling Techniques for Knowledge Representation of Expert System: A Survey. Journal of Applied Computer Science & Mathematics 2019; 13(28)
[http://dx.doi.org/10.4316/JACSM.201902006]

[52]   Shi F, Wang J, Shi J, *et al.* Review of artificial intelligence techniques in imaging data acquisition, segmentation and diagnosis for covid-19. IEEE Rev Biomed Eng 2020.
[http://dx.doi.org/10.1109/RBME.2020.2987975] [PMID: 32305937]

[53]   Casas L, Navab N, Demirci S. Patient 3D body pose estimation from pressure imaging. Int J CARS 2019; 14(3): 517-24.
[http://dx.doi.org/10.1007/s11548-018-1895-3] [PMID: 30552647]

[54]   Qi X, Jiang Z, Yu Q, *et al.* Machine learning-based CT radiomics model for predicting hospital stay in patients with pneumonia associated with SARS-CoV-2 infection: A multicenter study medRxiv 2020.
[http://dx.doi.org/10.1101/2020.02.29.20029603]

[55]   Zheng C, Deng X, Fu Q, *et al.* Deep learning-based detection for COVID-19 from chest CT using weak label medRxiv 2020.
[http://dx.doi.org/10.1101/2020.03.12.20027185]

[56]   Çiçek Ö, Abdulkadir A, Lienkamp SS, Brox T, Ronneberger O. 3D U-Net: learning dense volumetric segmentation from sparse annotation. In: International conference on medical image computing and computer-assisted intervention; 2016 Oct 17; Cham: Springer 424-32.

[57]   Milletari F, Navab N, Ahmadi SA. Fully convolutional neural networks for volumetric medical image segmentation. In: Proceedings of the 2016 Fourth International Conference on 3D Vision (3DV); ; 565-71.

[58]   Shan F, Gao Y, Wang J, *et al.* Lung infection quantification of covid-19 in ct images with deep learning 2020.

[59]   Zhou Z, Siddiquee MM, Tajbakhsh N, Liang J. Unet++: A nested u-net architecture for medical image segmentation.Deep Learning in Medical Image Analysis and Multimodal Learning for Clinical Decision Support. Cham: Springer 2018; pp. 3-11.
[http://dx.doi.org/10.1007/978-3-030-00889-5_1]

[60] Chen J, Wu L, Zhang J, *et al.* Deep learning-based model for detecting 2019 novel coronavirus pneumonia on high-resolution computed tomography: a prospective study MedRxiv 2020.
[http://dx.doi.org/10.1101/2020.02.25.20021568]

[61] Oktay O, Schlemper J, Folgoc LL, *et al.* Attention u-net: Learning where to look for the pancreas. 2018.

[62] Jin S, Wang B, Xu H, *et al.* AI-assisted CT imaging analysis for COVID-19 screening: Building and deploying a medical AI system in four weeks medRxiv 2020.
[http://dx.doi.org/10.1101/2020.03.19.20039354]

[63] Song Y, Zheng S, Li L, *et al.* Deep learning enables accurate diagnosis of novel coronavirus (COVID-19) with CT images medRxiv 2020.

[64] Shi F, Xia L, Shan F, *et al.* Large-scale screening of covid-19 from community acquired pneumonia using infection size-aware classification. 2020.

[65] Chen D, Liu F, Li Z. A Review of Automatically Diagnosing COVID-19 based on Scanning Image. 2020.

[66] Plummer MM, Pavia CS. Combining antigen detection and serology for the diagnosis of selected infectious diseases 2020.
[http://dx.doi.org/10.1016/bs.mim.2019.11.001]

[67] Wang S, Kang B, Ma J, *et al.* A deep learning algorithm using CT images to screen for Corona Virus Disease (COVID-19). MedRxiv 2020.
[http://dx.doi.org/10.1101/2020.02.14.20023028]

[68] Carver C, Jones N. Comparative accuracy of oropharyngeal and nasopharyngeal swabs for diagnosis of COVID-19. Centre for Evidence-Based Medicine 2020.

[69] Joung J, Ladha A, Saito M, *et al.* Point-of-care testing for COVID-19 using SHERLOCK diagnostics medRxiv 2020.
[http://dx.doi.org/10.1101/2020.05.04.20091231]

[70] Jia X, Zhang P, Tian Y, *et al.* Clinical significance of IgM and IgG test for diagnosis of highly suspected COVID-19 infection medRxiv 2020.
[http://dx.doi.org/10.1101/2020.02.28.20029025]

[71] Kashir J, Yaqinuddin A. Loop mediated isothermal amplification (LAMP) assays as a rapid diagnostic for COVID-19. Med Hypotheses 2020; 141: 109786.
[http://dx.doi.org/10.1016/j.mehy.2020.109786] [PMID: 32361529]

[72] Younes N, Al-Sadeq DW, Al-Jighefee H, *et al.* Challenges in Laboratory Diagnosis of the Novel Coronavirus SARS-CoV-2. Viruses 2020; 12(6): 582.
[http://dx.doi.org/10.3390/v12060582] [PMID: 32466458]

[73] Yang T, Wang YC, Shen CF, Cheng CM. Point-of-care RNA-based diagnostic device for Covid-19. Diagnostics (Basel) 2020; 10(3): E165.
[http://dx.doi.org/10.3390/diagnostics10030165] [PMID: 32197339]

[74] Traugott M, Aberle SW, Aberle JH, *et al.* Performance of SARS-CoV-2 antibody assays in different stages of the infection: Comparison of commercial ELISA and rapid tests. J Infect Dis 2020.
[http://dx.doi.org/10.1093/infdis/jiaa305]

[75] Li Y, Xia L. Coronavirus disease 2019 (COVID-19): role of chest CT in diagnosis and management. AJR Am J Roentgenol 2020; 214(6): 1280-6.
[http://dx.doi.org/10.2214/AJR.20.22954] [PMID: 32130038]

CHAPTER 15

Nucleic Acid-Based Detection of COVID-19

Abdul Basit[1], Ihtisham Ulhaq[2], Firasat Hussain[3], Zia-ud-Din[4] and Kashif Rahim[3,*]

[1] *Department of Microbiology, Faculty of Life Sciences, University of Okara, Pakistan*

[2] *Department of Biosciences, COMSATS University Islamabad (CUI) 45550, Pakistan*

[3] *Department of Microbiology, Cholistan University of Veterinary and Animal Sciences (CUVAS), Punjab, Bahawalpur-63100, Pakistan*

[4] *Department of Community Medicine, Kohat Institute of Medical Sciences (KIMS), Kohat, Pakistan*

Abstract: Current coronavirus disease-19 (COVID-19) pandemic is caused by a novel severe acute respiratory syndrome coronavirus-2 (SARS-CoV-2), posing a major health problem worldwide. Therefore, rapid and accurate identification of COVID-19 is playing an important role in preventing subsequent secondary spread from controlling this epidemic. Different diagnostic tools and nucleic acid (NA)-based technologies for COVID-19 have been adopted. Polymerase chain reaction (PCR) is widely used for molecular diagnosis at prime level. However, it exhibits low sensitivity and false-positive results in clinical applications. Therefore, loop-mediated isothermal amplification (LAMP) assay is considered a prominent NA amplification method for diagnosing COVID-19. Similarly, microarray and RNA-targeting clustered regularly interspaced short palindromic repeats (CRISPR) with advancements in instrumentation are recently adapted for rapid, high throughput, and portable sensing of COVID-19 NA detection. Besides, nanopore technology, rolling circle amplification-based method and silicon-based integrated point-of-need (PoN) transducer are also promising diagnostic tools for detecting COVID-19. This chapter will discuss the potential of all these latest technologies for COVID-19 diagnosis in detail.

Keywords: COVID-19, CRISPR, LAMP, Microarray, Nanopore Technology, Nucleic Acid-based Detection, PCR.

INTRODUCTION

Infectious diseases are a substantial burden on human health, safety, and economic stability. It accounts for about one-quarter of mortalities worldwide. Viral infectious diseases present growing challenges worldwide despite the

---

* **Corresponding author Kashif Rahim:** Department of Microbiology, Faculty of Veterinary Science, Cholistan University of Veterinary and Animal Sciences (CUVAS), Punjab, Bahawalpur 63100, Pakistan; E-mail: kashifrahim@cuvas.edu.pk

Kamal Niaz & Muhammad Farrukh Nisar (Eds.)
All rights reserved-© 2021 Bentham Science Publishers

significant advancement and efforts in the public healthcare systems [1]. An ongoing outbreak of highly pathogenic virus infection, a novel coronavirus disease-19 (COVID-19), has subsequently spread across the world. It outbreaks result in hundreds of thousands of confirmed cases and mortalities [2]. The novel COVID-19 has common flu-like symptoms such as soreness of the throat, dry cough, intermittent fevers, breathlessness, and fatigue. The disease is mild to severe, usually in the elderly and those with comorbidities. The majority of people are recorded as symptomatic, and this disease may cause pneumonia, severe respiratory issues, and multi-organ dysfunctions that lead to 2%-3% mortalities [3].

Coronaviruses are positive-sense enveloped RNA viruses that belong to the subfamily orthocoronavirinae and members of the family coronaviridae. The genome comprises about 27-34 kb and is attributed to the largest genome compared to related RNA viruses. Seven human coronaviruses (HCOVs) have been identified so far, such as HCOV-229E, HCOV-OC43, HCOV-HKU1, HCOV-NL63, severe acute respiratory syndrome coronavirus (SARS-COV), Middle East respiratory syndrome coronavirus (MERS-COV), and severe acute respiratory syndrome coronavirus-2 (SARS-CoV-2) [4]. SARS-COV, MERS-COV, and COVID-19 are associated with severe respiratory and mild to lethal neurological diseases. However, HCOV-229E, HCOV-OC43, HCoV-HKU1, and HCOV-NL63 commonly cause upper respiratory tract infection, which probably accounts for 15-30% similarity of catching a cold, especially in winters [4].

The emergence of COVID-19 infection during December 2019 and increasing mortalities around the globe have been challenging the public health communities worldwide. In this epidemic, the international caseload increases, and a comprehensive, accurate, and rapid diagnosis of COVID-19 is a dire need to combat this epidemic. The advanced molecular techniques, especially the nucleic acid-based detection methods are widely used as a key source to control the sources of infections and ultimately control the COVID-19 epidemic. Reverse transcription-polymerase chain reaction (RT-PCR) has been recommended for the examination of the COVID-19. RT-PCR is an efficient, rapid and economical testing method. However, it exhibits low sensitivity and false-positive/negative results in clinical applications. False-negative results certainly facilitate COVID-19 spread through delayed patient isolation from uninfected individuals, which ultimately affects the treatment and leads to the severity of the disease. Sequencing is another recommend and widely applied method for identifying, detecting, and monitoring of the evolution of COVID-19. However, sequencing probably unsuitable in conditions where crises due to the pandemic are at peak level. It sequencing requires more processing time and somewhat expensive to analyze the results. Moreover, targeting the specific RNA regions may affect viral detection due to mutation in targeted sites, limiting the target availability for their detection. Also, comprehensive and accurate analysis/detection of infecting viruses is important because certain other respiratory viruses may cause symptoms like pneumonia and fever. Therefore, other novel molecular methods for COVID-19 detection have been developed such as loop-mediated isothermal amplification (LAMP) assay, rolling circle amplification-based method, microarray-based method, RNA-targeting clustered regularly interspaced short palindromic repeats (CRISPR) diagnosis, and nanopore target sequencing (NTS) method Fig. (**1**). This chapter will describe the potential utilization of all these assays that could be used for COVID-19 diagnosis.

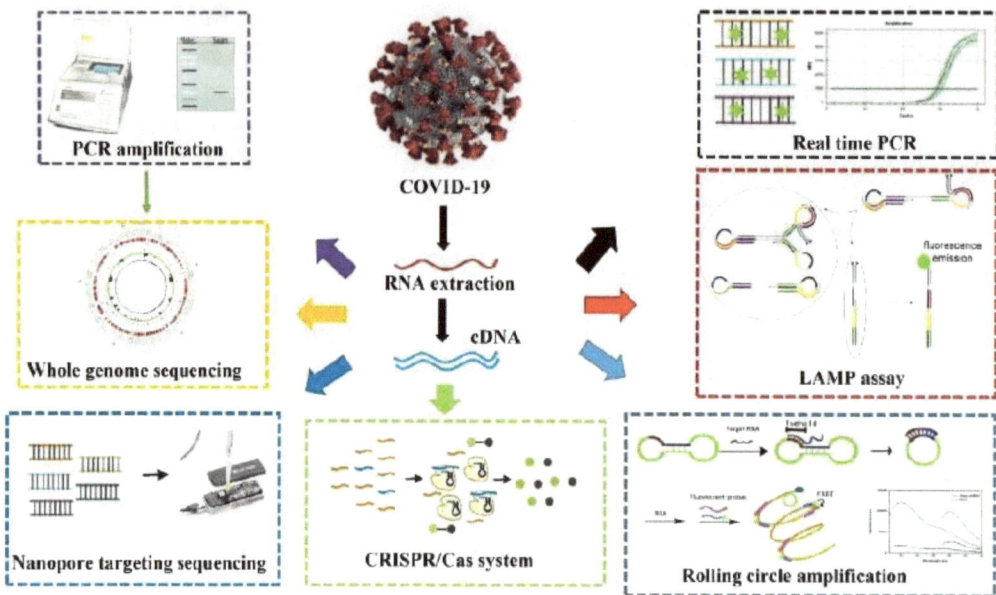

Fig. (1). The scheme for the nucleic acid-based detection of COVID-19.

Polymerase Chain Reaction (PCR) Based Method

Polymerase chain reaction (PCR)

The PCR has extensive use in molecular biology, which produces thousands to millions of DNA copies containing specific gene segments. It amplifies minute quantities of biological materials such as DNA which allows scientists to take a tiny sample of DNA. Its amplification provides sufficient evidence for detailed laboratory study later on. Due to its broader impact on the precise detection of diseases, the PCR-based methods have gained its importance as a routine and reliable method for identifying various diseases including COVID-19 [5, 6].

Generally, COVID-19 is an RNA virus, and can convert RNA into cDNA by reverse transcription using the reverse transcriptase enzyme. Subsequently, PCR amplifies the DNA sample using specific primers, followed by the gel electrophoresis visualization and gene sequencing of COVID-19 [7]. Although the conventional PCR method has been regarded as the recommended testing method for COVID-19 detection, certain limitations include low sensitivity and specificity, a time-consuming process, and often obtaining false-positive results due to cross-contamination.

Real-Time Reverse Transcriptase PCR

Real-time reverse transcriptase-PCR (RT-PCR) has superiority over the traditional PCR and widely used method for detecting COVID-19 due to its several advantages. RT-PCR is a simple quantitative assay and comparatively high sensitivity and specificity than the conventional PCR or RT-PCR [8]. The RT-PCR greatly helps in the diagnosis of COVID-19 in the early stage of infection. Therefore, it is still the most predominant method to be applied in numerous diagnostics [9]. Substantial efforts have been applied to further improve the RT-PCR assay towards a more advanced level. Because, there are several disadvantages of RT-PCR, including time-consuming for sample preparation, more chances of contamination during processing, and subsequent analyses [10]. One of the important disadvantages of this technique in the clinical diagnostics is the absence of positive controls because safe and accurate positive control has a key role in disease detection. To address this problem, Yu and colleagues [11] have recently established a real-time RT-PCR assay in which the armored RNA (aRNA) was used as a positive control for coronavirus detection. The aRNA is an engineered (inactivated or live RNA virus), quantifiable, and safe (noninfectious) technology designed to use as a positive control in COVID-19 detection. However, the rapid changes in viral genome sequences due to the mutating nature urge the need for precise detection of these genetically diverse virus strains. Therefore, the ability to precisely detect coronavirus has a vital role in reducing the risk of instigating false results made by the variations in the genome sequence. Studies also revealed that the establishment of multiplex real-time RT-PCR techniques for the accurate identification of coronavirus. It also displayed better sensitivity in multi-targeted coronavirus detection.

Quantitative RT-PCR (qRT-PCR) is an effective and frequently used molecular diagnostic tool in the detection of COVID-19 as well as for the diagnosis of many other infections. Single-step qRT-PCR with TaqMan chemistry can easily be applied as a routine diagnostic tool for COVID-19 detection with increased sensitivity and specificity. Real-time RT-PCR sensitivity has been further improved by using dual TaqMan probes [12]. Dual TaqMan probes have a broader range of applications, particularly where diagnostics tools' high sensitivity is required. As this technology is evolved, dual TaqMan probes can easily be performed due to its simple procedure. It requires specific primers and a pre-designed probe, while other components required for the reaction are the same as for other viruses (with or without slight modifications). Researchers also experienced RT-PCR SYBER green dye-based assay; however, their specificity was lower than the TaqMan probe-based assay [13].

In the recent outbreak of COVID-19, qRT-PCR assays remained in routine use for diagnostic purposes in the research laboratories and clinics. On the other hand, qRT-PCR probably disposed to false-negative results, leading to severe consequences, as discussed earlier. In the recent outbreak of COVID-19, five patients were tested negative by qRT-PCR. However, the chest examination *via* computerized tomography (CT) scan was found to be positive. Based on the results, samples were recollected and subjected to qRT-PCR, and all patients were confirmed positive for COVID-19 [14]. The sensitivity of qRT-PCR reported results were between 50-79%. It depended on the protocol, the number of samples, and the quality of samples (such as collection time and maintenance at low temperatures) [15, 16]. Besides the sensitivity, qRT-PCR has several other limitations that need to be considered, particularly bio-safety problems during sample transportation, sample processing procedures (RNA extraction), the requirement of a well-equipped laboratory, and availability of biosafety measures in the laboratory [17, 18].

Isothermal Nucleic Acid Amplification-Based Methods

Loop-Mediated Isothermal Amplification (LAMP) Assay

LAMP is a comparatively different nucleic acid amplification technique and is considered a prominent diagnosis method in the recent COVID-19 outbreak. LAMP is a rapid molecular amplification tool where amplification of genomic materials (DNAs or RNAs) occur in a shorter time with extreme sensitivity and specificity. This assay is based on the synthesis of target DNA using specially designed primers and DNA polymerase enzyme at a uniform temperature of 60-65°C which exhibits strand displacement activity rather than heat denaturation process as used in ordinary PCR [19]. Besides, due to its exponential amplification feature, it can identify six different targeted sequences using four different primers simultaneously [20]. LAMP assay amplifies the targeted sequence (more than 10^9 copies) of loop form DNA in an hour or even in a shorter time, with many inverted repeats as a final product. The application of LAMP assay does not require expensive reagents or instruments, therefore, a LAMP-based detection assay in clinical diagnostics was found to be cost-effective in the recent COVID-19 pandemic.

Gel electrophoresis is usually applied to analyze the amplified products acquired from the LAMP assay for endpoint detection. LAMP-based assay for the diagnosis of COVID-19 established effective viability of this technique by targeting and amplifying the ORF1b region of the coronavirus in the presence of 6 primers. Consequently, the displayed detection rate and sensitivity were found similar to the conventional PCR-based technique followed by the analysis of the amplified products on gel electrophoresis [21]. Similarly, Pyrc and colleagues [22] has established LAMP-based detection of human coronavirus (NL63) with favorable sensitivity and specificity. It amplifies products of clinical specimens and cell cultures to analyze *via* agarose gel electrophoresis. The amplification of the genomic material can be identified as the magnesium pyrophosphate precipitate. LAMP further employs in real-time by detection of the produced pyrophosphate turbidity. This technology of LAMP is found to be effective in avoiding the limitations of the COVID-19 endpoint detection. Modification in LAMP-based technology has been adopted and reported in many studies. RT-LAMP technology for the epidemiologic surveillance as well as diagnosis of human coronavirus was developed by Shirato and colleagues [23], which displayed the capability of detecting as few as 3.4 RNA copies of coronavirus. In addition, the high specificity and no cross-reaction with other respiratory viruses were also reported [23]. Sequence-specific LAMP-based method depends on non-specific signal transduction schemes. Double-stranded DNA amplicons intercalated with fluorescence dyes and polymerization to allows the release of pyrophosphates which caused the turbidity of the solution [24]. A quenching probe (QProbe) to monitor signals was also reported by Shirato *et al.* [23], which successfully improved RT-LAMP technology. In detecting human coronavirus, this method displayed the same efficient performance in line with the standard RT-PCR assay. Moreover, Huang and colleagues [25] have developed a technique in which the visualization of the nucleic acids of MERS-COV with naked eyes using a vertical flow visualization strip called RT-LAMP-VF (Fig. **2**). In this process, primers are labeled in isothermal amplification with fluorescein isothiocyanate (FITC) and biotin. Followed the amplification process, the biotin-labeled amplicons bind to the colloidal gold-labeled streptavidin to form a complex. This complex was afterward captured by an anti-FITC antibody coated on the strip and consequently forming a clear visible colored line [25].

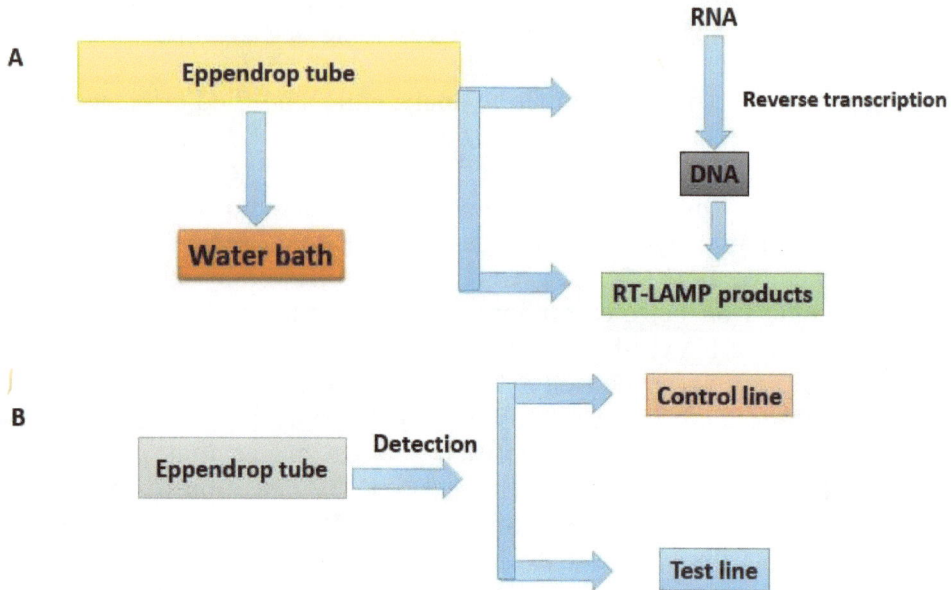

Fig. (2). Illustration of the RT-LAMP-VF assay. The figure was adapted from Huang *et al.* [25].

Another study was carried out where strand exchange signal transductions were developed using LAMP technology by combining it with thermostable invertase enzyme. MERS-COV template directly transduces the glucose signals, which can be detected on commercial glucometer easily, and have a sensitivity as low as 20-100 copies/μL [26]. Commercial kits are used for pregnancy testing in which human chorionic gonadotropin (hCG) signals are sensitively determined. The hCG is conjugated to site-specific DNA oligonucleotide, and the signal transduction is carried out through strand exchange, which can be determined by the capture and release of hCG [27]. Based on this principle, the LAMP-based virus detection method was adopted. The engineered hCG reporter protein was incorporated on commercially available pregnancy test strips to form LAMP-t--hCG signal transduction. This simple method can detect at least 20 copies of coronavirus templates in humans' blood serum and saliva. The detection of the COVID-19 can be adopted based on these developments for rapid and accurate detection keeping in view all the technological developments in LAMP assay.

Many studies revealed the broader impact of LAMP assays in the context of COVID-19 detection [22, 23]. However, as developing technology, there are certain limitations of LAMP-based assays. LAMP assay avoids the inclusion of an internal PCR inhibition control, which requires repeated reactions during testing. In addition, the apparent methodology complication, primer designing sometimes has difficulties, constrains the specificity or target site selection. Furthermore, the final product from the LAMP assay is usually a large fragment, due to which further cloning applications are limited. However, regardless of many disadvantages, LAMP is a highly sensitive nucleic acid amplification technique that identifies small amounts of DNA or RNA templates, even less than an hour. LAMP generally utilizes RT-PCR principal and has particular demands in the current situation of the COVID-19 pandemic due to rapid and reliable testing methods having better sensitivity. As the increasing numbers of suspected patients of COVID-19 remain a burden on hospitals, lots of suspects endure untested and hindering the control efforts in disease spread. Rapid and accurate diagnosis for COVID-19 is immediately needed, for which the LAMP method for coronavirus detection is highly recommended.

Rolling Circle Amplification-Based Methods

The efficacy of circular oligonucleotides, also known as padlock probes, has been established for the targeted nucleic acid sequence detection, which displayed better sensitivity than PCR [28, 29]. The rolling-circle amplification (RCA) technique displayed high sensitivity. DNA polymerase catalyzed the circularized DNA probe and created a rolling circle amplification (RCA) reaction template. DNA ligase is attached to both ends of the probe, followed by the targeted DNA or RNA sequence hybridization. The RCA assay has many advantages compared to other amplification methods, such as the ligation process entails the base pairing to both endpoints of the hybridized probe, which decreases the chances of non-specific binding with complementary strands. Besides, RCA allows the single-nucleotide polymorphism (SNPs) detection and avoids the amplifications with non-specificity as a result of PCR. RCA can be used for both DNA and RNA template recognition, which eliminates the RT-PCR requirement and thus provides a uniform assay platform for detecting both RNA and DNA [30]. Primers can easily bind single-strand DNA isolated from DNA polymerase, thus providing the potential for reactions to be carried out under thermal conditions and eliminating the need for thermocycler.

RT-PCR-based assays are widely used assay as a preliminary diagnostic tool, however, RT-PCR has the estimated sensitivity as low as 30%, depending on various factors such as type of specimens to be tested and collection time [29, 31]. Also, the amplification magnitude of RT-PCR is good. Still, the steps required for this process are time-consuming, such as RNA extraction, require expensive reagents, and a high-accuracy thermocycler. Cross-contamination leads to false-positive results as well. In contrast, RCA exhibit promising features and advantages, which depend on signal amplification instead of targeted amplification. Wang and colleagues [30] successfully established the RCA process for SARS-COV acquisition and demonstrated the broader impact of this diagnostic tool with greater sensitivity and specificity. RCA can sense at a single template level using artificial DNA templates in molecular modeling. Keeping in view all these demonstrated applications RCA has a potential role in the clinical diagnosis of SARS-COV. Additional work is still needed to improve the RCA requirements for COVID-19 acquisition for the development of a specific quantitative assay.

Nucleic Acid Hybridization through Microarray Technique

Microarray is a rapid diagnostic tool used to obtain high concentrations of coronavirus nucleic acid. Coronavirus RNA is converted into cDNA through the reverse transcription process, which is labeled with specific probes. These cDNA probes are then transferred into each well of microarray trays. Wells of the microarray plates contained oligonucleotides that are adhered to their surfaces. The hybridized probes remains bound followed by the washing steps several times. The unbound DNA will wash away, and thus, coronavirus has detected the existence of a virus-specific nucleic acid. Due to its beneficial aspects, the microarray assay can extensively be used in coronavirus detection [32].

Guo and co-workers [33] modified the microarray technique to detect SNP mutants with outstanding accuracy in the SARS-COV samples due to rapid genomic mutation. Since coronavirus potential got viral worldwide, diagnostic tools must be able to detect multiple strains of coronavirus and are implanted in or near a care setting (POC). Therefore, de Souza *et al.* [34] intended an oligonucleotide array with no fluorescence and low density, which can sense the whole coronavirus genus. The sensitivity of this technique in line with the sensitivity of the individual RT-PCR. New developments in the portable diagnostic platform were speculated where microarray chip technology was used and found effective in detecting the virus [35].

RNA-Targeting CRISPR Diagnosis

CRISPR a family of DNA sequence found in the genomic material of prokaryotic organisms such as bacteria and archaea. CRISPR-associated enzymes are the set of bacterial enzymes that recognize these sequences and cut at the specific sites on the DNA. CRISPR-associated protein 9 (Cas9), Cas12, and Cas13 are common examples of these enzymes. Cas12 and Cas13 enzyme families can be programmed to identify and cut the targeted viral RNA sequences [36]. Cas13 has recently been modified for the rapid sensing of nucleic acids [37].

The SHERLOCK (specific high-sensitivity enzymatic reporter unlocking) method has been established using Cas13 to cut down the sequences of reporter RNA, which is activated in response to COVID-19, the specific guided RNA [38]. The detector molecules specifically detect the cleavage of reporter RNA by cleavage enzyme, followed by isothermal amplification of the targeted viral RNA sequences, which can be visually apparent with a fluorophore [39]. These designed methods for CRISPR do not require complex equipment and can be studied using paper strips to detect COVID-19 with the utmost sensitivity. Both tests are relatively inexpensive and can be performed in less than an hour. RNA-targeting CRISPR diagnosis trials have great potential for POC diagnosis for the viral diseases [36]. CRISPR-based technology is also applicable in the detection of Dengue or Zika virus single-stranded RNA and their mutations in the samples. Their final COVID-19 agreements using CRISPR diagnostics have been developed to provide specific points for researchers interested in advancing. These diagnostic methods highlighting its potential as a unique, portable, quick, and multi-nucleic acid platform.

Nanopore Target Sequencing (NTS)

The NTS technology is based on the amplification of virulence gene fragments followed by sequencing the amplified fragment on the nanopore platform. A nanopore sequence platform can sense the long nucleic acid fragments and concurrently analyze data extraction in real-time. This method allows us to confirm the viral infection within a short time of sequencing by making a sequence map read on the virus genome and identifying the viral identity, authenticity, and display the output of the sequence results. The NTS method can detect multiple respiratory infections simultaneously, within 6-10 hours, and suitable for the modern diagnosis of COVID-19. However, the framework can be extended to detect different viral infections or pathogens [4].

The NTS is performed on a single MinION sequencer chip, which can apply to all testing samples, and bioinformatics channels analyzed the sequence data at systematic intervals (Fig. **3**). All high-grade readings are determined by mapping out the COVID-19 genome to increase the plasmid concentration. Like standard conventional PCR, NTS cannot detect a positive sample of infection by testing one or two sites [4, 40].

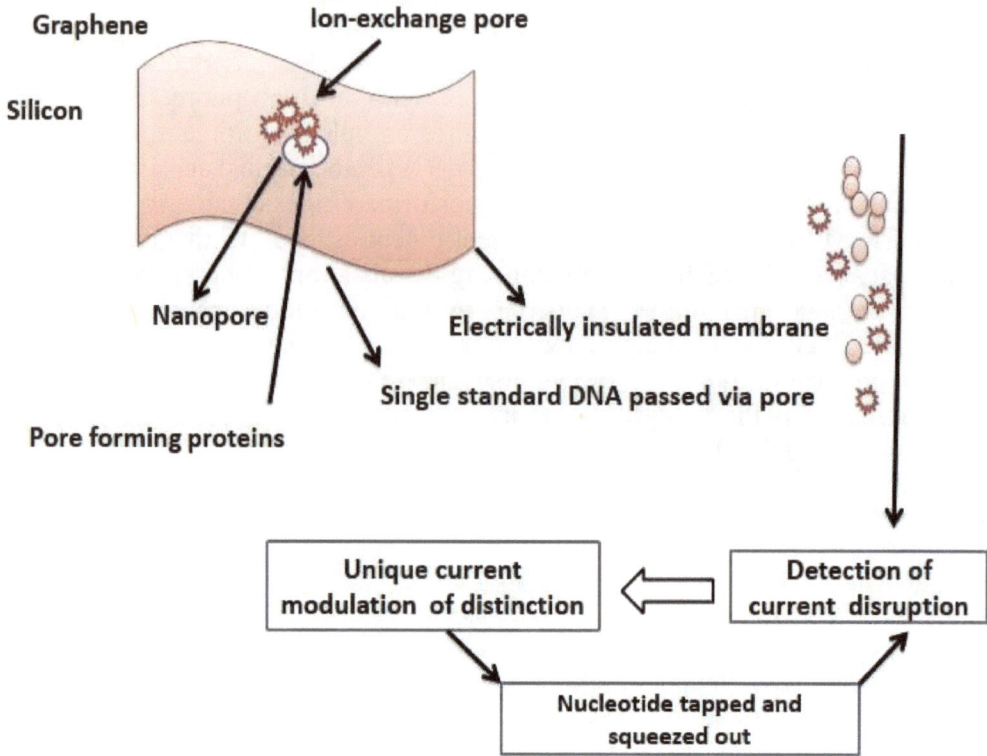

Fig. (3). An overview of the process for nanopore sequencing. (A) Preparation of DNA, (B) supplied with nanopore, (C) fixation on the MinION Flow cell membrane to generate ionic signals for sequencing (D) analysis and estimation of the DNA sequences. The figure was adopted from Bhattaru *et al.* [41].

Silicon-Based Integrated Point-of-Need (PON) Transducer

Despite the advancement of diagnostic tools in targeting nucleic acids, there is still a need for rapid screening at low cost with high sensitivity and testing of infectious diseases at PoN. Especially when dealing with highly infectious pathogens or disease-causing agents having no effective treatment such as COVID-19, which also shows no or similar symptoms to other disease/infection. Silicon-based-PoN transducers (TriSilix) can chemically enhance and detect the pathogen-related sequence of nucleic acids in real-time. Unlike other silicon-based technologies, TriSilix can be produced with the highest standard of a typical laboratory. A series of chemical-based methods for metal (water), electroplating, thermal bonding, and laser cutting to enable low-density fabric formation that does not require advanced semiconductor detection [42]. The proposed construction exploits the unique silicon properties and combines three modes of operation on a single chip to construct a low-cost device. Those modes include: 1). Electric heater (Joule), 2). A temperature sensor with negative confliction that can directly provide the temperature of the sample solution during the reaction, and 3). An electrochemical sensor to detect target nucleic acid sequences. Thus, TriSilix can tolerate disruptions in the global supply chain as the devices might be manufactured anywhere in the world [42].

TriSilix technology has several disadvantages. *i.e.,* TriSilix requires purified DNA samples for operation. Because the sample reservoir and polymer films are attached thermally at 110 °C, TriSilix cannot be operated beyond this temperature without causing the deboning of the layers and leaks from the sample reservoir. Usually, 110 °C is relatively high for nucleic acid amplification. The fabrication process would need to be modified in high temperatures, and thermoplastics with a higher melting point could be used [42].

CONCLUSION

The rapid and accurate diagnosis of COVID-19 is highly dependent on the availability of race-nucleic acid-based detection, and the race continues to develop an efficient and inexpensive diagnostic tool. This chapter provides a comprehensive review of the diagnosis of nucleic acid-based COVID-19 infection. Each method has its advantages and disadvantages. An important role of genetic testing is to confirm suspected cases because COV can be symptomatic or asymptomatic. RT-PCR has always been a commonly used method of detecting the genome virus, but there are limitations in terms of sensitivity and specificity of RT-PCR. Other nucleic acid-based assays, including LAMP, are a rapid molecular amplification tool in which amplification of genomic materials occurs in a shorter time with great sensitivity and specificity.

Similarly, the RCA technique and microarray are used for rapid high throughput detection of COV nucleic acid and displayed high sensitivity. Amplicon-based metagenomics sequencing and CRISPR-related technologies are also approved as the most effective techniques for COVID-19 detection. Applications of these molecular-based methods are combined to develop new technologies and methods.

CONSENT FOR PUBLICATION

Not Applicable.

CONFLICT OF INTEREST

The author confirms that this chapter contents have no conflict of interest.

ACKNOWLEDGEMENT

Declared none.

REFERENCES

[1]   Bloom DE, Cadarette D. Infectious disease threats in the twenty-first century: strengthening the global response. Front Immunol 2019; 10: 549.
[http://dx.doi.org/10.3389/fimmu.2019.00549] [PMID: 30984169]

[2]   Ming W. Nanopore target sequencing for accurate and comprehensive detection of SARS-CoV-2 and other respiratory viruses. medRvix 2020.

[3]   Singhal T. A review of coronavirus disease-2019 (COVID-19). Indian J Pediatr 2020; 87(4): 281-6.
[http://dx.doi.org/10.1007/s12098-020-03263-6] [PMID: 32166607]

[4]   Liu DX, Liang JQ, Fung TS. Human Coronavirus-229E,-OC43,-NL63, and-HKU1. Reference Module in Life Sciences 2020.
[http://dx.doi.org/10.1016/B978-0-12-809633-8.21501-X]

[5]   Balboni A, Gallina L, Palladini A, Prosperi S, Battilani M. A real-time PCR assay for bat SARS-like coronavirus detection and its application to Italian greater horseshoe bat faecal sample surveys. ScientificWorldJournal 2012; 2012: 989514.
[http://dx.doi.org/10.1100/2012/989514] [PMID: 22654650]

[6]   Uhlenhaut C, Cohen JI, Pavletic S, *et al.* Use of a novel virus detection assay to identify coronavirus HKU1 in the lungs of a hematopoietic stem cell transplant recipient with fatal pneumonia. Transpl Infect Dis 2012; 14(1): 79-85.
[http://dx.doi.org/10.1111/j.1399-3062.2011.00657.x] [PMID: 21749586]

[7]   Setianingsih TY, Wiyatno A, Hartono TS, *et al.* Detection of multiple viral sequences in the respiratory tract samples of suspected Middle East respiratory syndrome coronavirus patients in Jakarta, Indonesia 2015-2016. Int J Infect Dis 2019; 86: 102-7.
[http://dx.doi.org/10.1016/j.ijid.2019.06.022] [PMID: 31238156]

[8]   Noh JY, Yoon SW, Kim DJ, *et al.* Simultaneous detection of severe acute respiratory syndrome, Middle East respiratory syndrome, and related bat coronaviruses by real-time reverse transcription PCR. Arch Virol 2017; 162(6): 1617-23.
[http://dx.doi.org/10.1007/s00705-017-3281-9] [PMID: 28220326]

[9]   Corman VM, Landt O, Kaiser M, *et al.* Detection of 2019 novel coronavirus (2019-nCoV) by real-time RT-PCR. Euro Surveill 2020; 25(3): 2000045.
[http://dx.doi.org/10.2807/1560-7917.ES.2020.25.3.2000045] [PMID: 31992387]

[10]   van Elden LJ, van Loon AM, van Alphen F, *et al.* Frequent detection of human coronaviruses in clinical specimens from patients with respiratory tract infection by use of a novel real-time reverse-transcriptase polymerase chain reaction. J Infect Dis 2004; 189(4): 652-7.
[http://dx.doi.org/10.1086/381207] [PMID: 14767819]

[11]   Yu XF, Pan JC, Ye R, Xiang HQ, Kou Y, Huang ZC. Preparation of armored RNA as a control for multiplex real-time reverse transcription-PCR detection of influenza virus and severe acute respiratory syndrome coronavirus. J Clin Microbiol 2008; 46(3): 837-41.
[http://dx.doi.org/10.1128/JCM.01904-07] [PMID: 18160451]

[12]   Yip SP, To SS, Leung PH, Cheung TS, Cheng PK, Lim WW. Use of dual TaqMan probes to increase the sensitivity of 1-step quantitative reverse transcription-PCR: application to the detection of SARS coronavirus. Clin Chem 2005; 51(10): 1885-8.
[http://dx.doi.org/10.1373/clinchem.2005.054106] [PMID: 16189379]

[13]   Fajardo A, Pereira-Gomez M, Echeverria N, *et al.* Evaluation Of SYBR Green Real Time PCR For Detecting SARS-CoV-2 From Clinical Samples bioRxiv 2020.

[14] Xie X, Zhong Z, Zhao W, Zheng C, Wang F, Liu J. Chest CT for typical 2019-nCoV pneumonia: relationship to negative RT-PCR testing. Radiology 2020.: 200343.
[http://dx.doi.org/10.1148/radiol.2020200343]

[15] Yam WC, Chan KH, Poon LL, *et al.* Evaluation of reverse transcription-PCR assays for rapid diagnosis of severe acute respiratory syndrome associated with a novel coronavirus. J Clin Microbiol 2003; 41(10): 4521-4.
[http://dx.doi.org/10.1128/JCM.41.10.4521-4524.2003] [PMID: 14532176]

[16] Vogels CB, Brito AF, Wyllie AL, *et al.* Analytical sensitivity and efficiency comparisons of SARS-COV-2 qRT-PCR assays. medRxiv 2020.

[17] Chu DKW, Pan Y, Cheng SMS, *et al.* Molecular diagnosis of a novel coronavirus (2019-nCoV) causing an outbreak of pneumonia. Clin Chem 2020; 66(4): 549-55.
[http://dx.doi.org/10.1093/clinchem/hvaa029] [PMID: 32031583]

[18] Corman VM, Landt O, Kaiser M, *et al.* Detection of 2019 novel coronavirus (2019-nCoV) by real-time RT-PCR. Euro Surveill 2020; 25(3): 2000045.
[http://dx.doi.org/10.2807/1560-7917.ES.2020.25.3.2000045] [PMID: 31992387]

[19] Nagamine K, Hase T, Notomi T. Accelerated reaction by loop-mediated isothermal amplification using loop primers. Mol Cell Probes 2002; 16(3): 223-9.
[http://dx.doi.org/10.1006/mcpr.2002.0415] [PMID: 12144774]

[20] Francois P, Tangomo M, Hibbs J, *et al.* Robustness of a loop-mediated isothermal amplification reaction for diagnostic applications. FEMS Immunol Med Microbiol 2011; 62(1): 41-8.
[http://dx.doi.org/10.1111/j.1574-695X.2011.00785.x] [PMID: 21276085]

[21] Poon LL, Leung CS, Tashiro M, *et al.* Rapid detection of the severe acute respiratory syndrome (SARS) coronavirus by a loop-mediated isothermal amplification assay. Clin Chem 2004; 50(6): 1050-2.
[http://dx.doi.org/10.1373/clinchem.2004.032011] [PMID: 15054079]

[22] Pyrc K, Milewska A, Potempa J. Development of loop-mediated isothermal amplification assay for detection of human coronavirus-NL63. J Virol Methods 2011; 175(1): 133-6.
[http://dx.doi.org/10.1016/j.jviromet.2011.04.024] [PMID: 21545810]

[23] Shirato K, Yano T, Senba S, *et al.* Detection of Middle East respiratory syndrome coronavirus using reverse transcription loop-mediated isothermal amplification (RT-LAMP). Virol J 2014; 11(1): 139
[http://dx.doi.org/10.1186/1743-422X-11-139] [PMID: 25103205]

[24] Njiru ZK. Loop-mediated isothermal amplification technology: towards point of care diagnostics. PLoS Negl Trop Dis 2012; 6(6): e1572.
[http://dx.doi.org/10.1371/journal.pntd.0001572] [PMID: 22745836]

[25] Huang P, Wang H, Cao Z, *et al.* A rapid and specific assay for the detection of MERS-CoV. Front Microbiol 2018; 9: 1101.
[http://dx.doi.org/10.3389/fmicb.2018.01101] [PMID: 29896174]

[26] Du Y, Hughes RA, Bhadra S, Jiang YS, Ellington AD, Li B. A sweet spot for molecular diagnostics: Coupling isothermal amplification and strand exchange circuits to glucometers. Sci Rep 2015; 5(1): 11039.
[http://dx.doi.org/10.1038/srep11039] [PMID: 26050646]

[27] Du Y, Pothukuchy A, Gollihar JD, Nourani A, Li B, Ellington AD. Coupling sensitive nucleic acid amplification with commercial pregnancy test strips. Angew Chem Int Ed Engl 2017; 56(4): 992-6.
[http://dx.doi.org/10.1002/anie.201609108] [PMID: 27990727]

[28] Faruqi AF, Hosono S, Driscoll MD, *et al.* High-throughput genotyping of single nucleotide polymorphisms with rolling circle amplification. BMC Genomics 2001; 2(1): 4.
[http://dx.doi.org/10.1186/1471-2164-2-4] [PMID: 11511324]

[29]   Schweitzer B, Kingsmore S. Combining nucleic acid amplification and detection. Curr Opin Biotechnol 2001; 12(1): 21-7.
[http://dx.doi.org/10.1016/S0958-1669(00)00172-5] [PMID: 11167068]

[30]   Wang B, Potter SJ, Lin Y, *et al.* Rapid and sensitive detection of severe acute respiratory syndrome coronavirus by rolling circle amplification. J Clin Microbiol 2005; 43(5): 2339-44.
[http://dx.doi.org/10.1128/JCM.43.5.2339-2344.2005] [PMID: 15872263]

[31]   Peiris JS, Lai ST, Poon LL, *et al.* SARS study group. Coronavirus as a possible cause of severe acute respiratory syndrome. Lancet 2003; 361(9366): 1319-25.
[http://dx.doi.org/10.1016/S0140-6736(03)13077-2] [PMID: 12711465]

[32]   Chen Q, Li J, Deng Z, Xiong W, Wang Q, Hu YQ. Comprehensive detection and identification of seven animal coronaviruses and human respiratory coronavirus 229E with a microarray hybridization assay. Intervirology 2010; 53(2): 95-104.
[http://dx.doi.org/10.1159/000264199] [PMID: 19955814]

[33]   Guo X, Geng P, Wang Q, Cao B, Liu B. Development of a single nucleotide polymorphism DNA microarray for the detection and genotyping of the SARS coronavirus. J Microbiol Biotechnol 2014; 24(10): 1445-54.
[http://dx.doi.org/10.4014/jmb.1404.04024] [PMID: 24950883]

[34]   de Souza Luna LK, Heiser V, Regamey N, *et al.* Generic detection of coronaviruses and differentiation at the prototype strain level by reverse transcription-PCR and nonfluorescent low-density microarray. J Clin Microbiol 2007; 45(3): 1049-52.
[http://dx.doi.org/10.1128/JCM.02426-06] [PMID: 17229859]

[35]   Hardick J, Metzgar D, Risen L, *et al.* Initial performance evaluation of a spotted array Mobile Analysis Platform (MAP) for the detection of influenza A/B, RSV, and MERS coronavirus. Diagn Microbiol Infect Dis 2018; 91(3): 245-7.
[http://dx.doi.org/10.1016/j.diagmicrobio.2018.02.011] [PMID: 29550057]

[36]   Carter LJ, Garner LV, Smoot JW, *et al.* Assay techniques and test development for COVID-19 diagnosis 2020; 591-605.

[37]   Gootenberg JS, Abudayyeh OO, Lee JW, *et al.* Nucleic acid detection with CRISPR-Cas13a/C2c2. Science 2017; 356(6336): 438-42.
[http://dx.doi.org/10.1126/science.aam9321] [PMID: 28408723]

[38]   Zhang F, Abudayyeh OO, Gootenberg JS. A protocol for detection of COVID-19 using CRISPR diagnosticsA protocol for detection of COVID-19 using CRISPR diagnostics 2020; 8

[39]   Broughton JP, Deng X, Yu G, *et al.* CRISPR-Cas12-based detection of SARS-CoV-2. Nat Biotechnol 2020; 38(7): 870-4.
[http://dx.doi.org/10.1038/s41587-020-0513-4] [PMID: 32300245]

[40]   Yu L, Tong Y, Shen G, *et al.* Immunodepletion with Hypoxemia: A Potential High Risk Subtype of Coronavirus Disease 2019. medRxiv 2020.
[http://dx.doi.org/10.1101/2020.03.03.20030650]

[41]   Bhattaru SA, Tani J, Saboda K, *et al.* Development of a nucleic acid-based life detection instrument testbed. 2019.
[http://dx.doi.org/10.1109/AERO.2019.8742193]

[42]   Nunez-Bajo E, Kasimatis M, Cotur Y, *et al.* Ultra-low-cost integrated silicon-based transducer for on-site, genetic detection of pathogens. bioRxiv 2020.
[http://dx.doi.org/10.1101/2020.03.23.002931]

SUBJECT INDEX

A

ACE2 78, 103, 105, 114, 116, 117, 119, 150, 169, 199, 200, 201, 203, 204, 206, 208, 210, 211, 216, 226, 227, 234, 236
  binding receptor 78
  expression 116, 117
  for virus entry 200
  host cell receptor 105
  inhibitors 119
  upregulation 119
ACE2 receptor 74, 77, 104
  in epithelial cells 104
  molecule 74
  proteins 77
Acid 74, 123, 144, 210, 238, 239, 240, 241, 324, 396
  aspartic 123, 144
  canrenoic 241
  cimicifugic 239, 240, 241
  lipoic 74
  mycophenolic 324
  rosemarinic 239
  sialic 210
  viral nucleic 396
Activity 50, 87, 151, 175, 217, 229, 238, 239, 254, 323, 324, 330
  cellular kinase 87
  collagenolytic enzymes 238
  epigallocatechin 239
  exonuclease 229
Acute respiratory distress syndrome (ARDS) 119, 120, 151, 196, 316, 341, 351
African swine fever virus (ASFV) 86
Alkaline phosphatase 353
Amphiphysin 81, 82
Angiography 395
Angiotensin 103, 123, 143, 197, 200, 234, 251, 274, 316, 338
  converting enzyme 103, 123, 143, 197, 234, 251, 274, 316, 338
  receptor blockers (ARBs) 200

Antibodies 170, 171, 182, 195, 214, 217, 332, 344, 353, 410
  anti-FITC 410
  antigen-enzyme link 353
  cross-reactive 182
  enzyme-linked 344
  nucleocapsid protein 332
  polyclonal 170, 171, 182, 217
  therapeutic 195, 214
Antibody 320, 361
  assay 320
  based diagnosis 361
Antibody-dependent 323, 324
  cell-mediated cytotoxicity 323
  cellular cytotoxicity (ADCC) 323, 324
Antibody detection 276, 339, 345, 348
  assays 348
  rapid SARS-CoV-2 339
Antigenicity of spike protein 179
Antigens 150, 250, 252, 254, 257, 258, 259, 263, 264, 266, 267, 268, 316, 348, 350, 352, 353, 356, 397, 398
  capturing ELISA 263
  foreign 350, 356
  presenting cells (APCs) 150, 316, 350
  test 397
  viral 150, 264
Anti-inflammatory 241, 262
  effects 241
  pathways 262
Antiviral 238, 239, 242, 324
  activity 238, 239, 324
  drug discovery 242
Assays 250, 275, 276, 302, 331, 337, 339, 346, 347, 360
  antibody-based 360
  chemiluminescence 346, 347
  chemiluminescent 347
  enzyme-linked immunosorbent 276, 302, 331, 337, 339
  linked immunosorbent 250
  serological antigen-antibody reaction 275

www.ingramcontent.com/pod-product-compliance
Lightning Source LLC
Chambersburg PA
CBHW050758220326
41598CB00006B/56